Interventional Procedures for Adult Structural Heart Disease

Interventional Procedures for Adult Structural Heart Disease

John M. Lasala, MD, PhD
Professor of Medicine
Director, Interventional Cardiology
Medical Director, Cardiac Catheterization Laboratory
Barnes-Jewish Hospital
Washington University School of Medicine
St. Louis, Missouri

Jason H. Rogers, MD
Professor of Cardiovascular Medicine
Director, Interventional Cardiology and Cardiovascular Clinical Research Unit
Division of Cardiovascular Medicine
University of California–Davis Medical Center
Sacramento, California

ELSEVIER
SAUNDERS

1600 John F. Kennedy Blvd.
Ste 1800
Philadelphia, PA 19103-2899

ISBN: 978-1-4557-0758-4

Executive Content Strategist: Dolores Meloni
Content Development Specialist: Angela Rufino
Publishing Services Manager: Julie Eddy
Project Manager: Jan Waters
Design Direction: Louis Forgione

Printed in the United States of America

Last digit is the print number: 9 8 7 6 5 4 3 2 1

Working together
to grow libraries in
developing countries

www.elsevier.com • www.bookaid.org

To our patients, whose courage and consent have inspired these new procedures.
To our families, in recognition of their invaluable support and encouragement.
To our friendship, which inspires continued curiosity and innovation.

Contributors

Oluseun Alli, MD
Assistant Professor of Medicine
Director, Structural Heart Program
Section of Interventional Cardiology
University of Alabama at Birmingham
Birmingham, Alabama

Ehrin J. Armstrong, MD
Division of Cardiovascular Medicine
University of California Davis Medical Center
Sacramento, California

Vasilis Babaliaros, MD
Associate Professor of Medicine
Department of Medicine
Division of Cardiology
Emory University
Atlanta, Georgia

Richard G. Bach, MD
Associate Professor of Medicine
Department of Medicine
Washington University School of Medicine;
Director, Cardiac Intensive Care Unit
Barnes-Jewish Hospital
St. Louis, Missouri

David T. Balzer, MD
Professor of Pediatrics
Director, Cardiac Catheterization Laboratory
Department of Pediatrics
Division of Pediatric Cardiology
Washington University School of Medicine
St. Louis Children's Hospital
St. Louis, Missouri

Itsik Ben-Dor, MD
Department of Interventional Cardiology
Washington Hospital Center
Washington, DC

Lee N. Benson, MD
University Health Network
Toronto General Division
Department of Medicine
Division of Cardiology
The Labatt Family Heart Center
Department of Pediatrics
Division of Cardiology
The Hospital for Sick Children
University of Toronto School of Medicine
Toronto, Ontario, Canada

Stefan C. Bertog, MD
Assistant Professor
CardioVascular Center
Frankfurt, Germany;
Veteran Affairs Medical Center
University of Minnesota
Minneapolis, Minnesota

Ronald K. Binder, MD
Department of Cardiology
St. Paul's Hospital
University of British Columbia
Vancouver, British Columbia, Canada

Steven F. Bolling, MD
Division of Cardiac Surgery
University of Michigan
Ann Arbor, Michigan

David A. Burke, MD
Department of Internal Medicine
(Cardiovascular Division)
Beth Israel Deaconess Medical Center
Boston, Massachusetts

Qi-Ling Cao, MD
Rush Center for Congenital & Structural Heart Disease
Department of Pediatrics and Internal Medicine
Rush University Medical Center
Chicago, Illinois

John D. Carroll, MD
Professor of Medicine
Director, Cardiac and Vascular Center
Director, Interventional Cardiology
University of Colorado, Denver
Anschutz Medical Campus
Aurora, Colorado

Stacey D. Clegg, MD
Interventional Cardiology Fellow
Division of Cardiology
University of Colorado, Denver
Anschutz Medical Campus
Aurora, Colorado

Alain Cribier, MD
Professor of Medicine
Department of Cardiology
University Hospital Charles Nicolle
Rouen, France

Chethan Devireddy, MD
Andreas Gruentzig Cardiovascular Center
Division of Cardiology
Emory University Hospital
Atlanta, Georgia

Sammy Elmariah, MD, MPH
Interventional Cardiology and Structural Heart Disease
Massachusetts General Hospital
Harvard Medical School
Boston, Massachusetts

Ted E. Feldman, MD
Clinical Professor
Evanston Hospital
North Shore University Health System
Evanston, Illinois

Jennifer Franke, MD
Assistant Professor
CardioVascular Center
Frankfurt, Germany

Cindy J. Fuller, PhD
Swedish Heart & Vascular Institute
Swedish Medical Center
Seattle, Washington

Sameer Gafoor, MD
Andreas Gruentzig Cardiovascular Center
Division of Cardiology
Emory University Hospital
Atlanta, Georgia

Irvin F. Goldenberg, MD
Twin Cities Heart Foundation
Minneapolis, Minnesota

Ziyad M. Hijazi, MD, MPH
Director
Rush Center for Congenital and Structural Heart
   Disease
Rush University Medical Center
Chicago, Illinois

Ilona Hofmann, MD
Assistant Professor
CardioVascular Center
Frankfurt, Germany

David Holmes, Jr, MD
Professor of Medicine
Department of Cardiovascular Diseases
Mayo Clinic
Rochester, Minnesota

Noa Holoshitz, MD
Interventional Cardiology Fellow
Rush University Medical Center
Chicago, Illinois

Eric Horlick, MDCM
Director, Structural Heart Disease Intervention Program
Department of Medicine
Toronto General Hospital
Toronto, Ontario, Canada

Frank Ing, MD
Director, Cardiac Catheterization Laboratory
Associate Chief, Division of Cardiology
Children's Hospital, Los Angeles;
Clinical Professor of Pediatrics
Keck School of Medicine of the University of Southern
   California
Los Angeles, California

Samir R. Kapadia, MD
Director, Sones Catheterization Laboratories
Department of Cardiovascular Medicine
Cleveland Clinic
Cleveland, Ohio

Amar Krishnaswamy, MD
Associate Program Director
Interventional Cardiology Fellowship
Cleveland Clinic
Cleveland, Ohio

John M. Lasala, MD, PhD
Professor of Medicine
Division of Cardiology
Director, Interventional Cardiology
Washington University School of Medicine;
Medical Director
Cardiac Catheterization Laboratory
Barnes-Jewish Hospital
St. Louis, Missouri

D. Scott Lim, MD
Director, Heart Valve Center
Co-director, Adult Congenital Heart Disease Center
University of Virginia
Charlottesville, Virginia

C. Huie Lin, MD, PhD
Methodist DeBakey Heart and Vascular Center
Houston, Texas

Reginald I. Low, MD
Division of Cardiovascular Medicine
University of California Medical Center
Sacaramento, California

Ehtisham Mahmud, MD
Professor of Medicine/Cardiology
Chief, Cardiovascular Medicine
Director, Interventional Cardiology and Cardiac
   Catheterization Labs
Co-director, Sulpizio Cardiovascular Center
University of California–San Diego
San Diego, California

Ronan Margey, MD
Director, Structural Heart and Adult Congenital Heart
   Intervention
Hartford Cardiac Lab
Hartford Hospital
Hartford, Connecticut;
Assistant Professor of Medicine
Department of Medicine
University of Connecticut Medical School
Farmington, Connecticut

Jeffery Meadows, MD
Assistant Professor of Pediatric Cardiology
Pediatrics
University of California–San Francisco
San Francisco, California

Phillip Moore, MD, MBA
Professor of Pediatrics
Director, Pediatric Cardiac Catheterization Laboratory
Department of Pediatrics
University of California–San Francisco
San Francisco, California

Joshua Murphy, MD
St. Louis Children's Hospital
Washington University School of Medicine
St. Louis, Missouri

Mark Osten, MD
Department of Medicine
Division of Cardiology
University Health Network
Toronto General Division
Toronto, Ontario, Canada

Igor F. Palacios, MD
Director, Knight Catheterization Laboratory
Director, Interventional Cardiology
Institute for Heart, Vascular, and Stroke Care
Massachusetts General Hospital
Harvard Medical School
Boston, Massachusetts

Dhaval Parekh, MD
Associate Chief
Pediatric Cardiology
Children's Hospital, Los Angeles
Los Angeles, California

Mitul Patel, MD
Assistant Professor of Medicine
Sulpizio Cardiovascular Center
University of California–San Diego
San Diego, California

Wesley R. Pedersen, MD
Medical Director, Structural & Valvular Heart Disease
   Program
Minneapolis Heart Institute
Abbott Northwestern Hospital
Minneapolis, Minnesota

Jeffrey J. Popma, MD
Director, Interventional Cardiology Clinical Services
Beth Israel Deaconess Medical Center
Boston, Massachusetts

Robert A. Quaife, MD
Associate Professor of Medicine and Radiology
Director, Advanced Cardiac Imaging
University of Colorado, Denver
Anschutz Medical Campus
Aurora, Colorado

Nicolas T. Ramzi, MD
St. Louis Children's Hospital
Washington University School of Medicine
St. Louis, Missouri

Mark Reisman, MD
Swedish Heart & Vascular Institute
Swedish Medical Center
Seattle, Washington

Jason H. Rogers, MD
Associate Clinical Professor
Director, Cardiovascular Research Unit
Director, Interventional Cardiology
Department of Cardiovascular Medicine
University of California–Davis Medical Center
Sacramento, California

Ernesto E. Salcedo, MD
Professor of Medicine
Director of Echocardiography
University of Colorado, Denver
Anschutz Medical Campus
Aurora, Colorado

Shabana Shahanavaz, MD
Assitant Professor
Department of Pediatrics
Washington University
St. Louis, Missouri

Horst Sievert, MD
Assistant Professor
CardioVascular Center
Frankfurt, Germany

Gagan D. Singh, MD
Clinical Fellow
Division of Cardiovascular Medicine
University of California–Davis Medical Center
Sacramento, California

Harsimran S. Singh, MD, MSc
Assistant Professor of Medicine
Department of Internal Medicine
Weill Cornell Medical College–New York Presbyterian
   Hospital
New York, New York

Jeffrey A. Southard, MD
Associate Clinical Professor
Director, Transcatheter Aortic Valve Replacement
   Program
Division of Cardiovascular Medicine
University of California–Davis Medical Center
Sacramento, California

James Stewart, MD
Andreas Gruentzig Cardiovascular Center
Division of Cardiology
Emory University Hospital
Atlanta, Georgia

Vinod Thourani, MD
Division of Cardiothoracic Surgery
Emory University Hospital
Atlanta, Georgia

E. Murat Tuzcu, MD
Cleveland Clinic
Cleveland, Ohio

Laura Vaskelyte, MD
Assistant Professor
CardioVascular Center
Frankfurt, Germany

John G. Webb, MD
St. Paul's Hospital
Vancouver, British Columbia, Canada

Khung Keong Yeo, MBBS
Department of Cardiology
National Heart Centre Singapore
Singapore;
Department of Cardiovascular Medicine
University of California–Davis Medical Center
Sacramento, California

Alan Zajarias, MD
Assistant Professor of Medicine
Division of Cardiovascular Diseases
Washington University School of Medicine
St. Louis, Missouri

Preface

Interventional cardiology has experienced a renaissance in the past decade with the growth of interventional procedures for adult structural heart disease. Whereas numerous advances continue in the areas of coronary and peripheral vascular intervention, arguably the most notable and significant recent innovations have occurred in the arena of structural heart disease. Aortic and mitral balloon valvuloplasty were first popularized in the 1980s. Many developments followed in the 1990s, including the introduction of numerous occluder devices and improved imaging techniques. Since 2000, there has been an explosion of new technologies, including left atrial appendage occlusion, percutaneous treatments for mitral regurgitation, and transcatheter aortic valve replacement. The creative use of these technologies, in combination with improved understanding of structural disease states and marked advances in preprocedural and intraprocedural imaging, have all imparted significant momentum to this new field.

This first edition of *Interventional Procedures for Adult Structural Heart Disease* includes 23 chapters that cover a large number of topics relevant to the field. In each chapter, the goal was to include background, clinical presentation, and diagnostic findings, with particular emphasis on patient selection and indications for the procedure. We also attempted to spotlight practical technical procedural steps, equipment selection, tips and tricks, and important discussion of complications and management. Many figures and supplemental videos are included to illustrate this highly visual and three-dimensional specialty.

We believe this volume will be an indispensable resource for all those who take care of patients with structural heart disease, including referring cardiologists, cardiovascular imaging specialists, fellows in training, new interventional cardiologists, as well as structural interventionalists. Much of the information included in this volume is not easily retrieved from the published literature, and many of the "how to" components are not found anywhere else.

We thank our many friends, colleagues, and experts from around the globe who contributed to this volume, and without whose expertise this text could not have been completed. We thank the professional staff at Elsevier for their assistance in producing this text, especially Angela Rufino, Dolores Meloni, Louis Forgione, Mike Carcel, and Heather Krehling. Finally, we thank our families for their love, support, and inspiration.

John M. Lasala
Jason H. Rogers

Contents

Video Contents

Chapter 1

The Growing Specialty of Adult Structural Heart Disease

TED E. FELDMAN

The field of structural cardiac and cardiovascular intervention is relatively new. Some of the component procedures have been part of the interventional armamentarium for many years, but have never been grouped into a unified field. The development of new catheter technology for shunt closure, valve repair, and valve replacement has created this new subspecialty within interventional cardiology. Historically, the pediatric interventional community has performed many of these procedures, but their adaptation to adult patients and within adult cardiovascular programs is a relatively recent development.

There are currently no accredited training programs and structural interventional procedures and techniques, and there are no well-defined pathways for practicing interventional physicians to become involved with this field. As has been the case for every other major development in interventional cardiology, this first phase involves learning through both practice and trials. In contrast to the beginning era of angioplasty and early stent therapy for coronary artery disease, there is substantial experience to draw upon for creating paradigms for learning about structural intervention.

This chapter will review the knowledge base that has been defined for this field, some of the practical aspects of acquiring new procedural skills, and the landscape going forward for how these new therapies may impact interventional practice.

1.1 Core-Curriculum for Structural Intervention

The knowledge base in this growing field of structural intervention is not well defined. Many disciplines, including pediatric and adult interventional cardiology, cardiovascular and cardiothoracic surgery, vascular surgery, and interventional radiology are all spanned by the field. The knowledge base needed for practice is ideally the same for anyone who enters the field from among any of these varied disciplines. From a practical standpoint, the necessary new knowledge differs substantially depending on the prior experience and field of the operator, and especially on the interventions the operator intends to perform. At the beginning of an individual experience, the cardiologist specializing in adult intervention may have a large background with diagnostic catheterization and possibly balloon aortic valvuloplasty (BAV) for aortic stenosis. The knowledge base for further development of skills for percutaneous transcatheter aortic valve replacement (TAVR) would then be incremental.

In contrast, the needed skills for large-sized sheath insertion, removal, and complication management might come more easily to the physician with abdominal aortic stent graft experience and would require partnerships or additional experience for coronary interventional physicians with no experience with these large-sheath techniques. Management of congenital heart disease after prior surgical repair in adult patients requires a specialized background and is obviously better suited to the already-trained pediatric interventional practitioner.

There are no accreditation standards and no training programs for structural intervention. The Society for Cardiovascular Angiography and Interventions has published a core curriculum for structural heart interventions.[1-4] This will most easily be utilized by training programs, but it is a useful guide for the already-practicing interventional physician interested in this field. Structural procedures have been divided into basic and complex groups **(Boxes 1–1 and 1–2).** This division is a useful way to define which procedures might be adopted early in an operator's experience.

BOX 1–1

Interventions for Acquired Structural Cardiovascular Diseases

Basic Interventions
Transseptal left heart catheterization
Adult balloon aortic valvuloplasty
Ventricular septal ablation (chemical)

Complex Interventions
Transapical ventricular access
Adult mitral or tricuspid balloon valvuloplasty
Balloon pericardiotomy
Exclusion of the left atrial appendage
Closure of postinfarction ventricular septal defects
Closure of paravalvular leaks
Closure of ventricular pseudoaneurysms
Closure of endovascular endoleaks
Closure of aortic pseudoaneurysms
Transcatheter aortic valve replacement
Transcatheter mitral valve repair or implantation
Stenting pulmonary veins after ablation for atrial fibrillation

BOX 1–2

Interventions for Adult Congenital Cardiovascular Diseases

Basic Interventions
Closure of patent foramen ovale
Closure of simple atrial septal defect
Closure of patent ductus arteriosus
Pulmonary valvuloplasty

Complex Interventions
Closure of complex atrial septal defects
Closure of native, residual-patch, muscular, or perimembranous ventricular septal defects
Closure of coronary fistulas, pulmonary vascular malformations, and aorto-pulmonary collaterals
Angioplasty and stenting of pulmonary artery branch stenosis
Angioplasty and stenting for coarctation of the aorta
Angioplasty and stenting of pulmonary veins
Angioplasty and stenting of surgical conduits, baffles, and homograft
Angioplasty and stenting of interatrial septum and Fontan fenestrations
Transcatheter pulmonary valve implantation

Imaging modalities have become a critical part of the structural interventional knowledge base. Patient evaluation for valve and structural procedures is easily as important as performance of the procedure itself. The interpretation of computed tomography (CT) and magnetic resonance imaging, as well as cardiac and vascular studies are new for many interventional physicians, and experience with these studies is a key part of developing a structural program. The interpretation and use of transthoracic, transesophageal, and intracardiac echocardiographic studies is integral to this field. Most structural catheterization laboratories now have an additional permanent monitor screen in the procedure room for the display of echo imaging.[5] Although many interventional cardiologists have a strong background in imaging, just as many do not. The reliance on echocardiographic guidance for procedures for percutaneous mitral repair and especially for intracardiac shunt closure creates a substantial demand for this imaging skill set. Whereas courses exist for the acquisition of echo skills, the use of the imaging for interventional procedures is unique to the catheterization lab and requires an increasingly specialized background.

1.2 Acquiring Skills for Structural Intervention

How does one acquire basic skills? This question is complicated greatly by the wide variety of procedures that comprise this new and developing field. The basic skill sets for aortic valve, mitral valve, shunt closure, and atrial appendage occlusion are all different but, of course, interrelated. Some background in these areas as a diagnostic catheterizer is obviously helpful. The physician with a large background in balloon aortic valvuloplasty (BAV) will, of course, have experience that is helpful for entering the field of transcatheter aortic valve replacement (TAVR) therapy. Transseptal puncture is a basic building block for left atrial procedures, including all of those directed at the mitral valve, paravalvular leak closure, and left atrial appendage occlusion.

Transseptal puncture is not widely taught in basic fellowship programs, and most practicing interventional cardiologists do not have training or prior experience. The avenues to acquire skills are similar for all of these various background components and the new procedures themselves. Several courses for transseptal catheterization have been given and simulation has been helpful.

As new devices become approved, these therapies are now rolling out with training programs and on-site proctoring. These are invaluable aids to the acquisition of new procedural skills. The use of live case demonstrations at national and international meetings has been controversial but is also invaluable for understanding how these procedures are performed. The cross-pollination from one site to another that is facilitated by proctors teaching at new sites and live-case demonstrations at meetings cannot be replicated with taped cases.

One of the best pathways for entry into a particular procedure is to become involved in a research trial. The trial process provides training and provides a way into a procedure at a point when the playing field is level and no one has a substantial background in that specific procedure.[6]

A key part of training for many of the newer device trials has been simulation. Several companies have developed simulator equipment that allows practitioners to practice a new procedure. The haptics, or feel, of the procedure can be taught to some degree. The specifics of device preparation and use are easily incorporated into simulation programs. Decision making regarding the technique of the procedure or the management of a patient throughout the course of the procedure can be incorporated into

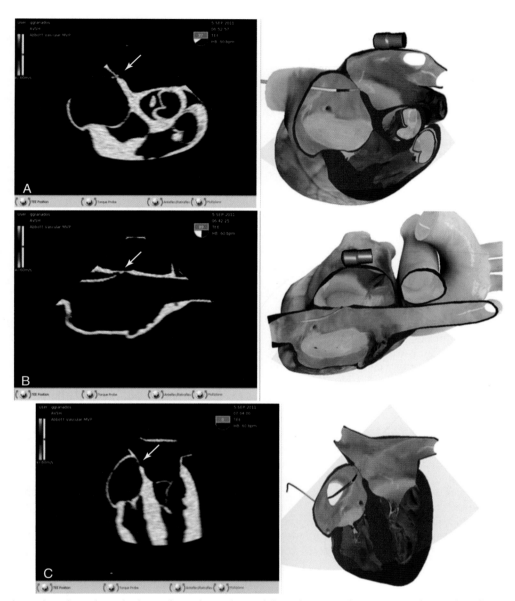

Figure 1–1   **A,** Software-based simulator displays echocardiographic and three-dimensional anatomic renderings that all move in synchrony as various procedure maneuvers are performed. This image shows a short-axis transesophageal echocardiography (TEE) view to guide transseptal puncture for percutaneous mitral repair. The *arrow* shows the tip of the transseptal needle "tenting" the atrial septum. The short axis identifies the anteroposterior location of the puncture. **B,** Bicaval TEE view demonstrates the superoinferior location of the puncture. As in **A,** the right-sided image is a three-dimensional rendering of where the echo plane is obtained. **C,** Four-chamber TEE view demonstrates the height of the puncture above the plane of the mitral valve.

simulation as well. A relatively new development has been the creation of a purely software-based simulator for training physicians in the use of percutaneous mitral repair. The simulator displays fluoroscopic, echocardiographic, and three-dimensional anatomic renderings that all move in synchrony as various procedure maneuvers are performed **(Figure 1–1).**

This latter software-based approach is especially useful, because the position trainees can bring the simulator home on a laptop computer and practice, whenever they might wish. In contrast, the more traditional simulator devices have a significant hardware component and are typically available in a much more limited way. Basic

skills such as transseptal puncture can also be taught using simulators.

Partnerships with other structural physicians are also useful. Many centers have pediatric interventional cardiologists who have all of the basic building block skills needed for structural interventions and are commonly heavily engaged in many of them in the pediatric population. The basic skills and procedural understanding for adult interventions are parallel to the pediatric skills.

There are no accredited trending programs for structural intervention. Structural experience is becoming an increasing part of interventional fellowship training in some centers. There are several challenges associated with training in structural intervention. Many programs are heavily weighted toward one or another type of structural intervention. For example, in some programs there may be great strength in aortic valve intervention and peripheral vascular intervention, whereas in others most of the structural interventions may be related to shunt closure or large-vessel stent grafting. Thus a single program where the broad, highly varied field of structural intervention can be taught would be unusual. There is also a challenge with the relationship between procedure volume and training. In percutaneous coronary intervention (PCI), 250 PCI procedures are required to meet training program requirements.[7,8]

If this volume-based model for credentialing and training is applied to structural intervention, structural interventions can be considered to be more complex and thus require an even higher volume to assure expertise from training. This is, of course, not possible since structural interventions are needed much less often than coronary and vascular interventional procedures. There is a further disconnect between the widely accepted assumption that there is a clear relationship between institutional and operator volume with clinical outcomes. The volume–outcome relationship is not always clear. To take bypass surgery (coronary artery bypass graft [CABG]) as an example, one widely cited report concludes that "hospital procedure volume is only modestly associated with CABG outcomes and therefore may not be an adequate quality metric for CABG surgery."[9]

A review of Medicare claims data on mortality examine six types of cardiovascular and eight types of cancer procedures. These investigators concluded, "Medicare patients undergoing selected … procedures can significantly reduce the risk of operative death by selecting a high-volume hospital." They also noted, "mortality decreased as volume increased for all 14 types of procedures, but the relative importance of volume varied markedly … differences in adjusted mortality rates between very–low-volume hospitals and very–high-volume hospitals range[d] from over 12% for some procedures to only 0.2% for others" and that "differences in adjusted mortality rates between very–low-volume hospitals and very–high-volume hospitals are greater than 5% for … replacement of an aortic or mitral valve and less than 2% for CABG and lower extremity bypass."[10]

1.3 Multidisciplinary Team and Interdepartmental Cooperation

The utilization of a team approach has been demonstrated to improve outcomes in these complex types of procedures.[11] The multidisciplinary team (MDT) necessary for a structural program goes beyond collaboration between cardiovascular disease interventional specialist and cardiothoracic surgical physician. Additional necessary components extend beyond the individual physicians to include several departments. On-site cardiac surgery is a necessary program component in order to enhance the overall care of the patients undergoing valvular therapies, less for the potential for emergency surgery than

for the quality of the preprocedure evaluation and decision making and for the intraprocedure and postprocedure care a patient is likely to receive in a center with an integrated program. For percutaneous procedures that do not directly involve the surgeon as a procedure operator, the role of the cardiac surgeon remains important. The surgeon has many roles, often as a patient advocate and commonly as a referring physician. The surgeon is a scientific study participant necessary in all of these device trials. Surgeons are familiar with established standards of care in surgery for comparison with percutaneous therapies and may often be the gatekeepers for assessment of high-risk patients for catheter therapy as an alternative to surgery.

After the postprocedure management phase, long-term follow-up for this select group of patients is also part of the MDT approach. Postapproval registries are likely to be requisite for many of the new transcatheter valve therapies. The existence of a research team is thus an important component.

For sites with no structural experience, the MDT can provide background from related procedures such as the insertion of ventricular assist devices and apical conduit therapy for aortic stenosis.

1.4 Facilities and Equipment

Any hospital planning a structural therapy program should have infrastructure that includes a dedicated cardiac procedure room or hybrid operating room. Use of mobile or free-standing C-arm x-ray machine in a conventional operating room does not provide adequate image quality for structural procedures. For TAVR the immediate availability of perfusion services for emergency femoral–femoral bypass is necessary. Retraining of catheterization lab staff to operating room standards of sterility and procedure conduct is necessary, because intravascular and intracardiac device implantations are common. At the same time, the catheterization lab should be recognized as a different environment than the operating room. A surgical recovery area and intensive care with staff experienced in caring for patients who have had cardiac surgical operations is necessary because many structural procedures are performed when the patient is under general anesthesia. Immediate access to vascular surgeons and interventional vascular specialists to deal with major peripheral vascular complications are all also requisite.

A large inventory of disposable equipment is required for the broad range of structural therapies. Intracardiac ultrasound is an absolute must. A dedicated echo machine for the catheterization lab that includes the console in addition to the disposable imaging transducers is critical. Three-dimensional echocardiography has now become a clear standard.

Although transesophageal echocardiography can be used in any situation that might require intracardiac imaging, the requirement for general anesthesia for transesophageal echocardiography adds a great deal of complexity and the need for heavier sedation for structural procedures. The use of intracardiac echocardiography simplifies this greatly.

Disposable equipment costs are considerable. An institutional commitment for a full range of sizes for atrial-septal defect (ASD)–closure devices may require a total investment of several-hundred thousand dollars, given that the cost per device is greater than $5000 and a size range spanning from 4 mm up to 38 mm is necessary for ASD occluders alone. Considering the need for vascular plugs, duct occluders, and ventricular septal defect occluders, as well as the potential to use several brands of septal closure devices, equipment costs can go up very quickly. The range of delivery sheaths and wires also greatly exceeds what might be found in a typical coronary interventional lab, spanning the range from 10F to 24F and sometimes larger. The inventory costs for percutaneous heart valves exceed $30,000 per device.

1.5 The Growing Landscape

The rapid increase in procedure numbers for TAVR internationally has created a dramatic expectation for structural-interventional procedure growth. A perspective regarding the volumes of structural procedures is necessary to understand the potential for the field overall. The volume of PCI in the United States approaches one million procedures annually. These procedures are performed by over 8000 board-certified interventional cardiology practitioners. The magnitude of volume for valve intervention is strikingly different. The total number of surgical aortic valve replacements annually in the United States is about 70,000. The numbers are similar for mitral valve repair and replacement combined. Other structural interventions are also performed in smaller volumes than PCI. The lack of clear definition of indications for closure for patent foramen ovale has minimized the potential for treatment of the tens of thousands of patients with cryptogenic stroke.

These considerations make it clear that structural interventions in the aggregate will grow steadily but do not have the same kind of likely total numbers that exist in the field of coronary therapy. The frequency of structural interventions can be substantial for individual practitioners. This is illustrated in a small way by the recent growth of BAV in the Medicare population. Clearly spurred by interest in TAVR, valvuloplasty has been recognized as the useful palliative therapy for many elderly patients with aortic stenosis who are reported as candidates for surgery and do not qualify for TAVR. BAV procedure volume is increasing **(Figure 1–2).**

The impact of new structural therapies on mortality and quality of life drives the uptake of the interventions. The rapid growth of TAVR internationally is based not only on the novel nature of the devices and procedures, but mostly on the mortality reduction and dramatic impact on quality of life. The slower uptake for mitral regurgitation interventions reflects in large part the complexity of the disease. The major factor in determining the number of structural procedures that ultimately will be performed is reimbursement. The approval of TAVR

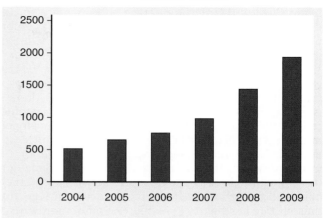

BALLOON AORTIC VALVULOPLASTY
Medicare volumes

Figure 1–2 There has been a steady increase in the volume of balloon aortic valvuloplasty procedures since 2008. This clearly reflects growing interest in transcatheter aortic valve replacement specifically and structural intervention in general.

with the immediate announcement of a National Coverage Decision by the Centers for Medicare and Medicaid Services makes it clear that there will be considerable pressure on the practitioner to use these procedures in patients for whom the trial data support their use, and that the pressure will be without latitude for off-label use.

The randomized trials for closure for patent foramen ovale are another example that has made it clear that evidence-based, randomized, trial-driven criteria will be used for patient selection for the range of structural interventions. It is likely that there will be this kind of development across the use of catheter-based therapies for aortic and mitral valve disease, as well as for shunt closure and atrial appendage occlusion.

1.6 Developing a Focus on Structural Intervention

A remarkable feature of practice in structural intervention as it has developed is the magnitude of time commitment necessary for these procedures. Because most of the structural interventions are in a trial phase, the screening for inclusion in the trials is highly rigorous. Most patients who come for evaluation have already had multiple studies including transthoracic and transesophageal echocardiograms, CT scans, and angiographic studies. The review of these multimodality studies and the assessment of clinical features of patients for appropriateness for these new therapies requires much more time than the typical and even highly complex coronary interventional patient. Compounding the time necessary to assess these patients is the challenge of the incompatibility of many of the imaging programs from one institution to another. In this author's practice, it is common to find compact disc (CD)-recorded imaging studies that will not play using any of several computers and programs. The fact that there is a Digital Imaging and Communications in Medicine imaging standard has been obfuscated by a whole variety of proprietary "imaging for dummies" formats used to create CD images for use outside of the institution that performed the initial study.

The acquisition of specific knowledge for each of the various device interventions contributes to this "structural intervention as full-time job" paradigm. Understanding the reading of cross-sectional CT angiographic images for assessment for TAVR, three-dimensional reconstruction of left atrial CT images to assess left atrial appendage size and morphology, and the utilization of intracardiac and transesophageal echocardiography for the evaluation for ASD closure represent the spectrum of cognitive skills that have to be incorporated into day-to-day practice in structural therapy. The time commitment is further compounded by patient evaluation after structural interventions, which also contributes to the level of dedication necessary to succeed in this new and rapidly developing field.

1.7 Summary

Starting a program in the growing field of structural heart interventions is a long-term project that requires a large personal and institutional commitment. A substantial and novel knowledge base, new skills, and a MDT are all essential elements. The path for developing a structural program is different for the various fields in the area; an adult cardiologist with experience in valve disease will not follow the same steps as someone with a coronary disease practice, and the surgeon with no catheter skills will similarly have different needs. Because the field is young, there are no defined training requirements or pathways. This new area of therapy is both a challenge and a great opportunity.

REFERENCES

1. Ruiz CE, Feldman TE, Hijazi ZM, et al: Interventional fellowship in structural and congenital heart disease for adults: core curriculum, *Catheter Cardiovasc Interv* E90-E105, 2010,
2. Ruiz CE, Feldman RE, Hijazi ZM, et al: Interventional fellowship in structural and congenital heart disease for adults. *JACC Cardiovasc Interv* 3:e1–e15, 2010.
3. Herrmann HC, Baxter S, Ruiz CE, et al: Results of the society of cardiac angiography and interventions survey of physicians and training directors on procedures for structural and valvular heart disease, *Catheter Cardiovasc Interv* 76(4):E106–E110, 2010.
4. Feldman T, Ruiz CE, Hijazi Z: The SCAI Structural Heart Disease Council: toward addressing training, credentialing, and guidelines for structural heart disease intervention, *Catheter Cardiovasc Interv* 76(4):E87–E89, 2010.
5. Feldman T: The increasing importance of echocardiographic guidance for structural heart intervention, *Catheter Cardiovasc Interv* 75:1141–1142, 2010.
6. Feldman T: Learning curve for transcatheter aortic valve replacement (TAVR), *Catheter Cardiovasc Interv* 78:985–986, 2011.
7. Hirshfeld JW Jr, Banas JS Jr, Brundage BH, et al: ACC training statement on recommendations for the structure of an optimal adult interventional cardiology training program: a report of the ACC task force on clinical expert consensus documents, *J Am Coll Cardiol* 34:2141–2147, 1999.
8. Pepine CJ, Babb JD, Brinker JA, et al: Guidelines for training in adult cardiovascular medicine. Core Cardiology Training Symposium (COCATS). Task Force 3: training in cardiac catheterization and interventional cardiology, *J Am Coll Cardiol* 25:14–16, 1995.
9. Petersen ED, Coombs LP, DeLong ER, et al: Procedure volume as a marker of quality for CABG surgery, *JAMA* 291:195–201, 2004.
10. Birkmeyer JD, Siewers AE, Finlayson EV, et al: Hospital volume and surgical mortality in the United States, *N Engl J Med* 346(15):1128–1137, 2002.
11. Neily J, Mills PD, Young-Xu Y, Carney BT, et al: Association between implementation of a medical team training program and surgical mortality, *JAMA* 304:1693–1700, 2010.

Chapter 2

Imaging in Structural Heart Disease

STACEY D. CLEGG • ERNESTO E. SALCEDO •
ROBERT A. QUAIFE • JOHN D. CARROLL

Transcatheter therapies for both congenital and noncongenital structural heart lesions continue to expand in both their scope and complexity. The evolution of percutaneous treatment options for structural heart disease (SHD) has also come with advances in the imaging techniques associated with successful outcomes. SHD intervention uniquely requires an understanding of anatomic relationships in three dimensions and soft-tissue visualization, necessitating the addition of echocardiography and more recently cardiac computed tomography (CT) and cardiac magnetic resonance (CMR) imaging to carry out the complex tasks required. Imaging has become an indispensable part of the SHD procedure from preprocedural planning and patient selection, intraprocedural guidance, postprocedural assessment of results, and finally, long-term follow-up care. The imaging techniques required for successful SHD interventions are often complex and require an expertise in several different imaging modalities. Additionally, these technologies must be brought directly into the cardiac catheterization lab. In this chapter the imaging modalities commonly used in SHD interventions and how they can be integrated into today's catheterization lab are discussed.

2.1 Imaging Modalities

The SHD interventionalist needs to be familiar with all the imaging modalities available and clearly understand the strengths and limitations of each technique. The fundamental SHD imaging modalities include: fluoroscopy and angiography; echocardiography, including two-dimensional (2D) and three-dimensional (3D) transthoracic echocardiography (TTE), intracardiac echocardiography (ICE), and transesophageal echocardiography (TEE); cardiac CT; and CMR imaging. **Table 2–1** outlines the basic imaging modalities used in SHD interventions and their respective strengths and weaknesses. Specific

examples of SHD interventions highlight each of the different imaging techniques, many of which require a multimodal approach. As technology continues to evolve there will likely be more multimodal imaging approaches as well as the expansion of hybrid imaging techniques that combine the familiarity and excellent device visualization of fluoroscopy with the soft tissue definition of 3D TEE, CT, and CMR imaging.

2.2 Imaging in the Catheterization Lab: Special Considerations

FACILITIES

The cardiac catheterization lab was introduced in the 1970s, a time when fluoroscopy was the only imaging modality employed in routine practice. The fluoroscopic C-arm remains the centerpiece of most cardiac catheterization labs. Fluoroscopy is a vital component of any laboratory; however, integration of other imaging modalities into this space must be a consideration in today's cardiac catheterization lab. SHD interventions often require real-time imaging guidance, often with TEE, ICE, or CT. Intravascular ultrasound, fractional flow reserve, and to a certain extent, ICE are conveniently designed as "plug and play" add-ons to the fluoroscopy system; however, this is not the case with the display and visualization components of TEE, CT, and CMR imaging. The modern cardiac catheterization lab should be large enough to accommodate the extra equipment and a team of sonographers and echocardiographers in addition to the interventional and anesthesia teams. The fluoroscopic C-arm is typically mounted at the head of the table where the echocardiographer and the anesthesiologist need access to the patient for their respective tasks. The room can often become crowded, and the various team members may not have an adequate view of the display monitors. When setting up an SHD laboratory of

TABLE 2–1
Strengths and Weaknesses of Imaging Modalities Used in Structural Heart Interventions

Imaging Modality	Strengths	Weaknesses	Preprocedure (pre cath lab)	Intraprocedure (in cath lab)	Postprocedure (in cath lab)
Fluoroscopy Angiography	Device and hardware visualization Familiar to interventionalist	2D only Soft-tissue visualization Radiation exposure	+	++++	++++
2D/3D TTE	Noninvasive and inexpensive Doppler hemodynamics Long-term follow-up care	Physical and sterile constraints of cath lab limit intraprocedural use	++++	+	+
2D TEE	Easily integrated in cath lab Spatial resolution Doppler hemodynamics	Invasive May require general anesthesia	+++	++++	+++
3D TEE	Easily integrated in cath lab Anatomic and soft-tissue visualization	Invasive May require general anesthesia Requires additional expertise	+++	++++	++++
ICE	Easily integrated in cath lab Spatial resolution No need for general anesthesia	Invasive Additional vascular access site Requires additional expertise	+	++++	+++
CT	Advanced structural characterization	Difficult to integrate in cath lab Requires additional expertise	+++	+	−
CMR/QCMR	Advanced structural characterization Hemodynamic characterization Shunt and regurgitant lesion evaluation	Difficult to integrate in cath lab Expensive Requires additional expertise	+++	−	−

2D, Two dimensional; *3D,* three dimensional; *CMR,* cardiac magnetic resonance; *CT,* computed tomography; *ICE,* intrathoracic echocardiography; *TEE,* transesophageal echocardiography; *TTE,* transthoracic echocardiography; *QCMR,* quantitative cardiac magnetic resonance.

the future, the imaging components should be considered as important as the fluoroscopy unit.[1]

The SHD lab or hybrid operating room should ideally be at least 800 square feet. The monitors should be large enough and mobile enough to provide adequate visualization for the interventionalist, as well as the echocardiographer, who usually is positioned at the opposite side of the table. The monitors should be capable of displaying a large number of inputs at a very high resolution. With the integration of advanced imaging techniques such as the importation of preprocedure CT and CMR images, there should be enough workstations with the appropriate software capabilities. Lastly there must be an integrated imaging archive system that can store intraprocedure imaging clips from several modalities in a composite "case" for postprocedure review.[1,2]

PERSONNEL, CORE KNOWLEDGE, AND TRAINING

In addition to the facilities, there are considerations with regard to the expertise that is available within the institution. Reading and interpreting imaging studies

for intervention is a markedly different task than reading studies for diagnostic purposes only. Preintervention studies focus on patient selection, device sizing and suitability, and intraprocedural strategy. For example, a preprocedural TEE for an atrial septal defect (ASD) closure is not simply to diagnose the ASD. Additional attention must be paid to size of the defect, the relationship and distance to surrounding structures, and adequate rims for seating of the closure device. These are not typically parameters recorded in a routine diagnostic study. A team of echocardiographers, imaging specialists, and radiologists who have a dedicated interest in SHD intervention is key to successful outcomes.

The increasing use of imaging in interventional cardiology may also change the paradigm of how future interventionalists are trained. The interventional cardiologist must be capable of interpreting imaging studies, including advanced modalities for which there may have been no formal training. The authors recommend that SHD training expand to include an imaging curriculum. At minimum, this would include instruction in ICE and TEE, including real-time 3D TEE (RT 3D TEE).

BOX 2–1

Imaging Considerations for the SHD Catheterization Lab

Facilities

Large room size

- Must accommodate imaging equipment and extra personnel (echocardiographer, sonographer, anesthesia team)

Monitors and displays

- Monitors visible to both imaging team and interventionalist
- Monitors large enough to display different imaging modalities simultaneously (i.e., fluoroscopy and echocardiography)

Integrated imaging equipment

- Embedded vascular access US, ICE, TTE, and TEE display
- Tableside controls

Computer imaging workstations
Imaging archiving and systems integration
Institutional requirements

- Must include CT, CMR imaging, and advanced echocardiography capabilities

Anticipate next-generation upgrades to imaging systems (i.e., rotational C-arm CT, larger displays, hybrid multimodality imaging)

Personnel

Dedicated imaging team with understanding of SHD intervention
Multidisciplinary team with expertise in echocardiography, CT, and CMR imaging

Core Knowledge and Experience

- Increasing reliance on imaging
- Interventional cardiology training often lacks the requisite imaging training for complex SHD interventions
- Imaging for SHD intervention differs in content and focus from diagnostic imaging

CMR, Cardiac magnetic resonance; *CT,* computed tomography; *ICE,* intracardiac echocardiography; *SHD,* structural heart disease; *TEE,* transesophageal echocardiography; *TTE,* transthoracic echocardiography; *US,* ultrasound.

Box 2–1 outlines the requirements for a successful integrated imaging and catheterization lab suite.

2.3 The Role of Imaging in SHD Intervention

The role of imaging in SHD intervention can be divided into three components: (1) preprocedural planning and patient selection, (2) intraprocedural imaging guidance, and (3) postprocedure assessment of results and long-term follow-up care.

PREPROCEDURAL IMAGING

Preprocedural planning often includes diagnostic imaging studies with a focus on interventional aspects of the procedure, including the type of defect, the vascular access, the navigation strategy, and any special equipment that may be required for the procedure. In advanced percutaneous valve interventions the preprocedural imaging is critical for patient selection and good outcomes. Preprocedural imaging often includes CT and CMR imaging as well as echocardiography. Nearly every patient who comes for a structural heart evaluation will have had some type of preprocedural imaging that includes baseline diagnostic studies. The key components of preprocedural imaging will be highlighted in several examples in this chapter.

INTRAPROCEDURAL IMAGING GUIDANCE

Intraprocedural guidance refers to physically bringing the imaging modality to the catheterization lab and actively using the images to navigate catheters, position and deploy devices, and immediately assess for complications. Although fluoroscopy provides important intraprocedure guidance, including the visualization of hardware, wires, and devices, the lack of soft-tissue definition and visualization of cardiac chambers has limited this modality in SHD interventions.

Intraprocedure imaging modalities must be portable, must not interfere with the set-up of the catheterization lab, and importantly, must provide real-time imaging that can be updated and changed as the procedure dictates. Imaging guidance has predominantly been an echocardiography-based task with ICE being the most familiar modality for navigation in the interventional lab. 2D TEE and, increasingly, RT 3D TEE are the preferred imaging modalities for complex SHD interventions. RT 3D TEE has been used to successfully guide most common percutaneous SHD interventions.[3-6] It provides the necessary soft-tissue definition and can be rapidly updated and repositioned for new views to optimize and tailor the image guidance.[7]

An example of the emergence of image guidance is provided in **Figure 2–1** depicting the transseptal puncture. This procedure was originally described by Ross, Braunwald, and Morrow over 50 years ago[8] and has been commonly performed with fluoroscopy alone, without the addition of expensive imaging equipment. However, safety and confidence can be enhanced with the echocardiographic imaging of the interatrial septum either with ICE or with 2D TEE or RT 3D TEE. The interatrial septum is visualized in several planes, with care to puncture at the site of the fossa ovalis, which is easily visualized as the thin portion of the septum. The Brockenbrough needle is pulled back from the superior vena cava to the right atrium, and the site of puncture is directly visualized. Simultaneous pressure monitoring also confirms successful crossing to the left atrium. With the advent of complex navigation requirements for mitral valve interventions there is increasing reliance on not only a safe transseptal puncture but also a strategic placement of the transseptal puncture. **Figure 2–2** shows the strategy of transseptal puncture for a MitraClip (Abbott Vascular Structural Heart, Menlo Park, Calif.) procedure. The correct alignment of the clip

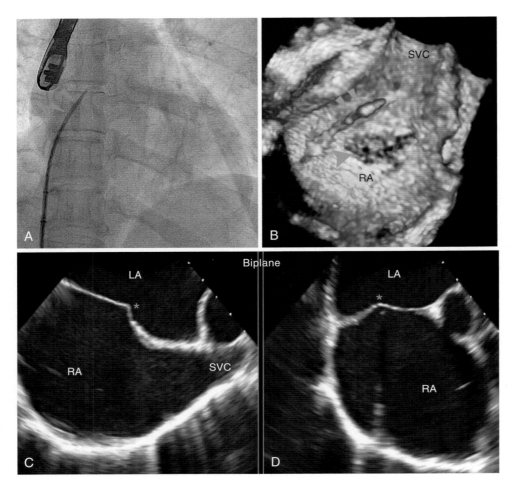

Figure 2–1 **Imaging guidance for transseptal puncture. A,** Fluoroscopic imaging of a transseptal puncture. In the anteroposterior position the wire (double red arrows) is pulled back from the superior vena cava *(SVC)* to the right atrium. Using a combination of tactile feedback and fluoroscopic orientation the septum is crossed. **B,** RT 3D TEE imaging during transseptal puncture. Note the wire (double red arrows) in the right atrium *(RA)*. The *arrowhead* points to the fossa ovalis, the thinnest area of the septum. The fossa can often have the appearance of a septal defect as a result of echo drop-out. **C** and **D** depict biplane TEE imaging of the transseptal puncture in the bicaval **(C)** and midesophageal 4-chamber **(D)** views. The catheter "tents" the septum *(*)* demarcating the position of puncture.

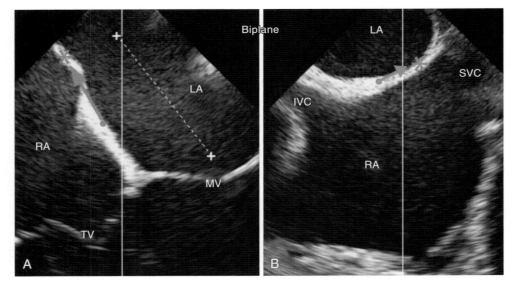

Figure 2–2 **Strategic transseptal puncture for Mitraclip procedure.** Biplane 2D TEE images of the interatrial septum. A midesophageal 4-chamber view **(A)** and the corresponding biplane bicaval view **(B)** of the interatrial septum. The *red arrows* demonstrate the direction of the ideal septal puncture site *(*)* compared to a standard septal puncture site *(•)*, ensuring more navigation room within the left atrium (LA). The additional anteroposterior navigation room within the LA is shown in **A** *(dashed white line)*.

delivery system perpendicular to the plane of the mitral valve orifice is critical and requires adequate navigation room within the left atrium. A strategic transseptal puncture must be performed posterior and superior from what might be considered the standard target puncture site.

Although image guidance is usually associated with a real-time imaging technology, CT is increasingly becoming an intraprocedure modality as well. CT has the benefit of excellent soft-tissue characterization and provides a full field of view. The limitation, however, is cardiac motion artifact and the need for electrocardiography (ECG)-gated

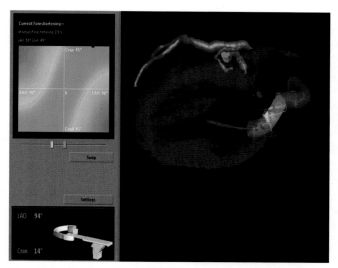

Figure 2–3   Cardiac CT fusion imaging for intraprocedural guidance. Fusion imaging of CT angiography (CTA) datasets with centerline data for preplanning the optimal fluoroscopic views at the time of percutaneous closure of a mitral paravalvular leak. Rotation of the image data provides the operator a 3D sense of the procedure. The gantry angulation can be predetermined, allowing for selection of an optimal perspective for target navigation without significant overlap of adjacent structures (LAO 94 CRAN 14 in this example). The left anterior descending coronary artery is shown on top *(red line)* for reference and orientation. The proposed pathway for closure is shown, with the paravalvular leak highlighted in *yellow.* Simultaneous RT TEE is used intraprocedure for wire positioning. This combined image guidance strategy provides maximal preprocedure and intraprocedural visualization to help successfully complete the task.

acquisitions. Preprocedure CT scans can be used to outline navigation strategies for complex procedures. The CT data set can be rotated into an orientation, mimicking the fluoroscopic C-arm projection and can provide a preplanned viewing angle for image guidance. **Figure 2–3** is an example of preplanning the intraprocedural navigation strategy for a mitral paravalvular leak closure using TrueView software (Phillips Medical, Andover, Mass.). The gantry position was predetermined for optimal viewing, and a roadmap of the catheter navigation to the mitral paravalvular leak was created. These data can then be imported into the angiographic suite and registered with fluoroscopy. As a result, the CT image will rotate with the C-arm during the procedure, providing real-time image guidance. This type of technology may limit radiation time and contrast dose and enhance procedural success. **Table 2–2** describes the modalities used for intraprocedural guidance. These techniques have fundamentally changed how SHD interventions are performed with an increased emphasis on safety and operator confidence.

POSTPROCEDURAL ASSESSMENT

Postprocedural assessment is often immediate and within the catheterization lab to assess the adequacy of device deployment and any immediate complications such as rupture, pericardial effusion, or device embolization. Long-term follow-up care includes routine TTE in almost all cases. CT may be of use in assessing for

residual prosthetic paravalvular leaks. CMR imaging may be necessary in complex congenital heart disease follow-up care, but with the *caveat* that in some cases shadowing and artifact from devices limits the use of CMR imaging once the procedure is completed.

2.4 Modality Selection

Modality selection is based largely on the procedure planned and the capabilities and expertise of the institution. In many scenarios more than one imaging modality is adequate and appropriate for the procedure, and local practices predict the modality of choice. Outlined here are the most common imaging modalities employed in SHD interventions with examples of their use. Each imaging modality has unique features and limitations. The major procedures covered in this book are listed in **Table 2–3** with the corresponding most appropriate and practical imaging modalities.

FLUOROSCOPY AND ANGIOGRAPHY

Despite a focus on the newer imaging techniques, fluoroscopy and angiography are still critical in every SHD intervention. Fluoroscopy provides a large field of view and excellent device and hardware definition based on the use of radio-opaque catheters and wires. The addition of iodinated contrast allows for cineangiography. These techniques have the advantage of being real time; however, they are limited in SHD because of the 2D projections and inability to navigate in a 3D space such as within cardiac chambers. The drawbacks of radiation and contrast can also limit the use of fluoroscopy and angiography in certain patient populations.

Vascular Closure Procedures

Fluoroscopy is the most familiar imaging modality to any interventional cardiologist, and the SHD interventionalist must recognize the fluoroscopic projections of radio-opaque interventional devices and wires used in all procedures. Angiography and fluoroscopy may be used alone for vascular closure procedures, including closure of coronary artery fistulas as well as other congenital or acquired vascular defects such as a patent ductus arteriosis or pulmonary arteriovenous malformations. In the case of coronary artery fistulae, a complete angiographic assessment to look for aneurismal dilations proximal to fistulae and the size of the vascular defect should take place. **Figure 2–4** shows a case where routine diagnostic angiography revealed a large coronary artery–to–pulmonary artery fistula. The lesion was successfully coiled with fluoroscopic guidance from an antegrade approach.

Alcohol Septal Ablation

Often angiography must be combined with other imaging modalities for guiding interventions. This is particularly the case with alcohol septal ablation for the treatment of hypertrophic cardiomyopathy. The angiographic imaging

TABLE 2–2

Image Guidance: Comparing ICE, RT 3D TEE, and Cardiac CT

	ICE	RT 3D TEE	Cardiac CT
Cost	Expensive, single use catheter	Equipment available in most institution Increased personnel and procedural time	Expensive, requires a preprocedural scan or rotational C-arm CT Special imaging equipment to import CT and integrate in cath lab
Safety	Potential complications of additional vascular access	General anesthesia or moderate sedation required	Additional ionizing radiation
Operator expertise	Interventionalist must manipulate and interpret images	Requires echo team with expertise in SHD and RT 3D TEE	Requires additional operator and institutional expertise in advanced cardiac imaging
Integration in cath lab	Good; often a built-in addition to cath lab	Fair; requires additional personnel, equipment, and space	Fair to poor; requires additional software and adequate displays
Personnel	Interventional team	Interventional team, echocardiography team, anesthesia team	Interventional team +/– advanced cardiac imaging team
Quality of image guidance	Excellent; limited to 2D	Excellent; includes 3D imaging, comprehensive evaluation of complex structures	Fair to good; good soft tissue delineation. Limited by cardiac and respiratory motion. Prospective gating within the cath lab is not yet feasible
Doppler capabilities	Excellent	Fair	No hemodynamic assessment possible
Procedural complexity	Minimal complexity; PFO and simple ASD closures	Complex; complex congenital and valvular SHD interventions	Complex; favors intervention on great vessels (nonmoving cardiac structures for C-arm CT) or preprocedure ECG gated CT for valvular intervention Images cannot be updated or manipulated in real time unless registered to fluoroscopy

2D, Two-dimensional; *3D,* three-dimensional; *ASD,* atrial septal defect; *CT,* computed tomography; *ECG,* electrocardiography; *ICE,* intracardiac echocardiography; *PFO,* patent foramen ovale; *RT 3D TEE,* real time three-dimensional echocardiography; *SHD,* structural heart disease.

must be correlated to the echocardiographic imaging to correctly target the site of septal ablation and avoid complications. Routine cineangiography is performed with special attention to the septal perforating vessels. The interventional cardiologist selects the septal vessel felt to supply the obstructive portion of the hypertrophic septum. Before alcohol injection, the interventionalist inflates a balloon to completely obstruct the septal perforating artery and then injects agitated saline contrast (in our laboratory this is an agitated cocktail of dilute contrast, a small amount of heme, and atmosphere) through the balloon catheter. The agitated saline contrast brightens the portion of the septum supplied by the target septal vessel as visualized by TTE or TEE. The distribution of contrast is examined in real time, assessing for size and location within the septum and for any signs of enhancement in the right ventricle or papillary muscles that might be associated with complications of transmural infarction or severe mitral regurgitation (MR). **Figure 2–5** shows an example of a patient with three large proximal septal perforating vessels. Each branch was assessed with the injection of agitated saline contrast. Once the appropriate septal perforator is determined, 100% alcohol is injected through the balloon catheter. Echocardiography is used to monitor the left ventricular outflow tract (LVOT) gradient and for reduction in systolic

anterior motion of the mitral valve. Continuous monitoring of the left ventricle for new wall motion abnormalities or significant MR should be performed, as it may suggest the presence of alcohol in another vascular distribution. Often the visualization of third-degree heart block with cardiac standstill is seen by the echocardiographer before the rhythm can be recognized.

ECHOCARDIOGRAPHY

There are four echocardiographic modalities related to SHD interventions to discuss, including: (1) ICE; (2) 2D TTE; (3) 2D TEE, and (4) RT 3D TEE. TTE is relatively limited in SHD because of the physical constraints of the catheterization lab, location of the C-arm relative to the patient and echocardiographer, and suboptimal views obtained with the patient flat on his or her back as opposed to in the left lateral decubitus position. Its use in these authors' laboratory is limited to alcohol septal ablation for defining the region of the septum to be targeted **(see Figure 2–5)**, although it may also be used to assess for aortic insufficiency after balloon aortic valvuloplasty and to assess the result after mitral balloon valvuloplasty. The other echocardiographic modalities have important strengths and weaknesses and are discussed in detail in the next paragraphs.

TABLE 2–3

Imaging Modalities for Structural Heart Interventions

Procedure	X-ray	TEE	ICE	CT	CMR	Notes
Valve Interventions						
Transseptal	++++	++++	++++	–	–	
Balloon aortic and pulmonic valvuloplasty	++++	+	–	–	–	
Transcatheter pulmonic valve implantation	++++	+	–	++	++	CT/CMR valuable in preprocedure and postprocedure evaluation.
Mitral balloon valvuloplasty	++++	++++	++	–	–	3D TEE preferable for image guidance
MitraClip	+++	++++	–	–	–	2D and 3D TEE imperative for image guidance and device deployment
Transcatheter aortic valve implantation	++++	++++	–	++++	–	Preprocedure patient selection with CT, TTE, TEE Intraprocedure guidance with 2D and 3D TEE
Mitral and aortic paravalvular leak closure	++++	++++	–	++++	–	Preprocedure strategy with CT 3D TEE preferable for image guidance
Structural Defect Interventions						
PFO closure	++++	+	++++	–	–	ICE generally preferred to TEE for convenience and efficiency
ASD closure	++++	++++	++++	–	–	Preprocedure CT/CMR if anatomy complex or ill-defined by TEE
VSD closure	++++	++++		+++	+++	Preprocedure strategy with CT/CMR Intraprocedure guidance with 2D and 3D TEE
PDA closure	++++	–	–	++	++	Preprocedure echo alone often is sufficient CT, CMR useful in adults with inadequate echo evaluation
Coronary fistula, PVM	++++	–	–	++	++	Preprocedure TTE with contrast for shunt assessment Preprocedure strategy with CT/CMR useful to identify PVM location, number, and size
Other Interventions						
Alcohol septal ablation	++++	++++	+	–	++++	TTE with contrast for intraprocedural guidance CMR for preprocedure and postprocedure assessment
LAA closure	++++	+++	+++	–	–	RT 3D TEE preferable for image guidance

2D, Two-dimensional; *3D,* three-dimensional; *ASD,* atrial septal defect; *CMR,* cardiac magnetic resonance; *CT,* computed tomography; *ICE,* intrathoracic echocardiography; *LAA,* left atrial appendage; *PDA,* patent ductus arteriosus; *PFO,* patent foramen ovale; *PVM,* pulmonary vascular malformation; *RT 3D TEE,* real time three-dimensional echocardiography; *TEE,* transesophageal echocardiography; *TTE,* transthoracic echocardiography; *VSD,* ventricular septal defect; *echo,* echocardiography.

Echocardiography is the predominant imaging modality in all aspects of SHD, including preprocedural assessment, procedural guidance, and follow-up care. Echocardiography is particularly powerful for imaging guidance because of its real-time acquisition, portability, and relative safety (no contrast or radiation).

INTRACARDIAC ECHOCARDIOGRAPHY

ICE is the only echocardiographic modality completely under the control of the interventional cardiologist without the need for other imaging personnel during the procedure. The interventionalist must be able to acquire, troubleshoot, and interpret the images. The most commonly used ICE catheters are 8F to 10F, 4.5 to 10 MHz phased-array transducers. The catheters typically have a depth of penetration of 10 to 20 cm making them well suited for near-field interventions such as ASD and patent foramen ovale (PFO) closures and less appealing for more distant structures such as the left atrial appendage (LAA). The ICE catheter is usually introduced via the femoral vein and positioned in the right atrium as the reference position. The catheter is maneuvered by rotation and flexion within the right atrium and right ventricle to acquire the diagnostic and navigational views. Its position can be locked to focus on a specific structure or target of intervention while the interventional cardiologist manipulates other wires and devices. The benefits of ICE are its good spatial and temporal resolution, Doppler capabilities, portability, and its "built-in" integration into the cardiac catheterization lab. Unlike TEE, there is no need for general anesthesia, keeping expense and procedure time

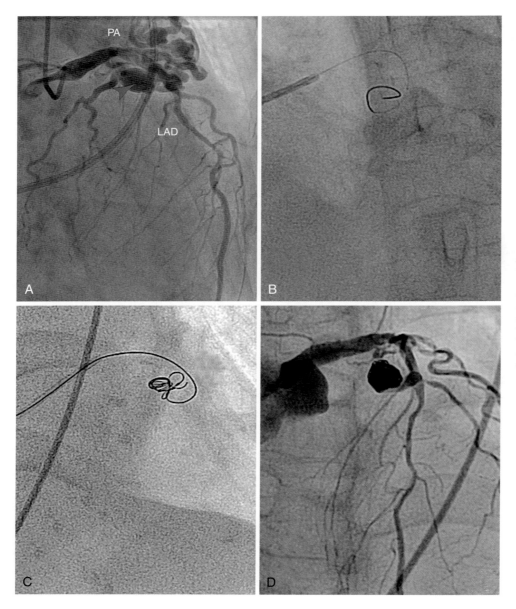

Figure 2–4 Coronary artery fistula closure. A, Diagnostic angiography reveals a large cavernous fistula *(arrowhead)* from the left anterior descending *(LAD)* to the pulmonary artery *(PA)*. Fluoroscopy and cineangiography are used alone to guide the radio-opaque coils into the fistula's feeder vessel via the antegrade approach (**B** and **C**). **D,** Complete closure of the fistula.

at a minimum; however, there is the risk of the additional vascular access site and the catheter itself is an expensive single-use device. First generation 3D-capable ICE catheters create a narrow-angle 3D volume set unlike the broad angle of RT 3D TEE.

Patent Foramen Ovale Closure

At our institution, University of Colorado Hospital, the ICE catheter is generally used for PFO closures and occasionally for simple ASD closures; however, its use has been validated in many other SHD interventions, including mitral balloon valvuloplasty, electrophysiology ablations, and LAA appendage occlusion.[9,10] It has been shown to be equally as effective as TEE in closing ASDs and PFOs without the need for anesthesia and additional operators.[11] PFO closure favors ICE because the disks of most devices usually adequately capture the septum primum and secundum without the worry of inadequate rim tissue. The

procedure can be performed efficiently without the need for general anesthesia. There are reports of safe PFO closure using only fluoroscopy[12]; however the PFO anatomy can vary widely with ranges of size, thickness of the septum secundum, presence of atrial septal aneurysm, or long tunnel length. All these anatomic variants can affect device seating,[13] and the use of echocardiographic guidance, either with ICE or TEE, is standard practice. **Figure 2–6** shows a PFO closure guided by ICE, illustrating the importance of echocardiographic guidance in this procedure for device sizing and complete closure.

TRANSESOPHAGEAL ECHOCARDIOGRAPHY

In many SHD cases there is already a need for general anesthesia, and as such, TEE is the imaging modality of choice for guiding structural heart interventions. In addition, it is often a preprocedure planning and diagnostic tool. The image quality of TEE is usually excellent, but

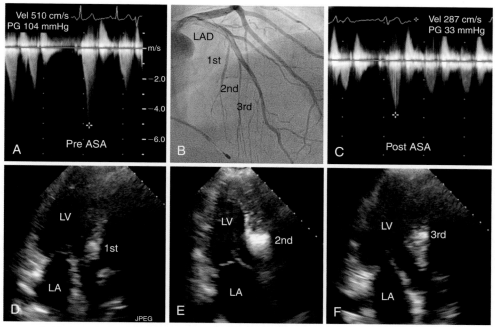

Figure 2–5 Alcohol septal ablation (ASA) in hypertrophic cardiomyopathy. A and **C** depict post-premature ventricular contraction (PVC) left ventricular outflow gradients before and after ASA. Note that the gradient decreased from 100 mmHg to 30 mmHg. **B** highlights the first, second, and third septal perforators on this right anterior oblique (RAO) left coronary arteriogram. **D, E,** and **F** illustrate septal enhancement at different levels of the interventricular septum corresponding to the septal perforator injected with contrast. Note that injection of the first septal perforator **(D)** produced enhancement of the septum near its membranous portion; this was considered inappropriately proximal for a successful ablation. The injection of the third septal perforator **(F),** was considered to be inferior, beyond the point of systolic anterior motion of the mitral valve (SAM). **E** depicts injection of the second septal perforator, which was at the level of SAM, and was chosen for alcohol ablation.

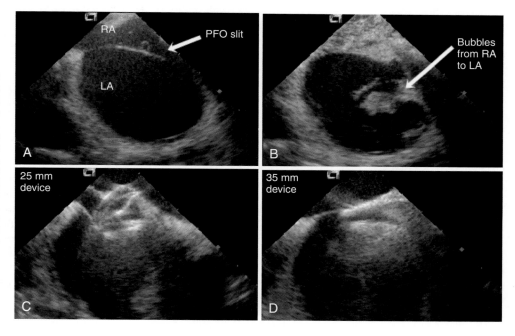

Figure 2–6 ICE guidance in PFO closure. A, ICE image of a large PFO showing the opening created by the thin septum primum unattached to the septum secundum. **B,** Agitated saline readily crosses from the right atrium (RA) into the left atrium (LA) via the PFO. **C,** A 25-mm Amplatzer PFO device is inserted; however, with pushing of the delivery cable, the right atrial disc prolapses into the PFO tunnel. **D,** A 35-mm device is inserted with good capture of the thick septum secundum, providing device stability and closure of the PFO.

limitations include the relatively narrow field of view and the varying echogenicity of catheters, wires, and devices, some of which may not be well visualized. TEE is generally favored over ICE for most SHD procedures predominantly because of the good image quality and the established safety and efficacy of 2D and RT 3D TEE in device sizing, navigation, deployment and assessment of postprocedure complications.[3,5,6,14]

The modern matrix-array TEE probes have capability of switching between biplane 2D TEE and RT 3D TEE. The matrix-array probe supports four different acquisition modes, including narrow sector (live 3D), wide-sector focused (3D zoom), large sector (full volume), and 2D simultaneous biplane (X plane) modes. **Table 2–4** outlines the different 3D TEE acquisition modes. The 2D-biplane mode has high spatial resolution and

TABLE 2–4

3D TEE Imaging Modes and Application in SHD Interventions

Data Set	Trade Name*	Dimensions	Real Time	Temporal Resolution	Spatial Resolution	Color Doppler	Application in SHD Interventions
Large sector	Full Volume	90° × 90° by 2D image depth	No	++++	+	Yes	Not for image guidance because of requirement for ECG gating and offline processing Useful in preprocedural planning: evaluation of LV size, function
Narrow sector	Live 3D	60° × 30° by 2D image depth	Yes	++++	++	Yes	Guiding catheters and devices Mimics 2D images; useful for evaluation for MV apparatus, LVOT, AoV
Wide sector focused	Live 3D Zoom	20° × 20° to 85° × 85° by variable height	Yes	+	++++	No	Guiding catheters and devices Detailed inspection of anatomy Image guidance of MV, LAA, interatrial septum, pulmonary veins
Simultaneous biplane	X-plane	2 planes at a 90° angle to each other	Yes	+++	+++	Yes	Guiding catheters and devices Doppler assessment of valve gradients, shunt lesions Image guidance of transseptal puncture, MV, LAA, interatrial septum, AoV

2D, Two-dimensional; *3D,* three-dimensional; *AoV,* aortic valve; *ECG,* electrocardiography; *LAA,* left atrial appendage; *LV,* left ventricle; *LVOT,* left ventricular outflow tract; *MV,* mitral valve; *SHD,* structural heart disease; *TEE,* transesophageal echocardiography.
*Philips Medical Systems, Andover, Mass.

provides color Doppler, which is critical in most cases. The live 3D mode acquires narrow-sector images equivalent to 2D TEE views. The live 3D zoom mode provides a magnified pyramidal volume focused on a region of interest with less depth. This mode is particularly useful for imaging specific cardiac structures during navigation of catheters and devices, for example, the mitral valve from the left atrial perspective (the surgeon's view), the interatrial septum, and the LAA with excellent spatial resolution. The acquired images are rotated and tilted to provide the ideal perspective. A systematic approach to 3D echo studies should be employed to provide a consistent and thorough analysis of the region of interest and to avoid getting "lost in 3D space" as the image is rotated and tilted during the interventional procedure.[15,16]

Atrial Septal Defect Closure

Transcatheter closure for hemodynamically significant secundum-type ASDs is now standard therapy with an excellent procedural success rate.[17,18] Candidates for transcatheter closure must have a thorough preprocedure imaging evaluation to assess the size of the defect, the adequacy of septal rims, and the relationship to adjacent structures such as the aortic valve and coronary sinus. Importantly, additional congenital defects including sinus venosus ASD and partial anomalous pulmonary venous return must be ruled out. This may require preprocedure TEE or CMR imaging to ascertain.

The size of the defect can be measured in two orthogonal planes using 2D TEE (bicaval view and

midesophageal four-chamber view). During the intervention, balloon sizing of the defect takes place to confirm measurements, with the *caveat* that oval defects will be converted to circular defects. Color Doppler is applied to demonstrate absence of interatrial shunting with balloon inflation. Several studies have shown the feasibility and usefulness of RT 3D TEE imaging in ASD closure and correlation between 2D TEE and balloon sizing of ASDs.[14,19] **Figure 2–7** shows the use of 2D TEE and RT 3D TEE in a secundum ASD closure with an Amplatzer (St. Jude Medical, St. Paul, Minn.) occluder device. 3D TEE is also useful in visualizing the shape of the defect, which is rarely a perfect circle. The interatrial septum is visualized from both the left and right atrial sides, and the diameter is measured easily; rims are identified by looking at the enface images. Encroachment of the device on surrounding structures and evidence of residual shunting is evaluated before device release.

Balloon Mitral Valvuloplasty

Evaluation and intervention on the mitral valve require a sophisticated and comprehensive imaging protocol. Mitral valve interventions often have complex navigation requirements that are performed in a stepwise fashion. Transseptal puncture is performed, followed by left atrial navigation, and then finally intervention within the mitral valve.

Balloon mitral valvuloplasty is performed based on preprocedure clinical and echocardiographic assessment. Candidates must have a favorable valve

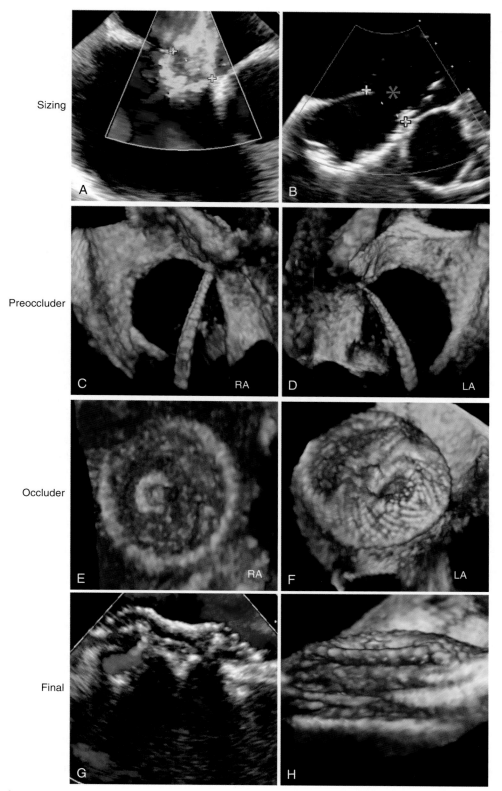

Sizing

Preoccluder

Occluder

Final

Figure 2–7 ASD closure. 2D and RT 3D TEE guidance of a secundum ASD closure. **A** and **B** depict sizing of the defect. **A,** 2D TEE image with color Doppler showing the defect in the septum and the presence of left-to-right shunt. A sizing balloon is inflated across the defect. The waist of the balloon (*) is measured while color Doppler confirms the absence of interatrial shunting. Measurements can be confirmed by viewing the enface images with RT 3D TEE. **C** and **D,** The right atrial *(RA)* and left atrial *(LA)* sides of the defect seen enface with an interventional wire crossing. An Amplatzer septal occluder covers the defect from the RA side **(E)** and LA side **(F).** The final occluder position is confirmed with both 2D **(G)** and 3D imaging **(H).** Note the absence of interatrial shunting with color Doppler and adequate capture of the surrounding rim tissue.

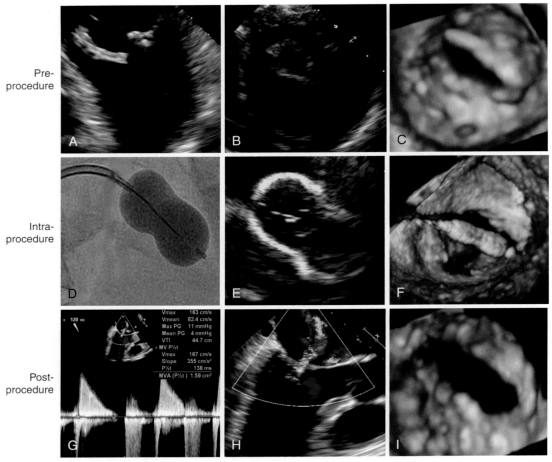

Figure 2–8   Mitral balloon valvuloplasty. A and **B,** 2D TEE images of the mitral valve showing typical thickened appearance of the valve leaflets and commissural fusion. **C,** 3D TEE image of the mitral valve in short axis. **D, E,** and **F,** Intraprocedural guidance of the Inoue balloon within the mitral valve orifice using three different imaging modalities. **D** depicts the fluoroscopic view, and **E** and **F** depict the 2D and 3D TEE views. Note that RT 3D TEE allows for accurate alignment of the balloon perpendicular to the valve plane unlike the other two modalities. **G, H,** and **I,** Postprocedure assessment of mitral stenosis by Doppler gradient **(G).** Color Doppler **(H)** looking for significant MR. Visual evidence of commissural splitting **(I).**

morphology based on the Wilkins score and absence of significant MR or LAA thrombus. Mitral valvuloplasty can be performed safely in suitable candidates with fluoroscopic guidance alone, but the addition of imaging helps direct the procedure in all steps, including guiding the transseptal puncture, navigating the catheter to the mitral valve orifice, avoiding the LAA, and aligning the catheter coaxial to the mitral valve. Immediately postprocedure the gradient and degree of MR is evaluated, and the operator looks for visual evidence of successful commissural splitting. The procedure concludes with a search for complications such as acute severe MR, pericardial effusion, or significant residual ASD. The imaging steps of TEE guidance for mitral balloon valvuloplasty are depicted in **Figure 2–8.**

Edge-to-Edge Repair for Mitral Regurgitation: MitraClip

Unlike mitral stenosis, MR has a more complex pathology and physiology. Until recently, invasive therapies for MR were limited to surgical valve repair or replacement. With the advent of new percutaneous therapies,

surgeons can now offer mitral valve regurgitation intervention to patients who are otherwise at high surgical risk. The MitraClip mimics the surgical Alfieri technique by clipping middle scallops of the anterior and posterior leaflets of the mitral valve, creating the typical "double orifice" mitral valve.[20,21] The EVEREST I and II studies showed the percutaneous method was technically safe and showed similar clinical outcomes when compared to traditional surgical intervention in high-risk patients.[21,22]

TEE is the central imaging modality for MitraClip procedures. Unlike any other interventional procedure, the use of real-time echocardiographic imaging guidance is critical, and the communication between the echocardiographer and interventional cardiologist must be clear. The recommendation is for an imaging protocol consisting of predetermined views for each step in the procedure.[23] Imaging guidance commences with the transseptal puncture. An ideal puncture site should be in the superior and posterior aspect of the interatrial septum (to achieve a height of 3.5 to 4.0 cm above the coaptation plane of the mitral leaflets), as depicted earlier in this chapter **(see Figure 2–2),** in order to provide enough navigation room within the left atrium.

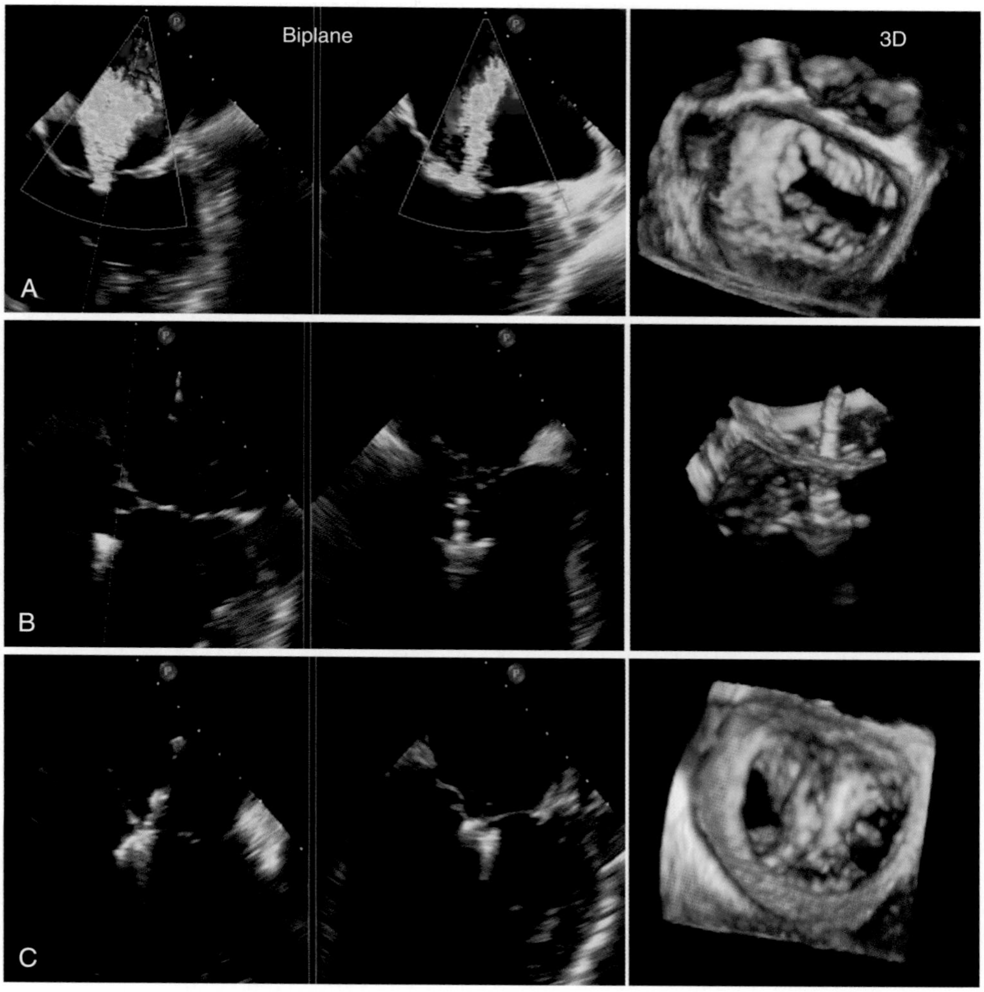

Figure 2–9 **Edge-to-edge repair with MitraClip.** Imaging steps for percutaneous mitral valve repair with a MitraClip using RT 3D TEE are shown at baseline (**A**) with biplane orthogonal images shown on the left and 3D images shown on the right. **B** shows positioning of the clip below the mitral valve both in biplane and 3D TEE. Note the left ventricular outflow view on the left and the commissural view on the right. **C** shows two clips in place after successful closure of the valve. Note in **C** the 3D TEE image from the left atrial perspective depicting the typical double orifice mitral valve.

The clip is then ideally positioned in the center of the regurgitant jet with the clip arms aligned perpendicular to the commissural line. The midesophageal left ventricular outflow view is used to guide anterior–posterior positioning, and the midesophageal commissural view guides medial–lateral positioning of the clip. Simultaneous biplane imaging is particularly useful **(Video 2–1).** Before and after clip release the degree of remaining MR and any evidence of clinical mitral stenosis is evaluated by Doppler echo **(Video 2–2).** If an additional clip is needed, the same views allow the medial–lateral and anterior–posterior positioning of a second clip relative to the first.

RT 3D TEE in conjunction with 2D TEE provides superior guidance of MitraClip procedures.[6] The 3D images of the mitral valve from both the left atrial and left ventricular sides provide better navigation, more accurate alignment of the clip at the middle scallops of the mitral valve, and easier visualization of clip arms perpendicular to the commissural line **(Videos 2–3, 2–4, 2–5).** Additionally the 3D view may facilitate communication between the interventional and echocardiography teams, because there is no need to mentally integrate two different imaging planes. **Figure 2–9** shows the use of both 2D and 3D TEE during a MitraClip procedure.

Left Atrial Appendage Occlusion

Atrial fibrillation is the most common cardiac arrhythmia, with a prevalence of over 10% in patients over the age of 75 years. The increased risk of stroke is felt to be attributable to thromboemboli originating from the LAA.[24] Medical therapy with oral anticoagulants reduces the stroke risk but is often underused and can be of high risk in the elderly. Closure of the LAA may represent another option for stroke prevention in these patients. Currently there are several LAA occluder devices available, including the WATCHMAN device (Atritech, Plymouth, Minn.) and the Amplatzer cardiac plug. TEE is used to rule out LAA thrombus before the procedure and to assess for left atrial enlargement and concomitant valve disease such as mitral stenosis. The LAA is characterized with attention to the number of lobes and its size and shape. Measurements are made in two orthogonal views for device sizing. Postdeployment the echocardiographer must monitor for pericardial effusion caused by LAA rupture, persistent flow within the LAA, and device embolization. **Figure 2–10** depicts the sizing and placement of an Amplatzer cardiac plug. RT 3D TEE is often employed for this procedure and is more accurate for sizing of the occluder device than 2D TEE when compared to preprocedure CT measurements.[25,26]

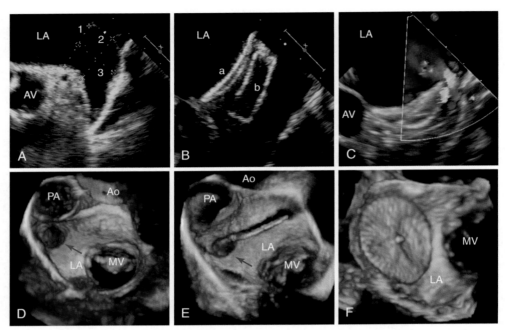

Figure 2–10   LAA occlusion. 2D and 3D TEE in a patient undergoing percutaneous LAA occlusion. **A,** The key required measurements of the LAA are illustrated. These are the diameter of the LAA os *(1)*, the neck diameter *(2)*, and the depth of the appendage neck. **B** illustrates the deployed device with the disk *(a)* facing the left atrium *(LA)* and the lobe or "puck" *(b)* facing the LAA. **C** illustrates with color Doppler the persistence of mild residual flow after deployment. **D** depicts an RT 3D TTE view of the LA as seen from the "surgeon's view," illustrating the relationship of the os of the LAA *(red arrow)* with the mitral valve *(MV)*, pulmonary artery *(PA)*, and aorta *(Ao)*. **E** illustrates the delivery catheter directed into the LAA. **F** illustrates the deployed device as seen from the LA with the expanded disc obliterating the os of the LAA.

CARDIAC COMPUTED TOMOGRAPHY

Cardiac multidetector CT (MDCT) offers several advantages over echocardiography, including a full field of view and excellent spatial resolution for displaying intracardiac structures. The temporal resolution of CT has been improved by the use of dual-source CT, implementation of multiphase contrast injectors, and the use of CT scanners with fast gantry rotation times. Cardiac motion artifact is overcome by ECG gating and heart-rate control. There are two types of ECG gating: (1) prospective and (2) retrospective. With prospective ECG gating, the acquisition is timed with the ECG and scanning takes place during a short portion of the R–R interval. An advantage of this method includes limited radiation exposure; however, this type of gating can be problematic in patients with arrhythmia, a common scenario in this patient population. Retrospective ECG gating requires continuous scanning throughout the entire R–R interval over several cardiac cycles. This uses much more radiation, because the scanner is "on" for the whole acquisition time. However, the images are more reproducible. Regardless of gating technique, a high-quality cardiac CT depends heavily on a slow heart rate, and usually β-blockers are used to achieve a goal heart rate of about 60 beats per minute.[27,28]

The images required for SHD interventions often require a dynamic CT evaluation, necessitating the highest temporal and spatial resolution. Additionally multiplanar and 3D volumetric reconstructions are particularly useful in SHD interventions to help visualize the important spatial and anatomic relationships. Typically retrospective ECG-gated MDCT with multiphase reconstruction is used for complex defects and in planning SHD interventions. Contrast injection protocols must also be tailored to the type of defect. For example, MDCT can have a role in detecting shunt directionality in ASDs, ventricular septal defects, and patent ductus arteriosis with the implementation of a triple phase contrast protocol.[29] It is important that pertinent clinical information is communicated to the imaging physician in order to optimize the CT protocol.

MDCT in SHD interventions is usually an adjunct to other imaging modalities, including echocardiography. The use of CT in multimodality imaging for SHD interventions is discussed in the Multimodality Imaging section. MDCT is rapidly becoming the gold standard for imaging of the aortic valve complex in transcatheter aortic valve replacement (TAVR) and is useful in defining complex anatomy in patients with congenital heart disease including ASD, persistent ductus arteriosis, ventricular septal defects, aortic coarctation, and pulmonic stenosis. The preprocedure use of cardiac CT for defining intraprocedural strategy is discussed in the following section with an example of prosthetic paravalvular leak closure.

Prosthetic Paravalvular Leak Closure

Paravalvular leaks can occur after surgical aortic or mitral valve replacements. This usually is caused by postoperative

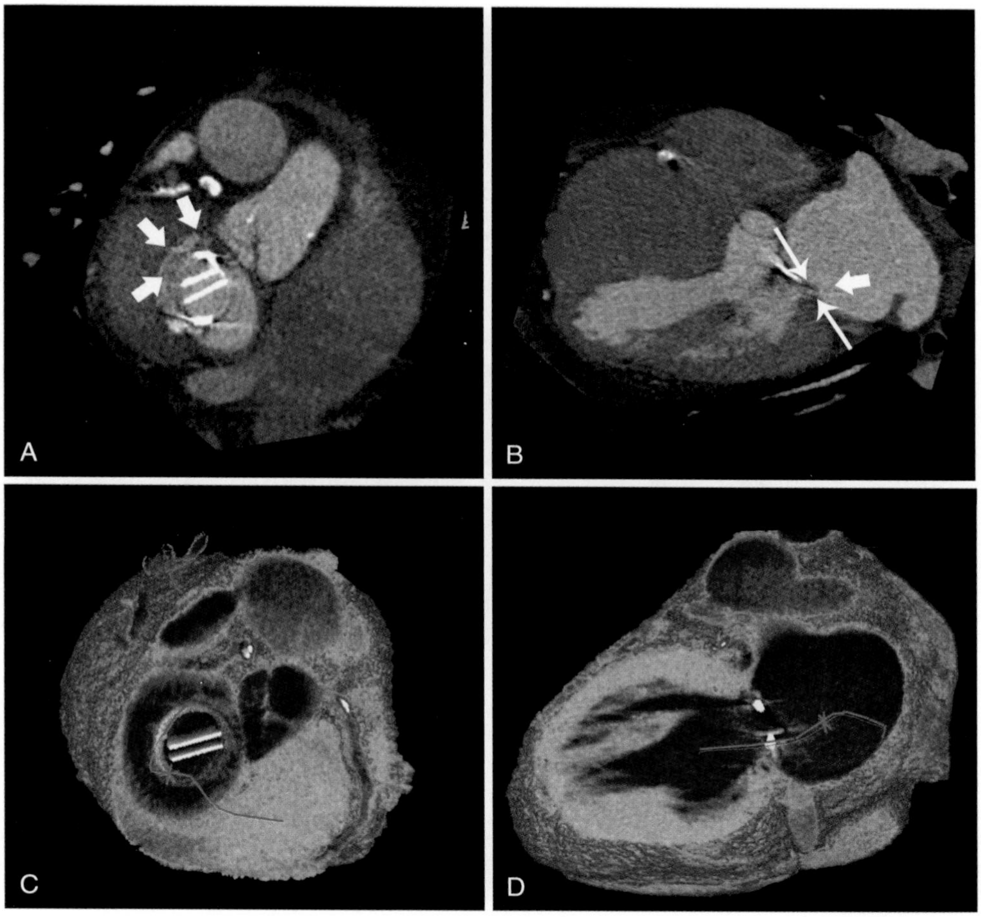

Figure 2–11 Cardiac CT in prosthetic mitral paravalvular leak closure. Images from a gated CTA depicting a prosthetic mitral valve with a periprosthetic valve leak (crescent shaped defect, *arrows* in **A** and **B**). Volumetric 3D images on the bottom show the proposed pathway for percutaneous closure of the leak. Note the lateral course (**C**) when viewed from the left atrial perspective. **D** shows the lateral perspective. The *red line* depicts the interventional course through the leak into the left ventricle beginning at the interatrial septum.

dehiscence of the sewing ring and can lead to significant valvular regurgitation, hemolysis, and heart failure. Percutaneous closure is an alternative to repeat surgery in patients for whom surgical valve repair or replacement is considered to be too high of a risk. Although paravalvular leaks can occur after TAVR, the use of transcatheter closure strategies for these leaks is in its infancy.

Preprocedural imaging using MDCT can be helpful in defining the anatomy of the leak and devising a preprocedural strategy for closure. Use of preprocedural CT scans may shorten procedural time and limit the radiation dose during these complex interventions. **Figure 2–11** shows preprocedure imaging in a case of a large mitral paravalvular leak using multiplanar and 3D reconstruction. Mechanical prostheses can cause significant artifacts, and the reconstruction kernel or filter must be adjusted to maximal sharpness to increase spatial resolution around the valve for accurate identification of the paravalvular leak. The use of nonstandard imaging planes is typical with paravalvular leaks in order to visualize the shape and location of these defects. The echocardiographic image guidance for the procedure is shown in **Figure 2–12.**

CARDIAC MAGNETIC RESONANCE IMAGING

CMR imaging is similar to cardiac CT in that it provides a large field of view and good spatial resolution with better temporal resolution. The use of CMR imaging in SHD has been more extensive in the pediatric population with complex congenital heart disease. CMR imaging has the benefit over cardiac CT in that it has the ability to quantify shunts, regurgitant volumes, and ventricular ejection fraction using phase contrast acquisitions. CMR imaging does not use ionizing radiation, an important consideration in young children and women of child-bearing age. Additionally, images of patients with congenital heart disease are often done with serial studies over the course of their lifetime, rendering the use of repeated CT imaging less attractive. Magnetic resonance imaging (MRI) also has several patient specific limitations. It is relatively contraindicated in patients with implantable defibrillators and pacemakers, and gadolinium contrast is contraindicated in patients with severe renal insufficiency because of the worry for nephrogenic systemic fibrosis.

CMR imaging is not yet a prime-time imaging guidance modality. Real-time MRI for guiding SHD procedures has been developed and used in isolated interventions,[30] but the expense and safety have not been fully evaluated. MRI does, however, allow for accurate definition of complex anatomy and can be used to diagnose and characterize ASDs and other complex shunt lesions for preprocedural planning.

The primary image sequences in CMR imaging can be categorized as bright blood cine, dark blood tissue

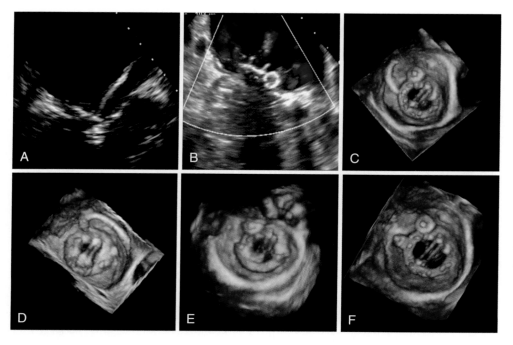

Figure 2–12 TEE in prosthetic mitral paravalvular leak closure. Placement of a vascular plug into a mitral prosthetic paravalvular leak. Planar 2D echo images are shown in **A** and **B**, with the first device placed and attached to the delivery cable **(A)** and subsequently released **(B)** with reduced leak. **C** and **D** show the wire crossing the paravalvular leak sites from the left atrial view using 3D TEE guidance. Note the previous vascular plug at 12 o'clock in **C. E** and **F** depict the final placement of the two vascular plugs.

specific, phase contrast velocity sensitive, MR angiographic, and delayed contrast enhancement. Similar to cardiac CT, cardiac gating and breath holding is required to reduce movement and enhance image quality. Bright blood images can be made into cine sequences to show cardiac motion and valve function. Black blood sequences are acquired at a single cardiac phase with bright soft-tissue structures and dark blood-filled structures (ventricles, atria and vessel lumen). Phase contrast sequences allow for the calculation of velocities, regurgitant volumes, and shunts by calculating the phase shift between moving spins and stationary spins. MR angiography can be done with or without gadolinium contrast. Contrast MR angiography is usually a non–ECG-gated scan employed for evaluation of the great vessels and pulmonary vasculature. Noncontrast T2 weighted scans can be an alternative to contrast MR angiography in patients with a contraindication to gadolinium contrast. MR angiography is the only sequence that allows for postprocessing into multiplanar and 3D reformatted images, often critical in SHD intervention planning. Delayed gadolinium enhancement involves a second pass T1 imaging approximately 10 to 30 minutes after administration of gadolinium contrast. Areas of scar, inflammation, or infection result in reduced contrast washout distinct from normal myocardium.[28,31]

Cardiac Magnetic Resonance Imaging in the Evaluation of Hypertrophic Cardiomyopathy

The details of imaging guidance for alcohol septal ablation for hypertrophic cardiomyopathy are discussed earlier in this chapter. The preprocedure assessment and postprocedure result are often studied by CMR imaging. CMR imaging provides an accurate measurement of wall thickness, degree of systolic anterior motion of the mitral

valve, and severity of outflow tract obstruction. Delayed gadolinium enhancement may also identify the degree of fibrosis within the left ventricle, a prognostic marker used to help assess the risk of sudden cardiac death. The use of CMR imaging after septal ablation evaluates the effectiveness of the procedure. The area of infarcted septal myocardium, degree of septal tissue regression, size of the LVOT and calculation of outflow tract gradient are used to quantify the efficacy of the septal ablation. **Figure 2–13** shows delayed gadolinium enhancement CMR images both before and after alcohol septal ablation. MRI should be performed 3 to 6 months postprocedure to allow time for septal remodeling. Often septal regression continues over time.[32,33]

MULTIMODALITY IMAGING

Despite the advantages of certain imaging modalities in particular SHD procedures, interventional cardiologists are increasingly relying on a multimodal approach. This specifically applies to patient selection and preprocedural planning. The best example of this multimodal imaging approach comes from transcatheter valve implantation therapies but applies to paravalvular leak closures, complex closures of ASDs, and complex shunt lesions as well.

Transcatheter Aortic Valve Replacement

With the commercial release of the Edwards SAPIEN (Edwards Lifesciences, Irvine, Calif.) transcatheter heart valve in November of 2011 and the ongoing trials of the Medtronic CoreValve (Medtronic CV) there has been a surge in the number of facilities that are now performing this procedure on a routine basis. The preprocedural patient selection is very rigorous. With regard to TAVR,

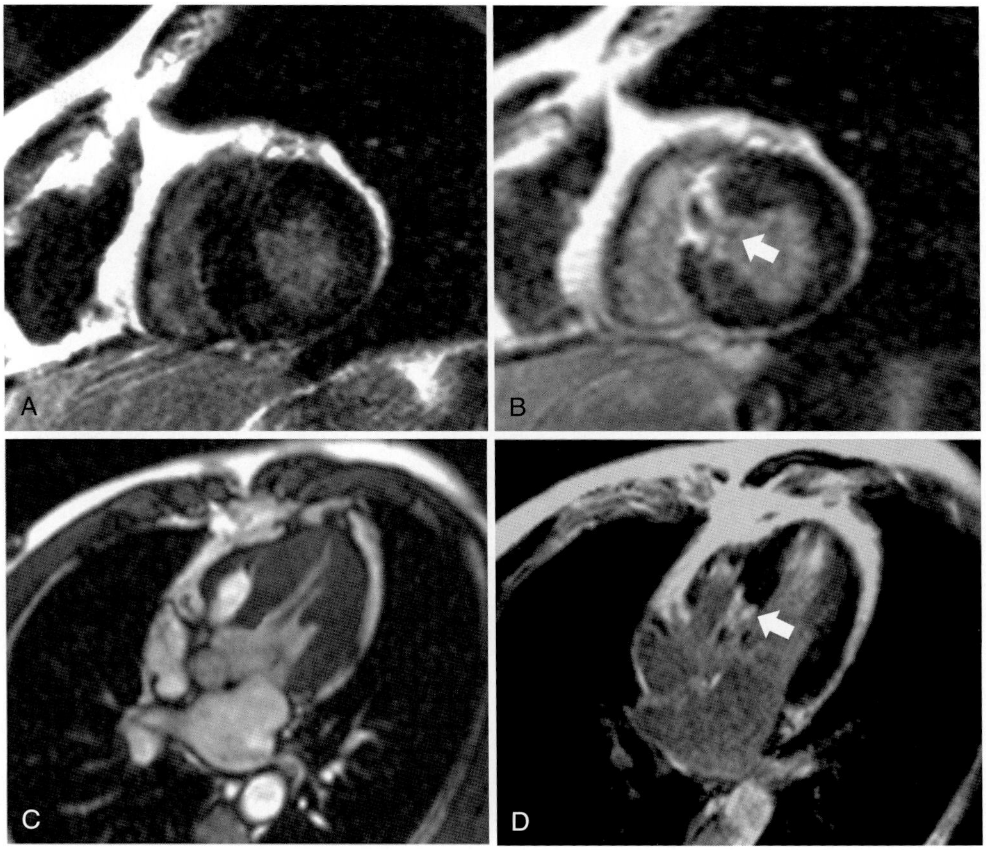

Figure 2–13 CMR imaging in hypertrophic cardiomyopathy. CMR images are shown with the baseline study on the left (**A** and **C**) and post–alcohol septal ablation procedure on the right (**B** and **D**). The short axis is on top and the 4-chamber view is on the bottom. The *arrows* show the delayed contrast enhancement from the septal ablation in the proximal anteroseptal myocardium.

patients must have severe symptomatic aortic stenosis (AS) and be deemed inoperable or prohibitive risk by a cardiothoracic surgeon after a thorough evaluation. Severe AS is defined as a transaortic peak gradient greater than 40 mmHg or a peak velocity greater than 4 m/sec. These parameters are usually readily attainable by TTE, and this often serves as the starting point for the evaluation. TTE provides routine assessment of left ventricle size and function as well as Doppler-derived transaortic gradients and any other regurgitant lesions such as severe aortic insufficiency or associated MR or stenosis. Careful attention must be paid not only to the gradients but also to the severity and distribution of calcium on the aortic valve and extension into the LVOT, the aortic annular dimension, as well as the shape of the LVOT and the ascending aorta.

The sophisticated positioning and navigation of the valve into the aortic annulus mandates a thoughtful and complete preprocedural evaluation of the aortic valve complex and the peripheral vasculature. In most cases this includes TTE and often TEE, cardiac CT angiography (CTA), coronary arteriography, and aortic and peripheral angiography. **Figure 2–14** outlines the multimodal imaging approach to preprocedure patient selection in TAVR. The use of these imaging techniques for patient selection and planning are key to success and accurately predict risk of postprocedure complications such as acute aortic regurgitation, vascular access complications, and device embolization.[34-36]

Once an initial echocardiogram is completed, attention is turned to the specific measurements related to TAVR. One of the primary roles of echocardiography is in the determination of the size of the aortic annulus. This is initially done by TTE; however, TTE may underestimate valve size, and TEE or CTA provide a more accurate assessment of the annular dimension. The best modality for imaging the aortic annulus is still under debate, and dimensions vary by technique; however, at this juncture TEE is considered the baseline measurement for determining valve sizing.[37] **Figure 2–15** shows the imaging techniques for accurate assessment of the aortic annulus. With TTE the annulus is viewed in the short axis and with biplane imaging the aortic valve is "cut" through the center to measure the annulus at its largest dimension in the corresponding 120-degree aortic outflow view. Measurement should be made from hinge-point to hinge-point of the aortic valve leaflets. This can be difficult to ascertain with the heavy shadowing from aortic valve calcification. CT measurements of the aortic valve are also shown in **Figures 2–15 and 2–16.** Several recent studies address the use of CT imaging of the aortic annulus for TAVR. Because of the calcification and shadowing with the use of echocardiography and the inability of 2D imaging to fully account for the elliptical shape of the aortic valve, TEE measurements may be less accurate in estimating valve size **(see Figure 2–16).** Annular measurement is critical, because underestimation of the

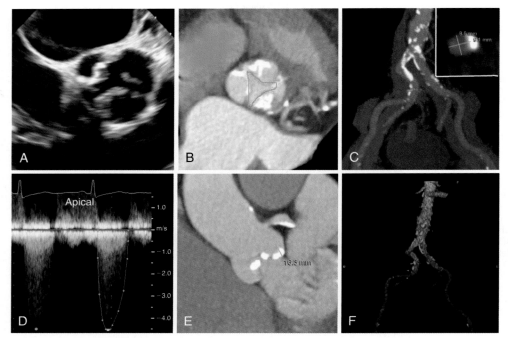

Figure 2–14 Multimodality Imaging in TAVR. Preprocedure patient selection requires TEE, TTE, and MDCT imaging. **A** and **D,** 2D TEE image of the aortic valve in short axis with attention to degree of calcification and valve dimensions. The corresponding transaortic valve Doppler gradient **(D)** indicates severe aortic stenosis with a peak velocity greater than 4 m/sec. **B** and **E,** Corresponding MDCT short axis image of the aortic valve **(B)** and coronal view of the aortic valve complex **(E)** showing the critical measurement from the annulus to the left main ostium. Note the more accurate demarcation of calcium in MDCT compared to TEE. **C** and **F,** MDCT of the peripheral vessels. Centerline measurements and cross sectional measurements **(C,** *insert)* should be performed for the entire length of the vessel to determine the true minimal luminal diameter. **F** shows a 3D reconstruction of the aortoiliac vessels, noting the degree of tortuosity and calcification that may impact sheath delivery.

valve size can lead to significant paravalvular leak and overestimation can lead to annular rupture.[38,39] CT may be the future gold standard for annular measurements and certainly provides additive information in conjunction with TEE.

Cardiac CTA also provides detailed characterizations of vascular anatomy, aortic root dimensions, sinotubular junction diameter, sinuses of Valsalva and ascending aorta, and the angle of the aortic valve plane. Additionally, coronal views measuring the distance from the valve annulus to the left main coronary artery and length and calcification of the left coronary cusp are required to assess risk of obstructing the left main ostium during implantation **(see Figure 2–14, E).** The specific measurements are unique to the type of aortic prosthesis.[34,36]

The large delivery system in the current generation of percutaneous valves requires a thorough assessment of the peripheral vascular access sites. In general, the peripheral vasculature must be large enough to accommodate up to a 24-French delivery system for the transfemoral approach. CTA is critical for providing cross-sectional images of the iliac vessels and determining the minimal luminal diameter and degree of calcification and tortuosity. In these authors' experience, the peripheral vasculature is the primary reason for exclusion from the transfemoral approach. It is expected that these exclusions will diminish as the delivery systems become smaller and/or with the adoption of the transapical or transaortic approach. **Table 2–5** summarizes

the key anatomic assessments for each of the requisite preprocedure imaging studies.

2.5 Future Directions

2D–3D REGISTRATION OF ECHOCARDIOGRAPHY AND FLUOROSCOPY

The newest advances in imaging guidance include not only a multimodality approach but also integrated, hybrid imaging. Recently, a prototype of an advanced x-ray–echo navigation system has been developed, allowing the registration of x-ray images with echocardiography. The 3D TEE probe is registered to the C-arm by its x-ray image orientation based on a 2D–3D image registration algorithm.[40] When the 3D TEE probe is activated for real-time acquisition, the 3D anatomic structures of the region of interest are presented simultaneously at three different viewing angles, including the sonographic, C-arm, and orthogonal views. As the C-arm is moved, the 3D TEE perspectives are updated and displayed based on the new gantry angle. The interventional cardiologist controls image cropping, marker placement, and orientation to tailor image guidance. The use of the landmark feature visible on both echo and fluoroscopy helps the operator mentally integrate the two modalities. This technology has been found to be most useful in complex navigation tasks such as paravalvular leak closures and MitraClip procedures.[41] **Figure 2–17** depicts the use

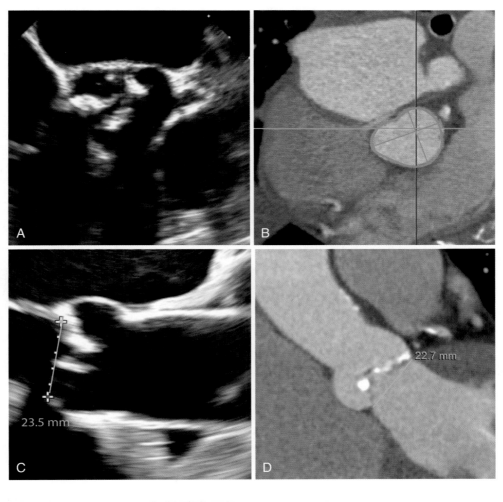

Figure 2–15 **Imaging the aortic valve annulus.** Annular dimension by TEE and MDCT. Accurate measurement of the aortic annulus with 2D TEE includes biplane imaging, bisecting the aortic valve in short axis **(A)** to ensure measurement of the maximal diameter in the corresponding 120-degree aortic outflow view **(C)**. Measurement should be made from hingepoint to hingepoint of leaflet insertion. The corresponding MDCT short-axis image is shown in **B** with the annular area outlined. The MDCT annular area can be used to determine appropriate valve size. **D** shows a coronal image of the aortic valve and annular dimension measurement. Both TTE and MDCT images of the aortic valve complex are used to determine accurate valve sizing.

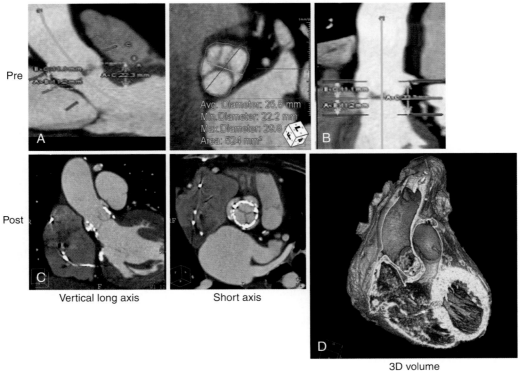

Figure 2–16 **MDCT measurements for TAVR.** Key measurements necessary for successful placement of a percutaneous aortic valve are shown in **A** and **B.** Note that the LVOT is elliptical with major and minor axes **(A).** The mean value is factored into selection of the correct valve size. The length of the left coronary cusp and left coronary leaflet are measured to prevent abrupt obstruction of the aortic valve during implantation **(B). C** depicts orthogonal MDCT images after successful placement of an Edwards SAPIEN aortic valve. **D** shows a 3D volume-rendered image. Notice that the stent portion of the valve straddles the annulus.

TABLE 2–5

Multimodality Imaging in TAVR Preprocedure Evaluation

Imaging Modality	Anatomic Evaluation	SAPIEN	CoreValve	Purpose
Aortography	Aortic dimensions Aortic valve plane	x	x	Sizing of prosthesis Determining optimal angle for valve deployment
Iliofemoral Angiography	Tortuosity, calcification, MLD	x	x	Suitability for vascular access
TTE	Annular dimension	x	x	Sizing of prosthesis
TEE	Annular dimension	x	x	Sizing of prosthesis
	Extent of calcification	x	x	Asymmetric bulky calcification may affect seating of valve, risks compromising coronary ostia
Cardiac CTA	Annular dimension	x	x	Sizing of prosthesis
	Sinotubular junction diameter		x	Assess risk of valve embolization
	Sinus of Valsalva diameter		x	Assess risk of compromising coronary ostia
	Ascending aorta	x	x	Assess for calcification, thrombus
	Aortic valve annulus to left main ostium	x	x	Asses risk of compromising coronary ostia
	Left ventricular septal thickness	x	x	Septal bulge may affect valve seating
	Aortic valve plane	x	x	Determining optimal angle for valve deployment
Peripheral CTA	Tortuosity, calcification, MLD	x	x	Suitability for vascular access Provides cross-sectional measurements of MLD

CTA, Computed tomographic angiography; MLD, minimal luminal diameter; TAVR, transcatheter aortic valve replacement; TEE, transesophageal echocardiography; TTE, transthoracic echocardiography.

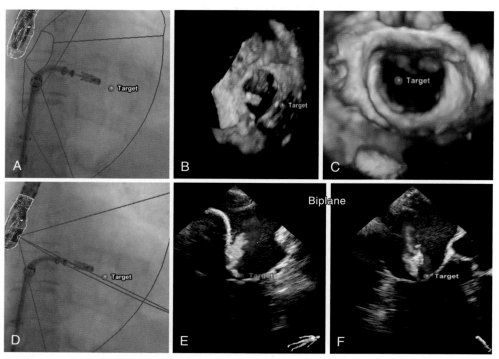

Figure 2–17   Integrated x-ray–echo navigation system. A, 2D–3D registration of x-ray and echocardiography used during a MitraClip placement. Note the image of the TEE probe. The probe image tracks the shape and orientation of the actual TEE probe, allowing for echocardiographic images corresponding to the x-ray gantry angle. **B** shows the echocardiographic version of the same shallow right anterior oblique projection with the mitral clip aligned with the mitral valve orifice. **C** shows simultaneous enface display of the mitral valve, providing a second view of the mitral valve *(Target)*. The landmark feature allows the interventionalist to mark the target on the TEE images with simultaneous display on the fluoroscopy screen (seen in all panels). **D, E,** and **F,** The operator has switched from 3D TEE to 2D biplane and aligns the clip with the regurgitant jet marked with the target.

Figure 2–18 **C-arm CT.** Rotational C-arm CT with timed contrast injection was used to create a 3D outline of the pulmonary artery for image guidance during a pulmonic valve implantation in a patient with pulmonic regurgitation. The 3D CT images are registered with fluoroscopy, and as a result, move simultaneously with the C-arm gantry. **A,** Deploying the Melody valve. **B,** The 3D image can be rotated to tailor image guidance. Note the simultaneous movement of the 2D fluoroscopic image with the 3D CT image. *(Courtesy of Dr. Thomas Fagan and Dr. Joseph Kay.)*

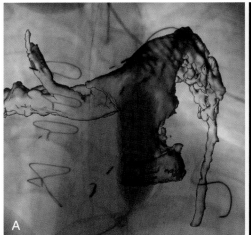 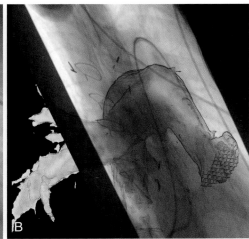

of the navigation system during a MitraClip procedure, demonstrating the simultaneous C-arm view and the working view. The landmark feature shows the "target" on both the fluoroscopic and the echocardiographic projections.

C-ARM COMPUTED TOMOGRAPHY

Real-time catheterization lab acquisitions of CT scans for interventional use have been limited because of cardiac and respiratory motion artifact and the need for ECG gating. However, new C-arm CT systems allow the flat panel C-arm to function as a CT scanner by performing a non–ECG-gated rotational acquisition that presents a CT-like projection. There are several commercially available rotational C-arm CT scanners that have been predominantly integrated into the neuroradiology and peripheral vascular interventional labs, but research is gradually moving this technology into the cardiac catheterization lab.[42]

The C-arm rotational scan is performed with a contrast medium injection timed to fill the cardiac chambers and allow for soft-tissue enhancement. The acquired images can be subsequently integrated with fluoroscopy to provide real-time image guidance **(Figure 2–18)**. During a pulmonic Melody (Medtronic CV) valve implantation a C-arm CT scan focused on the pulmonary arterial trunk was performed at the start of the procedure. The images were then registered with fluoroscopy and used to guide placement of the valve. The pulmonary arteries and great vessels have limited cardiac motion and are more amenable to non–ECG-gated scans. The use of this technology is limited for other intracardiac interventions because of motion artifact, but this is an exciting ongoing area of research.

2.6 Summary

The realm of imaging in SHD is a large topic and not all procedures could be covered in this chapter, but this serves as a framework for understanding the different modalities available and their key benefits and

limitations. The ideal choice of modality is based on the intervention planned, local expertise, operator confidence, training, and financial constraints. Preprocedure multimodal imaging studies serve as the starting point for appropriate patient selection and for defining the intraprocedural strategy. Fluoroscopy and echocardiography are the primary imaging modalities for guiding SHD interventions, but rapid advances in CT, MRI, and hybrid imaging with fluoroscopic registration are bringing more multimodal imaging to the catheterization lab.

REFERENCES

1. Chen SJ, Hansgen AR, Carroll JD: The future cardiac catheterization laboratory, *Cardiol Clin* 27:541–548, 2009.
2. Carroll JD, Mack M: Facilities: the structural heart disease interventional lab and the hybrid operating room. In Carroll JD WJ, editor: *Structural heart disease interventions*, Philadelphia, 2012, Lippincott, Williams and Wilkins, pp 9–26.
3. Balzer J, Kelm M, Kühl HP: Real-time three-dimensional transoesophageal echocardiography for guidance of noncoronary interventions in the catheter laboratory, *Eur J Echocardiogr* 10:341–349, 2009.
4. Balzer J, Kühl H, Rassaf T, et al: Real-time transesophageal three-dimensional echocardiography for guidance of percutaneous cardiac interventions: first experience, *Clin Res Cardiol* 97:565–574, 2008
5. Eng MH, Salcedo EE, Quaife RA, et al: Implementation of real time three-dimensional transesophageal echocardiography in percutaneous mitral balloon valvuloplasty and structural heart disease interventions, *Echocardiography* 26:958–966, 2009.
6. Altiok E, Becker M, Hamada S, et al: Real-time 3D TEE allows optimized guidance of percutaneous edge-to-edge repair of the mitral valve, *JACC Cardiovasc Imaging* 3:1196–1198, 2010.
7. Hudson PA, Eng MH, Kim MS, et al: A comparison of echocardiographic modalities to guide structural heart disease interventions, *J Interv Cardiol* 21:535–546, 2008.
8. Ross J Jr, Braunwald E, Morrow AG: Transseptal left heart catheterization: a new diagnostic method, *Prog Cardiovasc Dis* 2:315–318, 1960.
9. Green NE, Hansgen AR, Carroll JD: Initial clinical experience with intracardiac echocardiography in guiding balloon mitral valvuloplasty: technique, safety, utility, and limitations, *Catheter Cardiovasc Interv* 63:385–394, 2004.
10. Kim SS, Hijazi ZM, Lang RM, et al: The use of intracardiac echocardiography and other intracardiac imaging tools to guide noncoronary cardiac interventions, *J Am Coll Cardiol* 53(23):2117–2128, 2009.
11. Hijazi Z, Wang Z, Cao Q, et al: Transcatheter closure of atrial septal defects and patent foramen ovale under intracardiac echocardiographic guidance: feasibility and comparison with transesophageal echocardiography, *Catheter Cardiovasc Interv* 52:194–199, 2001.

12. Varma C, Benson LN, Warr MR, et al: Clinical outcomes of patent foramen ovale closure for paradoxical emboli without echocardiographic guidance, *Catheter Cardiovasc Interv* 62:519–525, 2004.

13. Carroll JD: PFO anatomy: 3D characterization and device performance, *Catheter Cardiovasc Interv* 71:229–230, 2008.

14. Taniguchi M, Akagi T, Watanabe N, et al: Application of real-time three-dimensional transesophageal echocardiography using a matrix array probe for transcatheter closure of atrial septal defect, *J Am Soc Echocardiogr* 22:1114–1120, 2009.

15. Salcedo EE, Quaife RA, Seres T, et al: A framework for systematic characterization of the mitral valve by real-time three-dimensional transesophageal echocardiography, *J Am Soc Echocardiogr* 22:1087–1099, 2009.

16. Hung J, Lang R, Flachskampf F, et al: 3D echocardiography: a review of the current status and future directions, *J Am Soc Echocardiogr* 20:213–233, 2007.

17. Warnes CA, Williams RG, Bashore TM, et al: ACC/AHA 2008 Guidelines for the Management of Adults with Congenital Heart Disease: a report of the American College of Cardiology/American Heart Association Task Force on Practice Guidelines (writing committee to develop guidelines on the management of adults with congenital heart disease), *Circulation* 118:e714–e833, 2008.

18. Du ZD, Hijazi ZM, Kleinman CS, et al: Comparison between transcatheter and surgical closure of secundum atrial septal defect in children and adults: results of a multicenter nonrandomized trial, *J Am Coll Cardiol* 39:1836–1844, 2002.

19. Lodato JA, Cao QL, Weinert L, et al: Feasibility of real-time three-dimensional transoesophageal echocardiography for guidance of percutaneous atrial septal defect closure, *Eur J Echocardiogr* 10:543–548, 2009.

20. Maisano F, Torracca L, Oppizzi M, et al: The edge-to-edge technique: a simplified method to correct mitral insufficiency, *Eur J Cardiothorac Surg* 13:240–245, 1998. discussion 5–6.

21. Feldman T, Wasserman HS, Herrmann HC, et al: Percutaneous mitral valve repair using the edge-to-edge technique: six-month results of the EVEREST Phase I Clinical Trial, *J Am Coll Cardiol* 46:2134–2140, 2005.

22. Feldman T, Foster E, Glower DD, et al: Percutaneous repair or surgery for mitral regurgitation, *N Engl J Med* 364:1395–1406, 2011.

23. Silvestry FE, Rodriguez LL, Herrmann HC, et al: Echocardiographic guidance and assessment of percutaneous repair for mitral regurgitation with the Evalve MitraClip: lessons learned from EVEREST I, *J Am Soc Echocardiogr* 20:1131–1140, 2007.

24. Stoddard MF, Dawkins PR, Prince CR, Ammash NM: Left atrial appendage thrombus is not uncommon in patients with acute atrial fibrillation and a recent embolic event: a transesophageal echocardiographic study, *J Am Coll Cardiol* 25:452–459, 1995.

25. Shah SJ, Bardo DM, Sugeng L, et al: Real-time three-dimensional transesophageal echocardiography of the left atrial appendage: initial experience in the clinical setting, *J Am Soc Echocardiogr* 21:1362–1368, 2008.

26. Nucifora G, Faletra FF, Regoli F, et al: Evaluation of the left atrial appendage with real-time 3-dimensional transesophageal echocardiography: implications for catheter-based left atrial appendage closure, *Circ Cardiovasc Imaging* 4:514–523, 2011. .

27. Flohr TG, Schoepf UJ, Ohnesorge BM: Chasing the heart: new developments for cardiac CT, *J Thorac Imaging* 22:4–16, 2007.

28. Quaife R, Carroll J: Cardiac CT and MRI in patient assessment and procedural guidance in structural heart disease interventions. In Carroll J, Webb J, editors: *Structural heart disease interventions*, Philadelphia, 2012, Lippincott, Williams and Wilkins.

29. Funabashi N, Asano M, Sekine T, et al: Direction, location, and size of shunt flow in congenital heart disease evaluated by ECG-gated multislice computed tomography, *Int J Cardiol* 112:399–404, 2006.

30. Krueger J, Ewert P, Yilmaz S, et al: Magnetic resonance imaging–guided balloon angioplasty of coarctation of the aorta, *Circulation* 113:1093–1100, 2006.

31. Chan FP: MR and CT imaging of the pediatric patient with structural heart disease, *Semin Thorac Cardiovasc Surg Pediatr Card Surg Annu*99–105, 2009.

32. van Dockum WG, Beek AM, ten Cate FJ, et al: Early onset and progression of left ventricular remodeling after alcohol septal ablation in hypertrophic obstructive cardiomyopathy, *Circulation* 111:2503–2508, 2005.

33. Valeti US, Nishimura RA, Holmes DR, et al: Comparison of surgical septal myectomy and alcohol septal ablation with cardiac magnetic resonance imaging in patients with hypertrophic obstructive cardiomyopathy, *J Am Coll Cardiol* 49:350–357, 2007.

34. Piazza N, de Jaegere P, Schultz C, et al: Anatomy of the aortic valvar complex and its implications for transcatheter implantation of the aortic valve, *Circ Cardiovasc Interv* 1:74–81, 2008.

35. Schoenhagen P, Kapadia SR, Halliburton SS, et al: Computed tomography evaluation for transcatheter aortic valve implantation (TAVI): imaging of the aortic root and iliac arteries, *J Cardiovasc Comput Tomogr* 5:293–300, 2011.

36. Tops LF, Wood DA, Delgado V, et al: Noninvasive evaluation of the aortic root with multislice computed tomography, *JACC Cardiovasc Imaging* 1:321–330, 2008.

37. Tzikas A, Schultz CJ, Piazza N, et al: Assessment of the aortic annulus by multislice computed tomography, contrast aortography, and transthoracic echocardiography in patients referred for transcatheter aortic valve implantation, *Catheter Cardiovasc Interv* 77:868–875, 2011.

38. Willson AB, Webb JG, LaBounty TM, et al: 3-Dimensional aortic annular assessment by multidetector computed tomography predicts moderate or severe paravalvular regurgitation after transcatheter aortic valve replacement, *J Am Coll Cardiol* 59(14):1287–1294, 2012.

39. Jilaihawi H, Kashif M, Fontana G, et al: Cross-sectional computed tomographic assessment improves accuracy of aortic annular sizing for transcatheter aortic valve replacement and reduces the incidence of paravalvular aortic regurgitation, *J Am Coll Cardiol* 59(14):1275–1286, 2012.

40. Gao G, Penney G, Ma Y, et al: Registration of 3D transesophageal echocardiography to x-ray fluoroscopy using image-based probe tracking, *Med Image Anal* 16:38–49, 2012.

41. Clegg S, Chen J, Salcedo E, et al: Integrated 3D echo-x-ray image guidance for structural heart interventions. American College of Cardiology 61st Annual Scientific Sessions, March 24-27, 2012, Chicago.

42. Wallace MJ, Kuo MD, Glaiberman C, et al: Three-dimensional C-arm cone-beam CT: applications in the interventional suite, *J Vasc Interv Radiol* 19:799–813, 2008.

Chapter 3

Vascular Access for Structural Heart Disease

JAMES STEWART • VASILIS BABALIAROS • CHETHAN DEVIREDDY •
VINOD THOURANI • SAMEER GAFOOR

Structural heart disease interventions require careful preprocedural planning. Imaging is the cornerstone for planning, particularly to determine whether the intervention is feasible and can be successful. The next critical step is to choose an approach that will maximize the chance of reaching the structural defect and provide enough support to deliver catheters and devices. This chapter discusses the vascular access for structural heart disease with emphasis on both percutaneous arterial/venous access and closure.

3.1 Arterial Access

Most of the renewed interest in arterial access has coincided with the advent of transcatheter aortic valve replacement (TAVR). Similar to the devices developed for endovascular aneurysm repair (EVAR), 16F to 24F sheaths are required to deliver transcatheter heart valves (THVs) from a retrograde transfemoral approach. Early in the experience of TAVR, a surgical cutdown with arteriotomy was often used for femoral arterial access and closure given the significant morbidity and mortality associated with vascular complications.[1] Smaller sheath sizes, advanced interventional techniques, and suture-mediated percutaneous closure devices have now made a completely percutaneous approach to TAVR and other structural heart disease procedures possible. This minimally invasive technique holds the most promise for the future of the procedure and, if done correctly, can dramatically decrease procedure time, postprocedure morbidity, and in some cases obviate the need for general anesthesia. Several steps are necessary to safely perform a completely percutaneous transfemoral TAVR: appropriate patient selection, proper procedural technique, and postprocedural management.

3.2 Patient Selection

Understanding which patients are candidates for a transfemoral approach to TAVR is the first step to a successful procedure. Large body mass index (BMI) or body surface area, high sheath–to–femoral artery ratio (SFAR), femoral artery calcification, peripheral arterial disease, and low operator experience have all been associated with high complication rates and poor outcome for a percutaneous transfemoral approach.[2–5] Patient-specific factors like BMI and prior peripheral arterial disease are known at the time of a clinic visit, but imaging is crucial for evaluating the vessel-specific factors of size, calcification, and tortuosity.

Imaging of the femoral and iliac vessels is performed by invasive angiography, contrast and noncontrast computed tomography (CT), magnetic resonance (MR) angiography, and intravascular ultrasound (IVUS). Though there is no consensus on which imaging modality is superior for TAVR planning, there is consensus that at least two modalities should be used for evaluation. At the Emory University Hospital in Atlanta, Ga., a bilateral lower extremity angiogram and noncontrast CT of the chest, abdomen, and pelvis are performed on all patients. The angiogram identifies stenoses, tortuosity, and aneurysms and allows for measurement of the true lumen diameter. Angiography should be done with digital subtraction angiography and a marker pigtail catheter (**Figure 3–1**). Rotational angiography has been advocated by some centers, but often a straight anteroposterior angiogram will allow for accurate calibration and measurements in both legs. The CT also helps confirm vessel size but primarily adds essential information about the location and extent of calcification in a vessel (**Figures 3–2 and 3–3**). For this reason it does not need to be done with contrast. Contrast CT can be performed in patients with adequate renal function and

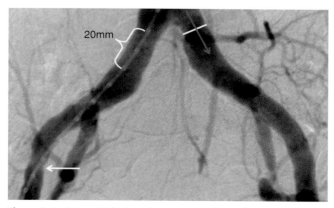

Figure 3–1 Proper technique for measuring the angiogram. Lower extremity angiography should be done using digital subtraction angiography. Zoom in on the area of interest and calibrate over two markers from the marker pigtail catheter *(bracket)* measuring leading edge to leading edge or lagging edge to lagging edge. Measure the diameter at the narrowest portion of the common iliac, external iliac *(white arrow)*, and common femoral arteries on each side, making sure the measurement *(white line)* is exactly orthogonal to the direction of blood flow *(red arrow)*.

adds additional certainty of vessel size when using a work station that can rotate images in three dimensions. MR angiography has been used, but the resolution is not as good as CT and invasive angiography. IVUS has been used to confirm lumen size in patients, but measurements may be confounded by catheter bias in tortuous vessels.

The next step in patient selection is to determine whether the available sheath/delivery system will pass through the patient's femoroiliac arteries. It has been determined that a noncalcified vessel will stretch up to 1 mm without rupture, although dissections can occur. SFARs above 1.05 have been associated with increased complications and mortality. A vessel with circumferential calcification will act like a rigid pipe and will not stretch beyond its nominal size without a significant risk of rupture. Noncircumferential calcification can cause significant drag on the delivery sheath, particularly in areas of high tortuosity such as the external iliac artery. Patients are often rejected for transfemoral approach if the external iliac arteries are calcified and the SFAR

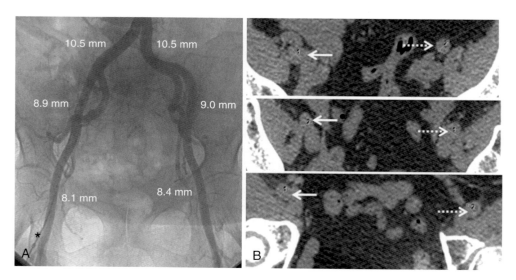

Figure 3–2 Excellent iliofemoral access for transcatheter aortic valve replacement in a patient with an aortic annulus measuring 21 mm (i.e., small transcatheter heart valve). The lower extremity angiogram **(A)** shows the vessels' lumen and tortuosity and allows precise measurement using a marker pigtail catheter *(asterisk)* for accurate calibration. Sequential axial cuts from the noncontrast computed tomography images **(B)** from the iliac to common femoral vessels on the right *(solid arrows)* and left *(dashed arrows)* show no calcification, indicating the vessel diameter will stretch up to 1 mm. The sheath–to–femoral artery ratio on the left is 0.83 for an 18F delivery system and approximately 1.0 for a 22F delivery system.

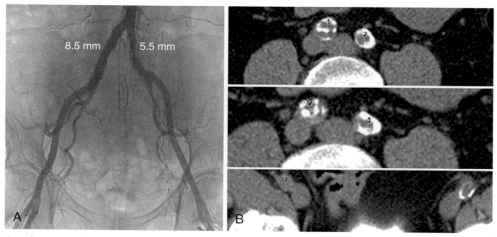

Figure 3–3 No options for transcatheter aortic valve replacement (TAVR) from a transfemoral approach. The lower extremity angiogram **(A)** shows obvious narrowing in the left common iliac artery, but the right common iliac artery appears to have an adequate diameter to accommodate an 18F to 22F sheath. Axial cuts from the noncontrast computed tomography **(B)** show a circumferentially calcified chronic dissection on the right that was not apparent on angiogram. The true lumen diameter is about 5 mm, illustrating the importance of using two different imaging modalities in concert when doing preprocedural planning. This patient had TAVR via a transapical approach.

is greater than 1.0. Calcium in the common iliac arteries is very common in transfemoral patients; the area is often straight with an SFAR of less than 1.0 and thus of no consequence.

Analysis of the angiography and noncontrast CT will usually reveal a preferred side for access, as well as the optimal part of the common femoral artery to puncture. The entry point into the common femoral artery should ideally be without calcification, even if this requires a "high" entry just distal to the inguinal ligament before the vessel dives into the pelvis. For patients over 100 kg, excessive scarring at or near the common femoral, or entry into the vessel at the area covered by the inguinal ligament, a surgical cut down should be considered. During preprocedure planning, the external or common iliac artery should be scrutinized for feasibility of an iliac conduit in case femoral access fails. If needed, this would be a Dacron graft anastomosis end-to-side to the external/common iliac artery, with the conduit externalized through the groin incision and the sheath inserted through the conduit. The minimum diameters accepted for 18F, 22F, and 24F sheaths are 6 mm, 7 mm, and 8 mm, respectively, in any part of the arterial tree.[6] Alternatively, the patient should be considered for a transapical, transaortic, or subclavian approach.

3.3 Description of Technique

Accessing the common femoral artery through 1) an anterior wall puncture at 2) a noncalcified site with 3) adequate size to accommodate the sheath and 4) a location that allows for proximal compression/control of the vessel is paramount to successfully performing a completely percutaneous TAVR. Meeting these four criteria often leaves only a short segment of femoral artery that would be acceptable for access. Adjunctive imaging with femoral ultrasound or angiographic road mapping of the femoral iliac vessels is helpful. At Emory University Hospital, experience with angiographic road mapping has been developed **(Figure 3–4).** First the femoral artery is accessed, a 6F sheath is inserted, and a JR4 catheter is advanced to the level of the distal aorta. The ostium of

the contralateral common iliac artery is engaged. The image intensifier is positioned over the contralateral femoral head, and a digital subtraction fluoroscopic road map image is taken using contrast injection. This creates an overlay of the contrast-filled lumen of the iliofemoral artery that remains on the screen during subsequent fluoroscopy.

The authors use a micropuncture system for access. The smaller needle is ideal, because it is often deflected by vessel calcification or dense fibrosis/scarring. This helps ensure that a soft portion of the anterior wall is punctured, and withdrawal after missed puncture is of no consequence. It is important to stay below the inguinal ligament, because passage of dilators and percutaneous closure may not be successful if the ligament is punctured. It is also important to make a shallow-angle entry into the vessel to minimize vessel trauma. The angle needs to be altered if the distance from the skin to vessel is longer than the needle length or if the needle needs to be hubbed to obtain access. If the access track is too long, subsequent percutaneous closure is likely to fail.

Once the vessel has been accessed, the micropuncture wire is inserted and a 1-cm skin incision is made to allow passage of a large-bore sheath. The track is dilated with an 8F and 10F dilator. After dilation, the vessel is preclosed with two Perclose ProGlide percutaneous suture devices (Abbott Laboratories, Abbott Park, Ill.). These pretied sutures are deployed at slight angulation from one another (10 o'clock and 2 o'clock positions), and care is taken not to pull on the sutures and tighten the knots down prematurely **(Figure 3–5).** For larger sheaths, some centers predeploy a third Perclose ProGlide device between the other two (12 o'clock position). Hemostats are used to clip the ends of the sutures together, and sutures are covered with a towel, keeping them hidden until the end of the procedure.

After deployment of the final Perclose ProGlide device, an Amplatz Extra Stiff Wire (Cook Medical, Bloomington, Ind.) is passed into the vessel. Sequential dilation of the vessel is performed using the hydrophilic coated dilators that come with the various THV introducer sheaths. Gentle rotation and firm pressure should be applied while watching the dilator advance fluoroscopically, and care

Figure 3–4 The roadmap image of the common femoral artery **(A)** and the corresponding fluoroscopic image **(B)** show the correct site of entry into the vessel *(asterisk)* below the pelvic rim and inguinal ligament at a compressible site without vessel calcification *(white arrow on computed tomography inset image)*. The correct trajectory of the needle from a shallow angle and parallel to the common femoral artery course *(white line)* ensures anterior wall puncture and minimal vessel trauma.

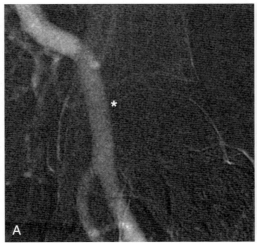
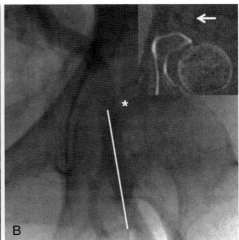

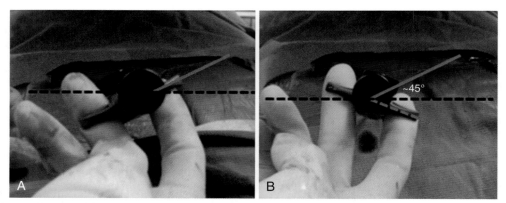

Figure 3–5   The first Perclose ProGlide suture **(A)** should be deployed at about 20 degrees *(solid red line,* 2 o'clock position) counterclockwise from level *(dashed black line),* and the second suture **(B)** should be deployed approximately at a 20-degree angle clockwise from level *(dashed red line,* 10 o'clock position). The 40- to 45-degree angulation from one to the other helps with vessel hemostasis but does not cause vessel stricturing and occlusion. In some cases, a third suture may be placed at the 12 o'clock position.

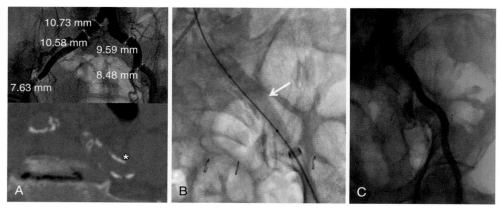

Figure 3–6   The preoperative angiogram **(A)** shows adequate vessel diameter on the left to accommodate the needed 22F sheath with a sheath–to–external iliac artery ratio of 0.97 but a tortuous, heavily calcified common iliac artery *(asterisk).* The large dilator would not pass, so balloon angioplasty of the left common and external iliac arteries **(B,** *arrow)* was performed from an ipsilateral retrograde approach. This fractured and straightened the calcification enough to pass the 22F sheath. The final angiogram after sheath removal **(C)** showed no vascular complication.

should be taken not to push too hard if the dilator does not advance, because this is a risk for vessel rupture. On rare occasions, performing balloon angioplasty of a focally stenotic, noncalcified lesion on the common or external iliac artery or of a large caliber but calcified and tortuous iliac system may be necessary to get the largest dilator to advance **(Figure 3–6).** Pre-stenting the iliac arteries is neither necessary nor desirable because of the risk of stent migration during sheath placement. Before placing the introducer sheath in the vessel, the vessel and tract should be dilated with a dilator that is equivalent in diameter to the outer diameter of the sheath being used. Sutures are used to secure the large sheath after it is deaired and flushed.

Once the TAVR has been successfully performed, safely removing the sheath requires coordination between at least two operators. The sheath should be wired so that access to the vessel is maintained at all times. The type of wire is less important, although the authors use a regular 0.035-inch exchange J-wire. One person is assigned to compress the vessel and control bleeding when the sheath is removed, and another person pulls the Perclose ProGlide sutures and tightens the knots down over the arteriotomy. Once both sutures have been tightened, an angiogram of the common iliac artery should be taken from the contralateral side. Most sheaths over 18F will require a third Perclose ProGlide suture placed after the angiogram. In rare instances, a balloon from the contralateral side may need to be inserted in the upstream external iliac and inflated to produce a bloodless field.

3.4 Postprocedural Management

Postprocedural management begins with the completion angiogram. If there is no evidence of vascular injury, the final Perclose ProGlide device is placed, and/or protamine is given to reverse anticoagulation. If there is vascular injury, the repair is addressed with endovascular techniques through the ipsilateral vessel, if possible **(Figure 3–7).** Endovascular repair combined with surgical repair can often save the patient from a major vascular surgery **(Table 3–1).** If the patients are selected carefully for transfemoral TAVR, vascular intervention of any kind is required in fewer than 5% of cases.

Patients are transferred back to the intensive care unit with compressive bandages over the access sites.

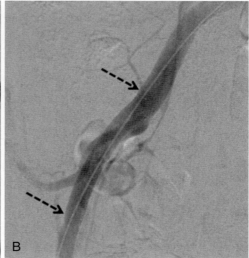

Figure 3–7 **A,** Completion angiogram after percutaneous transcatheter aortic valve replacement from the right shows a dissection flap *(solid arrows)* in the external iliac artery with no flow distally. **B,** This was repaired successfully with a self-expanding stent *(between dashed arrows)* from an ipsilateral approach with complete restoration of distal flow.

TABLE 3–1 ▬▬▬▬▬▬▬

Vascular Complications and Therapies after Transfemoral Transcatheter Aortic Valve Replacement

Non–Flow-Limiting Dissection	Avoid Reversing Anticoagulation
Flow-limiting dissection in common or external iliac artery	Peripheral stenting
Flow-limiting dissection in the common femoral artery	Open surgical repair
Vessel rupture	Proximal Coda balloon and covered stenting or open vascular surgical repair. Internal iliac artery may need to be percutaneously embolized to prevent back bleeding into the pelvis.

Coda; Cook Medical, Bloomington, Ind.

Patients remain on bed rest for longer than 4 hours but are allowed to sit up for extubation as soon as the general anesthesia wears off. Though late pseudoaneurysm or infections have been seen, they remain fairly uncommon. Management of these complications is consistent with the standard of care of the local institution.

3.5 Venous Access

Access to the venous system with large-caliber sheaths (up to 24F) is commonly necessary for percutaneous treatment of structural heart disease. One such procedure is transcatheter pulmonary valve replacement using either the Melody valve (Medtronic, Minneapolis Minn., 22F) or the Edwards SAPIEN valve (Edwards Lifesciences, Irvine Calif., 22F and 24F). Femoral vein access is obtained in a standard fashion and serially

dilated with care mostly directed to making an adequate subcutaneous tract and skin incision to accommodate the sheath. Vein closure and safe removal of large caliber sheaths often is more problematic than the access itself. Simple manual compression can be employed but requires delay until anticoagulation has worn off, prolonged compression times, and long periods of postprocedural bed rest. Dedicated venous closure devices do not exist, but adaptation of existing plug-and-suture–mediated arterial closure devices such as Angio-Seal (St. Jude Medical, St. Paul, Minn.) and Perclose ProGlide have been described.[7,8] Placement of these devices in veins is more difficult than in arteries because of the thin wall of the vessel that is difficult to feel upon pulling back and the low pressure flow that can be difficult to detect. A two-Perclose ProGlide predeployment technique performed without angulating the sutures has produced good results (both at approximately the 12 o'clock position). Other operators have used 10 o'clock and 2 o'clock positions with good results. In other cases, a temporary subcutaneous "figure-of-eight" suture can be used to achieve immediate hemostasis and sheath removal. This technique involves placing a continuous subcutaneous suture on either side of the venotomy by using two passes of the suture needle and then tying down the suture as the sheath is removed. This serves to pull the subcutaneous tissue together tightly and effectively compress just above the vein so as to achieve hemostasis without occluding or thrombosing the vein.[9] This technique can be safely employed over any shallow venous access such as the internal jugular or subclavian vein.

Adult patients with congenital conditions commonly have had multiple prior procedures, and femoral veins can become occluded. In such instances, approach from the internal jugular or subclavian vein may be appropriate as long as these conduits reach the area of interest and catheter manipulation from the chosen access is feasible. If femoral access is necessary, the occluded vein can be recannalized using a small 0.014- to 0.018-inch wire through a supportive 4F to 5F dilator to probe

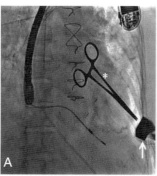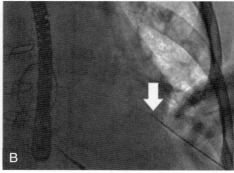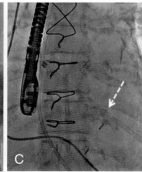

Figure 3–8   **A,** Percutaneous transapical approach guided by fluoroscopy using a hemostat *(asterisk)* to pick an optimal site to puncture the skin near the apex and just superior to a rib away from subcostal vascular structures, and transthoracic echocardiography *(solid arrow)* to avoid lung tissue and guide a path into the ventricle. **B,** A micropuncture needle and wire are used to access the ventricle *(wide arrow,* picture from different patient than shown in **A** and **C**). **C,** Once access was obtained, an 8F sheath *(dashed arrow)* was inserted to deliver a 10-mm muscular ventricular septal defect closure device. Access closure in this case was successfully achieved with an 8F Angio-Seal device with no bleeding complication.

the "beak" of the occluded femoral vein. A hand-injection angiogram in both the anteroposterior and lateral projections through the access needle will often be needed to identify the "beak," because venous collaterals commonly circulate into the iliac system or inferior vena cava and can obscure true femoral vein tract. Small incremental advancements followed by repeat hand injections through the dilator are used to monitor progress and see when free flow into the proximal patent vein is established. The occluded segment can then be wired and dilated, and a sheath at least the length of the segment can be inserted. The planned procedure should be done through this sheath first and then the femoral vein should be stented at the end of the procedure. This method resulted in long-term patency of the femoral vein in more than 85% of vessels.[10] Another alternative described mostly in pediatric patients is transhepatic venous access.[11] This approach is a feasible "last resort" option in the adult patient with no other venous access. Achieving hemostasis after transhepatic access can be problematic.

3.6 Transapical Access

In rare instances, a patient may have no vascular access options for a transcatheter structural heart procedure and may need a procedure (e.g., mitral paravalvular leak closure, left ventricle pseudoaneurysm closure, left ventricular outflow track access for electrophysiology procedures, or pulmonary vein access) for which direct left ventricular access is best suited. Lateral thoracotomy can easily be performed by the cardiac surgeon. Management of the ventriculotomy created by a large-bore sheath, however, is a skill that many cardiac surgeons do not have experience with (e.g., transapical TAVR). It is beyond the scope of this chapter to discuss surgical transapical access/closure for TAVR. Ventriculotomy with a sheath up to 16F should be manageable by the cardiac surgeon with a cardiologist.

Percutaneous left ventricular transapical access may be an option in some cases. The technique has recently been described using detailed CT angiography imaging

with overlay onto fluoroscopy to aid in puncturing near the left ventricular apex while avoiding coronary arteries and lung tissue.[12] At Emory University Hospital, angiography has been used to localize the coronary arteries and echocardiography has been used to select the trajectory of the needle puncture **(Figure 3–8).** Closure of the transapical puncture can be achieved successfully with manual pressure for small sheaths and devices ranging from coils to Amplatzer devices (St. Jude Medical, St. Paul, Minn.) for larger sheaths. Patients with multiple previous cardiac surgeries, particularly previous lateral thoracotomy, will have less issue with bleeding after sheath removal. Sheath removal in other patients may have unpredictable consequences and may require a chest tube, transfusion, and reversal of anticoagulation. One small series reports a 50% rate of bleeding complications after transapical access for mitral paravalvular leak closure.[13]

3.7 Summary

Vascular access strategies for structural heart disease should always be discussed during preprocedure planning. Several imaging modalities may be needed to decide on the appropriate approach, which can often dictate the success of the intervention. Though surgical access and closure can be considered the gold standard, percutaneous techniques are quickly being adopted for more than 95% of procedures. In the future, dedicated devices will simplify the percutaneous large-bore closure. Certainly, percutaneous transapical approaches will also be part of the armamentarium.

REFERENCES

1. Webb JG, Chandavimol M, Thompson CR, et al: Percutaneous aortic valve implantation retrograde from the femoral artery, *Circulation* 113:842–850, 2006.
2. Hayashida K, LeFevre T, Morice MC, et al: Transfemoral aortic valve implantation: new criteria to predict vascular complications, *JACC Cardiovasc Interv* 4:851–858, 2011.

3. Toggweiler S, Gurvitch R, Leipsic J, et al: Percutaneous aortic valve replacement: vascular outcomes with a fully percutaneous procedure, *JACC Cardiovasc Interv* 59:113–118, 2012.
4. Tchetche D, Dumonteil N, Sauguet A, et al: Thirty-day outcome and vascular complications after transarterial aortic valve implantation using both Edwards SAPIEN and Medtronic CoreValve bioprostheses in a mixed population, *EuroIntervention* 5:659–665, 2010.
5. Ducrocq G, Francis F, Serfaty JM, et al: Vascular complications of transfemoral aortic valve implantation with the Edwards SAPIEN prosthesis: incidence and impact on outcome, *EuroIntervention* 5:666–672, 2010.
6. Eltchaninoff H, Kerkeni M, Zajarias A, et al: Aortoiliac angiography as a screening tool in selecting patients for transfemoral aortic valve implantation with the Edwards SAPIEN bioprosthesis, *EuroIntervention* 119:3009–3016, 2009.
7. Shaw JA, Dewire E, Alan N, et al: Use of suture-mediated vascular closure devices for the management of femoral vein access after transcatheter procedures, *Catheter Cardiovasc Interv* 63:439–443, 2004.
8. Coto HA, Zhao D, et al: Closure of the femoral vein puncture site after transcatheter procedures using Angio-Seal, *Catheter Cardiovasc Interv* 55:16–19, 2002.
9. Cilingiroglu M, Feldman T, Zhao D, et al: Technique of temporary subcutaneous "figure-of-eight" sutures to achieve hemostasis after removal of large-caliber femoral venous sheaths, *Catheter Cardiovasc Interv* 78:155–160, 2011.
10. Ing FF, Fagan TE, Grifka RG, et al: Reconstruction of stenotic or occluded iliofemoral veins and inferior vena cava using intravascular stents: reestablishing access for future cardiac catheterization and cardiac surgery, *J Am Coll Cardiol* 37:251–257, 2001.
11. Shim D, Lloyd TR, Beekman RH: Transhepatic therapeutic cardiac catheterization: a new option for the pediatric interventionalist, *Catheter Cardiovasc Interv* 47:41–45, 1999.
12. Jelnin V, Dudiy Y, Ruiz C, et al: Clinical experience with percutaneous left ventricular transapical access for interventions in structural heart defects, *JACC Cardiovasc Interv* 4:868–874, 2011.
13. Nietlispach F, Johnson M, Moss R, et al: Transcatheter closure of paravalvular defects using a purpose-specific occluder, *JACC Cardiovasc Interv* 3:759–765, 2010.

Chapter 4

Transseptal Heart Catheterization

KHUNG KEONG YEO • JASON H. ROGERS • REGINALD I. LOW

4.1 Importance of Transseptal Puncture

The transseptal puncture has been in use since its description in 1959 by Drs. Ross, Braunwald and Morrow.[1] Until recently, transseptal puncture has been used relatively rarely, primarily for diagnostic purposes and percutaneous balloon mitral valvuloplasty (PBMV). In recent years, with the advent of complex structural heart interventions and electrophysiology ablation procedures, the use of transseptal puncture has increased.[2-4] In the arena of structural heart disease interventions, transseptal puncture is often a crucial initial part of the procedure. These procedures include PBMV, closure of the long-tunnel patent foramen ovale (PFO), atrial septostomy, left atrial appendage occlusion, percutaneous mitral valve repair (e.g., with MitraClip [Abbott Vascular Structural Heart, Menlo Park, Calif.]), mitral paravalvular leak closure, and many investigational mitral repair or replacement technologies.

In some procedures, the transseptal puncture is important primarily for access to the left atrium (LA), such as in PBMV for mitral stenosis. When the location of puncture is less important, experienced operators can easily perform blind puncture using fluoroscopic landmarks. However, in other procedures the precise location of the transseptal puncture is critically important, because it may either determine procedural safety (e.g., in atrial septostomy) or procedural success, such as in the MitraClip procedure or left atrial appendage closure. For procedures in which precise positioning is of utmost importance, some form of real-time echocardiographic imaging is essential.

4.2 Equipment

The transseptal puncture can be performed safely using standard equipment. This may include a Mullins sheath and dilator and a Brockenbrough needle (Medtronic,

Santa Rosa, Calif.) **(Figure 4–1).** However, there are more options available currently and operators may choose to use other commercially available needles and sheaths/dilators. These include the BRK series of transseptal needles and the SL series of transseptal sheaths (St. Jude Medical, St. Paul, Minn.) **(Figures 4–2 and 4–3).** Specific equipment for PBMV may also be used off-label. These include the "curly" left atrial guidewire (TORAYGUIDE Guidewire; Toray Industries, United States), which provides stable support in the LA.

In general, these authors recommend using the SL-0 sheath and dilator or the Mullins sheath with a BRK needle. The angle of the SL-0 sheath favors directing a wire towards the left upper pulmonary vein (LUPV). However, the Mullins sheath is also commonly used and may be useful if extra curve is required toward the mitral valve. The choice of the catheter is largely dependent on the specific patient anatomy, procedure type, and the preference of the operator. For example, a Mullins sheath may be particularly suitable in situations where there is a PFO or when the LA is large. Another important variation in the practice of transseptal punctures is that some operators use just the dilator with the BRK needle without the accompanying sheath. The Agilis NxT Steerable Introducers (St Jude Medical, St. Paul, Minn.) are specialized catheters with adjustable curves that may be particularly suitable for complex anatomy.

TRANSSEPTAL HEART CATHETERIZATION UNDER FLUOROSCOPIC GUIDANCE

Transseptal puncture under fluoroscopic guidance is usually performed for PBMV and other procedures in which precise location of the transseptal puncture is not crucial. Various methods have been described. The availability of advanced imaging technologies such as transesophageal echocardiography (TEE) and intracardiac echocardiography (ICE) have made the use of

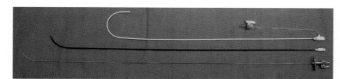

Figure 4–1 Components of a transseptal puncture system. *Top to bottom:* Mullins sheath, dilator, and transseptal needle.

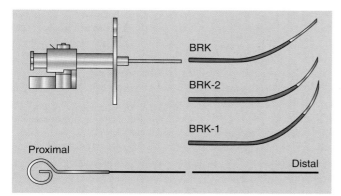

- **Curve options**
  - Available in three: two adult curves (BRK and BRK-1) and two pediatric (BRK and BRK-2)
- **Variety of length**
  - Three adult (71, 89, 98 cm) and one pediatric (56 cm)
  - The 98 cm needle designed for use with St. Jude Medical Agilis NxT steerable introducer

Figure 4–2 Some types of transseptal needles and catheters. *(Courtesy of St. Jude Medical, St. Paul, Minn.)*

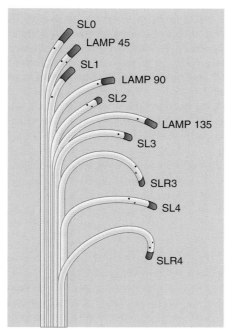

Figure 4–3 Different transseptal catheters are available with different curves and tip shapes. These are generally available in both 8F and 8.5F sizes. *(Courtesy of St. Jude Medical, St. Paul, Minn.)*

fluoroscopic maneuvers (including right atrial angiography) less common. Nonetheless, because PBMV is more commonly performed in developing countries, in which cost considerations of using these technologies may be important, it is important to understand the various techniques available using fluoroscopy to obtain a successful puncture.

"DROP" INTO THE FOSSA OVALIS

A transseptal puncture begins with access into the right femoral venous system. Although transseptal puncture is possible from the left femoral vein, the angulation is generally not favorable and therefore avoided if possible. A 0.032-inch guidewire is advanced from the inferior vena cava (IVC) into the superior vena cava (SVC), and the right femoral venous sheath is exchanged for a transseptal sheath and dilator (e.g., Mullins sheath or SL-0 catheter). The transseptal sheath is advanced into the SVC. Operators may, at the same time, choose to place a pigtail catheter in the ascending aorta to demarcate the position of the aorta on fluoroscopy **(Figure 4–4)**. This helps identify the aorta so that the operator may direct the transseptal needle away from it (appreciable primarily in the lateral fluoroscopic projection). In the meantime, the transseptal needle is flushed carefully and attached to a pressure transducer. Many operators will slowly continuously flush the needle with a saline infusion drip to prevent air from entering the system. The small saline flush that emanates from the tip of the sheath can also aid visualization if echocardiographic imaging is used. The needle is then advanced to the distal edge of the transseptal sheath, with the operator taking care to ensure that at least a distance of 1 cm is present between the needle and sheath tips. To do so, the needle is prevented from advancing forward by gripping it in the palm of the right hand while the thumb and index fingers hold the sheath and dilator system **(Figure 4–5)**. The orientation of the needle and sheath must be maintained by matching the metal arrow on the needle's hub to the direction of sheath's sidearm **(Figure 4–6)**. The operator ensures that that the needle does not slip forward inadvertently. The entire system of sheath, dilator, and needle is held as one unit and then gradually brought down to the level of the interatrial septum. This technique also maintains a constant and safe needle distance from the tip of the dilator. In a patient with normal or near normal anatomy, as the transseptal system is brought caudally (inferiorly), there is a "drop" into the fossa ovalis as the sheath cross the limbus. This is a tactile event and occasionally may also be appreciated on fluoroscopy as well.

At this point, the operator may puncture the septum by advancing the needle carefully out the end of the sheath **(Figure 4–7)**. By applying gentle forward pressure to the needle and transseptal sheath, the needle should cross in the LA easily. In some cases, as forward pressure is applied, the needle may slide cranially, and the original puncture location may be lost. In this case, it may be necessary to remove and reshape the needle to gain more purchase on the interatrial septum. In

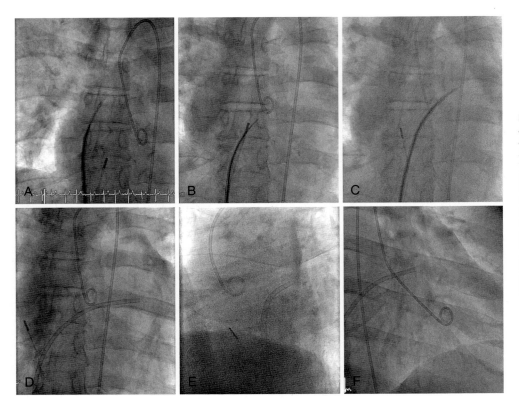

Figure 4–4 **Fluoroscopic appearance of transseptal puncture in anteroposterior (AP) projection.** **A,** Pigtail in aortic root, transseptal sheath in SVC. ICE catheter in RA. **B,** Transseptal sheath pulled back to RA, fossa engaged, and needle advanced. **C,** Transseptal sheath and dilator advanced over needle into LA. **D,** Dilator and needle withdrawn, sheath in LA. **E,** Lateral view showing transseptal sheath crossing posterior to aorta. **F,** Right anterior oblique (RAO) projection showing LA sheath and pigtail in left ventricle (LV).

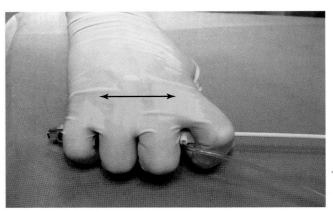

Figure 4–5 **Technique for holding the transseptal system.** The entire system is grasped within the hand to allow the system to move as one unit. The sheath and dilator and are grasped with the index finger and thumb, and the needle is grasped with the remaining fingers. This ensures a constant relationship between the needle and sheath *(two-headed arrow)*, and avoids inadvertent needle advancement.

addition, the wire mandril that comes with the Brockenbrough needle can also be used to "anchor" the needle into the septum and to assist in stabilizing the system as forward pressure is applied **(Figure 4–8).** As the needle crosses in the LA, the pressure transducer should show a left atrial pressure waveform. Importantly, the operator would hope not to see aortic pressure waveforms, which would indicate puncture of the aorta. The operator may also confirm that the needle is in the LA by aspirating blood backwards. Bright red blood will usually indicate that the needle is in the LA if pressure waveforms are consistent as well. An important cautionary note is to

avoid flushing the catheter if it appears that the needle has crossed but there is no waveform or if the waveform is dampened. This may represent a thrombus on the needle/catheter system. Flushing into the LA may result in a stroke. Gentle aspiration to remove the thrombus may help. Lack of any pressure may also indicate that the tip of the needle is in the wall of the LA, pericardial space, or other soft-tissue structure. If there is uncertainty as to the location of the needle, the transseptal sheath should never be advanced forward, and the entire system should be withdrawn into the right atrium (RA). There are times in which the needle appears to be clearly into the LA but there is no pressure waveform. This may occur especially if there is a very floppy septum or if an interatrial septal aneurysm is present. In such situations, although it may appear that the needle is very far into the LA on fluoroscopy, it may not have crossed the floppy septum. Adequate preprocedure echocardiography would be useful to identify the presence of a floppy septum or interatrial septal aneurysm. TEE guidance in such situations would be reassuring and would enhance patient safety.

Once across the interatrial septum, the needle is often directed posteriorly so a slight counterclockwise rotation will direct the needle away from the left atrial posterior wall. The dilator and sheath are carefully advanced over the needle and then just the sheath over the dilator to ensure that the sheath is well in the LA **(Figure 4–9).** The dilator and needle are then removed, and the sheath aspirated and flushed carefully. If there is difficulty aspirating, the operator needs to consider the presence of thrombus or that the sheath tip is impinging on the wall of the LA. In the latter case, the sheath may be rotated

Figure 4–6 The transseptal sheath and needle are moved as one system by rotating the hand. The arrow on the transseptal needle should be aligned with the sidearm of the sheath, which is oriented toward the curve of the transseptal sheath *(arrows)*. **A** and **B** show the system in the horizontal (3 o'clock) position. **C** and **D** show the system in the 4 o'clock position *(arrows)*, which is the preferred angle of crossing for the majority of structurally normal hearts. Note that this angle will change with RA or LA enlargement.

Figure 4–7 Needle advancement. **A** and **B** illustrate the relationship of the needle hub to the dilator when the needle is within the transseptal sheath dilator *(arrows)*. In **C** and **D,** the needle is advanced slightly out of the dilator, and the distance between the needle hub and dilator decreases *(arrows)*.

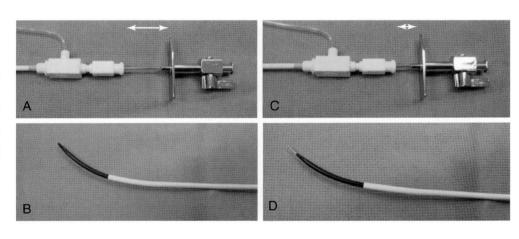

Figure 4–8 Use of microwire mandril to assist in transseptal puncture. In some cases the needle may slip when forward pressure is applied, and the desired location is not punctured. The wire mandril can be used to "stick" the septum, thereby fixing the needle in one position, and providing stabilization upon needle advancement. **A,** The needle alone with hub *(inset)*. **B,** The needle alone protruding from dilator. **C,** The needle with wire mandril advanced and hub detail (wire mandril shown by *arrows*). **D,** The needle and wire mandril advanced out of tip of dilator.

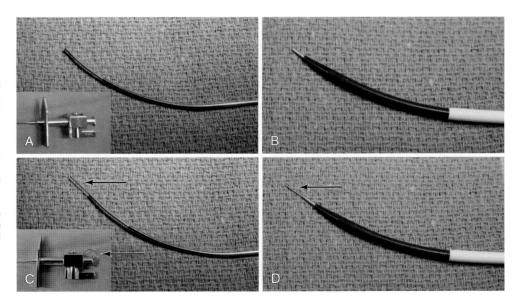

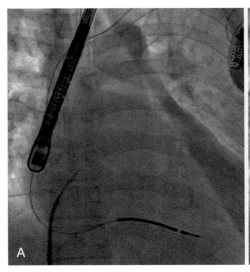
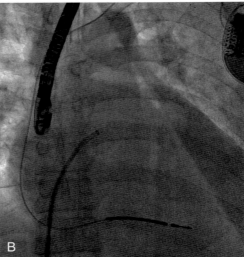

Figure 4–9 **A** shows the transseptal needle at the interatrial septum. **B** shows that the puncture has occurred and now the sheath is across the septum. The dilator and needle have been withdrawn back into the sheath.

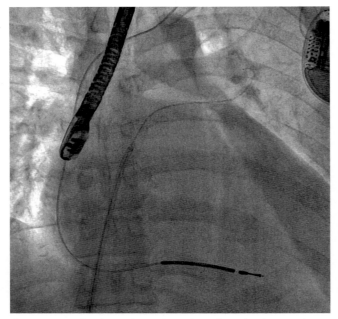

Figure 4–10 This shows the transseptal needle and catheter with successful puncture across the interatrial septum and a wire advanced to the LUPV.

either clockwise or counterclockwise to turn the sheath posteriorly or anteriorly away from the LA wall.

Depending on the procedure, a 0.035-inch stiff wire (e.g., Amplatz Super Stiff wire [St. Jude Medical, St. Paul, Minn.]) can be advanced to the LUPV and used as a rail for the delivery for equipment or devices **(Figure 4–10).** On occasion, a 6F or 7F multipurpose catheter may be used through the transseptal sheath to help guide the positioning of the wire in the LUPV.

4.3 Septal Flush or Staining Method

Some operators recommend the use of the "septal flush" or "stain" to demarcate the interatrial septum.[5] This may be done in conjunction with other fluoroscopic transseptal techniques. It is performed by injecting contrast against the interatrial septum. In the lateral projection, a vertical stain suggests dissection of the high septum. With tenting of the interatrial septum at the fossa ovalis, a triangular "tent" of contrast may be seen. These techniques are used when echocardiographic imaging may not be easily available.

FLUOROSCOPIC LANDMARKS

Before the advent of TEE and ICE, fluoroscopic landmarks were exclusively used in performing a transseptal puncture. These include the use of right atrial angiography, drawing imaginary lines on fluoroscopy stop-frame images, using a pigtail catheter on the ascending aorta, and recognizing the relative positions of the tricuspid valve, coronary sinus, and aorta. Amongst the key points to note is that it is important to avoid the aorta, which is an anterior structure **(Figure 4–11).** The pigtail catheter helps the operator avoid the aorta. A lateral projection can also help to identify the anterior/posterior direction of the transseptal needle. These techniques remain helpful, especially if imaging is not available. However, for complex structural heart interventions such as the MitraClip and atrial septostomy, or in patients who are at very high risk for transseptal complications (such as prior mitral valve surgery with atrial septal repair), the authors believe that it is essential to have imaging with either TEE or ICE. Fluoroscopy alone would be potentially risky in patients who cannot tolerate any hemodynamic embarrassment. Fluoroscopy would also be unable to determine a precise anatomic puncture site. Of note, electrophysiologists have used additional landmarking tools for transseptal punctures. These include the use of a catheter in the coronary sinus, which delineates the margin of the left atrial free wall; and a catheter at the bundle of HIS to identify the anterior aspect of the interatrial septum. Numerous techniques for transseptal puncture using fluoroscopy alone have been well described in the literature and will not be the focus of this chapter.

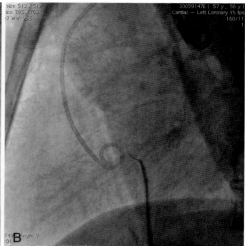

Figure 4–11 A shows the pigtail catheter in the ascending aorta with the transseptal needle/sheath at the interatrial septum, anteroposterior view. The needle is pointing in the right direction (assuming the patient has normal anatomy). **B,** Lateral view shows the pigtail anterior to the transseptal needle. The needle is pointing slightly too anteriorly.

PUNCTURING THE INTERATRIAL SEPTUM

Not uncommonly there may be difficulty in using the transseptal needle to puncture the interatrial septum. This may be because of a thickened or fibrosed septum, the presence of an interatrial septal aneurysm, or a PFO. In these situations, fluoroscopic guidance alone can be an uncomfortable experience, because the fluoroscopic appearance of the needle and catheter's position may lead one to believe that the puncture has already occurred. With echocardiographic guidance, the actual interaction between the catheter/needle apparatus is better appreciated. In such situations, an operator can patiently "lean" on the catheter/needle until it pops across the septum with the continuous motion of each heartbeat. Alternatively, the operator may use the back end of a 0.014-inch guidewire or the Brockenbrough stylet, which is usually stiff enough to puncture across the septum **(see Figure 4–8).** Gradual pressure with the needle after that is usually sufficient for crossing. Other operators have described the use of radiofrequency (RF) via a diathermy device (such as the Bovie; Bovie Medical Corporation, Clearwater, Fla.) to "cut" across the septum. Once the transseptal catheter and needle are in place at the fossa, the needle should be advanced to the tip of the dilator. The unipolar diathermy probe is then set at "cut" mode with an output of 15 to 40 W and touched to the metal hub of the transseptal needle for 1 to 2 seconds.[6-9] There are also dedicated RF transseptal needles (e.g., NRG RF Transseptal Needle, Baylis Medical, Quebec, Canada) in the market that may be used for the same purpose. Compared with standard electrophysiology ablation procedures, the Baylis system utilizes lower power (5 W vs. 35 to 50 W), short duration (1 sec vs. 60 to 90 sec), and high voltage (150 to 180 V vs. 30 to 50 V). The active tip is also smaller while ablation catheters tend to be larger in length and diameter. These devices may be useful in crossing floppy or thick septums **(Figure 4–12).**

TRANSSEPTAL HEART CATHETERIZATION FOR MITRACLIP PROCEDURE

More so than any other procedure, the transseptal puncture is a crucial part of the MitraClip procedure. It determines the height and position of the guiding catheter relative to the coaptation plane of the mitral leaflets and influences the maneuverability of the clip delivery system (CDS) and guiding catheter. The CDS with the MitraClip at its tip must be guided to the mitral valve for the proper placement of the clip. Because of the importance of the transseptal puncture in the MitraClip procedure, the steps involved in evaluating and selecting an ideal position has great learning value for transseptal punctures in general.

For the MitraClip procedure, a poorly positioned transseptal puncture will result in difficulty maneuvering the device in the LA. The guide may be too close to important structures such as the aorta by puncturing too anterior, or the guide may be directed toward the posterior wall of the LA by an inappropriately posterior puncture. The puncture may be too high above the valve coaptation plane, leaving insufficient height for the CDS and clip to reach and grasp the leaflets. Finally, the puncture may be too low, making it difficult to retract the CDS and grasp the leaflets.

A suboptimal transseptal puncture site may also limit the range of movement that is built into the MitraClip system. For example, an anterior puncture may result in an "aorta-hugger" scenario in which the CDS runs almost parallel to the aorta. In such a scenario, it is difficult for the CDS to orient perpendicular to the mitral valve.

4.4 Step-by-Step: Basic Transseptal Puncture

The next paragraphs provide a detailed step-by-step transseptal puncture technique for the MitraClip procedure, although the entire MitraClip procedure is discussed in more detail in Chapter 11 of this textbook. As discussed earlier, the transseptal puncture is critical and it is worthwhile to invest time and attention to obtain an ideal puncture. After right femoral venous access is obtained, a 0.032-inch wire is advanced to the SVC under fluoroscopic guidance. The venous sheath

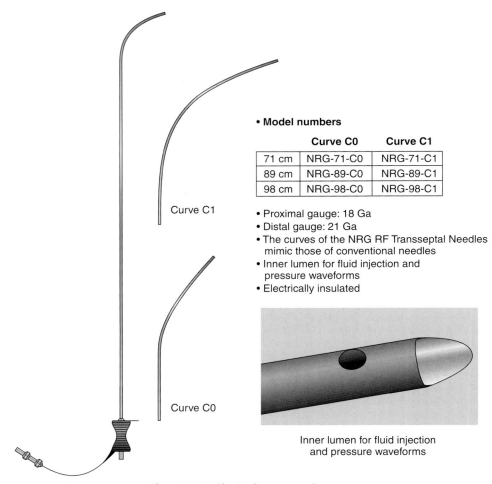

- **Model numbers**

	Curve C0	Curve C1
71 cm	NRG-71-C0	NRG-71-C1
89 cm	NRG-89-C0	NRG-89-C1
98 cm	NRG-98-C0	NRG-98-C1

- Proximal gauge: 18 Ga
- Distal gauge: 21 Ga
- The curves of the NRG RF Transseptal Needles mimic those of conventional needles
- Inner lumen for fluid injection and pressure waveforms
- Electrically insulated

Inner lumen for fluid injection
and pressure waveforms

Figure 4–12   The Baylis transseptal system.

is then exchanged for a transseptal sheath, such as the Mullins or SL-0 sheath, and dilator, which are advanced into the SVC. The wire is then removed and the transseptal needle is advanced to near the distal tip of the sheath and under fluoroscopic guidance (usually to ≈1 cm from the tip of the dilator). Under fluoroscopic and TEE guidance, the sheath and needle are slowly and carefully pulled back to the junction of the SVC and RA **(see Figure 4–4).**

From here, TEE almost completely guides the procedure. The first view is the bicaval view in which the superior–inferior orientation of the puncture is determined **(Figure 4–13)**. The ideal position in a routine EVEREST II-type procedure would be just slightly superior from the midpoint in this view **(Figures 4–13 to 4–15)**. The sheath dilator should be used to "tent" the septum **(Figure 4–16)**. Once this position is achieved, the echocardiologist obtains the short-axis view at the level of the aorta on TEE. This view provides an anteroposterior perspective on the transseptal location. To manipulate the transseptal needle and sheath posteriorly, the entire system is torqued clockwise; to turn anteriorly, the system is torqued counterclockwise. The ideal position is slightly posterior of the midline

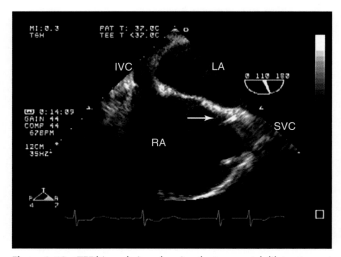

Figure 4–13   TEE bicaval view showing the transseptal dilator *(arrow)* at the junction of the SVC and RA as it is slowly pulled down from the SVC. *(With kind permission of Springer Science+Business Media. From Atlas of Percutaneous Edge-to-Edge Mitral Valve Repair. Chapter 3. Transseptal Puncture, Yeo, Rogers and Low. Jan 2013.)*

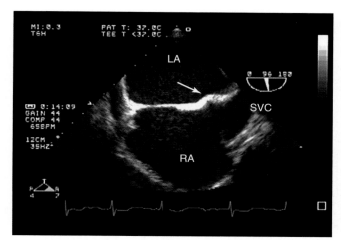

Figure 4–14 Bicaval view showing the transseptal dilator *(arrow* at site of tenting) now at the septum secundum. *(With kind permission of Springer Science+Business Media. From Atlas of Percutaneous Edge-to-Edge Mitral Valve Repair. Chapter 3. Transseptal Puncture, Yeo, Rogers and Low. Jan 2013.)*

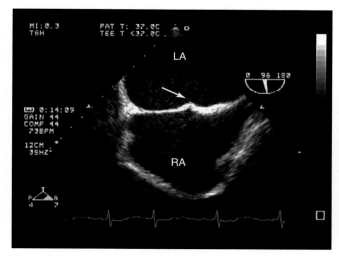

Figure 4–15 Bicaval view showing the transseptal dilator *(arrow)* at the limbus of the fossa ovalis. *(With kind permission of Springer Science+Business Media. From Atlas of Percutaneous Edge-to-Edge Mitral Valve Repair. Chapter 3. Transseptal Puncture, Yeo, Rogers and Low. Jan 2013.)*

(Figure 4–17). In some situations, clockwise or counterclockwise turning of the sheath may simply cause the tip of the sheath to pivot at the site of tenting. This happens when the dilator is tenting the septum too aggressively. It may therefore be necessary to slightly disengage (pull back) the catheter from the septum to allow repositioning. The same principle applies when adjusting the sheath in an anteroposterior direction by either advancing or withdrawing the catheter

The next view is the four- or five-chamber view in which the perpendicular (vertical) height of the transseptal tenting from the mitral valve is measured. This distance should be between 3.5 and 4.5 cm **(Figure 4–18).** The mitral valve reference point is either the mitral valve annular plane or the point of coaptation of the mitral valve leaflets. In patients who have mitral valve prolapse, the mitral annulus is usually a reasonable guide for height

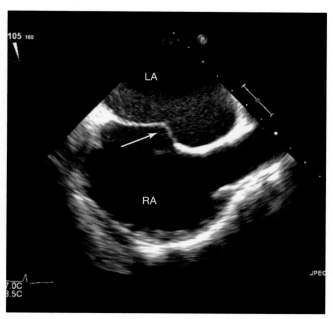

Figure 4–16 Bicaval view showing the transseptal dilator *(arrow)* tenting the fossa ovalis (septum primum) at a location near the midpoint. *(With kind permission of Springer Science+Business Media. From Atlas of Percutaneous Edge-to-Edge Mitral Valve Repair. Chapter 3. Transseptal Puncture, Yeo, Rogers and Low. Jan 2013.)*

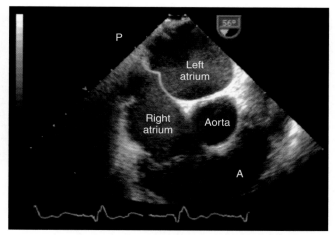

Figure 4–17 **Short-axis view at the level of the aorta.** The transseptal dilator should avoid the aorta. In an ideal position, the needle should tent the interatrial septum slightly posterior to the midpoint of the septum as seen in this view. Tenting too anteriorly may risk puncture of the aorta. Also, an anterior puncture may result in an "aorta-hugger" situation during steering of the device. In such a situation, it becomes difficult for the MitraClip to approach the mitral valve plane perpendicularly. *(Courtesy of Abbott Vascular. Copyright 2013 Abbott Laboratories. All rights reserved.)*

measurements. However, in patients with functional mitral regurgitation (MR), the point of coaptation is usually lower because of restricted leaflet mobility. Hence it is recommended to use the point of leaflet coaptation as a point of reference in patients with functional MR.

When making changes to the position of the sheath by manipulating the sheath/needle unit in one view, it is important to verify that the position in other planes has not been affected in an adverse manner. For example, since the fossa ovalis is shaped elliptically, movement of

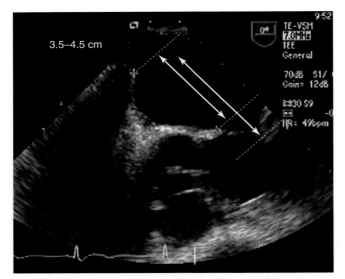

Figure 4–18   Four-chamber or five-chamber view. This view is meant for assessment of "height" above the mitral valve. This is the perpendicular distance from the tenting point *(shorter arrow)* to the mitral valve annulus. Some operators may choose to use the reference point as the point of mitral leaflet coaptation *(longer arrow)*. Regardless, the generally accepted distance is 3.5 to 4.5 cm, depending on the nature of the MR. *(Modified from images courtesy of Abbott Vascular. Copyright 2013 Abbott Laboratories. All rights reserved.)*

the sheath posterior may actually result in a more inferior position, so the operator should check orthogonal TEE views to ensure proper orientation in both planes before puncturing.

Once the suitability of the proposed transseptal puncture site has been confirmed as described, puncture across the septum is performed. This is performed by advancing the needle just beyond the tip of the dilator and exerting a gentle forward pressure. It is critical not to be too hasty in this part of the procedure. Excessive pressure can cause the needle tip to slide off its intended puncture spot. The needle should be connected to a pressure transducer to confirm entry into the LA by appearance of a venous waveform. Generally, a small "pop" is felt as the needle traverses the interatrial septum. Once the tip of the needle enters the LA, the needle and sheath should be rotated slightly counterclockwise to avoid inadvertent puncture of the posterior wall of the LA. The echocardiologist can also provide feedback on the location of the needle and dilator. The dilator and sheath are then advanced over the needle into the LA, and the sheath is then advanced over the needle and dilator. The needle and dilator are then carefully removed and the transseptal sheath is carefully aspirated and flushed to avoid any air entry or thrombus formation.

Once the transseptal puncture is done and the sheath or guide is across the interatrial septum, intravenous (IV) heparin to achieve an activated clotting time (ACT) greater than 250 sec is given. A 0.035-inch Amplatz Super Stiff guidewire is then advanced under fluoroscopic guidance to the LUPV (**see Figure 4–10**). Some operators have also used a short-tip 0.035-inch extra-stiff or short-tip wire. The advantage of the short tip is that it allows a longer segment of the stiff wire for use as a rail. However, the shorter tip can create a greater risk of perforation. Sometimes it is

necessary to use a nested catheter such as a multipurpose catheter through the transseptal sheath to guide the wire into the LUPV. Usually the echocardiologist will maintain real-time echo imaging of the left atrial appendage to warn the operator against advancing the wire into the appendage. At the same time, he or she can inform the operator if the wire is in the pulmonary vein. This is a useful and important step to prevent complications.

The transseptal sheath is then removed carefully, maintaining wire access in the LUPV. A 16F to 18F dilator is then used to dilate the femoral venous track. The MitraClip guide with its spiral dilator is then advanced slowly into the RA and against the interatrial septum. Gentle pressure is applied on the spiral dilator to cross the septum. It is important to do so cautiously though firmly. Overly aggressive pushing may tear the septum, resulting in significant interatrial shunting at the conclusion of the procedure. On rare occasions when the septum is thicker and the dilator does not easily cross, atrial septostomy with a balloon before MitraClip guide delivery has been reported.

Once the dilator and guide are across the septum, the dilator is withdrawn first into the guide and then the wire. The dilator and the wire are then both removed together from the guide while the operator aspirates gently with the wire well within the dilator. This is important, because the wire may damage the hemostatic valve of the guide if it is pulled through the guide outside of the dilator.

4.5 Special Transseptal Situations

TRANSSEPTAL CROSSING IN THE PRESENCE OF A PATENT FORAMEN OVALE

A PFO may potentially make it more difficult to perform a transseptal puncture. In situations where the purpose is simply access to the LA, crossing the interatrial septum via the PFO is acceptable. This may occur in examples of straightforward PFO closure or mitral valvotomy cases. However, for complex structural cases like the MitraClip procedure, it is not recommended to cross the PFO to enter the LA. The mobility of the PFO tract and its location often will result in a suboptimal position for the needle. For example, the PFO may bias the needle superiorly. If the needle or guide crosses at the PFO, it is often too "high" above the mitral valve plane and may limit steering of the device (**Figures 4–19 to 4–21**).

In the MitraClip and left atrial appendage closure cases, it is recommended to puncture the septum separately and avoid the PFO if possible. However, this is not always easily achieved. With a PFO or atrial septal aneurysm, it may be difficult for a transseptal dilator or needle to find purchase on the interatrial septum. Even if the ideal position is identified, when the operator advances the needle, it may slide out of position because of difficulty in creating a tent (**see Figure 4–21**). In this case, the tiny wire mandril that is packaged within the transseptal needle may be helpful if it is advanced through the needle into the interatrial septum, and it may provide additional fixation to allow controlled puncture (**see Figure 4–8**).

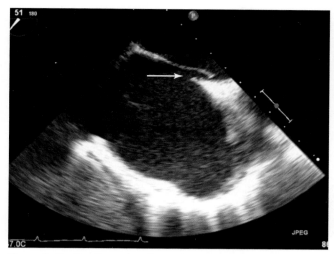

Figure 4–19 Baseline echo shows the presence of a PFO *(arrow)*. *(With kind permission of Springer Science+Business Media. From Atlas of Percutaneous Edge-to-Edge Mitral Valve Repair. Chapter 3. Transseptal Puncture, Yeo, Rogers and Low. Jan 2013.)*

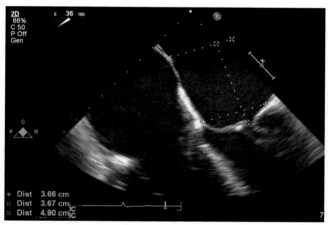

Figure 4–20 The transseptal puncture height is too high, with the PFO biasing the needle. *(With kind permission of Springer Science+Business Media. From Atlas of Percutaneous Edge-to-Edge Mitral Valve Repair. Chapter 3. Transseptal Puncture, Yeo, Rogers and Low. Jan 2013.)*

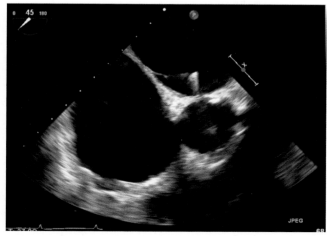

Figure 4–21 The transseptal needle has entered the LA via the PFO. *(With kind permission of Springer Science+Business Media. From Atlas of Percutaneous Edge-to-Edge Mitral Valve Repair. Chapter 3. Transseptal Puncture, Yeo, Rogers and Low. Jan 2013.)*

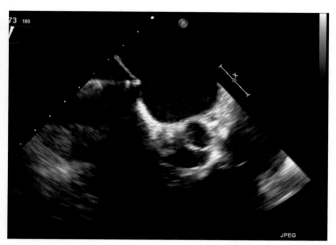

Figure 4–22 An attempt is made to puncture the septum separately from the PFO. In this case, the operator has angled the puncture site more posteriorly. The needle was reshaped gently to create the desired curvature. *(With kind permission of Springer Science+Business Media. From Atlas of Percutaneous Edge-to-Edge Mitral Valve Repair. Chapter 3. Transseptal Puncture, Yeo, Rogers and Low. Jan 2013.)*

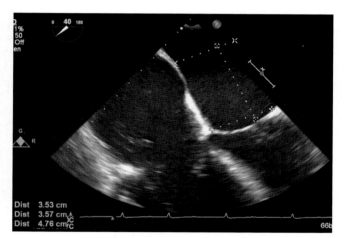

Figure 4–23 The new transseptal puncture height at 4.76 cm is not as high as the initial position. *(With kind permission of Springer Science+Business Media. From Atlas of Percutaneous Edge-to-Edge Mitral Valve Repair. Chapter 3. Transseptal Puncture, Yeo, Rogers and Low. Jan 2013.)*

Another way of obtaining adequate purchase on the septum is to use a transseptal sheath with greater curvature. For example, a Mullins sheath instead of an SR-0 or SL-0 catheter may provide greater angulation to "catch" on the interatrial septum **(Figures 4–22 and 4–23).** Similarly, a more curved transseptal needle may be required. For example, instead of the BRK needle, a BRK-1 needle may need to be used. The transseptal needles can also be carefully reshaped by hand slightly before use. A gentle curve added near the IVC–RA junction may allow the top of the dilator to exert more of a horizontal push vector against the septum.

In summary, it is important to identify the presence of a PFO before any transseptal procedure. In some cases, the PFO does not significantly impact the procedure. In others, such as atrial septal defect (ASD) closure, MitraClip, and left atrial appendage closure, precise location of the transseptal is more important. PFO location, tunnel length, diameter, and presence of a concomitant atrial septal aneurysm should be noted. Imaging with TEE or ICE should be used if the precise location of the puncture is required.

TRANSSEPTAL CROSSING IN THE PRESENCE OF AN ATRIAL SEPTAL DEFECT

An ASD obviates the need of a puncture if access to the LA is all that is required. However, for situations in which precise location of the puncture is crucial, like the Mitra-Clip procedure, the presence of an ASD severely limits the ability of the operator to determine the position of a transseptal puncture and therefore the ability to maneuver the device. The constraints of an ASD depend on its size, location, and whether it is single or fenestrated ASD. A very small ASD may not pose a significant problem. However, if a moderately sized ASD is present and in a suboptimal location, a transseptal puncture in the preferred location may result in a tear of the interatrial septum, causing massive left-to-right shunting.

If the ASD is in the ideal position, a left atrial appendage closure or MitraClip procedure may theoretically be performed through the defect. However, operators should be cognizant of the inability to properly evaluate the position of the equipment, because tenting with the transseptal needle is not possible. Furthermore, for the MitraClip procedure, advanced steering techniques may be required to position the CDS once in the LA.

TRANSSEPTAL PUNCTURE IN THE PRESENCE OF AN ATRIAL SEPTAL ANEURYSM

Transseptal puncture in the presence of an atrial septal aneurysm can be complicated because it is difficult to gain leverage on a floppy septum. This can result in difficulty in appreciating how much to push when viewed on fluoroscopy, because the needle may appear to have moved significantly into the LA but may still be in the RA. Inexperienced operators may use excessive force or manipulation of the transseptal needle, which can lead to complications such as perforation. The role of imaging is helpful in such situations because the operator can appreciate the degree of tenting. In these cases, as the transseptal puncture is attempted, the needle tents the interatrial septal aneurysm significantly. TEE in this case allows the operator to continue with confidence. With gentle forward pressure, puncture is achieved safely. Despite achieving LA access, the septal aneurysm continues to complicate the rest of this particular procedure, as in the case of a MitraClip procedure. The interatrial septal aneurysm may be so redundant that it is difficult to push the 22F MitraClip guide tip across the septum, resulting in tenting almost to the pulmonary vein orifice. As might be expected, doing such a procedure without appropriate echocardiographic guidance is difficult and likely to result in failure or complications.

Role of Intracardiac Echocardiography

ICE is a very useful tool in guiding transseptal punctures. Its use in guiding a transseptal puncture has been reported in the literature.[10,11] These authors find its use appealing because it does not require TEE, which can be uncomfortable in a conscious patient. The operator can perform imaging directly without involving another cardiologist. It can be used to guide transseptal puncture in unusual situations, such as when TEE may not offer adequate imaging of the septum (such as in a case of severe kyphoscoliosis or hiatal hernia). However, its use is limited by its two-dimensional functionality and absence of multiplane functionality (in commercial systems). In addition, it has limited field and depth of view and requires considerable expertise, which is difficult to obtain in daily work. This is as opposed to TEE, in which mastery is likely to be greater in view of its more widespread clinical application. For complex structural interventions like the MitraClip, ICE cannot replace TEE for the rest of the procedure after the transseptal puncture, because ICE currently cannot obtain some of the steering and assessment views required. Furthermore, commercial ICE systems do not yet possess three-dimensional capability. As such, ICE is not recommended for the entire MitraClip procedure at this time.

TRANSSEPTAL PUNCTURE FOR ATRIAL SEPTOSTOMY

In severe, late pulmonary hypertension in which right-sided pressures are near or at systemic pressures, the patient may suffer from symptoms of low cardiac output together with right ventricular volume and pressure overload. This is in part caused by severe underfilling of the left ventricle. Atrial septostomy is a palliative procedure that can help alleviate some of the manifestations of low cardiac output. By creating a right-to-left shunt via an iatrogenic ASD, left ventricular filling is improved, although at a cost of decreased systemic oxygen saturation. In severe, late pulmonary hypertension, the RA is usually large and compresses the LA. The severely deformed RA and LA make transseptal puncture potentially very difficult and dangerous. Although RA angiography may be performed to delineate the RA border, echocardiographic guidance is much preferred. **Figure 4–24** shows the almost slitlike LA compressed by the RA. As can be appreciated, an error during the transseptal puncture can result in inadvertent puncture of the walls of either atria or aorta. Using ICE, the LA and RA are well visualized. The interatrial septum with the transseptal needle can also be seen well. **Figures 4–25 and 4–26** show the visualization of the atrial septostomy on fluoroscopy and ICE. ICE is particularly useful for this procedure, because unlike TEE it is unlikely to result in respiratory embarrassment in these patients, who often have limited pulmonary reserve.

TRANSSEPTAL PUNCTURE FOR PATENT FORAMEN OVALE CLOSURE

In some cases, a PFO may have an excessively long tunnel that will not reduce sufficiently (or "accordion" out of the way) to allow full deployment and adequate seating of the transcatheter closure device. The technique of

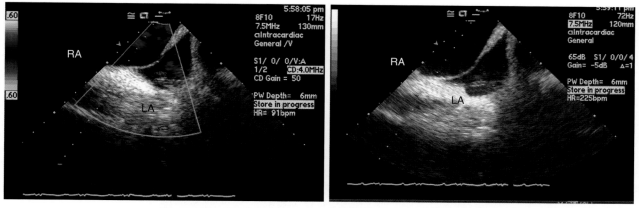

Figure 4–24 ICE shows the almost slitlike LA compressed by the RA.

Figures 4–25 This shows the visualization of the atrial septum on ICE (**A**) and fluoroscopy (**B**) with the atrial septostomy being performed.

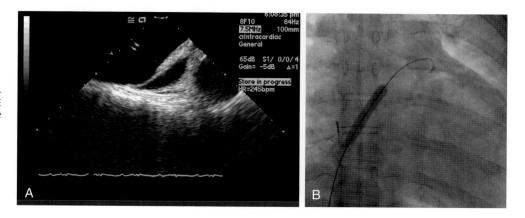

Figure 4–26 A shows a larger balloon being used as seen on fluoroscopy. **B** shows the right-to-left shunting seen across the newly created ASD. The 0.035-inch wire remains across the septum.

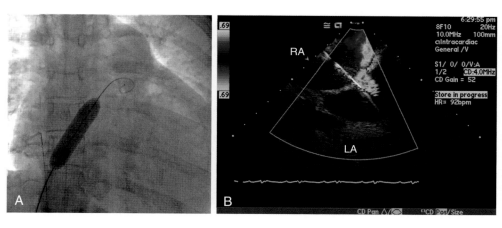

transseptal PFO closure (puncture technique) has been previously described.[12] In this technique, the septum primum is punctured at the limbus of the fossa ovalis to create a new small defect, through which the delivery sheath and closure device are delivered. In select cases, this approach can result in more effective compression of the septum primum against the septum secundum, with closure of the right-to-left shunt **(Figure 4–27).**

LOCATIONS FOR TRANSSEPTAL PUNCTURE

The ideal location for a transseptal puncture is different in different clinical scenarios, indications, and procedures. The operator should tailor his or her desired location accordingly. To illustrate the point, **Figure 4–28** shows the suggested locations for transseptal puncture in different clinical procedures. In general, for the MitraClip procedure, a desirable puncture is usually in the fossa, slightly superior, posterior, and with sufficient height above the mitral valve coaptation (≈3.5 to 4.5 cm). For left atrial appendage occluder device procedures, the puncture should ideally be posterior and slightly inferior (low) in the fossa. Where possible, the transseptal puncture should not be through a PFO in either procedure. For percutaneous closure of paravalvular leaks, the ideal puncture depends on the

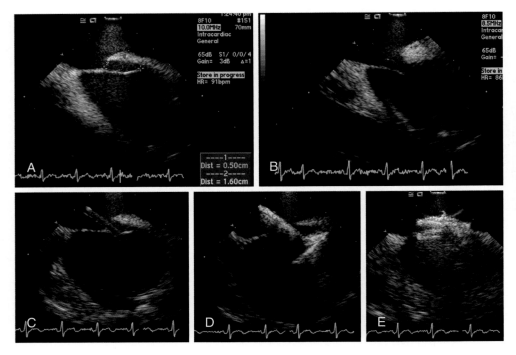

Figure 4–27 **Transseptal patent foramen ovale closure with intracardiac echocardiography guidance. A,** Long tunnel PFO (16 mm). **B,** Tenting of septum primum at limbus with transseptal needle. **C,** Delivery sheath in place after transseptal puncture. **D,** Left atrial disc of occluder device deployed. **E,** Final device appearance after right and left atrial disc deployment and release from delivery cable.

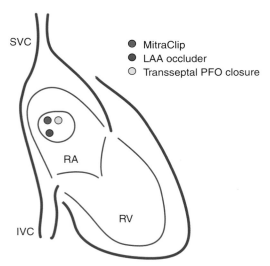

- ● MitraClip
- ● LAA occluder
- ○ Transseptal PFO closure

Figure 4–28 The interatrial septum has variable anatomy between patients, and different procedures require specific transseptal puncture sites. Familiarity with the techniques described in this chapter, use of intraprocedural imaging, and knowledge of the anatomic requirements of the procedure are all essential for success. Illustrated are suggested transseptal puncture sites for various procedures. (*IVC,* Inferior vena cava; *LAA,* left atrial appendage; *PFO,* patent foramen ovale; *RA,* right atrium; *RV,* right ventricle; *SVC,* superior vena cava.)

location of the leak as the operator needs to consider issues such as the curvature, trajectory, and reach catheters and sheaths used. For anterior paravalvular leaks, the puncture should be more posterior, whereas for lateral leaks a more superior puncture may be necessary. The overall size of the LA also affects the location of the transseptal puncture site.

4.6 Summary

The transseptal puncture is a critical skill for the structural heart interventionalist. Safe and efficient use of the transseptal puncture depends on the type of procedure, the patient's anatomy, and the availability of TEE and ICE as adjunctive imaging tools. When the anatomy is normal or near normal and the procedure is not dependent on precise localization of the transseptal puncture, fluoroscopy alone can be used to guide the puncture in experienced hands. However, when there is deformed atrial or interatrial septal anatomy, if the procedure is complex, or if the operator has limited experience, some form of echocardiographic guidance (TEE or ICE) in addition to fluoroscopy is strongly recommended. Echocardiographic guidance is mandatory for procedures like the MitraClip, left atrial appendage closure, and atrial septostomy. In performing a transseptal puncture, a step-by-step and methodical, patient approach is recommended. For complex structural heart procedures like the MitraClip procedure, a properly selected puncture location reduces procedure time and improves the chances of procedural success.

REFERENCES

1. Ross J Jr, Braunwald E, Morrow AG: Transseptal left atrial puncture; new technique for the measurement of left atrial pressure in man, Am J Cardiol 3:653–655, 1959.
2. Babaliaros VC, Green JT, Lerakis S, et al: Emerging applications for transseptal left heart catheterization old techniques for new procedures, J Am Coll Cardiol 51:2116–2122, 2008.
3. Schwagten B, Jordaens L, Rivero-Ayerza M, et al: A randomized comparison of transseptal and transaortic approaches for magnetically guided ablation of left-sided accessory pathways, Pacing Clin Electrophysiol 33:1298–1303, 2010.

4. Linker NJ, Fitzpatrick AP: The transseptal approach for ablation of cardiac arrhythmias: experience of 104 procedures, *Heart* 79:379–382, 1998.
5. Hung JS: Atrial septal puncture technique in percutaneous transvenous mitral commissurotomy: mitral valvuloplasty using the Inoue balloon catheter technique, *Cathet Cardiovasc Diagn* 26:275–284, 1992.
6. Knecht S, Jais P, Nault I, et al: Radiofrequency puncture of the fossa ovalis for resistant transseptal access, *Circ Arrhythm Electrophysiol* 1:169–174, 2008.
7. Bidart C, Vaseghi M, Cesario DA, et al: Radiofrequency current delivery via transseptal needle to facilitate septal puncture, *Heart Rhythm* 4:1573–1576, 2007.
8. McWilliams MJ, Tchou P: The use of a standard radiofrequency energy delivery system to facilitate transseptal puncture, *J Cardiovasc Electrophysiol* 20:238–240, 2009.
9. Capulzini L, Paparella G, Sorgente A, et al: Feasibility, safety, and outcome of a challenging transseptal puncture facilitated by radiofrequency energy delivery: a prospective single-centre study, *Europace* 12:662–667, 2010.
10. Shalganov TN, Paprika D, Borbas S, et al: Preventing complicated transseptal puncture with intracardiac echocardiography: case report, *Cardiovasc Ultrasound* 3:5, 2005.
11. Morton JB, Kalman JM: Intracardiac echocardiographic anatomy for the interventional electrophysiologist, *J Interv Card Electrophysiol* 13(Suppl 1):11–16, 2005.
12. Ruiz CE, Alboliras ET, Pophal SG: The puncture technique: a new method for transcatheter closure of PFO, *Catheter Cardiovasc Interv* 53:369–372, 2001.

Chapter 5

Aortic and Pulmonic Balloon Valvuloplasty

WESLEY R. PEDERSEN • IRVIN F. GOLDENBERG • ITSIK BEN-DOR • TED E. FELDMAN

5.1 Balloon Aortic Valvuloplasty

Balloon aortic valvuloplasty (BAV) for severe aortic stenosis (AS), a common disease of the elderly, was introduced by Dr. Cribier in 1986.[1] Initial experience demonstrated the technical feasibility, acceptable safety, and fairly modest improvement in valve areas. In spite of an only modest improvement in valve area, patients experienced significant symptomatic benefit, resulting in an initially enthusiastic embrace by interventional cardiologists. However, the subsequent recognition of high restenosis rates within a year of the procedure quickly tempered enthusiasm. Large series have demonstrated restenosis rates of 40% to 80% within 5 to 9 months and a failure to improve survival despite palliative benefits of BAV.[2-5] The clinical lag in symptomatic recurrence extends the palliative benefit 6 to 9 months beyond hemodynamic restenosis. Therefore an overall quality-of-life (QOL) benefit after BAV may last up to between 1 and 1.5 years in elderly patients who are generally less concerned about durable efficacy.[4]

BACKGROUND

Calcific AS is the most common expression of primary valvular heart disease in adults. Moderate to severe AS is observed in 4.6% of patients older than 75 years of age.[6] Surgical aortic valve replacement (AVR) is the preferred treatment strategy for patients of all age groups, although it has limitations in octogenarians and nonagenarians. Eight retrospective studies of patients over 80 years of age showed a pooled 30-day mortality rate of 9.2% for isolated AVR and 20.9% for combined AVR and coronary bypass grafting.[7] Transcatheter AVR (TAVR) has expanded the option for valve replacement therapy in elderly patients who are at high risk for surgery because of comorbidities and frailty. Although TAVR offers a more durable improvement for the treatment

of AS than BAV, BAV is being carried out with increasing frequency for a number of reasons. In the largest registry (i.e., National Heart, Lung, and Blood Institute [NHLBI]), outcomes of procedures performed in the late 1980s demonstrated the significant limitation in clinical benefit for younger patients in their late 70s, predominantly linked to restenosis. High complication rates were also reported in these early series (i.e., 25% in the NHLBI series; **Table 5–1**).[4,8]

The reemergence of BAV since 2000 resulted from a more clear definition of its palliative role in high-risk patient subsets, its requirement for predilation in TAVR, and its utility in clarifying the role of AS in symptomatic patients with multiple disease states before TAVR. In addition, broader adoption has resulted from improvements in technique. Recent series have highlighted improved outcomes and reduced complications **(Table 5–2)**.[9]

VALVE HISTOPATHOLOGY AND BALLOON AORTIC VALVULOPLASTY MECHANISM OF ACTION

Calcific AS is characterized by increased leaflet thickness, calcification, and rigid immobility, generally in the absence of commissural fusion. Until recently, calcific AS was considered to be histopathologically degenerative or passive in origin. It is now recognized as a complex, active, cellular process with features of atherosclerosis and biomineralization similar to osteogenesis in bone formation.[10]

The effects of BAV on stenosed aortic valves are poorly understood, but several mechanisms appear likely.[11] Primarily, balloon-induced fracturing of calcified nodules create hingepoints,[12] and along with the creation of cleavage planes in collagenous stroma, improve leaflet flexibility and valve opening. Separation of fused leaflets is uncommon given its infrequent occurrence

TABLE 5–1

NHLBI BAV Registry[4,8]

Demographics and Outcomes[4]		Complications During or Within 24 Hours After Valvuloplasty Procedure[8]	
Years enrolled	1987-89	**Complication**	**n (%)**
No. enrolled	674	Death	17 (3)
No. centers	24	Patients with any severe complication	167 (25)
Mean age	78 years	***Type of complication***	
Female	377 (56%)	Hemodynamic	
CAD	248 (43%)	Prolonged hypotension	51 (8)
Unknown	97 (15%)	CPR required	26 (4)
Presentation		Pulmonary edema	19 (3)
CHF NYHA class III/IV	76%	Cardiac tamponade	10 (1)
Angina class III/IV	23%	IABP use	11 (2)
Syncope/presyncope	34%	Aortic valvular insufficiency	6 (1)
Inappropriate for surgery	***80%***	Cardiogenic shock	15 (2)
Mean gradient (intraprocedural)	***Mean***	Neurological	
Baseline	55 mm Hg	Focal neurological event	13 (2)
Postvalvuloplasty	29 mm Hg	Respiratory	
Mean valve area (intraprocedural)		Intubation	28 (4)
Baseline	0.50 cm^2	Arrhythmia	
Postvalvuloplasty	0.80 cm^2	Treatment required	64 (10)
Follow-up (echocardiographic)	***N=182***	Persistent bundle-branch block	34 (5)
Baseline mean gradient	49 mm Hg	AV block requiring pacing	30 (4)
Gradient (mean or peak)	Mean	VF of VT requiring countershock	18 (3)
Postvalvuloplasty	38 mm Hg	Vascular	
6-Month follow-up	43 mm Hg	Vascular surgery performed	33 (5)
Valve area		Systematic embolic event	11 (2)
Baseline	0.57 cm^2	Transfusion required	136 (20)
Postvalvuloplasty	0.78 cm^2	Ischemic	
6-Month follow-up	0.65 cm^2	Acute myocardial infarction	10 (1)
Symptomatic improvement	***75% at 1 year***	Other severe complications	
Cause mortality		Pulmonary artery perforation	1 (0.1)
Procedure	3%	Acute tubular necrosis	1 (0.1)
At hospital discharge	10%		
30 Days	14%		
1 Year	45%		
2 Years	65%		
3 Years	77%		

AV, Atrioventricular; *CAD*, coronary artery disease; *CHF*, congestive heart failure; *CPR*, cardiopulmonary resuscitation; *IABP*, intraaortic balloon pump; *NHLBI*, National Heart, Lung, and Blood Institute; *NYHA*, New York Heart Association; *VF*, ventricular fibrillation; *VT*, ventricular tachycardia.

in nonrheumatic patients. Enhanced compliance or stretching of the adjacent annulus and calcified aortic root have also been suggested.[13]

Restenosis is generally believed to occur from scar tissue (cell-rich pattern of fibroblasts, capillaries, and inflammatory infiltrate) within small leaflet tears.[14] Heterotopic ossification (bone formation) was reported to occur in another small series.[15] On occasion, recoil of the elastic valve components may result in early valve renarrowing within hours to days.

PATIENT SELECTION

Current American College of Cardiology/American Heart Association (ACC/AHA) guidelines are listed in **Box 5–1**.[16] The substantial increase in BAV volumes over the past 5 to 10 years has come about for two primary reasons. The

first is based on a realization that an increasing population of elderly patients with comorbidities and who are at high risk or otherwise poorly suited for surgical AVR derive significant palliation. Multiple published experiences have shown a consistent reduction in New York Heart Association (NYHA) functional class, the preponderance improving from functional class III/VI to I/II.[8,17-19] The demonstrated safety in serial BAVs for patients with recurrent restenosis extends the opportunity for achieving longer periods of enhanced QOL. In general, these authors like to see at least 6 months of benefit before performing a subsequent BAV. In cases where this time is shorter, underdilation on the previous intervention may offer the opportunity for more aggressive increments in balloon sizing. Although unproven, some authors have suggested a survival benefit as well.[17,20] With improved technique, symptomatic AS patients who are not

TABLE 5–2

Two Large BAV Registry Experiences in U.S.[9] of Procedures Performed Since 2000

	Washington Hospital Center Jan. 2000-Dec. 2009	Minneapolis Heart Institute Jun. 2003-Feb. 2012
I. Demographics		
Patients	262	332
Procedures	301	412
Age (years)	81.7 ± 9.8	85.5 ± 6.6
STS score > 10 (%)	69.1	42.7
Female sex	145 (55.3%)	186 (56.0%)
Coronary artery disease	168 (64.1%)	184 (55.4%)
II. Patient BAVs		
Total number of patients	262	332
Patients with single BAV	223 (85.1%)	252 (75.9%)
Patients with 2 BAVs	29 (11.0%)	53 (16.0%)
Patients with 3 BAVs	8 (3.1%)	25 (7.5%)
Patients with 4 BAVs	2 (0.8%)	2 (0.6%)
III. A. Procedural Data		
Balloon size (mm)	22.9 ± 1.9	23.9 ± 1.2
# of Inflations	1.7 ± 0.9	3.2 ± 1.5
III. B. Combined BAV + PCI		
Total	**52 (17.2%)**	**56 (17.0%)**
PCI-1 vessel	44 (84.6%)	37 (66.1%)
PCI-2 vessel	6 (11.6%)	15 (26.8%)
PCI-3 vessel	2 (3.8%)	4 (7.1%)
IV. Intraprocedural Hemodynamics		
Mean gr pre-BAV (mmHg)	46.3 ± 19.7	49.8 ± 16.7
Mean gr post-BAV (mmHg)	21.4 ± 12.4	25.2 ± 10.4
AVA pre-BAV (cm^2)	0.58 ± 0.3	0.64 ± 0.2
AVA post-BAV (cm^2)	0.96 ± 0.3	N/A
V. Echocardiography		
Mean gr pre-BAV (mm Hg)	42.0 ± 13.9	43.55 ± 13.71
Mean gr post-BAV (mm Hg)	31.9 ± 11.8	26.78 ± 11.18
AVA pre-BAV (cm^2)	0.68 ± 0.15	0.61 ± 0.16
AVA post-BAV (cm^2)	0.87 ± 0.19	0.84 ± 0.30
LVEF pre-BAV (%)	45.4 ± 18.4	43.81 ± 12.84
LVEF post-BAV (%)	47.0 ± 18.0	45.74 ± 9.09
AR gr pre-BAV	0.8 ± 0.7	1.1 ± 0.8
AR gr post-BAV	1.0 ± 0.7	0.9 ± 0.6
MR gr pre-BAV	1.5 ± 1.2	2.4 ± 0.8
MR gr post-BAV	1.4 ± 1.0	2.2 ± 1.0
VI. Serious Adverse Events		
Intraprocedural death	5 (1.6%)	9 (2.2%)
Stroke	6 (1.99%)	5 (1.2%)
Coronary occlusion	2 (0.66%)	1 (0.2%)
Emergent interventions	Hypotension requiring CPR, intubation, cardioversion 5 (1.6%)	Intubations 7 (2.11%) Cardioversions 6 (1.81%) Emergent IABPs 5 (1.5%)
Tamponade	1 (0.3%)	2 (0.5%)
TPM	N/A	2 (0.5%)
PPM	3 (0.99%)	2 (0.5%)
Vascular complications	21 (6.9%) Requiring any intervention	3 (0.7%) Requiring surgical intervention

AR, Aortic regurgitation; *AVA,* aortic valve area; *BAV,* balloon aortic valvuloplasty; *CPR,* cardiopulmonary resuscitation; *gr,* grade; *IABP,* intraaortic balloon pump; *LVEF,* left ventricular ejection fraction; *MR,* mitral regurgitation; *PCI,* percutaneous coronary intervention; *PPM,* permanent pacemaker; *STS,* Society of Thoracic Surgery; *TPM,* temporary pacemaker.

BOX 5–1 ▰▰▰▰▰▰▰▰▰

2006 ACC/AHA Guidelines

Aortic Balloon Valvotomy

Class IIb

1. Aortic balloon valvotomy might be reasonable as a bridge to surgery in hemodynamically unstable adult patients with AS who are at high risk for AVR. (Level of Evidence: C)
2. Aortic balloon valvotomy might be reasonable for palliation in adult patients with AS in whom AVR cannot be performed because of serious comorbid conditions. (Level of Evidence: C)

Class III

Aortic balloon valvotomy is not recommended as an alternative to AVR in adult patients with AS; certain younger patients without valve calcification may be an exception.

ACC, America College of Cardiology; AHA, American Heart Association; AS, aortic stenosis; AVR, aortic valve replacement (surgical).

BOX 5–2 ▰▰▰▰▰▰▰▰▰

Candidates for Stand-Alone BAV in MHI's Adult Cardiology Practice in the TAVR Era

Patients with symptomatic AS poorly suited for eventual TAVR or AVR

High surgical risk profile secondary to comorbidities and/or frailty, plus one of the following:

1. Very limited longevity (<2 years)
2. Unsuitable cardiac or vascular anatomy for TAVR
3. No candidate for antiplatelet therapy secondary to bleeding risk

Bridge to TAVR or AVR

1. "Diagnostic" BAV in patients with severe AS and other potential causes for symptoms (i.e., lung disease)
2. Patients in which a significant degree of myocardial dysfunction, prerenal insufficiency, or other organ system dysfunctions that may be reversible with BAV
3. High risk for noncardiac surgery that is not elective
4. Patients requiring high-risk PCI before TAVR (combine BAV + PCI)
5. Acutely unstable patients

AS, Aortic stenosis; AVR, surgical aortic valve replacement; BAV, balloon aortic valvuloplasty; MHI, Minneapolis Heart Institute; PCI, percutaneous coronary intervention; TAVR, transcatheter aortic valve replacement.

candidates for surgical AVR or TAVR should be offered palliative BAV in place of medical therapy alone.

Second, the option for TAVR in poor–surgical-risk groups has had an explosive impact on the use of BAV that is not only essential for predilation, but has now been reported to successfully bridge patients to TAVR.[21] Patients initially too unstable in one series underwent successful TAVR after a mean interval of 59 ± 57 days. However, the precise role for BAV as a bridge requires further study. Many patients with severe AS and symptoms have other comorbidities such as severe lung disease that may play a significant role in their symptom complex. A "diagnostic" BAV can be performed to evaluate the role AS is playing, and if it is significant, BAV can then be followed by TAVR. Candidates in the current "TAVR era" for stand-alone BAV in the adult cardiology practice at Minneapolis Heart Institute (MHI) are shown in **Box 5–2.**

TECHNIQUE

BAV can be carried out using two different approaches that are well-described in the literature.[22-24] The most commonly used approach is the retrograde technique. The antegrade technique, which will be discussed in less detail, is predominantly indicated in patients with inadequate arterial access **(Figure 5–1).**

RETROGRADE APPROACH

Patient Preparation and Access

Over 50% of BAVs at MHI are performed electively by way of outpatient admission. Patients are pretreated with 325 mg of aspirin. A large-bore peripheral intravenous (IV) line and usually a Foley catheter are placed before transfer to the cardiovascular laboratory, especially in patients in whom postprocedure diuresis is anticipated. An intraaortic balloon pump (IABP) should be available

in the room for patients who are hemodynamically unstable or those with left ventricular ejection fraction (LVEF) less than 30%. Defibrillation patches are placed in the lateral chest positions where they will not interfere with imaging. The procedure is carried out under conscious sedation using IV midazolam and fentanyl.

Both right and left groins are prepped. The authors most commonly use just the right side for arterial and venous access. Six-French femoral arterial and 8F femoral venous sheaths are placed when the patient is under local anesthesia. Care is taken to document appropriate landmarks to ensure arterial access through the anterior wall of the common femoral artery. After confirming common femoral artery access with a contrast injection, the arterial access site is preclosed using two 6F ProGlide devices (Abbott Vascular, Abbott Park, Ill.).[25] Sutures are deployed sequentially at 90-degree angles to each other at the 10 o'clock and 2 o'clock positions and draped to either side with Kelly clamps. A 10F to 12F sheath is then exchanged for the initially placed sheath, depending on valvuloplasty balloon type and size. Alternatively, a single 10F Prostar device (Abbott Vascular, Abbott Park, Ill.) can be used. Patients are then given 70 units/kg of unfractionated IV heparin, which is titrated to achieve an activated clotting time (ACT) of 250 to 300 seconds.

Intraprocedural Diagnostic Evaluation

Coronary angiography is performed, most importantly, to rule out critical stenosis of the left main coronary artery before proceeding with BAV. An unprotected critical left main coronary artery, if anatomically suitable, should be stented before performing BAV. Other severe lesions felt to be clinically relevant can be treated safely after BAV as

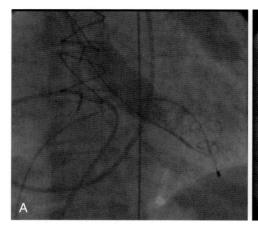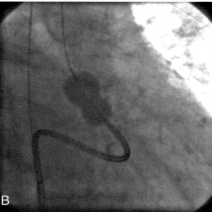

Figure 5–1 **A,** Retrograde arterial approach using a standard aortic balloon. **B,** Antegrade transseptal approach using an Inoue balloon *(Toray, New York, N.Y.).*

a combined procedure. See the subsequent discussion on combined coronary stenting and BAV.

Right heart catheterization is then performed with a Swan-Ganz catheter (Edwards Lifesciences, Inc., Irvine, Calif.). Given the incidence of disparity in cardiac outputs, the authors perform both thermodilution and estimated Fick outputs for use in the Gorlin formula when calculating the aortic valve area (AVA). The left heart catheterization is performed, and simultaneous left ventricular and aortic pressures using a dual lumen pigtail catheter are recorded to derive the mean valve gradient. Central aortic pressure from the ascending aorta should be sampled to prevent arterial amplification and a delay in the arterial waveform, which is seen when sampling from a peripheral site. It is imperative to place greater emphasis on the aortic valve index than the AVA when making treatment decisions. In large patients, AVA will significantly underestimate the severity of stenosis. A valve index greater than 0.6 cm^2/m^2 is severe.

Crossing the Aortic Valve and Guidewire Positioning

Patients undergoing BAV will be heparinized before the aortic valve is crossed. Nevertheless, it is important to routinely wipe wires and flush catheters with heparinized saline every 2 minutes during attempted crossing. Although one's choice of catheters for crossing the valve is somewhat personal, most operators use 6F Amplatz left (AL; Cordis Corporation; Bridgewater, N.J.) diagnostic catheters to best achieve a coaxial trajectory with a straight wire to access the left ventricle. A preferred choice has been an AL-1; however, an AL-2 configuration, especially in patients with a horizontal root and vertical valve, may be preferred.[24] The authors prefer to attempt crossing in a 20-degree to 40-degree left anterior oblique projection. A brief cine run for two to three cardiac cycles without contrast is first captured for defining the precise location of systolic leaflet separation. The catheter is then positioned within the systolic jet, which is confirmed fluoroscopically by visualizing catheter tip vibration. The softer end of the straight-tip wire is then used to gently probe the valve in the area where leaflet separation was documented. Clockwise and counterclockwise

catheter rotations are generally required to fall into the correct anteroposterior plane of the valve orifice. Once the valve is crossed, an attempt to fix the wire in the middle of the ventricular cavity is made, at which point the working view is switched to a right anterior oblique projection for further wire and catheter positioning **(Figure 5–2, A-E).** With the straight-tip wire fixed, the AL catheter is advanced into the left ventricle, avoiding advancement of the catheter tip and wire forcefully into the apex or other endocardial segments. Myocardial perforation can occur in this context. The catheter may be fixed in the mid-left ventricular chamber when removing the guide wire, allowing the broad secondary curve of the AL catheter tip to point back retrograde toward the aortic valve. A 0.035-inch J-tipped exchange wire can then be advanced through the AL catheter and easily draped in a broad curve across the anterior, apical, and inferior wall segments. A dual lumen pigtail catheter is then advanced into the left ventricle over the exchange wire, and simultaneous left ventricular and central aortic pressures are recorded to obtain a mean aortic valve gradient.

Rapid Ventricular Pacing

Rapid ventricular pacing has been invaluable for stabilizing balloon position across the aortic valve during inflation. The marked decrement in forward stroke volume with pacing significantly reduces the likelihood of the balloon being ejected into the aorta. A bipolar pacing lead is positioned in the right ventricle via the right femoral venous sheath, and stable capture thresholds are confirmed. Some operators have reported success in attaching an external pacemaker directly to the left ventricular wire and skin using alligator clips to achieve rapid pacing without the need for a transvenous pacemaker. A brief pacing run is carried out at 180 to 220 beats/min to ensure consistent 1:1 capture without intermittent loss of capture or 2:1 exit block. A drop in systolic blood pressure to less than 50 mmHg also needs to be confirmed with this rapid pacing sequence **(Figure 5–3).** In patients with severe left ventricular systolic dysfunction, pacing at add 180 beats/min is often adequate to achieve significant drop in blood pressure. Test runs should be kept to a minimum to avoid provoking a transient decrease in

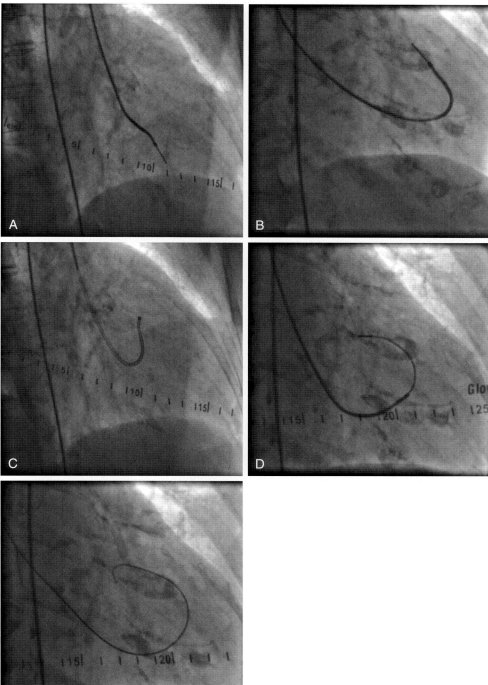

Figure 5–2 **A,** Amplatz diagnostic catheter with straight-tip wire positioned in mid-left ventricular (LV) cavity. **B,** The Amplatz catheter tip directed retrograde toward the aortic valve while removing the straight-tip guidewire. **C,** Amplatz catheter positioned in mid-LV cavity after removing straight-tip guidewire. **D,** 0.035-inch exchange wire being positioned in left ventricle and Amplatz catheter being withdrawn. **E,** 0.035-inch exchange wire draped in a broad curve across anterior and inferior LV wall segments before positioning the dual lumen pigtail catheter.

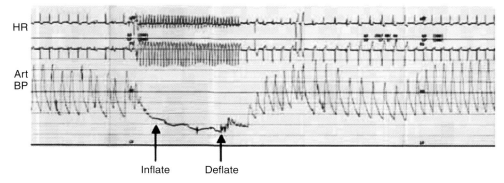

Figure 5–3 Rapid ventricular pacing. (*Art,* Arterial; *BP,* blood pressure; *HR,* heart rate.)

Inflate   Deflate

LVEF and more prolonged hypotension. These high pacing rate commands can be given only by pacing from the atrial (not ventricular) connection terminal on the pacing box. A lower rate limit of 60 beats/min is programmed for backup pacing if necessary.

Balloon Selection, Positioning, and Inflation

The authors use an Amplatz Extra Stiff 0.035-inch exchange wire for the balloon valvuloplasty. Before exchanging this wire through the double-lumen pigtail catheter (or other diagnostic catheter) in the left ventricle, a broad loop is shaped in the flexible end either using a dull instrument or finger tips **(Figure 5–4).** Broader loops should be made for larger left ventricles. The curve is generally begun just proximal to the stiffer shaft transition into the more flexible segment, thereby avoiding a potential acute angled buckle in the wire capable of perforating the ventricle. In a right anterior oblique fluoroscopic projection, the wire is advanced into the ventricle and with the aid of the indwelling pigtail catheter, can be easily draped across the anterior, apical, and inferior wall segments. It is important to preserve this distal wire curve and left ventricular relationship during balloon inflation to avoid left ventricular perforations, which can occur

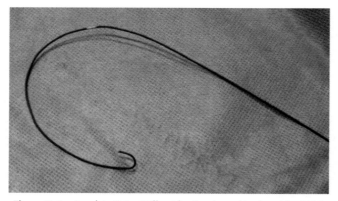

Figure 5–4 Amplatz Extra Stiff guidewire shaped by hand for BAV.

during subsequent balloon inflations if the distal wire tip or sharply angled bend is pointed into the apex or inferior wall **(Figure 5–5, A and B).**

Balloon sizing is generally more aggressive in stand-alone BAV than when predilation is carried out for TAVR. The authors use 4-cm noncompliant aortic balloons (e.g., Z-Med and Z-Med II [B. Braun Interventional Systems, Bethlehem, Pa.]) and generally begin with a balloon diameter-to-annulus ratio of 1:1 in stand-alone cases and 1 to 2 mm less when predilating for TAVR. The Maxi LD balloon (Cordis Corporation, Bridgewater, N.J.) is another popular choice; it is available in 4- or 6-cm lengths with a rated burst pressure of 5 to 6 atm and can be placed through smaller sheaths (8F to 12F) than the Z-Med balloons. More compliant balloons (e.g., Tyshak II [B. Braun Interventional Systems, Bethlehem, Pa.]) have the advantage of being lower in profile, and thus access sheaths ranging from 8F to 10F can be used. The more compliant balloons have less predictable inflation diameters, requiring the operator to use more conservative balloon diameters. In addition, rated burst pressures are just 2 atm or less. With these cylinder-shaped aortic balloons, antegrade migration can occur into the ascending aorta, even with rapid ventricular pacing. It is therefore important to choose a balloon diameter at least 1 to 2 millimeters less than the measured sinotubular junction diameter. Contrast used for balloon inflation is diluted to 1:8 or 1:10 to minimize viscosity and thus inflation/deflation times. The authors use a 60-cc handheld, disposable plastic syringe to inject the dilute contrast. Most balloons are filled using 20 to 30 cc of the dilute contrast. A 10-cc side syringe can be connected to a three-way stopcock on the balloon injection port to achieve more rapid filling or augment inflation volume. After positioning the uninflated balloon markers across the valve, rapid ventricular pacing is initiated. After confirming 1:1 capture and a systolic arterial blood pressure less than 50 mmHg, the balloon is inflated as rapidly as possible by the second operator or technician. The first operator holds the balloon catheter shaft, making adjustments under fluoroscopy to maintain a stable balloon position centered across

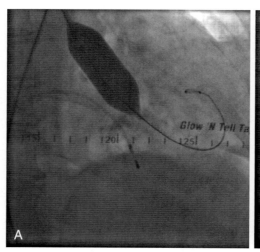

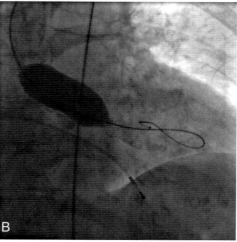

Figure 5–5 A, Correct wire position during balloon inflation. **B,** Example of incorrect wire position with balloon inflation that can result in stiff wire "sawing" through left ventricular apex.

the valve **(Figure 5–6).** The balloon is fully inflated for 2 to 3 seconds before deflation. Arterial pressure is monitored from the femoral arterial sheath side-arm. After balloon inflation, the contrast is aspirated as rapidly as possible, and the balloon pulled promptly back into the aorta. The pacer is not turned off until most of the contrast is removed from the balloon. Generally no more than 2 to 3 inflations are performed with each balloon size in stand-alone BAV. Subsequent inflations are not carried out unless the arterial blood pressure has completely returned to baseline. If necessary, we use 100 to 200 μ of phenylephrine in IV boluses to maintain systolic blood pressures greater than 100 mmHg. If there is difficulty squarely landing the inflated balloon on the valve, more rapid pacing rates may be beneficial, providing 1:1 capture is preserved.

After each set of inflations, the balloon catheter is exchanged for the double-lumen pigtail catheter, and an aortic valve gradient is remeasured. If hemodynamic targets are not achieved, a balloon that is 1 mm larger is used, and further dilations are carried out if the patient's condition remains stable. Over 90% of the balloon diameters used for aortic valvuloplasty at MHI range from 22 to 25 mm.

Intraprocedural Assessment and Goals

Initial subjective hemodynamic assessment often yields an obvious reduction in left ventricular systolic pressure and increase in aortic pressure (see **Figure 5–7, A and B** for pre-BAV and post-BAV gradients). In addition, the arterial waveform upslope is less delayed, demonstrating a more abrupt acceleration to peak systolic pressure.

The attempt is to achieve a 50% reduction in the mean transvalvular gradient. Confirmation of a successful result requires repeating cardiac outputs to determine the AVA. Optimally, the intraprocedural valve area should increase by 40% to 50% or better.

A significant drop in the aortic diastolic blood pressure, especially if accompanied by an increase in left ventricular end-diastolic pressure, is strongly suggestive of acute, severe aortic insufficiency (AI) **(Figure 5–8, A and B).** Under severe circumstances, the diastolic aortic–to–end-diastolic left ventricular gradient may be less than 10 mmHg. Severe insufficiency is poorly tolerated in these patients and can rapidly progress to cardiogenic shock. At MHI, aortography is not routinely performed after BAV; when the patient is hemodynamically unstable, emergent transthoracic echocardiography (TTE) is performed.

Intraprocedural Complications and Management

The most relevant procedural complications include intraprocedural death, stroke, and vascular complications. Intraprocedural mortality has remained stable over the past decade and is surprisingly low with improvement in BAV technique. Multiple series document mortalities of 1% to 3%.[9,17,19,26-28] Age or Society of Thoracic Surgery (STS) score does not appear to have a significant impact on this statistic.[29] Autopsy-confirmed series documenting the precise causes are not available. In general, the catastrophic events leading to abrupt hemodynamic collapse include aortic root and annular dissection, valve leaflet avulsion with wide-open AI, left ventricular perforation, severe left ventricular dysfunction, and pulmonary

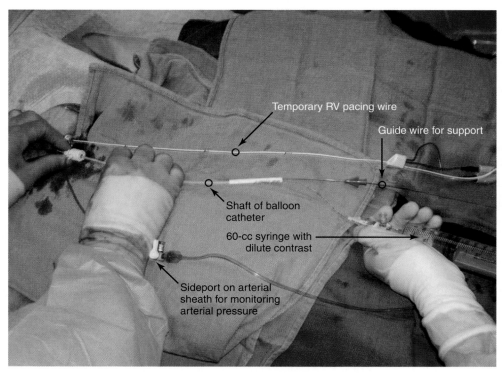

Figure 5–6 Catheter set up during balloon inflation.

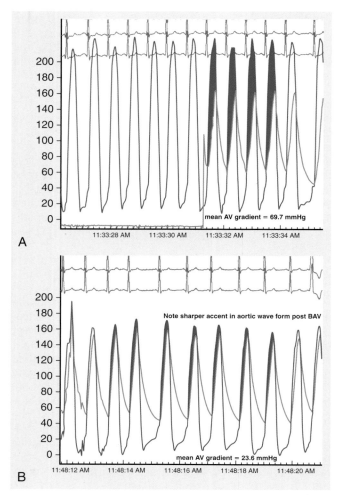

Figure 5–7 **A,** Pre-BAV simultaneous aortic and left ventricular pressure recordings, **B,** Post-BAV simultaneous aortic and left ventricular pressure recordings.

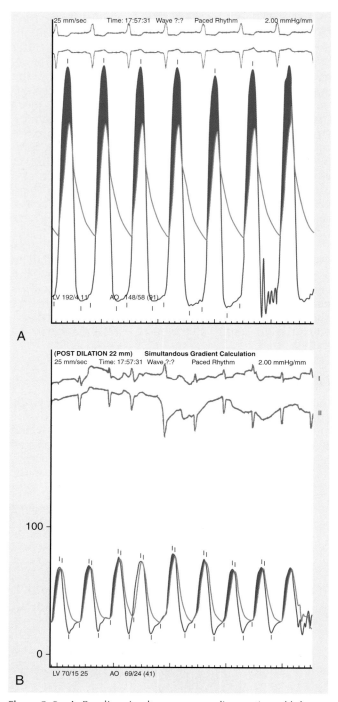

Figure 5–8 **A,** Baseline simultaneous ascending aortic and left ventricular pressure curves measured with a dual lumen pigtail catheter. Note severe aortic valve gradient before balloon valvuloplasty. **B,** Patient developed hemodynamic compromise after a single balloon inflation. Repeat simultaneous ascending aortic and left ventricular pressure measurements demonstrated significant reduction in the systolic gradient across the aortic valve; however, left ventricular end diastolic and aortic diastolic pressures are equal, characteristic of newly developed severe AI.

hemorrhage as a complication of right heart catheterization. Strokes are consistently reported to occur in 1% to 2% of patients, and again the precise embolic origin has not been defined.[17,26-28] Carotid protection devices should be of benefit to the extent that the embolic source would originate from the ascending and arch aorta or the aortic valve during the procedure. Severe AI is poorly tolerated in these patients with severe left ventricular hypertrophy and occurs consistently in 1% to 2% of BAVs.[9,17,26,27] Severe AI can often be temporarily managed with rapid pacing to limit diastolic regurgitation. In addition, severe AI sometimes improves over several hours, likely in part from annular recoil.

Vascular complications are considerably more variable, in part related to a previous lack of uniform definitions and poorly documented events in retrospective series. Vascular access site complications are now, however, clearly defined by the Valve Academic Research Consortium and divided into two broad categories: 1) major vascular complications and 2) minor vascular complications.[29] Serious vascular complications include: those leading to death, those needing blood transfusions greater than 4 units, those requiring unplanned surgical

TABLE 5–3

New AV Conduction Abnormalities After BAV at Minneapolis Heart Institute*

N=76	Maximal Balloon Diameter (mm)	Maximal Balloon/ LVOT Diameter Ratio	Number of Balloon Inflations
No new AV conduction abnormalities, n = 71 (93.4%)	23.6 ± 0.1	1.2 ± 0.1	3.9 ± 2.3
New AV conduction abnormalities, n = 5 (6.6%)	23.6 ± 0.2	1.2 ± 0.1	6.4 ± 3.2 (p = 0.02, no new vs. new AV abnormalities)
Primary AV block, n = 1 (1.3%)	25	1.3	5
Left bundle branch block, n = 3 (3.9%)	22.7 ± 0.1	1.2 ± 0.1	7.7 ± 3.8 (p = 0.008)
Complete heart block, n = 1 (1.3%)	25	1.3	4

Pedersen W, Dang M, Krueger D, et al: Intra and post procedural outcomes in severe aortic stenosis patients with left ventricular ejection fractions <20% undergoing balloon valvuloplasty, Abstract. *Catheter Cardiovasc Interv* 2011;77(Suppl):S136-S137.
AV, Atrioventricular; *BAV,* balloon aortic valvuloplasty; *LVOT,* left ventricular outflow tract; *MHI,* Minneapolis Heart Institute.
*Consecutive series of patients without permanent pacemakers.

repair, or those resulting in irreversible end-organ damage. Historically, complications requiring surgical intervention have occurred in at least 5% of BAV cases.[8,26] Vascular access complications requiring unplanned surgical repair have been significantly reduced with closure devices, occurring in fewer than 1% in one series of patients undergoing BAV.[25]

In cases where prolonged or refractory hypotension occurs immediately after BAV, potential causes include the following:

1. Acute left ventricular systolic failure (especially in patients with baseline LVEF < 30%)
2. Left ventricular perforation with tamponade
3. Aortic valve annulus dissection or ruptured proximal aorta (with or without tamponade)
4. Valve leaflet avulsion and severe AI
5. Acute severe mitral insufficiency (mitral apparatus disruption secondary to balloon trauma or guidewire entrapment)
6. Brisk bleeding from the access site into the retroperitoneum or into an expanding hematoma
7. Vagally mediated hypotension
8. Bradyarrhythmia secondary to balloon-induced atrioventricular conduction injury
9. Sustained ventricular tachyarrhythmia secondary to guidewire position, after rapid ventricular pacing or prolonged ischemia
10. Respiratory arrest

The etiology can generally be rapidly determined by assessing the rhythm, evaluating the arterial and venous pressure contours, and performing an emergent transthoracic echocardiogram. It is recommended to have a portable echocardiography machine in the room when performing BAV. Definitive management is directed by the urgent findings. Many of these patients are elderly, nonsurgical candidates, and the patient and family have often agreed before the BAV that rescue open-heart procedures or other heroic methods should not be pursued.

The incidence of complete heart block requiring permanent pacemaker implantation is very low, much less than in recent TAVR series and generally in fewer than 1.5% of BAV procedures. Of 76 consecutive patients

without a permanent pacemaker who underwent BAV at MHI, none required a permanent pacemaker in spite of the tendency to use large balloons and frequent dilations.[30] The mean maximal balloon diameter in the series was 23.6 ± 0.1 mm, the maximal balloon/left ventricular outflow tract (LVOT) diameter ratio was 1.2 ± 0.1, and the mean number of balloon inflations was 3.9 ± 2.3. Five of the 76 consecutive patients developed new atrioventricular conduction defects **(Table 5–3)**.[30] New atrioventricular conduction defects were associated with a greater number of balloon inflations but not maximal balloon size or balloon/LVOT ratio in this small series.

Access Site Management

Heparin reversal is carried out with IV protamine before removing the large-bore arterial sheath. It is also preferred to establish systemic arterial pressures below 150 mmHg using small increments of IV hydralazine or nitroglycerin. If preclosure sutures were deployed, the sheath is then removed over a guidewire, and knots from both sutures are alternately pushed down on the arteriotomy and the guidewire is removed when hemostasis is established. Patients are then maintained on bed rest for 3 to 4 hours. If manual compression is used, the arterial sheath is not pulled until an ACT of less than 140 seconds is documented. Graded manual compression is then applied for 40 minutes. Patients are subsequently maintained on bed rest for 4 to 6 hours.

In-House, Postprocedural Management

On the day after BAV, the arterial access site is carefully examined. An electrocardiograph, renal function parameters, and hemoglobin are also obtained. All patients undergo postprocedural (predischarge) echocardiograms after BAV to remeasure the baseline the LVEF, aortic valve gradient, and valve area and to quantitate any degree of AI. The mean aortic valve gradient may often be 5 to 10 mm higher than obtained intraprocedurally. This represents an element of recoil in the stenotic valve, but it may also reflect better left ventricular systolic function, which can be transiently impaired immediately after balloon inflations.

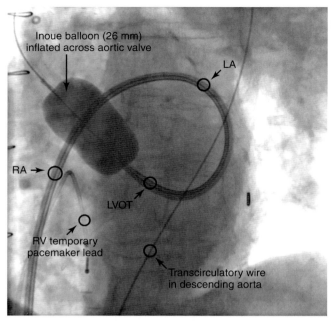

Figure 5–9 Antegrade BAV with Inoue balloon. (*LA,* Left atrium; *LVOT,* left ventricular outflow tract; *RA,* right atrium; *RV,* right ventricle.)

Although patients are often discharged the day after BAV, while they are still hospitalized, practitioners at MHI often take the opportunity to diurese those patients who had overt or decompensated heart failure and to further adjust ambulatory medications. An IV furosemide (Lasix) infusion is often started postoperatively to establish a consistent urine output (i.e., a net volume loss of 1000 to 2000 cc/day). Diuresis is titrated to examination findings, renal function, and brain natriuretic peptide (BNP). Patients are commonly discharged with their admission diuretic dose. Patients should be seen by their primary physician in 3 to 5 days with repeat labs. Providing they remain symptomatically stable, it is requested that they return to the valve clinic for a follow-up echocardiogram and BNP in 3 to 6 months. Alternatively, a follow-up examination may be requested in 4 to 6 weeks if bridging to surgical or TAVR is being considered.

ANTEGRADE APPROACH

The transfemoral antegrade approach requires transseptal access to the left heart and a transcirculatory wire loop for balloon delivery that is technically more demanding than the retrograde approach **(Figure 5–9).** The predominant advantage remains the ability to avoid placement of a large introducer sheath in diseased peripheral arteries. A transvenous delivery should result in fewer bleeding and ischemic complications. In addition, nonrandomized studies have shown a more effective valve opening with the antegrade approach when used in conjunction with the Inoue balloon (Toray, New York, N.Y.). It has been suggested that the bulbous distal balloon segment of this dumbbell-shaped balloon is able to hyperextend the valve leaflets more broadly into the aortic root sinuses of Valsalva creating broader hingepoints. One series reported a 20% greater valve area in patients undergoing

antegrade Inoue balloon valvuloplasty compared with a retrograde approach using standard aortic balloons.[22]

A 6F femoral arterial sheath is placed, through which a pigtail catheter is positioned in the ascending aorta. A transseptal puncture is then carried out with a transseptal needle and Mullins sheath (St. Jude Medical, St. Paul, Minn.) via a right femoral vein 14F sheath. A 7F balloon-tipped catheter is then advanced through the Mullins sheath and antegrade across the mitral valve. Simultaneous left ventricular and aortic pressure gradients are then measured. A 0.032-inch hydrophilic guidewire is then passed through the 7F balloon catheter and advanced across the aortic valve into the descending aorta. A 0.032-inch Amplatz Extra Stiff 360-cm guidewire is then exchanged for the hydrophilic wire and snared from a femoral artery providing a secure rail for the Inoue balloon delivery. Keeping a large loop of the guidewire in the left ventricle is very important throughout the procedure. If the guidewire is allowed to straighten between the mitral and aortic valve, severe mitral regurgitation may occur, resulting in abrupt hemodynamic collapse. In addition, irreversible trauma to the mitral valve apparatus may occur.

The Mullins sheath and 7F balloon-tipped catheter are then removed. A 26-mm Inoue valvuloplasty balloon (or standard aortic balloon) is delivered through the 14F venous sheath, over the transcirculatory wire rail. The aortic valve is then dilated sequentially with inflation diameters ranging from 24 to 26 mm to achieve an adequate reduction in the pressure gradient.

The balloon catheter is then withdrawn over the wire loop. The Mullins sheath is then replaced, and a 5F pigtail catheter is passed through the Mullins sheath over the wire and into the ascending aorta. The guidewire must be withdrawn through the protective covering of the pigtail catheter so that it does not have a "cheese cutter" effect, "sawing" through the aortic or mitral valve. After the guidewire has been removed from the pigtail catheter, the pigtail catheter is pulled back into the left ventricle, and transaortic valve pressures are recorded for the final intraprocedural mean aortic valve gradient.

CLINICAL OUTCOMES

Mortality

BAV is performed as a predominantly palliative procedure. It has never been proven to prolong survival as stand-alone therapy unless coupled as a bridge to eventual AVR. Medically treated patients with symptomatic AS have a 1-year survival rate of 60% and a 5-year survival rate of 32% in a recent series of 453 patients.[31] In a recently published series of 262 patients with inoperable AS who were undergoing BAV and had multiple comorbidities and a mean age of 81.7 ± 9.8 years, the 1-year mortality rate was almost 50%.[9] These patients were at very high risk with a calculated STS operative mortality of 13.3 ± 6.7% and logistic EuroSCORE of 45.6 ± 21.6. As expected, in patients who underwent BAV as a bridge to surgical replacement or TAVR, the outcome was much better than patients undergoing BAV alone (i.e., 25% mortality vs. 52.9% at a median follow-up of 181 days).

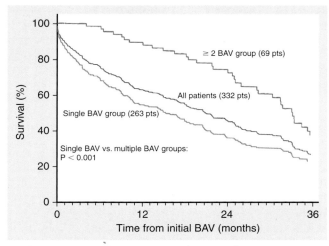

Figure 5–10 Kaplan-Meier survival estimate from MHI series.

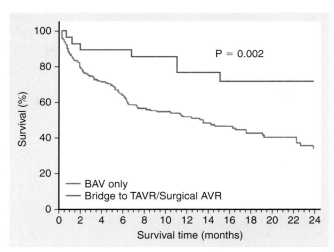

Figure 5–11 Kaplan-Meier survival curve of patients undergoing BAV only vs. BAV as a bridge to TAVR or surgical AVR. (*BAV*, Balloon aortic valvuloplasty; *TAVR*, Transcatheter aortic valve replacement; *AVR*, aortic valve replacement.)

Predictors of a lower survival after BAV also included final AVA of less than 1 cm², NYHA functional class IV, baseline renal insufficiency, and pulmonary hypertension. In the NHLBI registry, predictors of diminished survival included left ventricular dysfunction, decreased cardiac output, mitral insufficiency, renal insufficiency, NYHA class, and cachexia.[8] The overall survival rate in the NHLBI registry that included 674 patients with a mean age 78 years who were undergoing BAV was 55% at 1 year, 35% at 2 years, and 23% at 3 years.[8] In a single-center series with more experienced operators and 148 patients over 80 years of age, a mortality rate of 27% at 13 months was more favorable.[26] In the MHI series of 332 patients who were much older than those in the NHLBI registry with a mean age of 85.5 ± 6.6 years, the 1-year and 3-year survival rates were 56% and 25%, respectively. These data also precede the involvement in TAVR, thus resulting in higher long-term mortality rates in the absence of a TAVR option. A Kaplan-Meier survival curve for the patients undergoing BAV at MHI is shown in **Figure 5–10.** Ben-Dor et al., at the Washington Hospital Center, demonstrated in their BAV series the impact that bridging to TAVR or surgical AVR had with a graph that can be seen in **Figure 5–11.**[9]

Aortic Valve Area and Gradient Post–Balloon Aortic Valvuloplasty

Changes in mean aortic valve gradients and valve area with BAV have been reported in the literature either as acute changes derived by cardiac catheterization at the time of BAV or by echocardiography comparing baseline to predischarge findings 1 to 2 days after BAV. Changes documented by echocardiography as well as cardiac catheterization in several series are listed in **Table 5–4.**[8,9,32] In spite of the superior reduction in mean gradients and increase in AVAs reported by cardiac catheterization after BAV, the authors believe that the most reliable and clinically relevant data are derived from echocardiography when steady-state hemodynamics are in play 24 to 48 hours after the procedure.[32] Decreases in mean gradient ranging from 25 to 30 mm Hg and increases in AVA ranging from 0.30 to 0.50 cm² are reported from studies using intraprocedural (invasive) hemodynamics.[8,9,17,26,33]

In patient series using echocardiographic data, mean AV gradients are found to be increased by 10 to 15 mm Hg and AVAs are decreased by 0.20 to 0.30 cm². The authors believe that the postprocedural echocardiography data 24 to 48 hours post-BAV are most relevant and should be used as the standard outcomes reports. Factors that appear to influence post-BAV valve area include the nature of the underlying valve pathology, the severity of preoperative stenosis, the degree of calcification, and the aggressiveness in balloon sizing.

Functional Class

QOL indicators such as NYHA functional class and hospital readmissions are clearly improved with BAV. The only predictor of improvement in functional class has been a higher baseline level of functional impairment.[4] Eighty percent to 90% of patients undergoing BAV are NYHA functional class III to IV at baseline, the majority of whom experience improvement to class I to II.[4] In a series of nonagenarians undergoing BAV, NYHA functional class improved from 3.4 to 1.8.[19] In spite of restenosis in more than 80% of patients after 1 year, a symptomatic disconnect commonly results in a more sustained symptomatic improvement for up 1 to 1.5 years after BAV.[5] Furthermore, BAV may be repeated when symptoms recur at no additional risk of complication.[17] Repeat BAV serves to extend the QOL benefit seen after the initial intervention, even though it is less clear that there is a survival benefit.

Additional Perspectives

The authors have learned from experience with the very elderly patients at high surgical risk with NYHA class III-IV heart failure that they do not hope or even desire

TABLE 5–4

Early Echocardiographic vs. Invasive AV Hemodynamics (Pre-BAV to Post-BAV)

	NHLBI registry[4,8]	Washington Hospital Center[9]	MHI
Number of patients	674	262	332
Age (years)	78 ± 9	81.7 ± 9.8	85.5 ± 6.6
Echo			
Baseline AV mean gr. (mm Hg)	49 ± 16	42.0 ± 13.9	43.6 ± 13.7
Post BAV AV mean gr.	38 ± 14	31.9 ± 11.8	26.8 ± 11.2
Baseline AVA (cm^2)	0.57 ± 0.21	0.68 ± 0.15	0.61 ± 0.16
Post BAV AVA	0.78 ± 0.31	0.87 ± 0.19	0.84 ± 0.30
Baseline LVEF (%)	48 ± 19	45.4 ± 18.4	43.8 ± 12.8
Post BAV LVEF	N/A	47.0 ± 18.0	45.7 ± 9.1
Invasive			
Baseline AV mean gr. (mm Hg)	55 ± 21	46.3 ± 19.7	46.4 ± 17.7
Post BAV AV mean gr.	29 ± 13	21.4 ± 12.4	24.2 ± 9.1
Baseline AVA (cm^2)	0.5 ± 0.2	0.58 ± 0.3	0.64 ± 0.2
Post BAV AVA	0.8 ± 0.3	0.96 ± 0.3	N/A
Comparison of echo and invasive early results (Δ = pre to 24 to 72 hours post-BAV)			
ΔAV mean gr. (invasive)*	26 mm Hg	25 mm Hg	22 mm Hg
ΔAV mean gr. (echo)	11 mm Hg	10 mm Hg	16 mm Hg
ΔAVA (invasive)	0.30 cm^2	0.38 cm^2	n/a
ΔAVA (echo)	0.21 cm^2	0.19 cm^2	0.23 cm^2

AV, Aortic valve; *AVA,* aortic valve area; *BAV,* balloon aortic valvuloplasty; *gr.,* gradient; *LVEF,* left ventricular ejection fraction; *MHI,* Minneapolis Heart Institute; *N/A,* not applicable; *NHLBI,* National Heart Lung and Blood Institute.
*Invasively measured mean gr. and AVA appear much greater than echocardiographically measured values.

to achieve greater longevity. They are uniformly looking for a means to enhance their QOL via a low morbidity procedure. From the patient's perspective, BAV functions in this role quite well, providing the risk of stroke and other serious, nonreversible complications can be limited to 1% to 2%. It has been found that the option for repeated BAV for symptomatic restenosis after 1- to 2-years is well accepted by these patients, especially in the absence of any further increase in the procedural risk.

BAV IN UNIQUE CLINICAL SETTINGS

Balloon Aortic Valvuloplasty in Patients Requiring Noncardiac Surgery

In patients with severe AS who are being considered for elective, major noncardiac surgery, surgical AVR is generally recommended first, especially in patients who are symptomatic. Patients requiring nonelective surgery and thus less well-suited for undergoing AVR before surgery have been shown in two studies to be at an acceptable risk for their noncardiac surgery.[34] Although BAV has been shown to be safe in patients with severe AS before they undergo major noncardiac surgery,[35,36] in the absence of heart failure or baseline hemodynamic instability it would appear to be unnecessary.

It has been the approach at MHI to recommend BAV preoperatively in patients who are hemodynamically unstable, those with overt congestive heart failure and evidence of pulmonary edema, patients with severe left ventricular dysfunction, and patients with baseline NYHA class III or IV heart failure. There is a low threshold

to recommend monitoring these patients perioperatively with a Swan-Ganz catheter. In cases where severe blood loss may be expected, such as liver transplant, BAV should be strongly considered before surgery even in patients who are asymptomatic.

Balloon Aortic Valvuloplasty in Pregnancy

AS, when severe, is associated with an increased maternal and fetal risk. Neonatal complications in one study affected 25% of 49 pregnancies.[37] Conversely, 40% of pregnant women with severe AS, including patients who were asymptomatic, were documented to have complications.[38] The most common event was worsening of their heart-failure class. Many of those patients with severe AS can be managed medically. BAV has been effective and generally reserved for patients who have failed medical therapy.[39] Valve surgery during pregnancy is performed with a maternal mortality similar to that of nonpregnant women; fetal mortality, however, is between 12% and 20%.[40-42] It should be noted that AS in younger patients is often congenital or rheumatic in origin, thus resulting in more favorable or durable outcomes for BAV.

Balloon Aortic Valvuloplasty in Congenital Aortic Stenosis

An in-depth discussion of the management of congenital AS is beyond the scope of this chapter, and with the exception of an occasional patient with a bicuspid aortic valve, is rarely managed by the adult interventional cardiologist. In general, BAV of congenital bicuspid

TABLE 5–5

Difference in AVA Improvement Comparing Initial (First) and Subsequent (Second) BAV Invasive Hemodynamic Data

	Mount Sinai Hospital Series[17]	Washington Hospital Center[9]	University of Chicago
Number of patients	212	262	85
Number of BAV's	282	301	96
Age (years)	82 ± 8	81.7 ± 9.8	82 ± 6
AVA method	Invasive (Gorlin)	Invasive (Gorlin)	Invasive (Gorlin)
Baseline AVA (cm^2)	0.4 ± 0.19	0.58 ± 0.3	0.63 ± 0.23
AVA p 1st BAV (cm^2)	1.2 ± 0.3	0.96 ± 0.3	1.09 ± 0.32
ΔAVA p 1st BAV (cm^2)	0.59	0.41	0.45 ± 0.17
ΔAVA p 2nd BAV (cm^2)	0.56	0.28	0.20 ± 0.13

AVA, Aortic valve area; *ΔAVA*, improvement in AVA pre-BAV to post-BAV; *BAV*, balloon aortic valvuloplasty; *p*, post.

valve should be undertaken with reservation, given the increased likelihood of leaflet or annual disruption. Furthermore, symptomatic bicuspid aortic valve stenosis is more common after the fifth decade and best treated with surgical AVR.[43]

The pediatric interventional cardiologist has seen a rapid evolution in BAV technique for neonates, infants, and young children with AS. Procedural modifications have minimized vascular access complications and improved balloon stability, the postprocedural mean gradient, and AI. In the largest follow-up study available in the US, 509 patients were studied over a median of 9.3 years. Survival free from any aortic valve reintervention at 5 years was 72%, 54% at 10 years, and 27% at 20 years.[44]

Guidelines put forth by the AHA for BAV in patients with congenital AS includes the following Class I recommendations:[45]

1. Newborns with critical AS, who are by definition duct-dependent, regardless of the measured gradient across the aortic valve
2. Infants and children with depressed ventricular function regardless of the measured gradient across the aortic valve
3. Children with a resting peak systolic gradient of 50 mmHg or greater measured at catheterization
4. Children with a resting peak systolic gradient of 40 mmHg or greater measured at catheterization if there are symptoms of angina or syncope or ischemic ST-T wave changes on electrocardiography at rest or with exercise

Repeat Balloon Aortic Valvuloplasty in Aortic Valve Restenosis

With the option now of TAVR in patients who respond favorably to BAV, the likelihood of such a patient undergoing serial BAVs would seem to be diminished in favor of this more "definitive" therapy. Nevertheless, a significant experience in several labs with repeat BAV over the past decade has demonstrated this approach to be safe and effective. Demonstrated in several published experiences is a persistently low complication rate, unchanged for subsequent serial BAVs with the exception of an increased incidence of significant AI after three or more

BAVs. It is unclear if this is related to larger balloons in subsequent procedures. Findings with regard to a smaller increase in AVA with subsequent BAVs are conflicting (see **Table 5–5** for comparative data).[9,15,17]

One favorable series[17] demonstrated significant increase in AVA after BAV for both the first and second procedures (0.59 and 0.56 cm^2 respectively). The other two series demonstrated a significant drop off in AVA improvement after the second BAV.[9,15]

Details regarding balloon sizes, number of inflations, and diagnostic methodology are unavailable. More importantly, duration of symptomatic improvement between subsequent BAVs is not available. Collective experience indicates that the duration of symptomatic improvement is shorter after subsequent BAVs, but that it is substantial enough for many patients to elect undergoing a third or even fourth BAV. Repeat BAVs are generally discouraged at MHI if the duration of symptomatic benefit is less than 6 months.

Balloon Aortic Valvuloplasty in the Presence of Severe Left Ventricular Dysfunction

In the presence of congestive heart failure and advanced left ventricular dysfunction, the prognosis of patients with severe AS is poor and the risk of is AVR high.[46-49] Among the 674 patients of the NHLBI registry undergoing BAV, for those with mild, moderate, and severe left ventricular dysfunction, the 1-year survival rates were 59%, 50%, and 26%, respectively. In another series of 55 patients with a LVEF less than 40% who underwent BAV, the mean LVEF improved from 29 ± 7% to 34 ± 9%, and the 1-month, 6-month, and 12-month survival rates were 47%, 41%, and 36% respectively.[50] Contractile reserve on dobutamine stress echo (i.e., increase in stroke volume by ≥ 20%) identifies a group of patients with an improved operative mortality with surgical AVR but does not predict postoperative improvement in LVEF.[51,52]

The best management for an extremely high-risk subgroup of patients with an LVEF less than or equal to 20% who are predominantly denied both surgical AVR and TAVR is unknown. The risk of BAV in these patients and likelihood of improvement in LVEF has not been previously defined. BAV may serve as a diagnostic bridge to TAVR or surgical AVR if subsequent improvement

TABLE 5-6

BAV in Patients with Baseline LVEF < 20% MHI Experience[30]

Preoperative and Postoperative Echocardiographic Findings

	All Patients (16)	Group 1* EF < 20% (8)	Group 2† EF ≥ 20% (7)	P-Value
Pre-op LVEF (%)	16 ± 2.7	14.4 ± 2.7	17.4 ± 1.6	0.021
Post-op LVEF (%)	20.8 ± 4.8	17.1 ± 2.2	25.0 ± 3.2	<0.001
ΔLVEF	5.00 ± 3.5	2.75 ± 2.4	7.57 ± 2.7	<0.001
Pre-op mean AV gradient (mmHg)	33.1 ± 10.0	35.4 ± 10.2	31.5 ± 10.0	0.48
Post-op mean AV gradient (mmHg)	24.2 ± 11.7	21.9 ± 6.5	27.2 ± 15.7	0.4
Pre-op AVA (cm²)	0.59 ± 0.16	0.60 ± 0.12	0.60 ± 0.21	0.94
Post-op AVA (cm²)	0.85 ± 0.22	0.80 ± 0.21	0.92 ± 0.23	0.31
AVA percent increase (cm²)	45.3 ± 34.6	29.3 ± 20.7	66.7 ± 39.3	0.039
Patients with ΔAVA ≥ 0.2 cm² (%)	10 (66.7%)	3 (37.5%)	7 (100%)	0.026

AV, Aortic valve; AVA, aortic valve area; BAV, balloon aortic valvuloplasty; ΔAVA, increase in aortic valve area pre-BAV to post-BAV; EF, ejection fraction; LVEF, left ventricular ejection fraction; MHI, Minneapolis Heart Institute.
*Group 1 = patients whose LVEF remained <20% post-BAV.
†Group 2 = patients whose LVEF improved to ≥20% post-BAV.

in LVEF can be demonstrated. The greater majority of these patients have low flow–low gradient severe AS that should be confirmed if possible on preoperative dobutamine stress echocardiography.

Review of MHI's BAV database from January 2005 to December 2010 demonstrated 16 patients with an LVEF of less than 20% before BAV.[53] These 16 patients had a mean age of 83.1 ± 10.5%, and the mean LVEF was 16.0 ± 2.7%; 43.8% had coronary artery disease (CAD), and all 16 had NYHA class IV heart failure. Intraprocedural hemodynamics included mean arterial blood pressure of 85 ± 12.1 mmHg, pulmonary artery occlusion pressure of 25.7 ± 5.9 mmHg, and a cardiac index of 1.7 ± 0.4 L/min/m². An average of 3.3 ± 1.4 balloon inflations were carried out per BAV procedure, with a mean maximal balloon diameter of 23.6 ± 1.4 mm. Fifteen of the 16 patients had postprocedure echocardiograms and were divided into two groups:

Group 1: 8 patients (postoperative LVEF < 20%)
Group 2: 7 patients (postoperative LVEF ≥ 20%)

See **Table 5–6** and **Figure 5–12** for pre-procedural and postprocedural echocardiographic findings (postprocedural echocardiograms taken within 7 days of BAV).

Variables associated with a postprocedural LVEF greater than or equal to 20% included:

1. Absence of CAD (p = 0.041)
2. Higher preoperative LVEF (14.4 ± 2.7% vs. 17.4 ± 1.6%) (p = 0.02)
3. Post-BAV increase in AVA of 0.2 cm² or more (p = 0.026)

There were no intraprocedural mortalities, although four patients (25%) died during their index hospitalization. Twelve patients (75%) required IV phenylephrine and/or dopamine to maintain systolic blood pressure of 90 mmHg or greater. Two patients needed emergent intraaortic balloon pumps (IABPs) for prolonged hypotension after BAV. In short, BAV can be carried out with a low intraprocedural mortality. IV solutions of inotropic

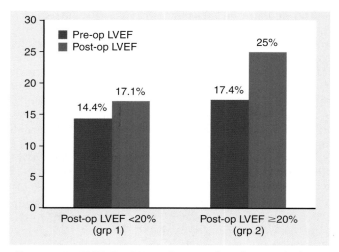

Figure 5–12 LVEFs Pre-BAV vs. Post-BAV from the MHI database.

and vasopressor agents should be prepared and hanging by each patient's side, and an IABP should be available in the CV room for possible emergent use. The incremental improvement in those patients with critically impaired left ventricular ejection fractions (LVEFs) (LVEF < 20%) is modest, but approximately 50% will improve to 20% (25.0 ± 3.2%) or better, and patients in this group may potentially became better candidates for surgical AVR or TAVR.

Balloon Aortic Valvuloplasty in Bioprosthetic Valve Aortic Stenosis

Although data is now emerging on favorable early outcomes for valve-in-valve transcatheter treatment of degenerative bioprosthetic aortic valve stenosis, there are no published clinical series large enough to understand the role for stand-alone BAV. The outcomes and incidence of complications with BAV is largely unknown and likely to remain that way in anticipation of a valve-in-valve strategy for nonsurgical candidates.

An interesting report on the findings after BAV on in-vitro degenerative bioprosthetic valves with stenosis that had been surgically explanted was published in the early years of BAV. An alarming list of ex-vivo adverse results were documented, including a high incidence of leaflet tears and perforations and dislodgement of calcific nodules. In this tabletop experiment, 20-mm balloons were inflated to 3 atm. The findings led the authors to strongly recommend avoiding BAV in bioprosthetic valve patients.[54] Successful outcomes with satisfactory reduction in mean valve gradients and improvement in functional class have been described in case reports, however.[55-57]

At least two reports of prosthetic leaflet disruption with hemodynamically significant AI have occurred, resulting in either death or surgical valve replacement.[57,58] At MHI, BAV has been performed in stenosed bioprosthetic aortic valves in three patients, all with successful short-term outcome and no complications. The balloon diameter is sized 1 mm less than the reported inner stent diameter for the specific valve type and size. These numbers are listed in a reference table available in an online appendix to a publication.[59]

Balloon Aortic Valvuloplasty in Patients with Aortic Insufficiency

BAV for AS is not significantly contraindicated by the presence of AI. This is quite different from the presence of moderate mitral regurgitation (e.g., in patients with mitral stenosis being considered for mitral valvuloplasty). Severe AI as a complication of BAV is rare (< 2.0%). When it does occur it can be catastrophic, and therefore patients with moderate AI are often inappropriately denied an effective treatment option. In the absence of severe AI as a contraindication, it is the practice at MHI to not restrict the use of BAV in those who would otherwise be an appropriate candidate. Patients with baseline 2+, and even 3+ AI on occasion, may actually be found to demonstrate a reduction in AI, resulting from enhanced leaflet mobility after BAV. A recent BAV series reported the outcome of 73 patients with moderate or severe AI.[60] After BAV, the degree of AI was improved or unchanged in 65 patients (89%) and only worsened by one grade in eight patients (11%). Only one patient died as a result of acute, severe AI. In five of these patients, severe AI was resolved in the cardiovascular laboratory. The cause of severe AI in these five patients was felt to be secondary to "a bent valve cusp stuck in the open position which was remobilized" through the manipulation of a pigtail catheter reinforced with a stiff guidewire. It should be noted that the operators predominantly use 20-mm balloons (98%), and in only three patients was the balloon size increased to 23 mm.

Combined Balloon Aortic Valvuloplasty and Percutaneous Coronary Intervention

Up to 50% of patients with symptomatic AS have significant CAD. Percutaneous coronary intervention (PCI) in the setting of severe AS has previously been limited to acute coronary syndromes. In stable patients who are not candidates for surgical AVR with coronary artery bypass, approaches are currently in evolution. Previously palliative BAV was performed, and if CAD was felt to be contributing to symptoms, PCI was offered in a staged fashion. It is known that untreated CAD in patients undergoing surgical AVR increases mortality.[61] The effect of untreated CAD on severe AS patients undergoing TAVR is unclear.

In an initial reported series of 17 patients who underwent combined coronary stenting and BAV, there was a 0% incidence of mortality, myocardial infarction (MI), stroke, or significant bleeding problems.[62] MHI has undertaken 56 cases of combined BAV and PCI with one perioperative MI and no mortalities; 37 patients (66%) underwent single-vessel stenting, 15 patients (27%) had double-vessel stenting, and four patients (7%) needed triple-vessel stenting. Complex lesions are generally avoided, and intervention is performed on stenosis subtending larger territories. Although initially coronary stenting was performed before BAV, the strategy has changed in favor of initially undertaking BAV followed by coronary stenting. In this respect, if transient closure should complicate coronary stenting, the risk for abrupt hemodynamic collapse should be reduced. Another recently published BAV series noted 52 patients (17.2% of the BAVs) underwent simultaneous BAV and PCI without any reported adverse events.[9]

BAV as a bridge has been undertaken simultaneously with PCI as an increasing common strategy in patients assessed as probable candidates for eventual TAVR. At the time of reevaluation in 1 to 3 months, the patient can potentially proceed to surgical AVR or TAVR. Prospective trials will need to be carried out demonstrating the benefit of performing simultaneous BAV and PCI as a bridge versus PCI alone before undergoing AVR or TAVR. PCI alone has been demonstrated in 254 patients with severe AS to be reasonably safe, resulting in a 4.3% mortality after 30 days.[63] Of note, however, within this group the 30-day post-PCI mortality was 5.4% when LVEF was less than or equal to 30% compared with 1.2% in patients with LVEF greater than 30% (p < 0.001). This raises the question of whether BAV performed with PCI in patients with significant left ventricular dysfunction would be safer. In general, the authors would perform simultaneous BAV in patients with overt or decompensated heart failure as well as in patients with severe reduction in left ventricular systolic function.

Balloon Aortic Valvuloplasty as a Bridge to Aortic Valve Replacement

In patients with severe symptomatic AS who are not candidates for surgical AVR or TAVR, BAV may be performed, preserving the option for subsequent surgical or transcatheter replacement in the presence of adequate clinical improvement. Long-term mortality is dramatically improved after BAV in patients who eventually undergo valve replacement.[9] There have now been several studies demonstrating the safety of performing BAV as a bridge to TAVR.[18,21,33,64-66] There are no randomized trials, however, demonstrating its relative benefits compared to proceeding directly to TAVR. Settings in which BAV have been carried out as an expectation for bridging to TAVR include: 1) severe left ventricular dysfunction; 2) marked frailty and generalized weakness; 3) unstable hemodynamics; 4) symptoms of uncertain origin (e.g., cardiac vs. pulmonary); 5) need to undergo PCI; 6) severe mitral regurgitation; 7) severe pulmonary hypertension; and 8) need for other evaluation before proceeding with TAVR (e.g., possible cancer).

Balloon Aortic Valvuloplasty for Transcatheter Aortic Valve Replacement Predilation

BAV in TAVR procedures serves to predilate the valve and thus enhance transcatheter delivery of the valve implant. Predilation is usually performed with balloons that are approximately 2 mm in diameter less than the annulus to minimize the likelihood of trauma with catastrophic consequences. BAV also offers the opportunity to minimize any likelihood of coronary occlusion and confirm annular size. Contrast injection through a pigtail catheter positioned in the aortic root with the balloon inflated determines, based on the absence of coronary filling, whether or not the patient is at risk for coronary occlusion with device implantation. If coronary obstruction is demonstrated, TAVR is either aborted or coronary access is preserved with a guidewire before TAVR to permit stent rescue. The balloon diameter should be the same as the proposed valve to be implanted.

There are at least two methods for using BAV to aid in TAVR sizing. In the first method, the operator observes for contrast regurgitation into the left ventricle with an aortic root injection while the valvuloplasty balloon of known diameter is inflated. If contrast spills into the left ventricle, a device of that balloon diameter would be undersized.[24] The second method, in brief, uses a noncompliant balloon in tandem with a pressure manometer on an Indeflator. On a sterile table, balloons are inflated to achieve 2 atm of intraballoon pressure, and the inflation volume is noted. Calipers are used to determine the balloon diameter achieved. The balloon is then deflated and positioned across the patient's aortic valve, after which it is reinflated with the same volume of dilute contrast. If just 2 atm of pressure are recorded, the balloon diameter is smaller than the annulus. On the other hand, if the intraballoon pressure exceeds 2 atm (i.e., additional intraballoon pressure), the annular size has been reached or exceeded by the balloon diameter.[67]

Future Perspectives in Aortic Valvuloplasty Technology

Balloons in current use for aortic valvuloplasty were not specifically designed for engaging this complex anatomy and none are approved by the U.S. Food and Drug Administration for this indication. In addition, the supportive guidewires currently used must be shaped at the distal end by the operator to prevent left ventricular perforation. With broader adoption of BAV among less-experienced interventionalists and cardiovascular surgeons, devices specifically designed for this purpose are greatly needed. The authors believe that geometric (i.e., "hour glass" balloon shapes) hold the promise of:

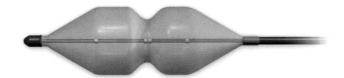

Figure 5–13 "Hour glass"-shaped aortic valvuloplasty balloon with a fixed reduction in the waist designed to prevent valve annulus over-dilation.

1) precise balloon positioning and stable fixation; 2) achieving greater AVAs with hyperextension of valve leaflets into the dilated sinus of Valsalva; and 3) achieving enhanced safety with a narrower balloon waist, reducing the likelihood of annular tears **(Figure 5–13)**. By combining a shorter aortic root segment with a method for fixation, aortic dissection at the sinotubular junction should be minimized. Additional balloon iterations should be tailored to achieve specific tasks (i.e., stand-alone BAV vs. predilation). Preshaped guidewires in several different sizes may achieve safer and more stable guidewire–left ventricular interface and reduce the likelihood of left ventricular perforation.

5.2 Pulmonic Valvuloplasty

VALVE PATHOLOGY AND MECHANISM OF ACTION

Pulmonic valve stenosis (PS) is congenital in 95% of patients, and 80% of those cases occur in isolation. Rarely, carcinoid or rheumatic valve disease may cause PS, but never in isolation. Congenital pulmonic valves are typically trileaflet with some degree of commissural fusion. The restricted valve leaflets have characteristic systolic doming on imaging and are rarely calcified. Acommissural, unicommissural, and bicuspid valves are uncommon. Congenital dysplastic valves are also less common and have thickened leaflets with a hypoplastic annulus. Dysplastic valves yield less favorable reductions in pulmonic gradients after balloon valvuloplasty. The mechanism of dilation for most congenital valves is thought to be separation of fused commissures, thus leaflets without fusion, such as dysplastic valves, generally yield poor results.

DIAGNOSIS

TTE is recommended for the initial diagnosis and serial follow-up care of PS. Echocardiography usually demonstrates a characteristic leaflet doming in systole. Stenosis severity is quantitated by the peak systolic valve gradient. During invasive pulmonic valve interrogation, the Gorlin formula is not used to determine valve area. Significant PS is determined by gradient only. Cardiac magnetic resonance (CMR) imaging is useful in ruling out subvalvular or supravalvular stenosis. In addition, CMR imaging is useful in quantitating associated abnormalities such as infundibular hypertrophy, pulmonary artery aneurysmic change, and pulmonary artery stenosis. The

2008 Updated ACC/AHA Guidelines for the Management of Valvular Heart Disease

6.6.3 Indications for balloon valvotomy in pulmonic stenosis

Class I

1. Balloon valvotomy is recommended in adolescent and young adult patients with pulmonic stenosis who have exertional dyspnea, angina, syncope, and an RV-to-pulmonary artery peak-to-peak gradient greater than 30 mm Hg at catheterization. (Level of Evidence: C)
2. Balloon valvotomy is recommended in asymptomatic adolescent and young adult patients with pulmonic stenosis and RV-to-pulmonary artery peak-to-peak gradient greater than 40 mm Hg at catheterization. (Level of Evidence: C)

Class IIb

1. Balloon valvotomy may be reasonable in asymptomatic adolescent and young adult patients with pulmonic stenosis and an RV-to-pulmonary artery peak-to-peak gradient 30 to 39 mm Hg at catheterization. (Level of Evidence: C)

Class III

1. Balloon valvotomy is not recommended in asymptomatic adolescent and young adult patients with pulmonic stenosis and RV-to-pulmonary artery peak-to-peak gradient less than 30 mm Hg at catheterization. (Level of Evidence: C)

ACC, American College of Cardiology; *AHA,* American Heart Association; *RV,* right ventricle.

authors have also used CMR imaging to measure pulmonic valve annulus diameter to assist in balloon sizing. Cardiac catheterization is not recommended for the initial diagnostic evaluation and is primarily performed in the setting of balloon valvuloplasty. The most important parameters measured are the pulmonic transvalvular gradient and right atrial pressure. The Gorlin formula in this setting has several problems, and the valve area does not improve the accuracy as an index of pulmonary stenosis severity.[68]

PATIENT SELECTION

Indications for balloon pulmonic valvuloplasty (BPV) of PS, as they appear from the 2008 updated ACC/AHA Guidelines for the Management of Valvular Heart Disease, are shown in **Box 5–3**.[69] These are guidelines that are adhered to at MHI and incorporated into the adult interventional practice.

Exercise testing is helpful in determining whether patients are truly asymptomatic. If the patient's exercise capacity is significantly limited, the algorithm for patients with symptoms should be considered. In patients who have PS with valve dysplasia, in spite of their tendency to result in only modest gradient reduction, balloon valvuloplasty is recommended as the initial treatment of choice. Unlike other congenital pulmonic valve lesions, balloons that are 1.4 to 1.5 times the annulus diameter

should be considered for use in dysplastic valves to achieve a good result.[70]

PROCEDURAL TECHNIQUE

BPV is performed in a standard cardiovascular laboratory suite with the patient under conscious sedation. All patients are pretreated with an aspirin and heparinized during the procedure to maintain ACTs of 200 to 250 seconds. Operators begin by placing a 5F sheath in the right femoral artery and an 8F sheath in the right femoral vein. A standard diagnostic right heart catheterization is then performed with a Swan-Ganz catheter. The Swan-Ganz catheter is then pulled back carefully across the pulmonic valve to obtain a systolic gradient. If the balloon tip accelerates through the right ventricular outflow tract (RVOT), preventing an accurate and sustained wave form tracing just below the pulmonic valve, operators position a second catheter (6F multipurpose) immediately under the pulmonic valve. Simultaneous pressures can then be recorded using the Swan-Ganz catheter positioned in the pulmonary artery. A Berman angiographic catheter (Arrow International) is then placed in the right ventricular apex. With the balloon inflated, biplane ventriculography is performed using a 10- to 15-degree left anterior oblique projection with 20 to 30 degrees of cranial angulation and a straight lateral projection. The authors generally use 35 cc of contrast delivered at 25 cc/sec. Ventriculography will confirm the site of obstruction and allow measurement of the pulmonic valve annulus in two orthogonal views **(Figure 5–14, A-D).**

The right femoral vein sheath is exchanged for a 12F sheath in the adult. We use a 5F or 6F multipurpose or right coronary diagnostic catheter that is then delivered into the right heart over a 0.035-inch J-tipped guidewire. After crossing the pulmonic valve, the catheter is then positioned in one of the lower segment pulmonary arteries for additional stability. A 0.035-inch Amplatz Extra Stiff or Super Stiff exchange-length guidewire is then exchanged with the J-tipped guidewire, over which BPV is performed.

Balloon Choice

Several balloon types are currently in use for BPV. Tyshak II, Z-Med, and Z-Med II balloons are commonly used. Tyshak II has the advantage of being lower in profile, but because it is more compliant, it has a less predictable inflated diameter. For this reason the less compliant Z-Med balloons are preferred. Recommended balloon/annulus diameter ratios have ranged from 1.2 to 1.4. Reports with long-term follow-up studies, however, have described a higher incidence of late pulmonary insufficiency with ratios of 1.3 or greater.[71-73] More recently, balloon/annulus ratios of 1.2 to 1.25 are thusly recommended.[74] The authors use balloons that are 4 cm in length, although some operators use balloons up to 6 cm in length to provide a longer landing zone for dilating the pulmonary valve. However, this may result in a greater likelihood of disrupting the tricuspid valve apparatus. In the adult group, larger venous access sheaths do not pose limitations, and with the larger balloon diameters available, the need for dilating with two

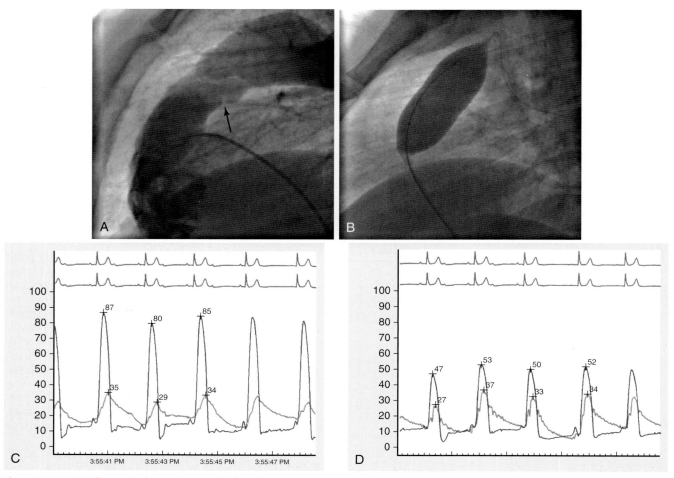

Figure 5–14 **A,** Right ventriculogram in a straight lateral projection. *Arrow* demonstrates position of pulmonic valve leaflets. **B,** Pulmonic valvuloplasty balloon inflated across pulmonic valve. **C,** Baseline transpulmonic peak valve gradient with simultaneous right ventricular and PA pressures. Peak gradient = 51.33 mmHg. **D,** Postvalvuloplasty transpulmonic peak valve gradient. Peak gradient = 17.75 mmHg.

balloons simultaneously has not been found. In addition, double-balloon valvuloplasty has not been demonstrated to yield superior results.[75,76] Nevertheless, if two balloons are used simultaneously, the following formula can be used to calculate the effective balloon diameter: 0.82 (D_1 + D_2), where D_1 and D_2 are the 2 balloon diameters. See **Figure 5–15** for a chart that can be used in deriving the effective diameter.

BALLOON VALVULOPLASTY

With selection of an appropriate balloon valvuloplasty catheter, it is advanced over the stiff guidewire and positioned across the pulmonary valve. A road map from the previously straight lateral right ventriculogram is placed on an adjacent monitor for landmarks. Useful landmarks include ribs, soft tissue densities, and catheter shafts. The balloon is inflated with 1:8 dilute contrast, and resolution of the balloon waist with full inflation should be documented. Two inflations are generally performed. If there is difficulty keeping the inflated balloon centered on the valve, rapid right ventricular pacing at 180 to 220 beats/min should mitigate this problem. The authors use a 60-cc disposable syringe for balloon inflation;

systemic arterial pressures are monitored at all times using the 5F right femoral artery sheath.

After valvuloplasty, the pressure gradient across the pulmonary valve is remeasured and cardiac output measurements are repeated to ensure that the drop in pressure gradient is not secondary to a drop in cardiac output. If sustained hypotension occurs secondary to dynamic RVOT obstruction, documented by careful pull-back pressures from the pulmonary artery to the right ventricle, fluid volume, IV phenylephrine, and β-blockers should be given. The negative inotropic effect of β-blockers results in reduced contractility and thereby a reduction in the dynamic obstruction at the RVOT level. Right ventriculography in a lateral projection may also be of assistance by documenting a dynamic RVOT obstruction **(see Figure 5–14, A).** This generally resolves over time with regression of the secondary hypertrophy.[77] Infundibular gradients occur in up to 30% of patients. It is more likely to occur in patients who are older and have more severe baseline obstruction.[78]

A satisfactory result is obtained when the peak-to-peak pressure gradient is reduced to less than 30 mmHg. In the absence of a good result, valvuloplasty is repeated with

EFFECTIVE DILATING DIAMETER (mm) USING DOUBLE BALLOON TECHNIQUE																					
5	6	7	8	9	10	11	12	13	14	15	16	17	18	19	20	21	22	23	24	25	
8.2	9.0	9.9	10.7	11.6	12.5	13.5	14.4	15.3	16.2	17.2	18.1	19.1	20.0	21.0	21.9	22.9	23.9	24.8	25.8	26.8	5
	9.8	10.7	11.5	12.4	13.3	14.1	15.1	16.0	16.9	17.8	18.7	19.7	20.6	21.6	22.5	23.5	24.4	25.4	26.5	27.3	6
		11.5	12.3	13.1	14.0	14.9	15.8	16.7	17.6	18.5	19.4	20.3	21.2	22.1	23.0	23.9	24.8	25.7	26.6	27.8	7
			13.1	13.9	14.8	15.6	16.5	17.4	18.5	19.2	20.1	21.0	21.9	22.8	23.7	24.7	25.6	26.5	27.5	28.4	8
				14.7	15.6	16.4	17.3	18.1	19.0	19.9	20.8	21.7	22.6	23.5	24.4	25.3	26.2	27.1	28.0	29.0	9
					16.4	17.2	18.0	18.9	19.7	20.6	21.5	22.4	23.3	24.2	25.1	26.0	26.9	27.2	28.8	29.7	10
						18.0	18.8	19.7	20.5	21.4	22.2	23.1	24.0	24.9	25.8	26.7	27.6	28.5	29.4	30.3	11
							19.6	20.5	21.3	22.1	23.0	23.9	24.7	25.6	26.5	27.4	28.3	29.2	30.1	31.0	12
								21.3	22.1	22.9	23.8	24.6	25.5	26.4	27.2	28.1	29.0	29.9	30.8	31.7	13
									22.9	23.7	24.6	25.4	26.3	27.1	28.0	28.9	29.7	30.6	31.5	32.4	14
										24.5	25.4	26.2	27.0	27.9	28.8	29.6	30.5	31.4	32.2	33.1	15
											26.2	27.0	27.8	28.7	29.5	30.4	31.2	32.1	33.0	33.9	16
												27.8	28.6	29.5	30.3	31.2	32.0	32.9	33.7	34.6	17
													29.5	30.3	31.1	32.0	32.8	33.6	34.5	35.4	18
														31.1	31.9	32.7	33.6	34.4	35.3	36.1	19
															32.7	33.6	34.4	35.2	36.1	36.9	20
																34.4	35.2	36.0	36.9	37.7	21
																	36.0	36.8	37.5	38.5	22
																		37.6	38.5	39.3	23
																			39.3	40.1	24
																				40.9	25

Figure 5–15 Chart that can be used in deriving the effective diameter.

a balloon diameter that is 1 to 2 mm larger. A portable echocardiography machine is kept in the cardiovascular laboratory during this procedure should the need for emergent imaging in the face of prolonged hypotension arise. This provides a quick screen for complications such as dynamic RVOT obstruction, pulmonary or tricuspid insufficiency, or pericardial effusion.

Patients are observed via telemetry overnight. A predischarge echocardiograph is performed the next day. Repeat echocardiography is obtained at 6 and 12 months.

OUTCOMES: RESULTS AND COMPLICATIONS

The highly favorable acute and long-term results after BPV in adolescents and adults make it the first line treatment. Surgical intervention is avoided in essentially all patients. The transpulmonary valve gradient usually decreases by two thirds of its baseline value. Hemodynamic outcomes from clinical trials are shown in **Table 5–7.** The Valvuloplasty and Angioplasty of Congenital Anomalies (VACA) registry reported on independent predictors of long-term

outcomes after BPV in 533 patients with a mean age of 3.7 years (range: 1 day to 55 years) at 22 institutions.[79] Independent predictors were: 1) study time interval; 2) annular diameter; 3) pulmonary valve gradient immediately postprocedure; and 4) balloon/annulus diameter ratio for nondysplastic valves.

Complications are rare with BPV. The VACA registry reported a 0.24% procedural mortality and a 0.35% major complication rate from 822 BAV procedures. Right bundle branch block, complete heart block, stroke, cardiac arrest, rupture of the tricuspid valve apparatus, pulmonary artery and valve tears, right ventricular perforation with tamponade, and ventricular tachycardia have all been reported but are rare. Residual pulmonary valve insufficiency is often present, although in the majority of cases, it is insignificant. Predictors of significant late follow-up pulmonic insufficiency are balloon valvuloplasty at a younger age and balloon/annulus ratio of 1.3 or greater. In both adult series with long-term follow-up studies listed in **Table 5–7,** there were no cases of restenosis or significant pulmonic insufficiency.[80-82]

TABLE 5-7 ▬▬▬▬
Hemodynamic Outcomes in Adolescent/Adult Patients after Balloon Pulmonary Valvuloplasty

	N	Age (Years)	Baseline Peak Gradient (mm Hg)	Postprocedure (mm Hg)	Long-Term Outcome (mm Hg)	Clinical Outcome
Sievert H, et al.[79]	24	39 (17-12)	92 ± 36	43 ± 19	N/A	
Teupe CH, et al.[80]	14	41 ± 14 (19-65)	82 ± 29	37 ± 14	31 ± 7 (mean f/u 6.5 yrs: range 4.5-9)	No restenosis 13/14 patients asymptomatic No "significant" PI
Chen C, et al.[81]	53	26 ± 11 (13-55)	91 ± 46	38 ± 32	19 ± 8 (mean f/u 6.9 ± 3.1 yrs; range 0.2-9.8)	No restenosis NYHA class improved from 1.9 ± 0.9 to 1.0 No "significant" PI

f/u, Follow-up; *N/A*, not applicable; *NYHA*, New York Heart Association; *PI*, pulmonic insufficiency.

REFERENCES

1. Cribier A, Savin T, Saondi N, et al: Percutaneous transluminal valvuloplasty of acquired aortic stenosis in elderly patients: an alternative to valve replacement? Lancet 1:63–67, 1986.
2. Safian RD, Berman AD, Driver DJ, et al: Balloon aortic valvuloplasty in 170 consecutive patients, N Engl J Med 319:125–130, 1988.
3. O'Neill WW: Mansfield Scientific Aortic Valvuloplasty Registry Investigators. Predictors of long-term survival after percutaneous aortic valvuloplasty registry, J Am Coll Cardiol 17:193–198, 1991.
4. Otto CM, Mickel MC, Kennedy JW, et al: Three-year outcome after balloon aortic valvuloplasty: insights into prognosis of valvular aortic stenosis, Circulation 89:642–650, 1994.
5. Rahimtoola S: Catheter balloon valvuloplasty for severe calcific aortic stenosis: a limited role, J Am Coll Cardiol 23(5):1076–1078, 1994.
6. Nkomo VT, Gardin JM, Skelton TN, et al: Burden of valvular heart disease: a population-based study, Lancet 368(9540):1005–1011, 1996.
7. Springs DC, Forfar JC: How should we manage symptomatic aortic stenosis in the patient who is 80 or older? Br Heart J 74:481–484, 1995.
8. NHLBI Balloon Valvuloplasty Registry Participants: Percutaneous balloon aortic valvuloplasty: acute and 30 day follow-up results in 674 patients from NHLBI balloon valvuloplasty registry, Circulation 84:2383–2397, 1991.
9. Ben-Dor I, Pichard AD, Satler LF, et al: Complications and outcomes of balloon aortic valvuloplasty in high-risk or inoperable patients, JACC Cardiovasc Interv 3(11):1150–1156, 2010.
10. Mohler ER III, Gannon F, Reynolds C, et al: Bone formation and inflammation in cardiac valves, Circulation 103:1522–1528, 2001.
11. Letac B, Gerber L, Koning R: Insight in the mechanism of balloon aortic valvuloplasty of stenosis, Am J Cardiol 62:1241–1247, 1988.
12. McKay RG, Safian RD, Lock JE, et al: Balloon dilatation of calcific aortic stenosis in elderly patients: post mortem, intraoperative, and percutaneous valvuloplasty studies, Circulation 74:119–125, 1986.
13. Hura H, Pedersen WR, Ladich E, et al: Percutaneous balloon aortic valvuloplasty revisited: time for a renaissance? Circulation 115:e334–e338, 2007.
14. van den Brand M, Essed CE, Di Mario C, et al: Histological changes in the aortic valve after balloon dilatation: evidence for a delayed healing process, Br Heart J 67:445–449, 1992.
15. Feldman T, Galgov S, Carroll JD: Restenosis following successful balloon valvuloplasty: bone formation in aortic valve leaflets, Catheter Cardiovasc Diagn 29:1–7, 1993.
16. Bonnow RO, Carabello BA, Chatterjee K, et al: American Heart Association Task Force on Practice Guideline (Writing committee to revise the 1998 guidelines for the management of patients with valvular heart disease). ACC/AHA 2006 guidelines for the management of patients with valvular heart disease: a report of the American College of Cardiology/American Heart Association Task Force on practice guidelines developed in collaboration with the Society of Cardiovascular Anesthesiologists endorsed by the Society for Cardiovascular Angiography and Interventions and the Society of Thoracic Surgeons, J Am Coll Cardiol 48:e1–148, 2006. Section 6.l.3.

17. Agarwal A, Kini AS, Attandi S, et al: Results of repeat balloon valvuloplasty for treatment of aortic stenosis in patients aged 59 to 104 years, Am J Cardiol 95:43–47, 2005.
18. Ussia GP, Capadanno D, Barbanti M, et al: Balloon aortic valvuloplasty for severe aortic stenosis as a bridge to high-risk transcatheter aortic valve implantation, J Invasive Cardiol 22:161–166, 2010.
19. Pedersen WR, Klaassen PJ, Boisjolie CR, et al: Feasibility of transcatheter intervention for severe aortic stenosis in patients >90 years of age: aortic valvuloplasty revisited, Catheter Cardiovasc Interv 70:149–154, 2007.
20. Rajani R, Buxton W, Haworth P, et al: Prognostic benefit of transcatheter aortic valve implantation compared with medical therapy in patients with inoperable aortic stenosis, Catheter Cardiovasc Interv 75:1121–1126, 2010.
21. Hamid T, Eichöffer J, Clarke B, et al: Aortic balloon valvuloplasty: is there still a role in high risk patients in the era of percutaneous aortic valve replacement? J Interv Cardiol 34(4):358–361, 2010.
22. Sakada Y, Syed Z, Salinger MH, et al: Percutaneous balloon aortic valvuloplasty: antegrade transseptal vs. conventional retrograde transarterial approach, Catheter Cardiovasc Interv 64:314–321, 2005.
23. Feldman T: Balloon aortic valvuloplasty: current techniques and clinical utility. In Huber C, Feldman T, editors: Transcatheter valve therapies, New York, 2010, Informa Healthcare, pp 40–57.
24. Cribier A, Eltechaninoff H: Preimplantation percutaneous aortic balloon valvotomy (retrograde approach). In Serryus P, Piazza N, Cribiera A, et al, editors: Transcatheter aortic valve implantation: tips and tricks to avoid failure, New York, 2010, Informa Healthcare, pp 161–170.
25. Solomon LW, Fusman B, Jolly N, et al: Percutaneous suture closure for management of large French size arterial puncture in aortic valvuloplasty, J Invasc Cardiol 13:592–596, 2001.
26. Eltchaninoff H, Cribier A, Tron C, et al: Balloon aortic valvuloplasty in elderly patients at high risk for surgery or inoperable. Immediate and mid-term results, Eur Heart J 16:1079–1084, 1995.
27. Agatiello C, Altchaninoff H, Tron C, et al: Balloon aortic valvuloplasty in the adult: immediate results and in-hospital complications in the latest series of 141 consecutive patients at the University Hospital of Rouen (2002-2005), Arch Mal Coeur Vaiss 99(3):195–200, 2006.
28. Anderson M, Schwartz RS, Pedersen C, et al: Severity of aortic stenosis, not STS score, predicts procedural mortality in elderly patients undergoing balloon aortic valvuloplasty, Cardiovasc Revasc Med 10:207, 2009. abstract.
29. Leon MB, Piazza N, Nikolsky E, et al: Standardized endpoint definitions for transcatheter aortic valve implantation clinical trials: a consensus report from the Valve Academic Research Consortium, J Am Coll Cardiol 57(3):253–269, 2011.
30. Pedersen W, Krueger D, Dang M, et al: Incidence of atrioventricular conduction abnormalities following balloon aortic valvuloplasty, Catheter Cardiovasc Interv 77(Suppl):S137–S138, 2011.

31. Yaradarajan P, Kapoor N, Bansal RC, et al: Clinical profile and natural history of 453 nonsurgically managed patients with severe aortic stenosis, *Ann Thorac Surg* 82:2111–2115, 2006.
32. Nishimura RA, Holmes DR Jr, Reeder GS, et al: Doppler evaluation of results of percutaneous aortic balloon valvuloplasty in calcific aortic stenosis, *Circulation* 78:791–799, 1998.
33. Shareghi S, Rasouli L, Shavelle DM, et al: Current results of balloon aortic valvuloplasty in high-risk patients, *J Invasive Cardiol* 19(1):1–5, 2007.
34. Raymer K, Yang H: Patients with aortic stenosis: cardiac complications in noncardiac surgery, *Can J Anaesth* 45:855–859, 1998.
35. Torsher LC, Shub C, Rettke SR, et al: Risk of patients with severe aortic stenosis undergoing noncardiac surgery, *Am J Cardiol* 81:448–452, 1998.
36. Roth RB, Palacios IF, Block PC: Percutaneous aortic balloon valvuloplasty: its role in the management of patients with aortic stenosis requiring major noncardiac surgery, *J Am Coll Cardiol* 13(5):1039–1041, 1989.
37. Siu SC, Sermer M, Colman JM, et al: Prospective multicenter study of pregnancy outcomes in women with heart disease, *Circulation* 104:515–521, 2001.
38. Silversides CK, Colman JM, Sermer M, et al: Early and intermediate-term outcomes of pregnancy with congenital aortic stenosis, *Am J Cardiol* 91:1386–1389, 2003.
39. Banning AP, Pearson JF, Hall RJ: Role of balloon dilatation of the aortic valve in pregnant patients with severe aortic stenosis, *Br Heart J* 70:544–545, 1993.
40. Mahli A, Izdes S, Coskun D: Cardiac operations during pregnancy: review of factors influencing fetal outcome, *Ann Thorac Surg* 69:1622–1626, 2000.
41. Pomini F, Mercogliano D, Cavaletti C, et al: Cardiopulmonary bypass in pregnancy, *Ann Thorac Surg* 61:259–268, 1996.
42. Parry AJ, Westaby S: Cardiopulmonary bypass during pregnancy, *Ann Thorac Surg* 61:1865–1869, 1996.
43. Roberts WC, Ko JM: Frequency of unicuspid, bicuspid and tricuspid aortic valves by decade in adults having aortic valve replacement for isolated aortic stenosis, *Circulation* 111:920–925, 2005.
44. Brown DW, Dipilato AE, Chong EC, et al: Sudden unexpected death after balloon valvuloplasty for congenital aortic stenosis, *J Am Coll Cardiol* 56:1939–1946, 2010.
45. Feltes TF, Bacha E, Beekman RH 3rd, et al: American Heart Association Congenital Cardiac Defects Committee of the Council on Cardiovascular Disease in the Young, Council on Clinical Cardiology, Council on Cardiovascular Radiology and Intervention. Indications for cardiac catheterization and intervention in pediatric cardiac disease: a scientific statement from the American Heart Association, *Circulation* 123:2607–2652, 2011.
46. Carabello BA, Green LH, Grossman W, et al: Hemodynamic determinants of prognosis of aortic valve replacement in critical aortic stenosis and advanced congestive heart failure, *Circulation* 62:42–48, 1980.
47. Kennedy JW, Doces J, Steward DH: Left ventricular function before and following aortic valve replacement, *Circulation* 56:944–950, 1977.
48. Smith N, McAnulty JH, Rahimtoola SH: Severe aortic stenosis with impaired left ventricular function and clinical heart failure: results of valve replacement, *Circulation* 58:255–264, 1978.
49. Connolly HM, Oh JK, Orzulak TA, et al: Aortic valve replacement for aortic stenosis with severe left ventricular dysfunction: prognostic indicators, *Circulation* 95:2395–2400, 1997.
50. Berland J, Cribier A, Savin T, et al: Percutaneous balloon valvuloplasty in patients with severe aortic stenosis and low ejection fraction: immediate results and 1-year follow-up, *Circulation* 79:1189–1196, 1989.
51. Quere JP, Monin JL, Levy F, et al: Influence of preoperative left ventricular contractile reserve on postoperative ejection fraction in low-gradient aortic stenosis, *Circulation* 113:1738–1744, 2006.
52. Clavel MA, Fuchs C, Burwash JG, et al: Predictors of outcomes in low-flow, low-gradient aortic stenosis: results of the multicenter TOPAS Study, *Circulation* 118(Suppl 14):S234–S242, 2008.
53. Pedersen W, Dang M, Krueger D, et al: Intra- and postprocedural outcomes in severe aortic stenosis patients with left ventricular ejection fractions <20% undergoing balloon valvuloplasty, *Catheter Cardiovasc Interv* 77(Suppl):S136–S137, 2011.
54. Waller BF, McKay C, Van Tassel J, et al: Catheter balloon valvuloplasty of stenotic porcine bioprosthetic valves. Part II. Mechanisms, complications, and recommendations for clinical use, *Clin Cardiol* 14:764–772, 1991.
55. Dejam A, Hokinson M, Laham R: Repeated successful balloon valvuloplasty of a bioprosthetic aortic valve in a nonagenarian, *Catheter Cardiovasc Interv* 77:589–592, 2011.
56. Orbe LC, Sobrino N, Maté I, et al: Effectiveness of balloon percutaneous valvuloplasty for stenotic bioprosthetic valves in different positions, *Am J Cardiol* 68(17):1719–1721, 1991.
57. McKay CR, Waller BF, Hong R, et al: Problems encountered with catheter balloon valvuloplasty of bioprosthetic aortic valves, *Am Heart J* 115:463–465, 1988.
58. Kirwan C, Richardson G, Rothman MT: Is there a role for balloon valvuloplasty in patients with stenotic aortic bioprosthetic valves? *Catheter Cardiovasc Interv* 63:251–253, 2004.
59. Piazza N, Bleiziffer S, Brockmann G, et al: Transcatheter aortic valve implantation for failing surgical aortic bioprosthetic valve: from concept to clinical application and evaluation. Part 1, *JACC Cardiovasc Interv* 4(7):721–732, 2011.
60. Saia F, Marrozzini C, Ciuca C, et al: Is balloon aortic valvuloplasty safe in patients with significant aortic valve regurgitation? *Catheter Cardiovasc Interv* 79(2):315–321, 2012.
61. Mullany CJ, Elveback LR, Frye RL, et al: Coronary artery disease and its management: influence or survival in patients undergoing aortic valve replacement, *J Am Coll Cardiol* 10:66–72, 1987.
62. Pedersen W, Klassen P, Pedersen C, et al: Comparison of outcomes in high risk patients >70 years of age with aortic valvuloplasty and percutaneous coronary intervention versus aortic valvuloplasty alone, *Am J Cardiol* 101:1309–1314, 2006.
63. Goel SS, Agarwal S, Tuscu M, et al: Percutaneous coronary intervention in patients with severe aortic stenosis. Implications for TAVR, *Circulation* 125:1005–1013, 2012.
64. Kapadia SR, Goel SS, Yuksel U, et al: Lessons learned from balloon aortic valvuloplasty experience from the pre-transcatheter aortic valve implantation era, *J Interv Cardiol* 23(5):499–508, 2010.
65. Tissot C-M, Attias D, Himbert D, et al: Reappraisal of percutaneous aortic balloon valvuloplasty as a preliminary treatment strategy in the transcatheter aortic valve implantation era, *EuroIntervention* 7(1):49–56, 2011.
66. Saia F, Marrozzini C, Moretti C, et al: The role of percutaneous balloon aortic valvuloplasty as a bridge for transcatheter aortic valve implantation, *EuroIntervention* 7(6):723–729, 2011.
67. Babaliaros V, Junagadhwalla Z, Lerakis S, et al: Use of balloon aortic valvuloplasty to size the aortic annulus before implantation of a balloon-expandable transcatheter heart valve, *JACC Cardiovasc Interv* 3:1114–1118, 2010.
68. Ellison RC, Freedom RM, Keane JF, et al: Indirect assessment of severity in pulmonary stenosis, *Circulation* 56(I):114–I20, 1977.
69. Bonnow RO, Carabello BA, Chatterjee K, et al: ACC/AHA Practice Guideline: 2008 focused update incorporated into the ACC/AHA 2006 Guidelines for the Management of Patients with Valvular Heart Disease, *J Am Coll Cardiol* 52:1–142, 2008.
70. Rao PS: Balloon dilatation in infants and children with dysplastic pulmonary valves. Short-term and intermediate-term results, *Am Heart J* 116:1168–1173, 1998.
71. Rao PS, Galal O, Patnana M, et al: Results of three-to-ten-year follow-up of balloon dilatation of the pulmonary valve, *Heart* 80:591–595, 1998.
72. Rao PS: Long-term follow-up results after balloon dilatation of pulmonary stenosis, aortic stenosis and coarctation of the aorta: a review, *Prog Cardiovasc Dis* 42:59–74, 1999.
73. Garty Y, Veldman G, Lee K, et al: Late outcomes after pulmonary valve balloon dilatation in neonates, infants and children, *J Invasive Cardiol* 17:318–322, 2005.
74. Rao PS: Percutaneous balloon pulmonary valvuloplasty: state of the art, *Catheter Cardiovasc Interv* 69:747–763, 2007.
75. Rao PS, Fawzy ME: Double balloon technique for percutaneous balloon pulmonary valvuloplasty: comparison with single balloon technique, *J Interv Cardiol* 1:257–262, 1988.
76. Rao PS: Balloon pulmonary valvuloplasty: a review, *Clin Cardiol* 12:55–72, 1989.

77. Fontes VF, Esteves CA, Eduardo J, et al: Regression of infundibular hypertrophy after pulmonary valvotomy for pulmonic stenosis, Am J Cardiol 62:977–979, 1988.

78. Thapar MK, Rao PS: Significance of infundibular obstruction following balloon valvuloplasty for valvar pulmonic stenosis, Am Heart J 118:99–103, 1989.

79. McCrindle B: Independent predictors of long-term results after balloon pulmonary valvuloplasty: Valvuloplasty and Angiography of Congenital Anomalies (VACA) registry investigators, Circulation 89:1751–1759, 1994.

80. Sievert H, Kober G, Bussman WD, et al: Long-term results of percutaneous pulmonary valvuloplasty in adults, Eur Heart J 10:712–717, 1989.

81. Teupe CH, Burger W, Schräder R, et al: Late (five to nine years) follow-up after balloon dilation of valvular pulmonary stenosis in adults, Am J Cardiol 80:240–242, 1996.

82. Chen C, Cheng TO, Huang T, et al: Percutaneous balloon valvuloplasty for pulmonic stenosis in adolescents and adults, N Engl J Med 335:21–25, 1996.

Chapter 6

Transcatheter Aortic Valve Replacement: Edwards SAPIEN Valve

ALAN ZAJARIAS • ALAIN CRIBIER

Aortic stenosis (AS) remains the most common form of adult acquired valvular heart disease in developed countries, increasing in prevalence with age.[1] As noted by Ross and Braunwald,[2] the natural history of symptomatic AS carries a poor prognosis. Medically treated patients with symptomatic AS have 1 and 5 year survival rates of 60% and 32% respectively.[3] Aortic valve replacement (AVR) is the only effective treatment for symptomatic AS that alleviates symptoms and improves survival. In the ideal candidate, surgical AVR has an estimated operative mortality of 4%.[4] However, the operative mortality and incidence of postoperative complications increases with age, becomes significantly higher when surgery is done urgently, and when preexistent comorbidities such as coronary artery disease (CAD), poor left ventricular function, renal insufficiency, pulmonary disease, and diabetes are present.[5,6] These factors are considered to be the main reasons that one third of patients with valve disease are not referred for surgery.[7] Transcatheter aortic valve replacement (TAVR) has opened the possibility for treating patients who have been left untreated because it was believed that their operative mortality outweighed the benefits offered by traditional AVR.

The concept of catheter-based valve therapies dates to the 1970s with the development of experimental approaches for the treatment of aortic insufficiency (AI).[8-10] In 1989 Henning-Rud Andersen[11] first implanted an original model of a balloon-expandable, catheter-mounted stented valve within the aortas of pigs, using a handmade mesh containing a porcine valve. Andersen's and others' experimental concepts emerged in the early 1990s but were not followed with human application.[11-14] In 2000 Philip Bonhoeffer developed a stented valve made of a bovine jugular vein conduit inserted in a platinum-iridium stent, which was implanted in the pulmonary arteries of lambs.[15] Bonhoeffer performed the first human implantation of this device in a right ventricle–to–pulmonary artery conduit in 2000,[16] marking the beginning of the era of transcatheter valve replacement.

TAVR was introduced in 2002 by Dr. Alain Cribier[17] and utilized a bioprosthetic valve made of equine pericardium mounted on a balloon-expandable stainless steel stent. The first procedure was done via an antegrade approach in a subset of patients with severe AS who were not surgical candidates for reasons of compassion.[17-20] Moderate to severe aortic insufficiency, valve embolization, and procedural complexity limited diffusion of the procedure. Significant technical and prosthetic modifications solved the previously encountered limitations. To reduce the degree of perivalvular regurgitation, valves were oversized in relation to the aortic annulus, and a second prosthesis size, 26 mm, became available. The transverse diameter of the aortic annulus at the level of aortic leaflet insertion was identified for appropriate valve sizing. In addition the necessary landmarks for valve positioning were recognized, decreasing the risk of valve embolization. A catheter with a manually activated deflectable tip (Retroflex catheter; Edwards LifeSciences, Irvine, Calif.) that aids in the atraumatic passage across the aortic arch and in centering the guidewire through the aortic commissures facilitated the valve delivery through the retrograde approach. Modifications in the delivery sheath also reduced vascular complications. Sheath length was increased to deliver the catheter/valve ensemble directly in the descending aorta, decreasing the risk of vascular injury.[21] Multicenter registries from the United States (REVIVAL II), the European Union (REVIVE II), and Canada (Canadian Special Access) included patients with a valve area less than 0.8 cm^2 and a high predicted operative mortality (logistic European System for Cardiac Operative Risk Evaluation [EuroSCORE] >20%) to continue to evaluate procedural safety and efficacy. New valve modifications were added to improve long-term function; these included use of

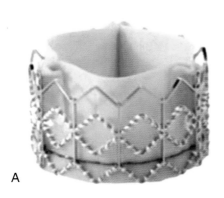
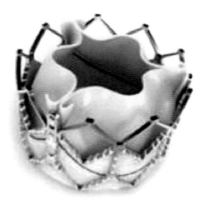

Figure 6–1 **A,** The Edwards SAPIEN valve is a trileaflet bovine pericardial valve mounted on a balloon-expandable stainless steel stent that is placed in the subcoronary position. A positron emission tomography (PET) skirt is placed around the ventricular third of the valve to decrease perivalvular insufficiency. **B,** The second generation SAPIEN XT valve has a new bovine pericardial leaflet design, is mounted on a cobalt chromium stent that reduces its profile, and has a longer skirt to minimize perivalvular insufficiency.

bovine pericardium, elongation of the skirt to decrease perivalvular insufficiency, and the addition of an anticalcification treatment, culminating in the prosthesis that is currently used **(Figure 6–1).** The series of retrograde implantation published by Webb et al[21] showed initial procedural success of 78%, which increased to 96% after the first 25 cases, reflecting an important learning curve.[22] Observed 30-day mortality was 12%, and the expected 30-day mortality was 28%. At median follow-up examination, there was no evidence of valve deterioration, migration, restenosis, or central valvular insufficiency. Moderate perivalvular leaks were seen in three cases at 1 month. Perivalvular AI was mild, clinically inconsequential, and stable during follow-up study in the majority of the patients. This information led to the approval and valve commercialization in Europe in the fall of 2007.

Minimal arterial diameter, vessel tortuosity, and vessel calcification were still the major limiting factors. For these patients the transapical (TA) approach was envisioned. Initial experience in an animal model has been extrapolated to early human experience with promising results.[23,24] The first published data related to the TA approach was from Lichtenstein et al[23] and consisted of 7 high-risk patients with AS. Valve implantation was successful in all with no procedural deaths. Transvalvular gradient and aortic valve area improvement was seen in all patients, and the results were consistent with those found after retrograde implantation. Observed 30-day mortality was lower than the expected mortality (14% vs. 35%).[25] Published multicenter experience using this innovative approach has been growing. Walther et al.[26] reported 93.2% successful implantations with a conversion rate to traditional AVR of 6.8%.

Procedural success continues to improve as the procedure becomes more refined and patient selection is perfected. The completion of the first randomized trial using TAVR in high-risk or otherwise inoperable patients (Placement of AoRTic TraNscathetER Valve [PARTNER]) has established TAVR as part of the treatment armamentarium. With current results, TAVR carries the potential of offering a therapeutic option to patients who, until recently, have been left untreated and also to revolutionize the treatment of severe AS and prosthetic dysfunction.

The remainder of the chapter addresses patient selection, technique, vascular access management, and complications and reviews the most recent body of literature surrounding TAVR.

6.1 Patient Selection for Transcatheter Aortic Valve Replacement

Transfemoral (TF)–TAVR was the first approved route for TAVR in the United States for patients with severe symptomatic AS who have a prohibitive surgical risk as documented by two independent surgeons. TAVR via the TA approach, or the use of TAVR (irrespective of the approach), in patients with severe AS who have a high surgical risk is commercially available outside of the United States and was approved by the FDA for use in the United States in 2012. Patient selection is critical for procedural and clinical success and will be discussed in detail in the following section.

RISK STRATIFICATION

Patients are considered to have a high operative risk when their projected mortality is in the upper decile or have a 30-day mortality greater than 15%. Surgical risk is most commonly estimated by the Society of Thoracic Surgery Predicted Risk of Mortality (STS-PROM) and the EuroSCORE. The EuroSCORE has been validated in patients undergoing valvular surgery.[27,28] However, this algorithm has been shown to persistently overestimate the mortality rate.[29,30] The STS-PROM score is derived from the STS database, a voluntary registry of practice outcomes, and estimates the risk of mortality, morbidity, renal failure, and length of stay after valvular and nonvalvular cardiac surgery.[31] This score has been shown to underestimate the true mortality rate after cardiac surgery, but it more closely reflects the operative and 30-day mortality for the patients having AVR who are at the highest risk.[32]

The STS-PROM and the EuroSCORE provide an objective way to quantify risk. Although thorough, these risk scores do not include certain characteristics that would complicate surgery and increase the operative mortality such as previous mediastinal irradiation, the presence of a severe calcification in the thoracic aorta (porcelain aorta), anatomic abnormality of the chest wall, history of mediastinitis, liver cirrhosis, or patient's frailty. In addition, the algorithms were calculated from patients who underwent surgery, thus limiting their applicability to patients who were not considered surgical candidates. Clinical judgment and the patient's level of independent function are subjective parameters that influence outcomes after cardiac surgery but are difficult to measure.[33] Judicious use of TAVR is recommended in order to maximize appropriate outcomes.

6.2 Patient Screening

The evaluation of all patients undergoing TAVR should include:

1. A screening echocardiogram to document the severity of AS, verify the absence of other severe valvular disease, describe the valve anatomy and calcium distribution, and determine aortic annular diameter and left ventricular function. The presence of a protuberant septum at the level of the left ventricular outflow tract is important to note, because its presence may impede appropriate valve deployment.
2. Right and left catheterization to determine the presence of pulmonary hypertension and concomitant CAD, which may need to be treated before valve implantation.
3. Aortic angiography to note the correct orientation of the image intensifier during valve positioning and to determine potential complicating factors in the aortic arch that may interfere with the procedure.
4. Thoracoabdominal computed tomography (CT) angiography with iliofemoral runoff to determine the anatomy of the aorta, the vessel diameter, calcification, and tortuosity.

VASCULAR SCREENING

After the screening process has been completed and the patients have been deemed eligible for TAVR, the route of implantation needs to be determined. There are two implantation routes available for the Edwards SAPIEN (Edwards Lifesciences, Irvine, Calif.) valve: (1) TA and (2) TF. Both delivery methods are comparable in success and complication rates. Selection depends on tortuosity, calcification, and internal diameter of the femoral, external iliac, and common iliac arteries. The presence of abdominal aortic aneurysms or history of their repair would favor the use of a TA or subclavian approach. Vascular complications have been associated with significant mortality and may be prevented with appropriate screening.[34] Safety should not be sacrificed if both approaches are available and patients are considered good candidates.

Contrast angiography provides an appropriate screening tool for route selection[35]; however, it does not provide a detailed determination of the vascular anatomy. The presence of an outer sheath diameter–to–femoral artery minimal luminal diameter ratio of 1.05 or greater is a predictor of major vascular complications and 30-day mortality.[36,37] By inserting a guidewire across the iliac arteries, one can evaluate the degree that the vessels will

TABLE 6–1 ▮

Minimal Vessel Diameter Requirements for Arterial Transcatheter Aortic Valve Replacement

Valve Size	Sheath Size	Minimal Arterial Diameter
SAPIEN		
23 mm	22F	7 mm
26 mm	24F	8 mm
SAPIEN XT		
23 mm	18F	6 mm
26 mm	19F	6.5 mm

straighten; if the arteries persist with significant tortuosities after insertion of a stiff guidewire, a TA approach is preferred. Multislice computed tomographic angiography (MSCTA) allows for precise determination of the degree, extent, and localization of vascular calcification. In addition, three-dimensional vessel reconstruction and cross-sectional imaging allow for precise determination of vessel luminal diameter. The minimal luminal diameter and the length of the segment with the minimal luminal diameter are the main considerations for selecting the delivery approach. Contrasted MSCTA is preferred; however, if chronic renal insufficiency precludes the use of a fully contrasted study, then intraarterial administration of a small contrast bolus[38] or a noncontrasted CT may provide appropriate images for the necessary measurements. The use of intravascular ultrasound provides an invasive way of measuring the arterial diameter; however, it may provide unreliable dimensions because of image obliquity.

The first generation Edwards SAPIEN valve requires minimal luminal diameters of 7 and 8 mm to allow for the 22F and 24F sheaths that are required for valve delivery. The new Edwards SAPIEN XT valve allows for use in vessels of 6 and 6.5 mm, requiring 18F and 19F sheaths, respectively **(Table 6–1)**. Special attention needs to be given at the level of the aortoiliac and internal–external iliac artery bifurcations, because these areas tend to be involved in vascular complications.

Aortic Annulus Diameter and Prosthetic Sizing

The aortic annulus diameter can be measured with different imaging modalities: transthoracic echocardiogram (TTE), transesophageal echocardiogram (TEE), contrast angiography, multislice computed tomography (MSCT), or magnetic resonance imaging (MRI). The diameter is measured in midsystole at the level of leaflet insertion. Because of the lack of a sewing ring, catheter-based prostheses need to be oversized by 5% to 30% relative to the aortic annulus in order to ensure valve stability and diminish AI. The aortic annulus appears to be noncircular, which may lead to underestimation by planar imaging. MSCT provides coronal, sagittal, and axial images of the annulus and aortic root, allowing the determination of the minimal and maximal diameter, annular circumference, and area.[39,40] Annular determinations by TTE or TEE appear to be most commonly obtained. However, as the annular

TABLE 6–2

Baseline and Follow-up Characteristics of Patients Undergoing TAVI with the Edwards SAPIEN Valve

Study	Patients	Age (years)	Logistic EuroSCORE (%)	STS Score (%)	Procedural Success (%)	AVA Pre (cm²)	AVA Post (cm²)
Canada	339	81 ± 8	NR	9.8	93.3%	0.63 ± 0.17	1.55 ± 0.41
Source	1038	81.2	27.4	NR	93.8	0.59	1.7
Partner	358	83.1 ± 8	26.4 ± 17.2	11.6 ± 6	96.6	0.6 ± 0.2	1.5 ± 0.5

AVA, Aortic valve area; *LVEF,* left ventricular ejection fraction; *NR,* not reported; *NYHA,* New York Heart Association classification; *TAVI,* transcatheter aortic valve implantation.

determination becomes more uniform, it is expected that MSCT will be the primary sizing modality **(Table 6–2).**

CORONARY DISEASE

Patients with concomitant CAD have higher operative mortality risk scores and associated comorbidities than those without CAD. It is recommended to revascularize the vessels that supply a large area of myocardium at risk while disregarding the smaller branches before TAVR.[41-43] The timing of revascularization is controversial. Patients enrolled in the PARTNER trial required a minimum of 30 days between coronary revascularization and valve implant. Revascularization is generally preferred before TAVR if the amount of myocardium at risk is large. It can be done in the same setting before TAVR or a couple of days earlier in order to minimize radiation and contrast exposure and other potential complications.

CEREBROVASCULAR DISEASE

Patients considered for TAVR are generally elderly and have multiple comorbidities (CAD, peripheral vascular disease, hypertension, previous stroke or transient ischemic attacks [TIAs]) that predispose them to cerebrovascular events with AVR. Heavy atheromata of the ascending aorta or transverse arch and bulky calcium or mobile debris on the aortic valve are also considered risk factors for neurologic complications with TAVR. Patients at risk should undergo carotid Doppler examination, and lesions that are flow-limiting or with high-risk characteristics should be considered for treatment before TAVR.

CHRONIC OBSTRUCTIVE PULMONARY DISEASE

Severe pulmonary disease and AS are commonly manifested with dyspnea. In patients with concomitant severe AS and severe pulmonary disease being considered for TAVR, it must be emphasized that symptom improvement after valve replacement may be limited to the reversible component caused by AS. Symptoms of heart failure may be misdiagnosed as a chronic obstructive pulmonary disease (COPD) exacerbation or progression. Careful evaluation to clarify the origin of the symptoms will ensure better clinical outcomes after TAVR.

6.3 The Edwards SAPIEN Valve

The Edwards SAPIEN valve consists of a bioprosthetic valve, the balloon catheter on which it is mounted, the Retroflex catheter, and the crimping tool.

THE EDWARDS SAPIEN VALVE

The Edwards SAPIEN Valve **(see Figure 6–1)** is a trileaflet bioprosthesis made of bovine pericardium that is mounted in a balloon-expandable stainless steel stent. It has been pretreated to decrease calcification and functional deterioration. The stent has a fabric cuff placed in the ventricular side that covers one half of the frame, limiting stent expansion and decreasing perivalvular insufficiency. Because of the lack of a sewing ring, the valve is oversized to the aortic annulus to ensure postdeployment stability and is currently available in two sizes: 23 mm and 26 mm. In bench-top testing, its durability is greater than 10 years. The SAPIEN valve provides a larger effective orifice area and lower hemodynamic profile than corresponding surgically implanted valves but have a higher incidence of perivalvular insufficiency.[44]

The new generation device, the Edwards SAPIEN XT valve, is commercialized in Europe and made of a cobalt–chromium alloy that provides the same radial strength yet reduces the valve profile. This valve is available in 20-mm, 23-mm, 26-mm, and 29-mm sizes. The ongoing PARTNER II Trial is designed to evaluate this valve technology **(see Figure 6–1).**

THE BALLOON CATHETER

The valve is mounted on a custom made balloon that is 30 mm in length with balloon diameters that correspond to the prosthesis size. The balloon ends in a nose cone that facilitates crossing the native valve **(Figure 6–2).** Its inflation profile decreases movement during inflation.

THE CRIMPING TOOL

A crimping tool **(see Figure 6–2)** is used to manually and symmetrically compress the overall diameter of the transcatheter heart valve (THV) from its expanded size to its minimal delivery profile. A measuring ring is used to calibrate the balloon inflation to its desired size and to determine the volume of saline/contrast mixture in

Mean gradient Pre (mmHg)	Mean gradient Post (mmHg)	NYHA III/IV Pre (%)	NYHA III/IV Post (%)	LVEF Pre (%)	LVEF Post (%)	Survival 1 year (%)
46 ± 17	10 ± 4	90.9	NR	55 ± 14	NR	76
53.5	3.95	79.2	10	NR	NR	NR
44.5 ± 15.7	11 ± 6.9	92	16.7	53.9	57.2	69.3

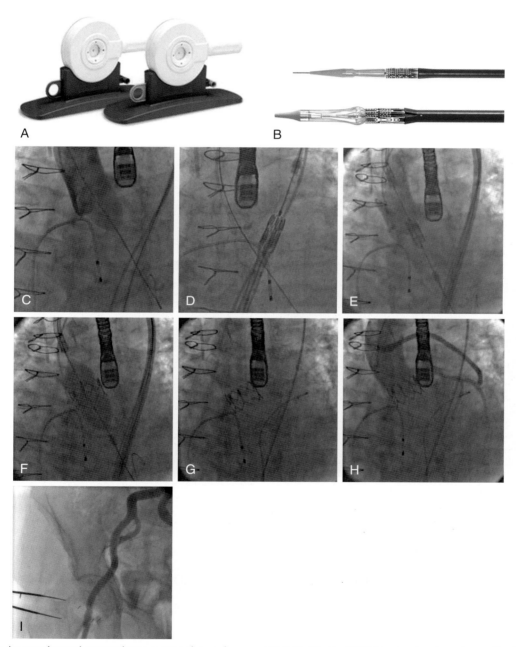

Figure 6–2 For the transfemoral transcatheter aortic valve replacement (TAVR) **(A)**, the SAPIEN valve is crimped over the delivery catheter **(B)**. Supraaortic angiography is performed in a view that places all three coronary cusps in the same plane. **C**, A balloon aortic valvuloplasty (BAV) is performed to facilitate valve positioning. The delivery catheter is advanced through the descending aorta **(D)**. The retroflex catheter is activated to allow the passage of the valve through the aortic arch. Correct valve position is confirmed by echo and angiography **(E)**, the valve is deployed during rapid ventricular pacing (RVP) **(F)**. Aortic angiography confirms valve position, lack of aortic insufficiency, and unrestricted flow through native coronary arteries and bypass grafts (**G** and **H**). The delivery sheath is removed and iliofemoral angiography is performed to confirm the absence of vascular complications **(I)**.

the syringe necessary for the proper inflation at the time of deployment.

THE RETROFLEX GUIDING CATHETER AND THE ASCENDRA DELIVERY SYSTEM

The Retroflex catheter has a deflectable tip that changes direction when activated by the rotation of an actuator incorporated in the handle, facilitating the passage of the THV across the aortic arch from the retrograde approach[45] **(see Figure 6–2).** The catheter is used to direct the valve delivery system through the arterial system, around the aortic arch, and across the aortic valve, providing a less traumatic passage. The Retroflex catheter assists in centering and supporting the valve as it crosses the calcified and stenotic native valve. This system also provides precise positioning at the aortic annulus. The Novoflex catheter (Edwards Lifesciences, Irvine, Calif.) is a newer generation catheter that allows

loading the Edwards SAPIEN XT prosthesis onto the balloon while it is in the body, decreasing the sheath size dramatically.

The Ascendra delivery system (Edwards LifeSciences, Irvine, Calif.) is the delivery catheter used for the TS route **(Figure 6–3).** This catheter allows for easy valve manipulation to improve the prosthetic orientation.

DELIVERY SHEATH

The THV assembly and deflecting guiding catheter are introduced through a 25-cm hydrophilic coated sheath that extends into the abdominal aorta to decrease vascular complications. The TF delivery system for the SAPIEN valve requires 22F and 24F sheaths for the 23- and 26-mm valves, respectively. With the introduction of SAPIEN XT and Novoflex, the insertion sheath has decreased to 18F and 19F, respectively. The sheath is equipped with a hemostatic mechanism to decrease blood loss. For the

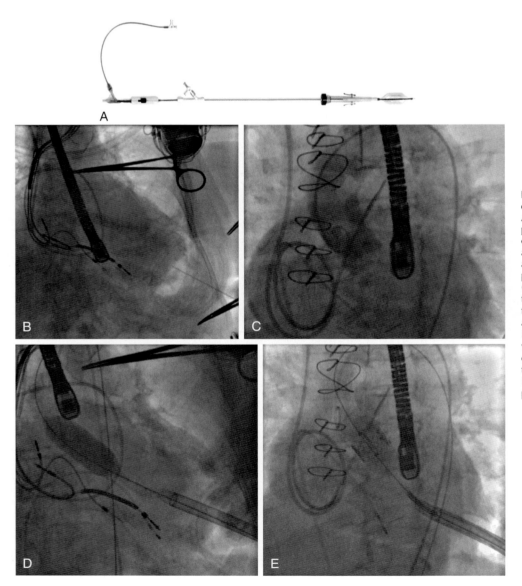

Figure 6–3 Transapical delivery of the SAPIEN valve requires the Ascendra delivery system **(A).** The procedure starts with a lateral thoracotomy. After the heart is exposed and a purse string suture is placed around the puncture site, a needle is placed in the left ventricle (LV) apex **(B)** to mark the trajectory. **C,** An aortic angiogram is performed to align the aortic cusps in the same plane, and the delivery sheath is inserted into the LV cavity. **D,** A balloon valvuloplasty is performed through the delivery sheath during rapid ventricular pacing (RVP). **E,** The valve is then advanced to its appropriate position and deployed during RVP.

23-mm THV, the introducer sheath has an outer diameter of 7.2 mm (21.6F) and an inner diameter of 6 mm (18F). For the 26-mm THV, the introducer sheath has an outer diameter of 7.5 mm (22.5F) and inner diameter of 6.3 mm (19F). Other improvements in the access sheath include the development of the eSheath (Edwards Lifescience, Irvine, Calif.). The eSheath has a dynamic expansion mechanism that allows the sheath to transiently expand as the Novoflex delivery system is pushed forward and then recoil to its nominal diameter. The eSheath has an inner diameter of 5.3 mm (16F) and outer diameter of 6.6 mm (20F) for implantation of the 23-mm THV and an inner diameter of 6.0 mm (18F) and outer diameter of 7.2 mm (21 to 22F) for implantation of the 26-mm THV.

The transapical (TA) delivery sheath is 26F in diameter, is shorter, and has a flexible tip to decrease trauma when placed in the left ventricle (LV).

6.4 Transfemoral Valve Implantation

ROOM REQUIREMENTS

TF–TAVR can be performed in the cardiac catheterization lab or in the hybrid operating room, provided that the room is equipped with a fixed fluoroscopy unit that provides high image quality and the ability to store reference images for road-mapping. There must be enough room for operators to work comfortably and the circulators to move freely. A cardiopulmonary bypass machine should be accessible if complications arise. Equipment to treat peripheral vascular or coronary complications should be stocked in the room and available on demand (see Figure 6–2).

ANESTHESIA

The procedure can be done when the patient is under general anesthesia[46,47] or conscious sedation. General anesthesia is preferred if a TEE is performed simultaneously during the procedure. If not, conscious sedation and local anesthesia may provide enough relief during the procedure. Continuous invasive hemodynamic monitoring should be used throughout the procedure.

INFECTION AND ANTITHROMBOTIC PROPHYLAXIS

In order to decrease the risk of prosthetic infection, measures to reduce infection are taken. Patients are given procedural antibiotics as dictated by local practice. Aspirin (325 mg) and clopidogrel (300 mg) are administered 24 hours before the procedure.

VENOUS AND ARTERIAL ACCESS

In the ipsilateral leg, femoral arterial access is obtained for aortic angiography with a 5F to 6 F pigtail catheter, and a venous sheath is inserted for rapid ventricular pacing (RVP). The contralateral artery is cannulated percutaneously or by surgical cutdown. If accessed percutaneously, it can be preclosed with two suture mediated devices (10F Prostar; Abbott Vascular, Abbott Park, Ill.). If a surgical cutdown is performed, the common femoral artery should not be completely dissected in the posterior aspect, because the sheath insertion is easier when the vessel is partially anchored.

AORTIC ANGIOGRAPHY

Ascending aortic angiography is performed in a projection that places all aortic cusps in line and perpendicular to the image intensifier. The ideal projection should have been previously determined using CT angiography or coronary angiography in order to minimize the radiation and contrast exposure.

TEMPORARY PACEMAKER PLACEMENT

A temporary transvenous pacemaker is placed in the right ventricle. After testing for appropriate capture, an RVP test is performed at a rate of 180 to 220 beats per minute (BPM).

If the pacemaker is unstable, then inserting it over a Mullins Sheath should be considered.

CROSSING THE AORTIC VALVE

Once the patient's blood is anticoagulated with heparin and a therapeutic activated clotting time (ACT) is confirmed (>300 sec), the native aortic valve is crossed using an Amplatz AL-2 catheter and a straight guidewire. The previously shaped Amplatz Extra Stiff 0.035-inch guidewire is then exchanged through the AL-2, and the catheter is withdrawn while maintaining the distal wire position in the LV. Simultaneous aortic and ventricular pressures are obtained for aortic valve area calculation.

DELIVERY SHEATH INSERTION

With the guidewire coiled in the LV apex, the previously inserted 8F sheath is removed. Serial dilation of the femoral and iliac arteries is performed with arterial dilators of increasing size (16F to 25F). The delivery sheath is then inserted and positioned in the descending aorta. If there is severe vascular tortuosity, the insertion of a supportive wire before the insertion of the delivery sheath minimizes complications.

BALLOON AORTIC VALVULOPLASTY

Balloon aortic valvuloplasty (BAV) is performed during RVP before TAVR. A 20-mm or 23-mm Retroflex balloon (Edwards LifeSciences, Irvine, Calif.) are used for placement of a 23-mm or 26-mm SAPIEN prosthesis. The valve prosthesis should be ready to be inserted before the completion of the BAV because of the possibility that severe AI and hemodynamic instability develops.

VALVE INSERTION AND DEPLOYMENT

The SAPIEN prosthesis and the delivery system are then inserted in the sheath over the Ampltaz Extra Stiff wire.

Once the delivery system reaches the aortic arch the Retroflex catheter is activated, allowing the safe passage of the delivery system across the aortic arch. The system is then advanced until it reaches the ascending aorta. In the predetermined reference projection (aortic annulus perpendicular to the screen, the valve is positioned in the aortic position, maintaining a 60% to 40% ratio of ventricular/aortic positioning. After confirmation of the appropriate location with angiography (and TEE if available), the valve is deployed during RVP. The valve is deployed after the confirmation that the systemic blood pressure has reached and maintained its nadir. Balloon inflation is held 3 to 5 seconds before deflation and then RVP is stopped in order to avoid traction on the prosthesis while the balloon catheter is being withdrawn. The RVP run generally does not last longer than 15 seconds. The delivery system is straightened and withdrawn. The transvalvular gradient is measured, and paravalvular leaks are evaluated by angiography and echocardiography. If the amount of perivalvular AI is significant, then postdilation with the same delivery balloon adding 1 to 2 cm of volume is considered.

Delivery of the SAPIEN XT valve requires other steps, because the valve prosthesis is loaded and fully crimped inside the body. After sheath insertion, the Novoflex catheter is advanced until it is positioned in the descending aorta. Once positioned in a straight portion of the aorta, valve alignment and loading onto the balloon is obtained with catheter manipulation. The valve is then advanced across the aortic arch while activating the Retroflex component and positioned as desired. The valve is deployed under RVP. Once the delivery system is being retrieved, it is crucial to dearticulate the Novoflex catheter, preventing vascular injury.

SHEATH REMOVAL AND ARTERIOTOMY CLOSURE

The sheath is withdrawn with careful monitoring of blood pressure and simultaneous contrast administration through the pigtail catheter placed at the level of the iliac bifurcation. A precipitous drop in the blood pressure or extravasation of contrast media indicates a vascular rupture. This complication should be treated appropriately and expeditiously using a covered stent or surgical repair. Immediate tamponade of the ruptured vessel with the large sheath and/or closure of the iliac artery or abdominal aorta with a large-size balloon can be urgently performed before arterial repair. A covered stent is recommended when there is vessel rupture or extravasation of contrast. A noncovered stent is aimed at patients with dissection that does not penetrate the vessel or in the presence of a bifurcating vessel. The arteriotomy site is then closed surgically or percutaneously with the previously placed preclosure device.

If percutaneous closure is performed, it is recommended that a guidewire is advanced from the contralateral side up to the superficial femoral artery to ensure access to this site if a vascular complication occurs. It is recommended to occlude the iliac artery with a vascular balloon in order to assist in obtaining hemostasis at the site of large-bore catheter insertion.[48] After hemostasis is confirmed, the balloon is deflated and removed. Control angiography should be performed to confirm vessel patency and rule out vascular injury.

TRANSAPICAL APPROACH

The procedural steps of valve deployment are relatively similar to the TF route, and as such only the differences will be illustrated[25] **(see Figure 6–3).** Femoral arterial and venous access is obtained for aortic root angiography and RVP as previously described. A small left lateral thoracotomy is performed. The planes are dissected until the LV apex is visualized. A purse string suture is placed in a muscular segment of the apicolateral wall that was selected via TEE guidance. Once the patient's blood has been anticoagulated and the ACT is therapeutic, a direct puncture of the LV is performed and a 7F or 8F sheath is inserted into the LV. Guided with a Judkins right (JR) curve catheter, a 0.035-inch J-tipped wire is then advanced through the valve into the descending aorta. The wire must be free of the papillary muscles and mitral chordal structures in order to avoid complications with the insertion of the delivery sheath. Once in the descending aorta, the wire is exchanged for an extra-stiff wire, (such as the 0.035-inch Amplatz Super Stiff guidewire; Boston Scientific, Minneapolis, Minn.) and the JR catheter is removed. The sheath is exchanged for a 26F delivery sheath that is inserted 3 to 4 cm into the LV cavity. Under RVP a BAV is performed with a 20-mm Retroflex balloon. The Ascendra delivery system is advanced into the sheath and deaired. The valve/catheter ensemble is advanced into the aortic position, maintaining a ratio of 50:50 aortic/ventricular position. After confirmation of the appropriate position by TEE and angiography, RVP and a patient breathhold is begun. The valve is deployed as the blood pressure is at its nadir, and the balloon is deflated and withdrawn. Once the degree of AI is assessed and the valve position has been confirmed by TEE, the ventricular sheath can be removed.

If the valve needs to be postdilated, then this procedure follows. If no further intervention is needed, then the delivery sheath is removed (under RVP), the puncture site is repaired, and the anticoagulation is reversed. The thoracotomy is closed over a drain.

The transaortic approach requires the puncture in the ascending aorta and is being evaluated in the PARTNER II trial.

MANAGEMENT OF VASCULAR ACCESS

Selecting the appropriate site for TF access is critical for successfully replacing the aortic valve and avoiding vascular complications. The arterial puncture site selection will depend on the artery that: 1) has the largest lumen, 2) has the least amount of calcification at the puncture site, 3) has the least amount of tortuosity, and 4) is the most accessible. For the insertion of larger delivery systems, it is recommended to obtain surgical exposure of the vessel with appropriate distal and proximal arterial control with vessel loops. The vessel is then palpated to select the appropriate puncture site and note the presence of atherosclerotic plaque in the area adjacent to the site of sheath entry. A smaller sheath (5F to 7F) is inserted initially using the standard Seldinger technique. A supportive wire (Amplatz Extra Stiff or Lundequist [Cook Medical, Bloomington, Ind.]) is used to facilitate arterial dilation and navigate the vessel tortuosity. It is important to minimize dwell time of the sheath in order to prevent the adhesion of the endothelium to the hydrophilic coating of the sheath, which would precipitate complications during sheath removal.

During the insertion of the 22F or 24F sheath, it is important to visualize the insertion point of the sheath into the artery. Particular attention should be placed to the transition point of the dilator and sheath, because it may "catch" on the vessel wall as it is being inserted. If the sheath is unable to be inserted past this point, then it may be helpful to use a Cook sheath (Cook Medical, Bloomington, Ind.) of the same size, which facilitates a smoother transition from dilator to sheath.

With the smaller and newer delivery systems, using a preclosure system is helpful.[48] The puncture site is selected by ultrasound guidance or placing a pigtail catheter at the desired puncture site from the contralateral groin. Once access is obtained, then two Pro-Glide closure devices (Abbott Medical, Abbott Park, Ill.) are placed at 90 degrees from each other. Without losing wire access, an 8F sheath is then used to maintain access while crossing the aortic valve and performing the valve replacement as noted earlier. Access from the contralateral groin is exchanged for a 7F 45-cm Flexor sheath (Cook Medical, Bloomington, Ind.) that is advanced across the aortoiliac bifurcation, and a 0.018-inch guidewire is advanced and maintained in the superficial femoral artery. After valve replacement, a peripheral angioplasty balloon sized to the iliac arterial lumen is inserted over the 0.018-inch guidewire. Once the balloon is in place in the external iliacs, the delivery sheath is removed as the balloon is expanded, occluding flow distal to the iliac and femoral artery. The preclosure knots are secured, and once hemostasis is obtained the balloon is deflated to ensure hemostasis.

Contrast angiography then confirms blood flow and lack of extravasation of contrast. If complications are observed (dissections, avulsions, or vessel interruptions) then the necessary steps for percutaneous or open treatment are followed. The use of an aortic occlusion balloon is lifesaving in the setting of vascular perforation, rupture, or avulsion.

OUTCOMES

The results of TAVR for severe AS are encouraging. The majority of the data has been driven by postmarketing registries and one randomized multicenter clinical trial evaluating the Edwards SAPIEN valve. As the field of TAVR expands, it has become apparent that a standardized method of assessing efficacy and safety of this new technology is necessary. As a result, the Valvular

Academic Research Consortium (VARC)[49] was established with the goals of:

1. Determination of homogenous clinical endpoints reflecting safety and efficacy.
2. Standardization of definition of endpoints in valve-related clinical trials.

A brief synopsis of the most important trials and registry data utilizing the SAPIEN valve follows.

Placement of AoRTic TraNscathetER Valve (PARTNER) U.S. Trial

The PARTNER U.S. trial was the first prospective, randomized, multicenter trial for THVs. Patient evaluation and selection was required by a heart valve team consisting of surgeons and cardiologists who deemed patients suitable for inclusion. The trial consisted of two individually powered patient cohorts with severe symptomatic AS:

1. Cohort A[5] included patients with high estimated surgical mortality (STS risk score >10%) and randomized them 1:1 to AVR vs. TAVR using the Edwards SAPIEN prosthesis.
2. Cohort B[51] included inoperable patients whose life expectancy was longer than 1 year and randomized them to optimal medical therapy (including BAV) vs. TAVR using the Edwards SAPIEN valve.

Cohort A

In the high-risk operable arm, TAVR was noninferior when compared with surgical AVR at 1 year for all-cause mortality (24% vs. 27%, $p = .001$ for noninferiority). When compared with surgery, TAVR was associated with a higher rate of stroke and TIAs at 30 days (5.5% vs. 2.4%, $p = .04$) and at 1 year (8.3% vs. 4.3%, $p = .04$).[50] Both treatments resulted in important improvements in patients' quality of life at a 1-year follow-up examination.[51] For patients eligible for the TF approach, TAVR resulted in substantial quality of life benefit over surgical AVR at 1 month, with similar benefits at 6-month and 1-year follow-up examinations. For patients eligible only for the TS approach, there was no benefit of TAVR over surgery at any time point, and quality of life tended to be better in the surgical group at 1 and 6 months follow-up examination.

Cohort B

All-cause mortality (30.7% vs. 50.7%, $p < .001$), cardiovascular mortality (19.6% vs. 41.9%, $p < .001$), repeat hospitalization (22.3% vs. 44.1%, $p < .001$), and the composite endpoint of death or repeat hospitalization (42.5% vs.71.6%, $p < .001$) was seen less often in patients randomized to TAVR. In follow-up studies, there was no evident degeneration of the valvular prosthesis or restenosis. Heart failure symptoms were less severe in patients treated with TAVR. Patients treated with TAVR had a higher incidence of major vascular complications

TABLE 6–3

Procedural Characteristics and Complications of Patients Undergoing TAVI with the Edwards SAPIEN Valve

Study	Procedural Mortality (%)	30-Day Mortality (%)	Valve in Valve (%)	Conversion to Open AVR (%)	AI > 2+ (%)
Canada TF	1.8	9.5	2.4	1.2	6
Canada TA	1.7	11.3	2.8	2.3	6
Source TA	NR	10.3	0.03	3.5	2.3
Source TF	NR	6.3	0.006	1.7	1.5
PARTNER	1.1	5.0	1.7	0	12

AI, Aortic insufficiency; *AVR,* aortic valve replacement; *NR,* not reported; *PARTNER,* Placement of AoRTic TraNscathetER Valve; *TAVI,* transcatheter aortic valve implantation; *TA,* transapical; *TF,* transfemoral.

(16.2% vs 1.1%, $p < .001$), major bleeding (22.3% vs. 11.2%, $p < .001$), and of major strokes (5.0% vs. 1.1%, $p = .06$).[52] In patients with severe AS who are not suitable for AVR, TAVR should be the new standard of care. The survival advantage continues to 2 years.[53] Improvement in the quality of life was apparent in patients at 30 days and 1 year compared with the control group,[54] and the procedure appeared to be cost effective.[55]

Canadian Edwards Registry

The Canadian Registry of the Edwards SAPIEN valve from 2005 to 2009 in six centers enrolled 339 patients with severe AS and high surgical risk treated with TA-TAVR (50.4%) and TF-TAVR (49.6%).[56] The procedural success was 93.3% with a 30-day mortality of 10.4%. Mortality was 22% at a mean follow-up study of 8 months with periprocedural sepsis, need for hemodynamic support, chronic kidney disease, and COPD as independent predictors of late mortality regardless of the approach. Patients with porcelain aorta and frailty had acute outcomes similar to the overall cohort, and patients with porcelain aorta had as good or better survival rates at a 1-year follow-up examination **(Table 6–3).**

SOURCE Registry

The Edwards SAPIEN Aortic Bioprosthesis European Outcome (SOURCE) Registry included 1123 consecutive patients who underwent TAVR in 32 centers across Europe and was created for postmarketing surveillance. Seventy-two of the enrolling centers had no prior experience with the SAPIEN valve and underwent a structured training program. Procedural success was 93.8% with a 30-day mortality of 6.3%.[57] Single-center experience noted a 30-day mortality as low as 3.6%.[58] At 30 days, functional improvement was dramatic (NYHA class I/II at baseline; 19% vs. 86% at 30 days, $p < .001$), and mean survival at 224 days was 74%.

Symptomatic improvement persists during follow-up care without evidence of valve structural deterioration, progression of AI, or restenosis. The complication rates have decreased since the original experience: major vascular complications in 8% of the TF implantations, tamponade in 4%, permanent pacemaker in 4.4%, infection in 2.4%, and stroke in 5.3% **(see Table 6–3).**[57] Although vascular injury was less common in the TA group, when present it was associated with a higher mortality rate.

The 30-day and 1-year mortality rates in the TA group are higher when compared with the TF group; however this is likely the result of a selection bias. Patients who undergo the TA approach are generally older, have a higher degree of comorbidities, and have a higher EuroSCORE. In addition, the procedure is more invasive and has a steeper learning curve. To date, TF valve implantation is the default strategy, and the TA approach is only offered to those who do not qualify for the TF approach. Nonrandomized comparisons of patients at high risk undergoing surgical AVR vs. TA-TAVR show similar operative mortality rates, similar 1-year survival rates, shorter intensive care unit (ICU) stays, and shorter duration of mechanical ventilation.[59,60] In general, the TA approach is complementary to the TF approach because a number of patients are not candidates to the TF approach as a result of the presence of peripheral vascular disease; up to 70% are not considered surgical candidates and would remain untreated.[56]

FRANCE Registry

In November 2009, the results of the French Aortic National CoreValve and Edwards (FRANCE) Registry were released from 19 sites. Patients in this registry had similar baseline demographics to the European PARTNER registry, but patients in this registry received either the Edwards SAPIEN valve or the Medtronic CoreValve (Medtronic, Luxembourg).[61] Patients had severe AS with valve areas less than 0.6 cm^2/m^2, NHYA scores greater than 2, high surgical risk with EuroSCORE greater than 20% (STS >10%), or a contraindication for surgery. Patients were treated with either the Edwards SAPIEN valve (TF 39%, TS Edwards 29%) or the CoreValve (27% TF, 5% subclavian). Procedural success was seen in 97% of patients. Major complications of death at 30 days, stroke, vascular complications, and transfusions of more than 1 unit occurred in 13%, 4%, 7%, and 21%, respectively. There were little differences in mortality, stroke, or vascular complications between groups. Higher logistic EuroSCORE, NYHA class III or IV symptoms, TA-TAVR, and paravalvular AI were all associated with decreased survival.[62]

Major CVA/TIA (%)	Major Vascular Complications (%)	MI (%)	Acute Kidney Injury (%)	Pacemaker (%)	Major Bleeding (%)
0.6	13.1	0.6	1.8	3.6	NR
0.6	13	1.7	3.4	6.2	NR
2.6	2.4	0.6	7.1	7	9.9
2.4	10.6	0.6	1.3	7	8.9
5/0	16.2	0	1.1	3.4	16.8

6.5 TAVR in Special Subgroups

FAILING SURGICAL BIOPROSTHETIC VALVES

The operative mortality for an elective redo aortic valve surgery for a degenerated bioprosthesis ranges from 2% to 30% depending on the comorbidities and clinical status.[63-65] Placing a catheter-based prosthesis to alleviate bioprosthetic valve dysfunction (stenosis or regurgitation) is possible (valve in valve [VIV]). Understanding the dimensions, structure, and size of surgical prostheses is crucial for valve selection.[66] The mechanism of failure, fluoroscopic identification of the sewing ring, and determination of the internal diameter of the failed prosthesis is fundamental for VIV implantation. Successful VIV implantations have been reported with the Edwards SAPIEN THV for failing stented and stentless surgical bioprostheses.[67] The resultant transvalvular gradient appears to be higher than in native AS.

BICUSPID VALVES

Although congenital or acquired bicuspid aortic valve stenosis is considered a contraindication to transcatheter aortic valve implantation, several successful case reports have been documented in high-risk individuals.[68-70] Anecdotally, stenotic bicuspid aortic annuli are usually larger and more eccentric than stenotic tricuspid aortic valves.[71,72] As such, three-dimensional imaging is strongly advised for transcatheter aortic valve sizing.

LOWER SURGICAL RISK PATIENTS

TAVR was originally envisioned to open therapeutic options for patients who were otherwise untreated. With the improving safety, efficacy, and ease of delivery, it has become apparent that an increasing number of TAVR procedures are being performed in patients who have a lower risk profile than the patients initially evaluated. The treatment of patients at lower risk has improved clinical outcomes when compared to the higher risk groups.[73] The current treatment of this patient group should be reserved to clinical trials only, because there is no evidence available to endorse this practice. Ongoing trials such as the PARTNER II trial and the SURgical

AVR versus Transcatheter Aortic Valve Implantation (SURTAVI) trial will evaluate TAVR in a group of patients who have severe AS and are at moderate risk.

6.6 Complications

CARDIAC COMPLICATIONS

Heart Block and Arrhythmias

Conduction abnormalities are commonly seen in the patients undergoing TAVR. It is estimated that atrial fibrillation is seen in approximately 12% after TA procedure. The incidence of conduction abnormalities in patients undergoing TAVR with the SAPIEN prosthesis are: 1) complete heart block requiring a pacemaker, 5.7%; 2) left bundle branch block, 12%; and 3) first-degree atrioventricular block, 15%.[74] The presence of a preexisting right bundle branch block is a predisposing factor to pacemaker dependency. Conduction defects are transient when related to trauma to the conduction tissue; however, if there is myocyte necrosis in the interventricular septum then new atrioventricular block will likely develop.[75,76] With the CoreValve revalving system, the insertion depth into the LV cavity and a smaller aortic annulus is associated with complete heart block.[77]

Life-threatening cardiac arrhythmias (e.g., ventricular fibrillation/tachycardia) associated with TAVR can occur in up to 4% of patients.[21]

Cardiac Perforation

Cardiac perforation has been reported in 2% to 4% of patients undergoing TAVR.[78] Cardiac perforation may be the consequence of ventricular injury by the temporary pacemaker lead or stiff guidewire. Small, hypertrophic LV cavities (commonly seen in elderly females) or inadequate preshaping or positioning of the LV support wire may increase the risk for this complication. Procedural TEE can easily detect a pericardial effusion **(Figure 6–4)**.

Severe Aortic Insufficiency

Severe AI is a rare event. According to its etiology it may be categorized as valvular or perivalvular. Valvular

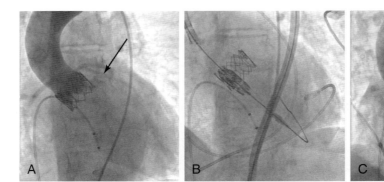

Figure 6–4 A 92-year-old woman with severe aortic stenosis and an aortic annulus of 21 mm underwent placement of a 26-mm SAPIEN XT valve. **A,** After valve implantation she developed chest pain and became progressively hypotensive. Aortic angiography noted an annular rupture *(arrow)*. **B,** Emergent pericardiocentesis was performed relieving the effusion; however, there was persistent reaccumulation. **C,** As a result, a second valve was deployed to "plug the hole," and repeat angiography confirmed the lack of communication with the pericardial space.

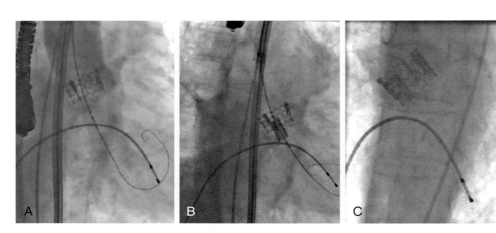

Figure 6–5 An 85-year-old man with severe aortic stenosis and a 20.6 mm aortic annulus underwent placement of a 23-mm SAPIEN XT valve. A, Control aortography demonstrated that the valve was positioned too high (toward the aortic side) with severe paravalvular insufficiency. **B,** A second valve was positioned inferiorly to secure the other valve and correct the paravalvular leak. **C,** Control aortography demonstrated lack of aortic insufficiency and stable position.

(central) AI is most commonly caused by the guidewire and disappears once the wire is removed. It is rarely caused by prosthetic malfunction or when the native leaflets interfere with prosthetic function. This is treated with placement of a new valve inside the previously placed valve **(Figure 6–5).** Perivalvular insufficiency is a result of: 1) inappropriate sizing, 2) malposition, or 3) stent underexpansion. For underexpansion, or malapposition, valve postdilation may be performed cautiously by adding 1 or 2 cc to the same balloon catheter that must be centered within the valve. Because the stent has a skirt that does not allow further expansion, postdilation with a larger balloon will cause flaring of the aortic portion of the stent, changing the conformation of the ventricular portion and worsening the AI. If the valve is inappropriately positioned, then placing a new valve or snaring the prosthesis may limit the amount of AI. The presence of AI has been associated with worse outcomes and, as a result, should be minimized.

Valve Embolization

Valve embolization is generally the result of malposition, undersizing the prosthesis, or inappropriate capture during RVP. Valvular embolization to the LV cavity is uniformly fatal. If aortic embolization occurs, it is imperative not to remove the guidewire from across the

prosthetic valve until it is anchored in the distal aorta, because this prevents it from turning. A balloon catheter is placed in the proximal end of the valve, and the valve is then pulled until it can be deployed or fully expanded after the left subclavian artery. After the embolized valve is fixed, then a new valve can be placed in the aortic position while correcting the original cause of the complication. If the guidewire is removed before the valve is fixed in place, the valve may become inverted, not allowing the passage of blood through it. Unless the valve can be opened with a stent or surgically, this complication is also uniformly fatal. Aortic angiography is recommended after valve embolization to rule out aortic dissection **(Figure 6–6).**

Coronary Obstruction

The SAPIEN prosthesis in placed in the subcoronary position and should not interfere with the coronary ostia or future attempts of percutaneous revascularization.[79] Coronary obstruction occurs in 0.6% of the cases and is seen in patients with effacement of the sinotubular junction, which causes the coronary ostia to migrate.[58] Determination of the distance of the ostia to the aortic annulus by CT angiography is routinely performed during patient screening. Coronary obstruction may be inconsequential if patients have

Figure 6–6 An 84-year-old man with severe aortic stenosis and a 20-mm aortic annulus underwent placement of a 23-mm SAPIEN valve. **A,** After valve deployment the valve embolized to the aorta. **B,** The deployment balloon was advanced proximal to the valve and inflated. **C,** Once inflated, the valve was then pulled to the descending aorta where it was anchored distal to the origin of the left subclavian artery. A new valve was then inserted and positioned appropriately.

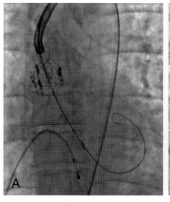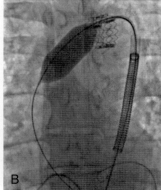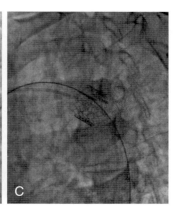

Figure 6–7 An 85-year-old man with severe aortic stenosis and a 24-mm aortic annulus was planned for transfemoral transcatheter aortic valve replacement with a 26-mm SAPIEN valve. **A,** Because of iliac tortuosity, a Lunderquist wire was advanced and serial dilation of the iliac arteries was performed. **B,** Angiography was performed after the 25F dilator and showed external iliac rupture with contrast extravasation *(arrow)*. **C,** A balloon was used to obstruct flow in the distal aorta, allowing placement of a covered stent graft.

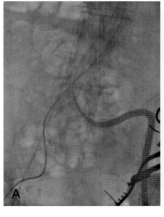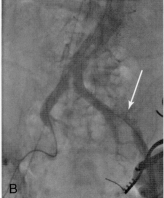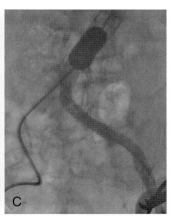

functioning coronary artery bypass grafts. If occlusion occurs, emergency percutaneous revascularization can be performed.

Vascular Complications

Vascular complications occur in 6.6% of cases. They more commonly occur in the TF approach (8% vs. 3.6%),[57] but are more likely to be fatal in the TA approach. Vascular complications include dissection, vascular perforation, and vessel avulsion. Prevention is preferred; hence the importance of vascular screening and the determination of the appropriate luminal diameter and absence of luminal calcification. Although previously associated with higher mortality, with increasing experience, vascular complications are easy to prepare for, thus decreasing their mortality. They may arise from difficult sheath insertion or prolonged sheath time as the adluminal surface adheres to the endothelium **(Figures 6–7 and 6–8).** They are easily recognized by sudden onset of hypotension. Aortic occlusion balloons should be accessible to minimize bleeding while stabilizing the patient. Aortic root dissections may occur if the native valve is not appropriately predilated and the passage of the prosthesis is vigorous, or after attempts to capture an embolized valve. Aortic annular tear is seen in patients with a heavily calcified aortic root and can be avoided by limiting the degree of prosthesis oversizing.

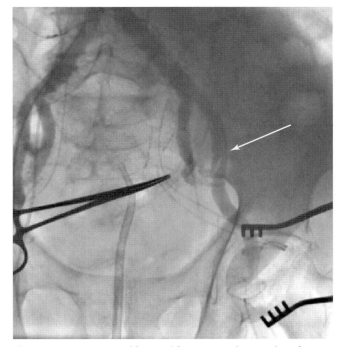

Figure 6–8 An 89-year-old man with severe aortic stenosis underwent placement of a 26-mm SAPIEN valve. After procedure completion, an angiogram of the distal aorta demonstrated a non–flow-limiting retrograde dissection *(arrow)* of the external iliac artery (sheath insertion site) that was treated conservatively. Follow-up arterial Doppler study demonstrated normal arterial blood flow to the distal left lower extremity.

NONCARDIAC COMPLICATIONS

Renal Dysfunction

Acute kidney injury post-TAVR is not uncommon and has an incidence of 12% to 28% and may progress to the need for renal replacement therapy in 1.4% of cases. The presence of hypertension (odds ratio [OR] = 4.66), chronic obstructive pulmonary disease (COPD) (OR = 2.64), transfusion requirement (OR = 3.47), and preexisting renal disease are important risk factors for its development.[80,81] The presence of acute kidney injury is associated with mortality (28% vs. 7%).[82-84] When compared to surgery, acute kidney injury (9.2% vs 25%) and need for dialysis (2.5% vs. 8.7%) is less common in patients undergoing TAVR.[85]

Stroke

The general incidence of clinically significant stroke is 2.5% to 6%.[86-89] The cerebrovascular event rate (cerebrovascular accident [CVA] and TIA) in the PARTNER trial was double in the TAVR group as compared to the surgical arm. The highest stroke rate occurs within the first 24 hours; however, one half to one third of the remaining events occur between days 2 and 30.[86] It was originally postulated that the rate of CVA was going to be lower in the TA approach, because the aortic arch was not manipulated. However, the incidence appears to be similar.[87] Recent studies suggest a higher incidence of subclinical perfusion abnormalities documented by MRI.[88,89] Cerebral embolization can occur during the passage of the valve across the aortic arch when the surgeon is trying to traverse the aortic valve to gain access into the LV and during BAV and valve implantation. The use of cerebral embolic protection devices during TAVR is currently being evaluated.[90,91] Antiplatelet regimens are not standardized for TAVR and are inappropriate.

6.7 Summary

TAVR has proven to be an effective therapy for the treatment of severe symptomatic AS in a select patient population. Improvements in catheter design yielding smaller delivery systems and easier deployment techniques have improved the procedural safety. The results of the ongoing PARTNER II trial, which will evaluate the treatment of patients with a lower risk profile and the use of TAVR for the treatment of degenerated bioprosthetic valves, will likely continue to expand the indications and use of this technology. A very exciting and promising future will follow the field of TAVR.

REFERENCES

1. Lindroos M, Kupari M, Heikkila J, et al: Prevalence of aortic valve abnormalities in the elderly: an echocardiographic study of a random population sample, J Am Coll Cardiol 21:1220–1225, 1993.
2. Ross JJR, Braunwald E: Aortic Stenosis, Circulation 38(1Suppl):61–67, 1968.
3. Varadarajan P, Kapoor N, Bansal RC, et al: Clinical profile and natural history of 453 nonsurgically managed patients with severe aortic stenosis, Ann Thorac Surg 82:2111–2115, 2006.
4. Edwards FH, Peterson ED, Coombs LP, et al: Prediction of operative mortality after valve replacement surgery, J Am Coll Cardiol 37:885–892, 2001.
5. Society of Thoracic Surgeons, STS National Database, STS U.S. Cardiac Surgery Database: Aortic valve replacement patients: preoperative risk variables. Chicago, 1997, Society of Thoracic Surgeons. 2000.
6. Otto C: Valvular aortic stenosis: disease severity and timing of intervention, J Am Coll Cardiol 47:2141–2151, 2006.
7. Iung B, Baron G, Butchart EG, et al: A prospective survey of patients with valvular heart disease in Europe: The Euro Heart Survey on Valvular Heart Disease, Eur Heart J 24:1231–1243, 2003.
8. Davies H: Catheter-mounted valve for temporary relief of aortic insufficiency, Lancet 285:250, 1965.
9. Moulopoulos SD, Anthopoulos L, Stamatelopoulos S, et al: Catheter-mounted aortic valves, Ann Thorac Surg 11:423–430, 1971.
10. Phillips SJ, Ciborski M, Freed PS, et al: A temporary catheter-tip aortic valve: hemodynamic effects on experimental acute aortic insufficiency, Ann Thorac Surg 21:134–137, 1976.
11. Andersen HR, Knudsen LL, Hasenkam JM: Transluminal implantation of artificial heart valves: description of a new expandable aortic valve and initial results with implantation by catheter technique in closed chest pigs, Eur Heart J 13:704–708, 1992.
12. Moazami N, Bessler M, Argenziano M, et al: Transluminal aortic valve placement: a feasibility study with a newly designed collapsible aortic valve, ASAIO J 42:M381–M385, 1996.
13. Pavcnik D, Wright KC, Wallace S: Development and initial experimental evaluation of a prosthetic aortic valve for transcatheter placement: work in progress, Radiology 183:151–154, 1992.
14. Sochman J, Peregrin JH, Rocek M, et al: Percutaneous transcatheter one-step mechanical aortic disc valve prosthesis implantation: a preliminary feasibility study in swine, Cardiovasc Intervent Radiol 29:114–119, 2006.
15. Bonhoeffer P, Boudjemline Y, Saliba Z, et al: Transcatheter implantation of a bovine valve in pulmonary position: a lamb study, Circulation 102:813–816, 2000.
16. Bonhoeffer P, Boudjemline Y, Saliba Z, et al: Percutaneous replacement of pulmonary valve in a right-ventricle to pulmonary-artery prosthetic conduit with valve dysfunction, Lancet 356:1403–1405, 2000.
17. Cribier A, Eltchaninoff H, Bash A, et al: Percutaneous transcatheter implantation of an aortic valve prosthesis for calcific aortic stenosis: first human case description, Circulation 106:3006–3008, 2002.
18. Cribier A, Eltchaninoff H, Tron C, et al: Early experience with percutaneous transcatheter implantation of heart valve prosthesis for the treatment of end-stage inoperable patients with calcific aortic stenosis, J Am Coll Cardiol 43:698–703, 2004.
19. Bauer F, Eltchaninoff H, Tron C, et al: Acute improvement in global and regional left ventricular systolic function after percutaneous heart valve implantation in patients with symptomatic aortic stenosis, Circulation 110:1473–1476, 2004.
20. Cribier A, Eltchaninoff H, Tron C, et al: Treatment of calcific aortic stenosis with the percutaneous heart valve, J Am Coll Cardiol 47(6):1214–1223, 2006.
21. Webb JG, Chandavimol M, Thompson CR, et al: Percutaneous aortic valve implantation retrograde from the femoral artery, Circulation 113:842–850, 2006.
22. Webb JG, Pasupati S, Humphries K, et al: Percutaneous aortic valve replacement in selected high risk patients with aortic stenosis, Circulation 116:755–763, 2007.
23. Lichtenstein SV, Cheung A, Ye J, et al: Transapical transcatheter aortic valve implantation in humans: initial clinical experience, Circulation 114:591–596, 2006.
24. Dewey TM, Walther T, Doss M, et al: Transapical aortic valve implantation: an animal feasibility study, Ann Thorac Surg 82:110–116, 2006.
25. Ye J, Cheung A, Lichtenstein AV, et al: Six month outcome of transapical aortic valve implantation in the initial seven patients, Euro J Cardiothorac Surg 31:16–21, 2007.
26. Walther T, Simon P, Dewey T, et al: Transapical minimally invasive aortic valve implantation. Multicenter experience, Circulation 116(suppl I), 2007. I-240-I-24.
27. Collart F, Feier H, Kerbaul F, et al: Valvular surgery in octogenarians: operative risk factors, evaluation of EuroSCORE and long term results, Eur J Cardiothorac Surg 27:276–280, 2005.

28. Roques F, Michel P, Goldstone AR, et al: The logistic EuroSCORE, Eur Heart J 24:882–883, 2003.
29. Pinna-Pintor P, Bobbio M, Colangelo S, et al: Inaccuracy of four coronary risk adjusted models to predict mortality in individual patients, Eur J Cardiothorac Surg 21:199–204, 2002.
30. Gossi EA, Schwartz CF, Yu PJ, et al: High risk aortic valve replacement: are the outcomes as bad as predicted? Ann Thorac Surg 85:102–107, 2008.
31. Shroyer AL, Coombs LP, Peterson E, et al: The Society of Thoracic Surgeons: 30-day operative mortality and morbidity risk models, Ann Thorac Surg 75:1856–1865, 2003.
32. Dewey TM, Brown D, Ryan W, et al: Reliability of risk algorithms in predicting early and late operative outcomes in high risk patients undergoing aortic valve replacement, J Thorac Cardiovasc Surg 135:180–187, 2008.
33. Piazza N, Wenaweser P, Van Gameren M, et al: Relationship between the logistic EuroSCORE and the Society of Thoracic Surgeons Predicted Risk of Mortality score in patients implanted with the CoreValve Revalving System—a Bern Rotterdam study, Am Heart J 159:323–329, 2010.
34. Masson JB, Kovac J, Schuler G, et al: Transcatheter aortic valve implantation: a review of the nature, management, and avoidance of procedural complications, JACC Cardiovasc Interv 2:811–820, 2009.
35. Eltchaninoff E, Kerkeni M, Zajarias A, et al: Aortoiliac angiography as a screening tool in selecting patients for transfemoral aortic valve implantation with Edwards SAPIEN bioprosthesis, EuroIntervention 5:438–442, 2009.
36. Hayashida K, Lefevre T, Chevalier B, et al: Transfemoral aortic valve implantation: new criteria to predict vascular complications, JACC Cardiovasc Interv 4:851–858, 2011.
37. Piazza N, Serruys PW, Lange R: Getting safely in and out of a transcatheter aortic valve implantation procedure vascular complications according to the valvular academic research consortium criteria, JACC Cardiovasc Interv 4:859–860, 2011.
38. Joshi SB, Mendoza DD, Steinberg DH, et al: Ultra–low-dose intra-arterial contrast injection for iliofemoral computed tomographic angiography, JACC Cardiovasc Imaging 2:1404, 2009.
39. Ng AC, Yiu KH, Ewe SH, et al: Influence of left ventricular geometry and function on aortic annular dimensions as assessed with multidetector row computed tomography: implications for transcatheter aortic valve implantation, Eur Heart J 32:2806–2813, 2011.
40. Schultz C, Moelker A, Tzikas A, et al: The use of MSCT for the evaluation of the aortic root before transcutaneous aortic valve implantation: the Rotterdam approach, EuroIntervention 6:505–511, 2010.
41. Masson JB, Lee M, Boone RH, et al: Impact of coronary artery disease on outcomes after transcatheter aortic valve implantation, Catheter Cardiovasc Interv 76:165–173, 2010.
42. Wenaweser P, Pilgrim T, Guerios E, et al: Impact of coronary artery disease and percutaneous coronary intervention on outcomes in patients with severe aortic stenosis undergoing transcatheter aortic valve implantation, EuroIntervention 7:541–548, 2011.
43. Dewey TM, Brown DL, Herbert MA, et al: Effect of concomitant coronary artery disease on procedural and late outcomes of transcatheter aortic valve implantation, Ann Thorac Surg 89:758–776, 2010.
44. Clavel MA, Webb JG, Pibarot P, et al: Comparison of the hemodynamic performance of percutaneous and surgical bioprosthesis for the treatment of severe aortic stenosis, J Am Coll Cardiol 53:1883–1891, 2009.
45. Covello RD, Ruggeri L, Landoni G, et al: Anesthetic management for percutaneous aortic valve implantation: an overview of worldwide experience, Minerva Anestesiol 76:100–108, 2010.
46. Motloch LJ, Rottlaender D, Reda S, et al: Local versus general anesthesia for transfemoral aortic valve implantation, Clin Res Cardiol 101:45-53, 2011.
47. Covello RD, Landoni G, Zangrillo A: Anesthetic management of transcatheter aortic valve implantation, Curr Opin Anaesthesiol 24:417–425, 2011.
48. Sharp AS, Michev F, Taramasso M, et al: A new technique for vascular access management in transcatheter aortic valve implantation, Catheter Cardiovasc Interv 75:784–793, 2010.
49. Leon MB, Piazza N, Nikolsky E, et al: Standardized endpoint definitions for transcatheter aortic valve implantation clinical trials: a consensus report from the Valve Academic Research Consortium, Eur Heart J 32:205–217, 2011.
50. Smith CR, Leon MB, Mack MJ, et al: Transcatheter versus surgical aortic-valve replacement in high-risk patients, N Engl J Med 364:2187–2198, 2011.
51. Reynolds MR, Magnuson EA, Wang K, et al: Health-related quality of life after transcatheter or surgical aortic valve replacement in high risk patients with severe aortic stenosis, J Am Coll Cardiol 60:548–558, 2012.
52. Leon MB, Smith CR, Mack M, et al: Transcatheter aortic-valve implantation for aortic stenosis in patients who cannot undergo surgery, N Engl J Med 363:1597–1607, 2010.
53. Makkar RR, Fontana GP, Jilaihaiwi H, et al: Transcatheter aortic valve replacement for inoperable severe aortic stenosis, N Engl J Med 366:1696–1704, 2012.
54. Reynolds MR, Magnuson EA, Lei Y, et al: Health-related quality of life after transcatheter aortic valve replacement in inoperable patients with severe aortic stenosis, Circulation 124:1964–1972, 2011.
55. Reynolds MR, Magnuson EA, Wang K, et al: Cost effectiveness of transcatheter aortic valve replacement compared with standard care among inoperable patients with severe aortic stenosis: results from the placement of aortic transcatheter valves (PARTNER) trial (cohort B), Circulation 125:1102–1109, 2012.
56. Rodes-Cabau J, Dumont E, Dela Rochelliere R, et al: Feasibility and initial results of percutaneous aortic valve implantation including selection of the transfemoral or transapical approach in patients with severe aortic stenosis, Am J Cardiol 102:1240–1246, 2008.
57. Thomas M, Schymik G, Walther T, et al: Thirty-day results of the SAPIEN aortic bioprosthesis European Outcome (SOURCE) Registry: a European registry of transcatheter aortic valve implantation using the Edwards SAPIEN valve, Circulation 122:62–69, 2010.
58. Webb JG, Altwegg L, Boone RH, et al: Transcatheter aortic valve implantation: impact on clinical and valve-related outcomes, Circulation 119:3009–3016, 2009.
59. Walther T, Schuler G, Borger MA, et al: Transapical aortic valve implantation in 100 consecutive patients: comparison to propensity-matched conventional aortic valve replacement, Eur Heart J 31:1398–1403, 2010.
60. Zierer A, Wimmer-Greinecer G, Martens S, et al: Is transapical aortic valve implantation really less invasive than minimally invasive aortic valve replacement? J Thorac Cardiovasc Surg 138:1067–1072, 2009.
61. Eltchaninoff H, Pratt A, Gilard M, et al: Transcatheter aortic valve implantation: early results of the FRANCE (French Aortic National CoreValve Edwards) Registry, Eur Heart J 32:191–197, 2011.
62. Gilard M, Eltchaninoff H, Iung B, et al: Registry of transcatheter aortic valve implantation in high risk patients, N Engl J Med 366:1705–1715, 2012.
63. Jamieson WR, Burr LH, Miyagishima RT, et al: Reoperation for bioprosthetic aortic structural failure: risk assessment, Eur J Cardiothorac Surg 24:873–878, 2003.
64. Vogt PR, Brunner-LaRocca H, Sidler P, et al: Reoperative surgery for degenerated aortic bioprostheses: predictors for emergency surgery and reoperative mortality, Eur J Cardiothorac Surg 17:134–139, 2000.
65. Christiansen S, Schmid M, Autschbach R: Perioperative risk of redo aortic valve replacement, Ann Thorac Cardiovasc Surg 15:105–110, 2009.
66. Piazza N, Bleiziffer S, Brockmann G, et al: Transcatheter aortic valve implantation for failing surgical aortic bioprosthetic valve: from concept to clinical application and evaluation. Part 1, JACC Cardiovasc Interv 4:721–732, 2011.
67. Piazza N, Bleiziffer S, Brockmann G, et al: Transcatheter aortic valve implantation for failing surgical aortic bioprosthetic valve: from concept to clinical application and evaluation. Part 2, JACC Cardiovasc Interv 4:733–742, 2011.
68. Kochman J, Huczek Z, Koltowski L, et al: Transcatheter implantation of an aortic valve prosthesis in a female patient with severe bicuspid aortic stenosis, Eur Heart J 33:112, 2012.
69. Ferrari E, Locca D, Sulzer C, et al: Successful transapical aortic valve implantation in a congenital bicuspid aortic valve, Ann Thorac Surg 90:630–632, 2010.
70. Wijesinghe N, Ye J, Rodes-Cabau J, et al: Transcatheter aortic valve implantation in patients with bicuspid aortic valve stenosis, JACC Cardiovasc Interv 3:1122–1125, 2010.
71. Unsworth B, Malik I, Mikhail GW: Recognising bicuspid aortic stenosis in patients referred for transcatheter aortic valve implantation: routine screening with three-dimensional transoesophageal echocardiography, Heart (British Cardiac Society) 96:645, 2010.

72. Delgado V, Tops LF, Schuijf JD, et al: Successful deployment of a transcatheter aortic valve in bicuspid aortic stenosis: role of imaging with multislice computed tomography, *Circ Cardiovasc Imaging* 2:e12–e13, 2009.

73. Lange R, Bleiziffer S, Mazzitelli D, et al: Improvements in transcatheter aortic valve implantation outcomes in lower surgical risk patients: a glimpse into the future, *J Am Coll Cardiol* 59:280-287, 2011.

74. Sinhal A, Altwegg L, Pasupati S, et al: Atrioventricular block after transcatheter balloon expandable aortic valve implantation, *JACC Cardiovasc Interv* 1:305–309, 2008.

75. Godin M, Eltchaninoff H, Furuta A, et al: Frequency of conduction disturbances after transcatheter implantation of an Edwards SA-PIEN aortic valve prosthesis, *Am J Cardiol* 106:707–712, 2010.

76. Gutierrez M, Rodes-Cabau J, Bagur R, et al: Electrocardiographic changes and clinical outcomes after transapical aortic valve implantation, *Am Heart J* 158:302–308, 2009.

77. Bleiziffer S, Ruge H, Horer J, et al: Predictors for new onset complete heart block after transcatheter aortic valve implantation, *JACC Cardiovasc Interv* 5:524–530, 2010.

78. Lange R, Bleiziffer S, Piazza N, et al: Incidence and treatment of procedural cardiovascular complications associated with trans-arterial and transapical interventional aortic valve implantation in 412 consecutive patients, *Eur J Cardiothorac Surg* 40:1105–1113, 2011.

79. Zajarias A, Eltchaninoff H, Cribier A: Successful coronary intervention after percutaneous aortic valve replacement, *Catheter Cardiovasc Interv* 69:522–524, 2007.

80. Nuis RJ, Piazza N, Van Mieghem NM, et al: In-hospital complications after transcatheter aortic valve implantation revisited according to the valve academic research consortium definitions, *Catheter Cardiovasc Interv* 78:457–467, 2011.

81. Nuis RJ, Van Mieghem NM, Tzikas A, et al: Frequency, determinants, and prognostic effects of acute kidney injury and red blood cell transfusion in patients undergoing transcatheter aortic valve implantation, *Catheter Cardiovasc Interv* 77:881–889, 2011.

82. Bagur R, Webb JG, Nietlispach F, et al: Acute kidney injury following transcatheter aortic valve implantation: predictive factors, prognostic value, and comparison with surgical aortic valve replacement, *Eur Heart J* 31:865–874, 2010.

83. Sinning JM, Ghanem A, Steinhauser H, et al: Renal function as predictor of mortality in patients after percutaneous transcatheter aortic valve implantation, *JACC Cardiovasc Interv* 3:1141–1149, 2010.

84. Tamburino C, Capodanno D, Ramondo A, et al: Incidence and predictors of early and late mortality after transcatheter aortic valve implantation in 663 patients with severe aortic stenosis, *Circulation* 123:299–308, 2011.

85. Arregger F, Wenaweser P, Hellige GJ, et al: Risk of acute kidney injury in patients with severe aortic valve stenosis undergoing transcatheter valve replacement, *Nephrol Dial Transplant* 24:2175–2179, 2009.

86. Tay EL, Gurvitch R, Wijesinghe N, et al: A high-risk period for cerebrovascular events exists after transcatheter aortic valve implantation, *JACC Cardiovasc Interv* 4:1290–1297, 2011.

87. Astarci P, Glineur D, Kefer J, et al: Magnetic resonance imaging evaluation of cerebral embolization during percutaneous aortic valve implantation: comparison of transfemoral and transapical approaches using Edwards SAPIENS valve, *Eur J Cardiothorac Surg* 40:475–479, 2011.

88. Kahlert P, Knipp SC, Schlamann M, et al: Silent and apparent cerebral ischemia after percutaneous transfemoral aortic valve implantation: a diffusion-weighted magnetic resonance imaging study, *Circulation* 121:870–878, 2010.

89. Ghanem W, Muller A, Nahle CP, et al: Risk and fate of cerebral embolism after transfemoral aortic valve implantation, *J Am Coll Cardiol* 55:1427–1432, 2010.

90. Nietlispach F, Wijesinghe N, Gurvitch R, et al: An embolic deflection device for aortic valve interventions, *JACC Cardiovasc Interv* 3:1133–1138, 2010.

91. Macdonald S: New embolic protection devices: a review, *J Cardiovasc Surg* 52:821–827, 2011.

Chapter 7

Self-Expanding Transcatheter Aortic Valve Replacement Using the CoreValve Transcatheter Heart Valve

JEFFREY J. POPMA • DAVID A. BURKE

7.1 Key Points

- Transcatheter aortic valve replacement (TAVR) using the self-expanding Medtronic CoreValve Revalving System (Medtronic, Maple Grove, Minn.) transcatheter heart valve (THV) provides an alternative to surgical aortic valve replacement (SAVR) in patients who are poor candidates for surgery.

- Unique features of the CoreValve design are its ability to conform to the eccentric annulus, a supraannular location of the low-profile porcine pericardial valve with a long commissural length to reduce stress, a constrained region of the nitinol frame to access the coronary arteries, and an outflow region that orients the valve to provide maximal flow.

- Preprocedural evaluation using echocardiography and multidetector computed tomography (MDCT) imaging allows patient selection and optimal sizing for the CoreValve THV. Patients who have unsuitable iliofemoral anatomy can be treated by means of a subclavian or direct aortic approach.

- Optimal CoreValve implantation technique includes positioning of the CoreValve frame less than 6 mm below the aortic annulus; evaluation for postimplantation paravalvular regurgitation using echocardiography, hemodynamics, and aortography; and monitoring for conduction system abnormalities.

- Complications of TAVR include stroke, conduction system abnormalities, paravalvular regurgitation, and vascular complications and may be minimized with comprehensive preprocedural planning and optimal implantation technique.

Aortic stenosis is the most common valve disorder in developed countries.[1] The recommended therapy for the majority of patients with symptomatic aortic stenosis is SAVR.[1,2] Surgical risk assessment is most often obtained through a thorough review of the patient's clinical history and physical examination, aided by use of the Society for Thoracic Surgery Predicted Risk of Mortality (STS-PROM) score estimated 30-day mortality rate[3] or other scores that provide a quantitative assessment of outcome. A number of clinical and anatomic factors are considered by the surgical team that may render the patient an unsuitable candidate for SAVR, including aortic calcification[4,5] **(Figure 7–1, A-F)**, hostile mediastinum related to the crossing of the left internal mammary artery (LIMA) across the midline of the chest **(Figure 7–1, G)**, severe lung or liver disease, frailty, and renal failure.[6-10] In patients who are deemed unsuitable or "high risk" for sAVR because of underlying comorbidities, TAVR has been used as an alternative for symptom relief and extension of life.[11-15] Sustained improvement after CoreValve TAVR three years after implantation has been reported.[16]

7.2 CoreValve ReValving System

The 18F Medtronic CoreValve ReValving System is a THV comprised of a self-expanding nitinol support frame that anchors a trileaflet porcine pericardial

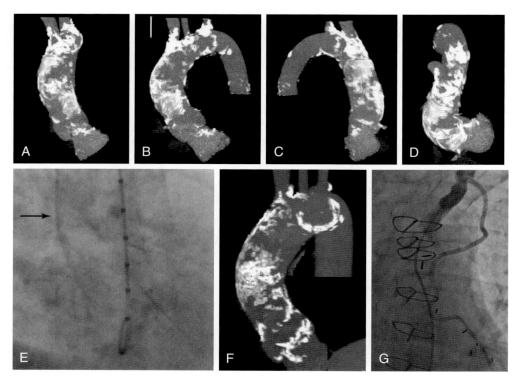

Figure 7–1 Porcelain aorta and hostile mediastinum. A-D, Rotational CT of the aortic root demonstrates diffuse calcification of the ascending aorta precluding cross-clamping during surgical aortic valve replacement. **E,** Cineangiography of the aortic root during cardiac catheterization reveals dense calcification of the aortic root *(arrow).* **F,** Another example of a densely calcified aorta is shown. **G,** A left internal mammary artery that transverses beneath the sternum renders the patient at prohibitive risk for repeat surgery.

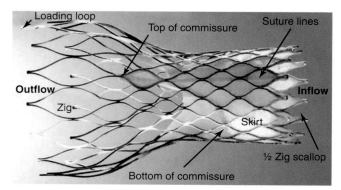

Figure 7–2 **CoreValve ReValving System.** The CoreValve transcatheter heart valve frame is comprised of a series of staggered nitinol zigs (or cells) that are 8 mm in length at the level of the inflow. The inflow portion of the frame provides radial expansive strength at the annulus to secure its location within the left ventricular outflow tract and aortic annulus. There is a 12-mm skirt that is constructed of porcine pericardium that prevents leaking around the valve frame. The central (or constrained) portion of the frame contains the trileaflet porcine pericardial valve and allows access to the coronary arteries. The leaflet commissures are longer than standard surgical valves to distribute the diastolic load along the length of the valve rather than at its posts. *(Reproduced from Michiels, R. CoreValve ReValving system for percutaneous aortic valve replacement. In Serruys PW, Piazza N, Cribier A, et al., editors.* Transcatheter aortic valve implantation: tips and tricks to avoid failure, *New York: Informa Healthcase, 2010, with permission).*

tissue valve, an 18F delivery catheter, and a valve loading system **(Figure 7–2).** The nitinol frame was designed with three levels of radial and hoop strength. The frame inflow exerts high radial expansive force to secure the frame within the aortic annular location, allowing the frame to partially conform to the noncircular shape of the aortic annulus. The "constrained"

center portion of the frame has high hoop strength that resists compression and shape deformation, which is critical as this portion of the frame contains the "supraannular" valve porcine leaflets. The constrained portion of the frame is concave to avoid the coronary ostia, allowing coronary artery cannulation after CoreValve implantation. The outflow portion of the frame serves to orent the frame to the aorta parallel to flow through the valve.

The porcine pericardium was selected because of its lower profile (compared with bovine pericardium) and for its long-term durability. The zigs (or cells) of the frame are 8 mm in length and are connected in their central portion **(Figure 7–3).** When the frame is constrained in its delivery sheath, the joint distances are separated by 4 mm, providing radiopacity to aid in the positioning of the device as the constraining membrane of the delivery sheath is withdrawn. Optimal positioning for the CoreValve THV is at a depth of 4 to 6 mm below the aortic annulus. The CoreValve THV is available in 23-mm (for use with aortic annular diameters between 18 and 20 mm), 26-mm (annular diameters between 20 and 23 mm), 29-mm (annular diameters between 24 and 27 mm), and 31-mm (annular diameters between 26 and 29 mm) sizes **(Figure 7–4).**

7.3 The Heart Team

A collaborative and multidisciplinary approach to the evaluation and management of patients with complex aortic valve disease has led to the crucial development of the "heart team." **(Table 7–1).**[17,18] The heart team is

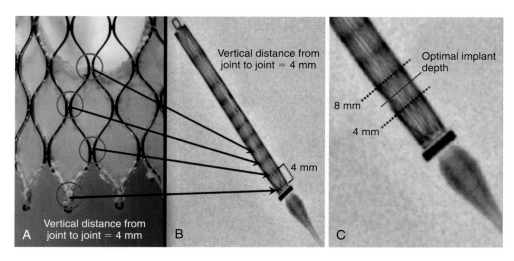

Figure 7–3 Magnified view of the CoreValve frame. A, The zigs (or cells) at the inflow region are 8 mm in length and staggered with a vertical distance from joint to joint of 4 mm. **B,** Constrained within the delivery sheath, there are radiopaque lines every 4 mm. **C,** The radiopaque marker at the distal tip of the retaining membrane provides guidance for optimal implantation 4 to 6 mm below the noncoronary sinus of Valsalva.

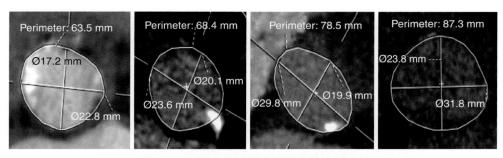

Figure 7–4 Multidetector computed tomography perimeter sizing for the aortic valve. Perimeter measurement for the various CoreValve sizes from 23 mm to 31 mm. Valve perimeters are obtained from the inflow portion of the frame with optimal oversizing between 10% and 20%.

Valve size	23	26	29	31
Annular perimeter	63.5	68.4	78.5	87.3
Valve perimeter	72.2	81.6	91.1	97.3
% oversize	12%	16%	14%	10%

composed of cardiac surgeons, interventional cardiologists, cardiac anesthesiologists, imaging specialists, electrophysiologists, neurologists, heart failure cardiologists, and geriatricians.[19] Vascular surgeons may be needed for complex access and management of vascular complications after the procedure. Nursing services provide critical support services in the preoperative and postoperative periods, as well as coordination of outpatient care after TAVR.

The primary purpose of the heart team is to coordinate the risk assessment of the patients and to facilitate the preoperative and postoperative care. The primary tool for the assessment of 30-day cardiac surgical mortality in the United States is the STS-PROM score.[3] Although the STS-PROM score remains a key component in assessing risk for sAVR, it is supplemented by additional factors affecting outcomes after surgery that are not included in the STS-PROM. Additional risk factors termed STS *Plus* are being used as part of the CoreValve US Pivotal Trial and take into account factors such as degree of aortic calcification, pulmonary hypertension, liver disease, chest deformity, hostile mediastinum, severe chronic obstructive pulmonary disease, home oxygen or continuous positive airway pressure (CPAP), and markers of frailty (body mass index [BMI] <21, albumin <3.3, wheelchair bound, and not living independently). The importance of the heart-team approach has been endorsed by several recent multispecialty guidelines.[20,21] Training standards for the structural heart disease heart team have been established.[20,21]

PATIENT SELECTION

Patients enrolled in regulatory trials in the United States that have evaluated the CoreValve THV and the Edwards SAPIEN balloon-expandable THV (Edwards Lifesciences, Irvine, Calif.) have met strict risk-assessment criteria for enrollment.[11,12] All patients were required to be symptomatic from their aortic stenosis and have New York Heart Association class II or greater heart failure symptoms. "Inoperable" (or "extreme risk") patients are those who have been assessed by two cardiac surgeons and are deemed to have greater than a 50% risk of mortality or irreversible morbidity within 30 days after sAVR.[11] "High-risk" patients are those deemed to be at substantial risk for sAVR based on an estimated 30-day mortality rate of 15% or more.[12] This has generally been established as an STS-PROM score

TABLE 7–1

The Multidisciplinary Transcatheter Aortic Valve Replacement Team

	Preprocedural Assessment	Implantation Procedure	Postoperative Care
Core Implanting Team			
Cardiac surgeon	Surgical risk assessment Hemodynamic assessment Vascular assessment	Transapical or direct aortic access TAVR implantation	Postoperative management
Interventional cardiologist	Medical risk assessment Hemodynamic evaluation Noninvasive assessments Vascular assessment	TAVR implantation	Postoperative management
Cardiac anesthesiology	Anesthesia risk	Conscious sedation General anesthesia Transesophageal echocardiography	Postoperative ICU management
Imaging Specialists			
Echocardiography	Annular sizing Biventricular and valvular function	Transthoracic or transesophageal echocardiography	Postoperative valve function
CT angiography	Aortic annular sizing Aortic root and sinus assessment Subclavian and iliofemoral assessment		
Cardiac MRI	Annulus and root assessment in patients with prohibitive renal disease		
Supporting Specialists			
Electrophysiology	Conduction system assessment with EPS as indicated for AV block		Permanent pacemaker placement (if required)
Neurology	Neurologic evaluation		Neurologic evaluation
Heart failure service	Assessment of systolic and diastolic function		Heart failure management
Pulmonary	Preoperative assessment for patients with severe lung disease		Postoperative ventilator and outpatient management
Geriatric service	Dementia and frailty assessment Medication review		Medical management
Vascular surgery	Vascular assessment	Vascular access in complex cases	Complication management
Nursing Services			
Case management	Case coordination		Rehabilitation assessment

AV, Atrioventricular; CT, computed tomography; EPS, electrophysiological service; ICU, intensive care unit; MRI, magnetic resonance imaging; TAVR, transcatheter aortic valve replacement.

of 8 or higher and consideration for other factors that contribute to surgical mortality.

Echocardiographic criteria for enrollment in clinical trials in the United States have included an aortic valve area of 0.8 cm^2 or less (or index $\leq$0.5 cm^2) associated with a mean gradient greater than 40 mmHg or peak gradient greater than 4 m/sec shown with at-rest echocardiography. In patients with reduced left ventricular function, these measurements can be augmented by dobutamine infusion at the time of the echocardiogram or simultaneous measurement during cardiac catheterization.[11,12] These criteria have been liberalized for CoreValve commercial use outside the United States (aortic

valve area < 1.0 cm^2 and no minimal gradients or jet velocities). Patients with severely reduced left ventricular ejection fraction (LVEF <20%); outflow tract gradients caused by basal septal hypertrophy; severe mitral regurgitation; low-gradient, low output aortic stenosis without contractile reserve; and bioprosthetic valve failure were excluded from the clinical trials in the United States.[11,12]

Expanded clinical use outside the United States with the CoreValve THV has also included a number of clinical subsets, including patients with bioprosthetic valve failure,[22,23] reduced left ventricular function,[24] and aortic regurgitation,[25] as well as those with low-gradient, low flow aortic stenosis,[26,27] severe mitral regurgitation,[28] bicuspid valves,[29] and underlying coronary artery disease.[30]

ANATOMIC CRITERIA

The design of the CoreValve THV requires that there is careful evaluation of the aortic valvar complex with imaging studies before the procedure, most often with MDCT **(Table 7–2)**. Accurate and reliable aortic annular measurements are key to determining the size of device used, and also in reducing the impact of paravalvular regurgitation **(Figure 7–5)**.[31] Owing to the eccentric geometry of the aortic annulus, correlative studies have shown a systematic underestimation of the annular size by two-dimensional echocardiography alone.[32-34] MDCT provides a better estimate of the long- and short-axis diameters of the aortic annulus, surface area, and perimeter measurements,[32,35,36] and has been used extensively for annular sizing in the United States for the CoreValve THV. Oversizing of the THV and excessive calcification may result in aortic annular rupture.[37,38] Three-dimensional imaging using transesophageal echocardiography may provide accurate assessments of the aortic annulus.[39]

Annular diameters outside the range of smaller than 18 mm or larger than 29 mm cannot be treated with the current generation of the CoreValve device **(Table 7–3)**. Adequate sinus of Valsalva width (>25 mm for the 23-mm valve; >27 mm for the 26-mm valve; and >29 mm for the 29-mm and 31-mm valves) **(Figure 7–6)** and Sinus of Valsalva height (>15 mm) is required to avoid coronary occlusion. Determination of the height of the coronary arteries is important to understand the potential displacement of the leaflets during CoreValve THV deployment **(Figure 7–7)**. The ascending aortic diameter should be less than 40 mm for the 26-mm valve and less than 43 mm for the 29-mm and 31-mm valves **(Figure 7–8)**. Other anatomic criteria include an adequate aortoventricular angle smaller than 70 degrees for the iliofemoral and left subclavian access routes and smaller than 30 degrees for the right subclavian approach **(Figure 7–9)**, and the estimation of the extent and distribution of annular calcification may be reliably assessed **(Figure 7–10)**. Dense calcification of the left coronary sinus, aortomitral curtain, and mitral valvular calcification should be avoided because of the potential for the inability to fully expand the frame **(Figure 7–11)**.

VASCULAR CRITERIA

The 18F CoreValve Revalving System is advanced through an 18F sheath, requiring that the access vessel diameter is 6 mm or greater in a noncalcified vessel and 7 mm or greater for a severely calcified vessel **(Figure 7–12)**. Although initial studies used aortography to select patients for CoreValve placement, more recent screening procedures have included MDCT of the abdomen and pelvis, including the ascending and descending aorta and peripheral run-off vessels (subclavian, iliac, and femoral arteries).[40]

7.4 CoreValve Procedure

PREPROCEDURAL PREPARATION

Patients should be pretreated with 325 mg of aspirin and 300 mg of clopidogrel at least 24 hours before the procedure. Prophylactic antibiotic coverage should be administered at least 1 hour before the procedure, similar to patients undergoing surgical AVR. β-Blockers and diuretics in the absence of decompensated heart failure should be withheld on the morning of the procedure.

PROCEDURE LOCATION

TAVR performed by the femoral access route can be performed in either a cardiac catheterization lab or a hybrid operating room. The benefit of the hybrid suite is that its size allows all members of the interventional team and circulating staff sufficient space to work comfortably, allows seamless transition to treat vascular or coronary complications if these arise, and provides accessibility to cardiopulmonary bypass.

The procedure can be performed using either general anesthesia or conscious sedation with local anesthesia. General anesthesia affords the benefit of using transesophageal echocardiography during the procedure, which can assist in optimal valve positioning and evaluating paravalvular regurgitation.

VASCULAR ACCESS

Common femoral arterial and venous access is obtained on the contralateral side to the planned site for advancement of the CoreValve THV. Although an open surgical approach can be used for borderline arterial diameters or extensive calcification, percutaneous suture closure with ProStar or ProGlide suture-based closure devices and the "preclose" technique is the most commonly performed. A single-wall puncture of the common femoral artery selected for the 18F sheath should be performed, guided by selective angiography or vascular ultrasound. The latter method allows localization of the common femoral artery (proximal to the bifurcation of the superficial femoral artery and profundis) as well as calcification (which can be avoided with arterial puncture).[41] After the vascular access has been obtained, anticoagulation using unfractionated heparin or bivalirudin should be administered to achieve an activated clotting time longer than 250 seconds. The CoreValve THV can be prepared once femoral access has been obtained.[42] The femoral artery sheath should be progressively dilated with 14F-22F dilators, and then the 18F sheath can be advanced under fluoroscopic guidance to the central aorta.

COREVALVE IMPLANTATION

From the contralateral artery, a 5F marker pigtail catheter is advanced to the ascending aorta and the distal tip of the catheter is positioned in the noncoronary aortic cusp. The posterior location of the noncoronary cusp is best performed in the right anterior oblique projection.

TABLE 7–2

Anatomic Criteria for Placement of the CoreValve Transcatheter Heart Valve

Diagnostic Findings	NONINVASIVE			ANGIOGRAPHY			SELECTION CRITERIA	
	Echo	CT/MRI	LV	Ao Root	CAG	Vascular	Recommended	Not Recommended
Left ventricular hypertrophy	X						≤1.6 cm	≥1.7 cm
Atrial or ventricular thrombus	X						Not present	Present
Subaortic stenosis	X						Not present	Present
LVEF	X						≥20%	<20% with Reserve
Mitral regurgitation	X		X				≤ Grade 2	> Grade 2
Coronary artery disease		X			X		None, Mid >70%	Proximal >70%
Aortic arch angulation		X		X	X		Large radial turn	Sharp turn
Aortoventricular angle		X		X	X		<70°	>70°
Vascular access diameter		X				X	≥6 cm	<6 cm
Aortic and vascular disease		X		X		X	None to moderate	Severe
23-mm CoreValve								
Annular diameter		X					18-20 mm	<18 mm or >20 mm
Sinus of Valsalva width		X			X		≥25 mm	<25 mm
Sinus of Valsalva height		X			X		≥15 mm	<15 mm
Ascending aortic diameter		X			X		≤34 mm	>34 mm
26 mm CoreValve								
Annular diameter		X					20-23 mm	<20 mm or >23 mm
Sinus of Valsalva width		X			X		≥27 mm	<27 mm
Sinus of Valsalva height		X			X		≥15 mm	<15 mm
Ascending aortic diameter		X			X		≤40 mm	>40 mm
29 mm CoreValve								
Annular diameter		X					24-27 mm	<24 mm or >27 mm
Sinus of Valsalva width		X			X		≥29 mm	<29 mm
Sinus of Valsalva height		X			X		≥15 mm	<15 mm
Aortic root diameter		X			X		≤43 mm	>43 mm
31 mm CoreValve								
Annular diameter		X					26-29 mm	<26 mm or >29 mm
Sinus of Valsalva width		X			X		≥29 mm	<29 mm
Sinus of Valsalva height		X			X		≥15 mm	<15 mm
Ascending aortic diameter		X			X		≤43 mm	>43 mm

Ao, Aortic; CAG, coronary angiography; CT/MRI, computed tomography/magnetic resonance imaging; LV, left ventricle; LVEF, left ventricular ejection fraction.

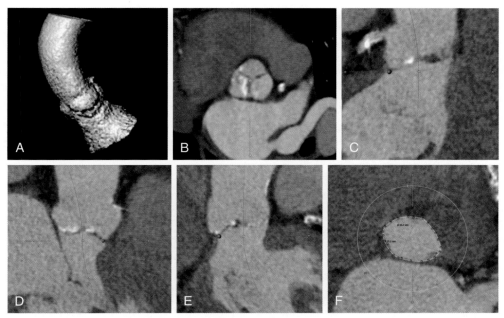

Figure 7–5 **Multidetector computed tomography assessment of annular sizing. A,** The aorta valvar complex is constructed by identification of a centerline that begins in the left ventricular outflow tract through the aortic annulus and extending into the ascending aorta. **B,** A cross-section of the sinus of Valsalva is obtained from the centerline. **C,** The basal locations of the left coronary sinus, right coronary sinus **(D),** and noncoronary sinus **(F)** are identified *(dots)*.

TABLE 7–3

Annular Diameters for the CoreValve Transcatheter Heart Valve

Valve Size	Annular Diameter, mm	Annular Perimeter, mm	Ascending Aorta, mm
23 mm	18-20	56.5-62.8	≤ 34 mm
26 mm	20-23	62.8-72.3	≤ 40 mm
29 mm	23-27	72.3-84.8	≤ 43 mm
31 mm	26-29	81.6-91.1	≤ 43 mm

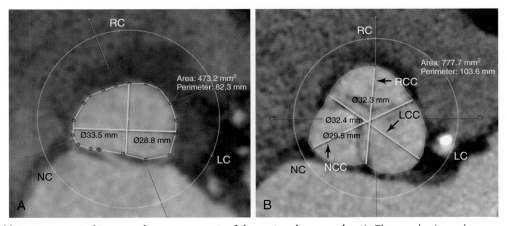

Figure 7–6 **Multidetector computed tomography measurements of the aorta valvar complex. A,** The annulus is used to measure the maximum annular diameter, perpendicular to the maximum diameter, and the annular area and annulus. The maximum length is 28.8 mm and the length perpendicular to the maximum length is 19.6 mm. The area was 473.2 mm^2, and the perimeter was 82.3 mm. **B,** The maximum sinus of Valsalva diameters are comprised of the maximum diameter of the left coronary sinus (32.4 mm), right coronary sinus (29.5 mm), and noncoronary sinus (32.8 mm). The area of the sinus of Valsalva is 777.7 mm^2, and the perimeter is 103.6 mm.

After positioning the pigtail catheter, the gantry position is optimized to allow visualization of all three coronary sinuses in the same plane, most often in a shallow left anterior oblique projection. MDCT imaging is useful for determining the optimal angulation to minimize contrast use during the procedure **(Figure 7–13).** Ideally, the basal portions of all three coronary sinuses should be visualized.

A 5F balloon-tipped temporary pacemaker is positioned in the right ventricular apex from either the internal jugular or femoral vein. Pacing and sensing

thresholds are tested, and blood pressure response to rapid ventricular pacing at 180 beats/min is tested to achieve a peak arterial pressure less than 60 mmHg. If this is not achieved, higher pacing rates can be used. Some patients develop heart block at fast pacing rates; in this case, pacing can be started at a slower rate and increased at increments of 10 beats/min until the peak arterial pressure is less than 50 mmHg.

An Amplatz-1 (AL-1) angiographic catheter is advanced through the 18F sheath over a standard, J-tipped 0.035-inch guidewire and positioned in the

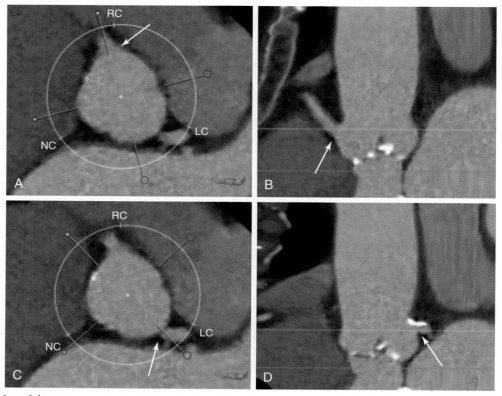

Figure 7–7 **Location of the coronary arteries. A,** The height of the right coronary artery is identified *(arrow).* **B,** The height of the right coronary artery *(arrow)* from the annular base is 18.1 mm. **C,** The location of the left coronary artery is identified *(arrow).* **D,** The height of the left coronary artery *(arrow)* from the basal annulus is 15.2 mm.

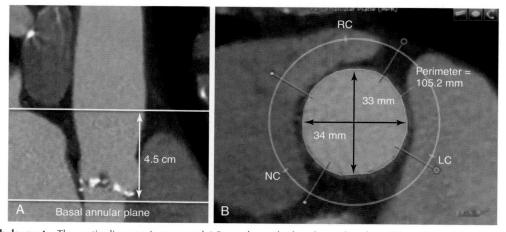

Figure 7–8 **Tubular aorta.** The aortic diameter is measured 4.5 cm above the basal annular plane **(A),** and the diameters are measured **(B).**

ascending aorta in the sinus of Valsalva. The wire is exchanged for a straight-tipped 0.035-inch guidewire that is used to cross the native aortic valve, typically in a shallow left anterior oblique projection. Once the guidewire is across the aortic valve, the AL-1 catheter is gently advanced into the left ventricle. A 0.035-inch exchange-length J-wire is advanced through the AL-1 catheter and positioned in the apex of the left ventricle. The AL-1 catheter is exchanged for a pigtail catheter so that aortic valve gradients can be measured across the aortic valve. An 0.035-inch Amplatz Super Stiff exchange

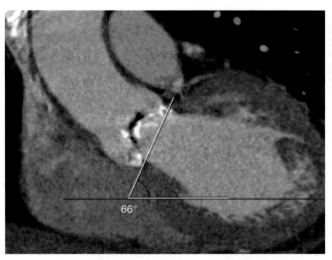

Figure 7–9 Determination of the aortoventricular angle. The angle of the horizontal plane and the aortic annulus is measured at 66 degrees.

guidewire is advanced through the pigtail catheter and carefully positioned in the apex of the left ventricle along the inner wall of the left ventricle, making sure to avoid the mitral valve apparatus. Careful shaping and "coiling" of the transition zone of the stiff and floppy parts of the wire prevents inadvertent perforation **(Figure 7–14).** The position of the guidewire should be fluoroscopically visualized and confirmed during the procedure.

BALLOON AORTIC VALVULOPLASTY

Balloon aortic valvuloplasty should not be performed until the CoreValve THV has been prepared. Balloon aortic valvuloplasty is then performed using a short, straight, and noncompliant balloon sized approximately 1 mm smaller than the minor axis of the aortic annulus. The balloon should be at least 18 mm but not larger than 25 mm in diameter.

VALVE DEPLOYMENT

After valvuloplasty, the CoreValve THV delivery catheter is loaded over the wire and is advanced and positioned across the native valve. Aortography is used to identify the most inferior aspect of the valvular plane in the non-coronary cusp **(Figure 7–15, A).** After the delivery catheter is advanced across the aortic valve, the X-ray gantry can be readjusted caudally to visualize the deployment sheath marker ring en-face.

The CoreValve THV is then positioned with the inflow portion within the aortic annulus (less than 4 to 6 mm

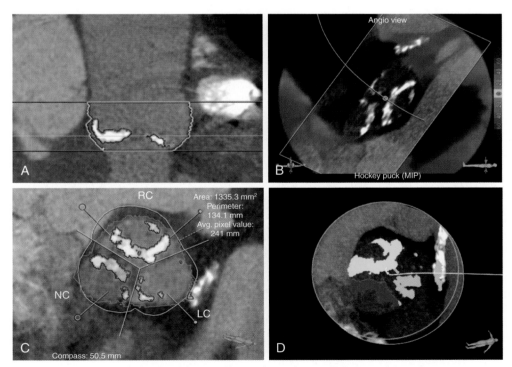

Figure 7–10 Assessment of aortic valve calcification. The stretch view shows dense calcification of the right coronary cusp, noncoronary cusp, and left coronary cusp. The stretch view **(A),** angiographic overlay **(B),** cross-sectional view **(C),** and "hockey puck" view **(D)** allow quantification of the calcium in the aortic valve.

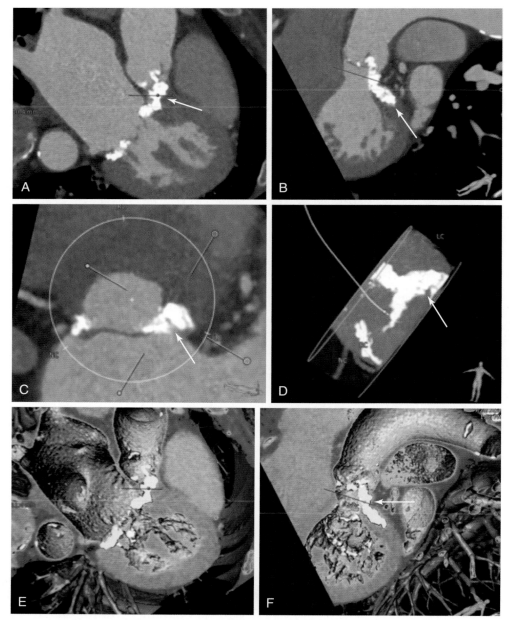

Figure 7–11   Mitral annular calcification. Dense calcification of the left coronary annulus is seen (**A-D,** *arrows*). Volume rendering of the mitral valve shows dense calcification extending from the left coronary sinus to the mitral annulus (**E** and **F**). This extent of calcification would be suboptimal for CoreValve transcatheter heart valve placement.

below the annulus) and the shaft of the THV is aligned so that the marker is perpendicular to the aortic root and parallel to the plane of the aortic annulus **(Figure 7–15, B).** Once the position of the CoreValve THV has been confirmed, the "microknob" at the distal end of the delivery catheter is turned slowly in a clockwise motion, which gradually withdraws the sheath covering the valve positioned across the native aortic valve. The microknob is turned until the sheath is retracted to position 0. Aortography is then performed to confirm correct positioning. The microknob is turned further to retract the sheath to position 1 with further aortography to optimize positioning. With further turns of the microknob, the sheath is retracted to between

positions 2 and 3, and the inflow portion of the valve frame begins to flare. Adjustments can be made to the depth of the prosthesis in relation to the aortic annulus. Once satisfactory position has been achieved, fast pacing may be carried out at 120 beats/min to blunt cardiac output, and the microknob is turned rapidly until the valve is two thirds deployed. Fast pacing is particularly useful for patients with aortic regurgitation, hypertension, or large annular diameters. Repeat aortography is performed to confirm correct positioning of the CoreValve THV **(Figure 7–15, C).** If the position is appropriate, the pigtail catheter is withdrawn from the noncoronary cusp to the aortic arch, and the microknob is turned to fully release and deploy the valve.

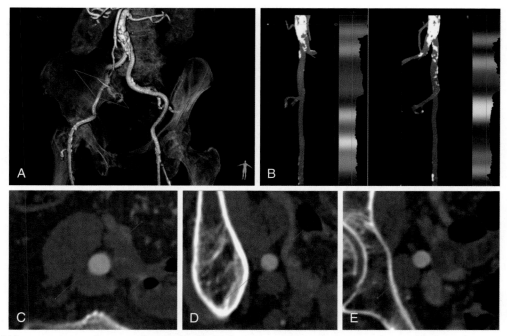

Figure 7–12 **Multidetector computed tomography peripheral vascular assessment. A,** A reconstructed view of iliofemoral anatomy with slight obliquity shows the vessel tortuosity. **B,** The stretched views with overlay of calcification and vessel diameter allow determination of the minimal lumen diameters. **C,** Based on centerline reconstructions, the common iliac, external iliac **(D),** and proximal common femoral arterial **(E)** measurements are obtained.

After deployment of the CoreValve device, the capsule is withdrawn into the delivery catheter to the descending aorta.

There are specialized requirements for implantation of the 31-mm device. The target implantation depth is 4 mm below the annulus, understanding that the 31-mm device moves forward within the left ventricle during deployment. The position of the CoreValve THV should be adjusted accordingly before the engagement of the CoreValve frames with the annulus. The 31-mm valve should be released very slowly during the first third of the deployment, with frequent pauses to release the radial force. It is important to release the tension on the guidewire and slightly push forward on the catheter to remove any tension placed on the valve by the catheter before final deployment.

Once the CoreValve frame has been deployed, the contralateral pigtail catheter is repositioned in the aortic root, and aortography is performed to assess the degree of aortic regurgitation **(Figure 7–15, D)**. A pigtail catheter is then readvanced and positioned in the left ventricle, and simultaneous pressures are recorded across the aortic valve prosthesis and the transvalvular gradient is assessed. Simultaneous aortic and left ventricular hemodynamics recordings are invaluable in determining the presence, degree, and severity of aortic regurgitation.

Additional balloon postdilation of the valve frame may be necessary in the event of significant paravalvular regurgitation caused by incomplete frame expansion but should be used judiciously.[43] After the aortic THV placement has been completed and the clinical result is deemed acceptable, the 18F sheath is withdrawn over a hydrophilic wire under fluoroscopic guidance. The introducer sheath can be reintroduced in the setting of significant vascular disease and resistance to sheath withdrawal. A "cross-over" wire technique can be performed to provide balloon occlusion of the iliac artery during sheath removal to decrease the arterial pressure. After suture ligation of the arteriotomy site, angiography also assists in making certain that there is no vascular injury.

TEMPORARY PACEMAKER PLACEMENT

Patients should be observed with a temporary pacemaker in place in a cardiovascular intensive care unit for 48 hours to monitor for conduction system disturbance. If these are not are observed, the patient is monitored for an additional 72 hours and discharged. Indications for permanent pacemaker placement are discussed below.

DISCHARGE MEDICATIONS

The patient should be continued on dual antiplatelet therapy (aspirin and clopidogrel) for 3 months after the procedure. In the presence of atrial fibrillation or other indications for system anticoagulation, warfarin and either aspirin or clopidogrel can be continued indefinitely. As these elderly patients are often at risk for gastrointestinal bleeding after the procedure, use of a proton pump inhibitor may be useful.

NONILIOFEMORAL ACCESS

In patients with iliofemoral vasculature unable to accommodate an 18F access sheath, the procedure can be performed via alternate access routes **(Figure 7–16).** Subclavian or axillary arterial access involves a surgical cut down to the artery in a subclavicular position.[44-47]

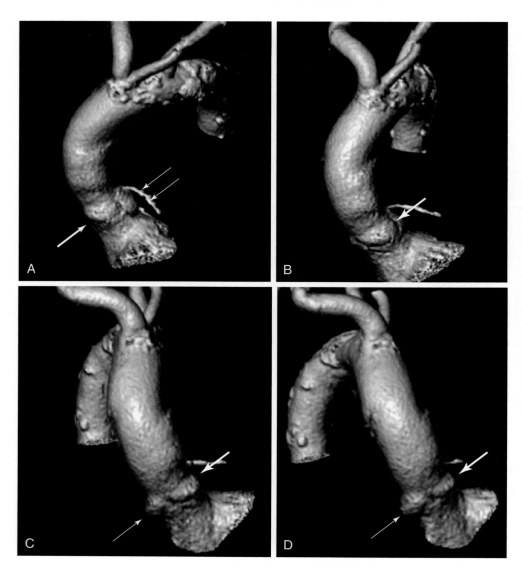

Figure 7–13 **Optimal implantation angulation for transcatheter heart valve implantation.** The location of the right and noncoronary cusps can be identified in the steep left anterior oblique (bold arrow, right coronary cusp; double arrow, left coronary artery) **(A)**, shallow left anterior oblique **(B)**, anteroposterior (bold arrow, right coronary cusp; double arrow, left coronary artery) **(C)**, and right anterior oblique projections **(D)**. The basal plane is more caudal in the right anterior oblique projections and slightly more cranial in the left anterior oblique projections. Separation of the right coronary and noncoronary sinus is best seen in the right anterior oblique projection **(D)**.

Although it is not an absolute contraindication, in patients with previous coronary bypass grafting and LIMA graft, the left subclavian approach is preferably avoided. Arterial dimensions are the same for the femoral approach, with a minimal luminal diameter of 6 mm for noncalcified vessels and 7 mm if vessels are calcified. The left subclavian approach allows for a straighter route to the aortic valve with less angulation, and the aortoventricular angle should be no more than 30 degrees for a right subclavian approach. The pigtail catheter for aortography can be inserted via radial or brachial arterial sheath if there is occlusive iliofemoral disease.

The direct aortic access route involves surgical right thoracotomy or hemisternotomy and direct visualization of the ascending aorta **(Figure 7–17)**.[48-50] Aortography before ascending aortic cannulation aids in optimal positioning to ensure access a minimum of 6 cm above the aortic annulus to allow sufficient room for valve detachment without removing the tip of the sheath from the artery **(Figure 7–18)**. A purse-string suture is placed in the ascending aorta before directly visualized puncture and wiring.

7.5 Complications

A unique series of complications have been observed after placement of the CoreValve THV. The Valve Academic Research Consortium (VARC) has provided standardized definitions for outcome reporting of these adverse events.[51] A central focus of ongoing device development and procedural improvement involves decreasing rates of TAVR-related complications, with the ultimate goal of expanded use to lower risk patients.

STROKES AND TRANSIENT ISCHEMIC ATTACKS

A central theme after TAVR has been the detection and prevention of neurologic disturbances after

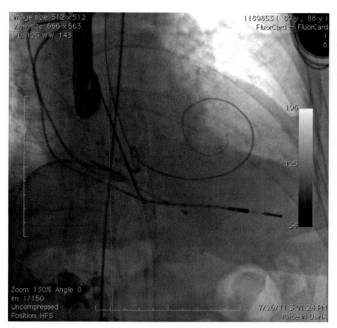

Figure 7–14   Guidewire positioning in the left ventricle. A 0.035-inch Amplatz Extra Stiff or Super Stiff guidewire is shaped so that there is a smooth curve in the left ventricle.

transcatheter therapy. The VARC has defined a stroke as any neurologic defect that persists over 24 hours or any transient (<24 hours) neurologic abnormality that is associated with a structural defect on brain imaging.[51-53] A disabling stroke is defined as a modified Rankin Score of 2 or higher.[52]

Neurologic disturbances after TAVR may result from atheroembolism of friable material with device movement around the aortic arch and across the aortic valve during TAVR, hemorrhage resulting from systemic anticoagulation, and thrombotic embolization caused by underlying atrial fibrillation.[54,55] Approximately 25% to 50% of the events occur after TAVR.[12,56]

Although the overall incidence of stroke has been relatively low (2% to 4%) immediately after the procedure,[56,57] higher rates of major stroke have been reported at 12 months (5.1% to 8.4%).[11,12] In a meta-analysis of 53 studies that includes 10,037 patients undergoing TAVR, procedural (<24 hours) stroke occurred in 1.5 ± 1.4% of patients, and the 30-day stroke or transient ischemic attack (TIA) rate was 3.3 ± 1.8%,[58] with the majority being major strokes (2.9 ± 1.8%).[58] During the first year after TAVR, stroke and TIA increased up to 5.2 ± 3.4%.[58] Thirty-day mortality was 3.5-fold higher in patients when compared with those without stroke (25.5 ± 21.9% vs. 6.9 ± 4.2%).[58] A similar relationship with late mortality has been reported by others.[56] Predictive factors for stroke include repeated

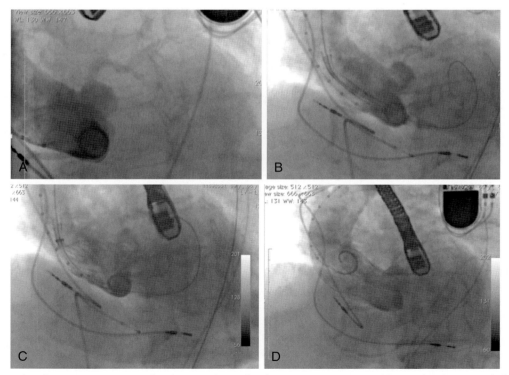

Figure 7–15   CoreValve placement. A, A 5F pigtail catheter is advanced to the noncoronary sinus to delineate the alignment of all three coronary sinuses, and to confirm the optimal angiographic deployment angle for the CoreValve device. **B,** The CoreValve device is then advanced across the aortic valve with careful positioning of the inflow portion of the frame just below the coronary sinuses. **C,** The delivery sheath is then slowly withdrawn, allowing the inflow portion of the frame to open and fix in the aortic annulus. The CoreValve is fully functioning once the sheath is withdrawn approximately two thirds of its length. **D,** The CoreValve frame is then released. Final aortography shows a well-positioned frame and no paravalvular regurgitation.

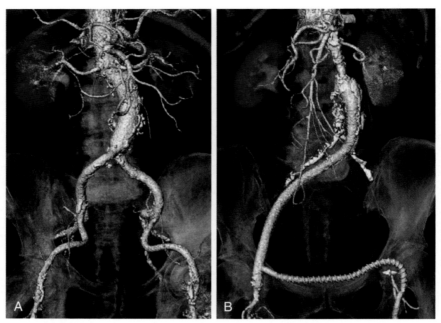

Figure 7–16   Prohibitive iliofemoral anatomy. Examples of prohibitive vascular anatomy for an iliofemoral approach include an abdominal aortic aneurysm **(A)** and a femoral–femoral bypass graft **(B)**. These patients are candidates for a direct aortic approach using the CoreValve devices.

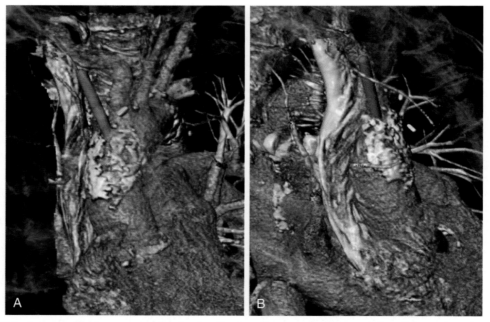

Figure 7–17   Multidetector computed tomography planning for direct aortic approach. The angulation of the aortic arch and aortic annulus is used to determine the optimal approach using a right thoracotomy **(A)** and median sternotomy **(B)**.

device implantation attempts,[56] BMI less than 25 kg/m^2,[56] transapical approach,[59] a history of a recent neurologic events,[59] and advanced functional disability.[59]

In addition to clinically apparent stroke, cerebral perfusion abnormalities manifest by defects in diffusion-weighted magnetic resonance imaging may occur in up to 70% to 80% of patients after TAVR.[60] Transcranial Doppler has demonstrated embolic events during TAVR,[61] most often during manipulation of the aortic valve. Novel embolic protection devices have been developed

to lessen the incidence of stroke and cerebral perfusion abnormalities after TAVR.[62]

PARAVALVULAR AORTIC REGURGITATION

Aortic regurgitation may be present in up to 25% of patients after TAVR.[31,63,64] Moderate to severe paravalvular regurgitation may occur in up to 15% of patients after CoreValve TAVR and has been associated with a worse late mortality rate.[24] The aortic regurgitation

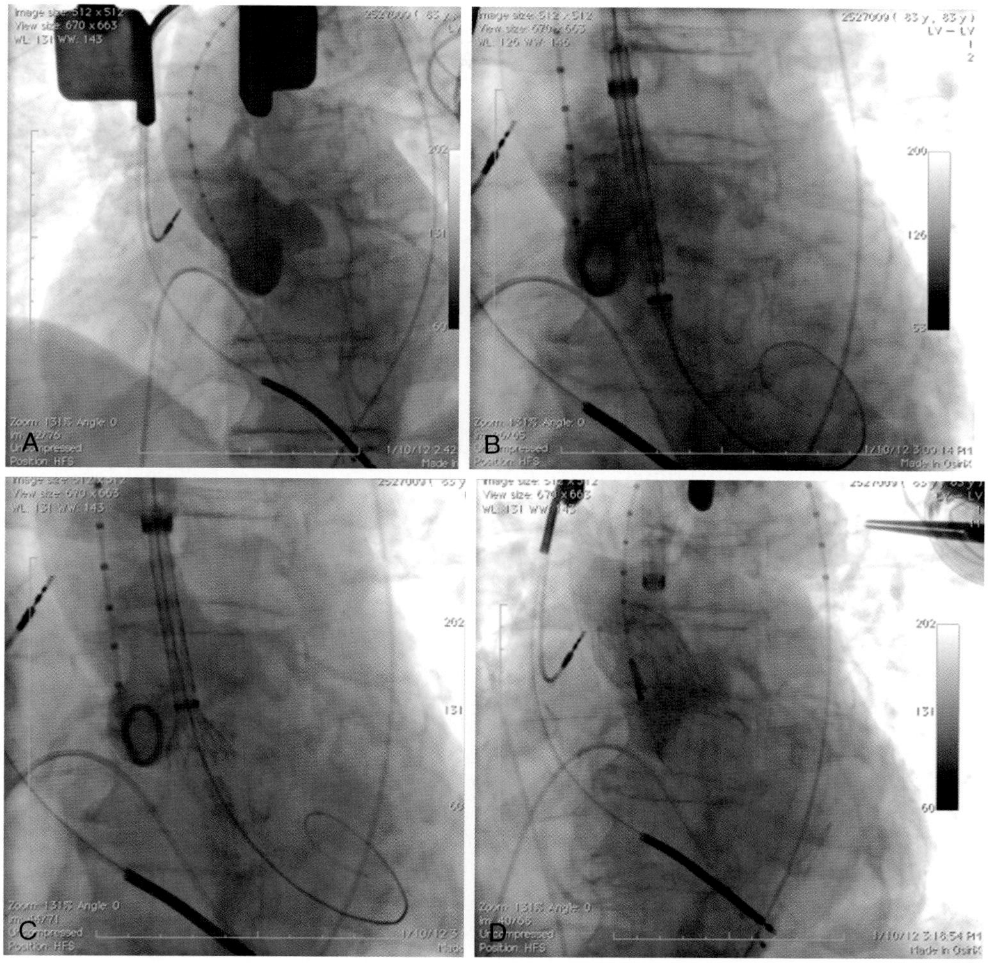

Figure 7–18 Direct aortic approach. A, A 5F pigtail catheter is advanced from the femoral artery and used for aortography to align the basal annular plane. **B,** The CoreValve device is then advanced across the aortic valve with careful positioning of the inflow portion of the frame just below the coronary sinuses. **C,** The delivery sheath is then slowly withdrawn, allowing the inflow portion of the frame to open and fix in the aortic annulus. **D,** The CoreValve is fully functioning once the sheath is withdrawn approximately two thirds of its length. The CoreValve frame is then released. Final aortography shows a well-positioned frame and no paravalvular regurgitation.

(AR) index is calculated as the ratio of the difference between the diastolic blood pressure (DBP) and left ventricular end-diastolic pressure (LVEDP) to systolic blood pressure (SBP):

$$[(DBP - LVEDP)/SBP] \times 100$$

A low (<25) aortic regurgitation index has been associated with a higher 1-year mortality.[65]

A detailed assessment of the degree of paravalvular regurgitation is performed using aortography, echocardiography, and hemodynamic assessment of the end-diastolic aortic and left ventricular pressures. Concordance of the findings suggesting significant aortic regurgitation may determine whether additional interventions are needed. There are a number of potential etiologies for paravalvular leak (PVL), primarily related to low positioning of the CoreValve frame, incomplete expansion of the frame into the eccentrically shaped aortic annulus, rigidity of the underlying aortic annulus because of calcium,[64,66] or undersizing of the valve relative to the aortic annular size.

When the CoreValve frame is incompletely expanded, postdeployment balloon valvuloplasty may useful, and when the CoreValve frame is positioned too low in relation to the aortic annulus after deployment, retraction of

the frame loops using a retrieval snare may allow appropriate positioning, although it may prove technically difficult. In the event that balloon aortic valvuloplasty is needed, it is recommended that a short, nontapered, and noncompliant balloon is used. The size of the postdilation balloon should be 1 to 2 mm smaller than the annular size, but it should be no larger than a 25-mm balloon for a 26 mm-CoreValve THV or a 28-mm balloon for the 29-mm and 31-mm CoreValve THVs. On occasion, valve-in-valve therapy is required.

Despite the potential benefit of balloon postdilation on the reduction of aortic regurgitation, adjunctive measures should be performed judiciously. In a series of 211 patients, balloon postdilation was performed for significant PVL in 28% of patients, leading to a reduction in at least 1 degree of aortic regurgitation in 71% of patients, with residual aortic regurgitation less than 2 degrees in 54% of the patients.[43] Predictors of the need for a balloon postdilation were the degree of valve calcification and transfemoral approach. Patients who underwent balloon postdilation had a higher incidence of cerebrovascular events at 30 days (11.9% vs. 2.0%, p = 0.006), with most events (83%) within the 24 hours after the procedure occurring in patients undergoing TAVR.[43]

CONDUCTION SYSTEM DISTURBANCES

The proximity of the interventricular membranous septum and the left bundle branch adjacent to the junction of the right coronary and noncoronary cusps renders patients susceptible to conduction system abnormalities after TAVR, particularly with self-expanding stent designs.[67] In early series, a new left bundle branch block occurred in 45.8% to 55% of patients, and complete atrioventricular block requiring permanent pacemaker implantation occurred in approximately 20% of patients.[67] In a meta-analysis of 7 national registries with 2,156 patients, there was a permanent pacemaker requirement of 28.7% (18.5% − 41.1%).[42]

A new left bundle branch block has been reported in up to 34% of patients who have had TAVR, including 51.1% of patients undergoing CoreValve TAVR and 12.0% undergoing balloon-expandable TAVR, respectively (p < 0.001).[68] All-cause mortality was 37.8% in patients with left bundle branch block and 24.0% in patients without left bundle branch block (p = 0.002); independent predictors for all-cause mortality were TAVR-induced left bundle branch block, chronic obstructive lung disease with LVEF 50% or less, and baseline renal dysfunction.[68] More favorable outcome data in patients with new left bundle branch block after TAVR are forthcoming. Patients who received permanent pacemakers for conduction disturbances had similar late mortality as those patients who did not receive a pacemaker.[69] Important predictors of need for permanent pacemaker placement include baseline right bundle branch block,[70] small interventricular septal thickness,[18] and the distance between the noncoronary sinus and the depth of implantation.[18,71]

A judicious approach to the implantation of a pacemaker based on symptoms and current indications has been proposed.[72] With better implantation techniques, including those that reduce the injury at the time of balloon aortic valvuloplasty,[73] and higher implantation methods facilitated by the CoreValve delivery catheter, permanent pacemaker rates of fewer than 20% have been reported.[42]

VASCULAR ACCESS COMPLICATIONS

Because of the relatively large (18F) caliber sheath required for placement, vascular complications may occur during and after CoreValve placement[74] with an incidence that varies between 4% to 13%. Careful preprocedural screening using CT angiography, use of vascular ultrasound guidance for arterial access,[41] and the use of alternative (e.g., subclavian) access have provided better case selection in attempts to avoid vascular complications. The majority of vascular complications can be managed via transcatheter techniques.[74]

7.6 Summary

The CoreValve ReValving system is a valuable alternative to sAVR in patients who are poorly suited for conventional cardiac surgery. The CoreValve design has particular advantages of a broad range of sizes (annular diameter 18 to 29 mm), supraannular location of the valve to allow conformability to the eccentric annulus, and a lower profile owing to the porcine pericardial valve. Complications, including stroke, PVL, conduction system abnormalities, and vascular complications are a central focus for future improvements of the CoreValve design.

REFERENCES

1. Carabello BA, Paulus WJ: Aortic stenosis, Lancet 373(9667):956–966, 2009 Mar 14.
2. Bonow RO, Carabello BA, Chatterjee K, et al: ACC/AHA 2006 guidelines for the management of patients with valvular heart disease: a report of the American College of Cardiology/American Heart Association Task Force on Practice Guidelines (writing Committee to Revise the 1998 guidelines for the management of patients with valvular heart disease) developed in collaboration with the Society of Cardiovascular Anesthesiologists endorsed by the Society for Cardiovascular Angiography and Interventions and the Society of Thoracic Surgeons, J Am Coll Cardiol 48(3):e1–e148, 2006 Aug 1.
3. O'Brien S, Shahian D, Filardo G, et al: The Society of Thoracic Surgeons 2008 cardiac surgery risk models. Part 2. Isolated valve surgery, Ann Thoracic Surg 88:S23–S42, 2009.
4. Bittner HB, Savitt MA: Management of porcelain aorta and calcified great vessels in coronary artery bypass grafting with off-pump and no-touch technology, Ann Thoracic Surg 72(4):1378–1380, 2001 Oct.
5. Byrne JG, Aranki SF, Cohn LH: Aortic valve operations under deep hypothermic circulatory arrest for the porcelain aorta: "no-touch" technique, Ann Thorac Surg 65(5):1313–1315, 1998 May.
6. Boeken U, Schurr P, Feindt P, et al: Cardiac valve replacement in patients with end-stage renal failure: impact of prosthesis type on the early postoperative course, Thorac Cardiovasc Surg 58(1):23–27, 2010 Feb.
7. Boulton BJ, Kilgo P, Guyton RA, et al: Impact of preoperative renal dysfunction in patients undergoing off-pump versus on-pump coronary artery bypass, Ann Thorac Surg 92(2):595–601, 2011 Aug.
8. Brinkman WT, Williams WH, Guyton RA, et al: Valve replacement in patients on chronic renal dialysis: implications for valve prosthesis selection, Ann Thorac Surg 74(1):37–42, 2002 Jul.
9. Bloomstein LZ, Gielchinsky I, Bernstein AD, et al: Aortic valve replacement in geriatric patients: determinants of in-hospital mortality, Ann Thorac Surg 71(2):597–600, 2001 Feb.
10. Bose AK, Aitchison JD, Dark JH: Aortic valve replacement in octogenarians, J Cardiothorac Surg 2:33, 2007.
11. Leon MB, Smith CR, Mack M, et al: Transcatheter aortic-valve implantation for aortic stenosis in patients who cannot undergo surgery, N Engl J Med 363(17):1597–1607, 2010 Oct 21.
12. Smith CR, Leon MB, Mack MJ, et al: Transcatheter versus surgical aortic-valve replacement in high-risk patients, N Engl J Med 364(23):2187–2198, 2011 Jun 9.
13. Makkar RR, Fontana GP, Jilaihawi H, et al: Transcatheter aortic-valve replacement for inoperable severe aortic stenosis, N Engl J Med 366(18):1696–1704, 2012 Mar 26.
14. Kodali SK, Williams MR, Smith CR, et al: Two-year outcomes after transcatheter or surgical aortic-valve replacement, N Engl J Med 366(18):1686–1695, 2012 Mar 26.
15. Stortecky S, Schmid V, Windecker S, et al: Improvement of physical and mental health after transfemoral transcatheter aortic valve implantation, EuroIntervention 8(4):437–443, 2012 Aug 25.
16. Ussia GP, Barbanti M, Petronio AS, et al: Transcatheter aortic valve implantation: 3-year outcomes of self-expanding CoreValve prosthesis, Eur Heart J 33(8):969–978, 2012 Jan 12.
17. Holmes DR, Mack M, Kaul S, et al: 2012 ACCF/AATS/SCAI/STS expert consensus document on transcatheter aortic valve replacement, J Am Coll Cardiol 59(13):1200–1254, 2012 Mar 27.
18. Seipelt RG, Hanekop GG, Schoendube FA, et al: Heart team approach for transcatheter aortic valve implantation procedures complicated by coronary artery occlusion, Interact Cardiovasc Thorac Surg 14(4):431–433, 2012 Apr.
19. Stortecky S, Schoenenberger AW, Moser A, et al: Evaluation of multidimensional geriatric assessment as a predictor of mortality and cardiovascular events after transcatheter aortic valve implantation, JACC Cardiovasc Interv 5(5):489–496, 2012 May.

20. Tommaso CL, Bolman RM, Feldman T, et al: Multisociety (AATS, ACCF, SCAI, and STS) expert consensus statement: operator and institutional requirements for transcatheter valve repair and replacement. Part 1. Transcatheter aortic valve replacement, *Catheter Cardiovasc Interv* 143(6):1254–1263, 2012 Mar 1. epublication.

21. Bakaeen FG, Kar B, Chu D, et al: Establishment of a transcatheter aortic valve program and heart valve team at a Veterans Affairs facility, *Am J Surg* 204(5):643–648, 2012 Aug 23.

22. Ong SH, Bauernschmitt R, Schuler G, et al: Short- and mid-term safety and effectiveness of transcatheter aortic valve implantation in a failing surgical aortic bioprosthesis, *Eur J Cardiothorac Surg* 42(2):268–276, 2012 Aug.

23. Buellesfeld L, Grube E: A permanent solution for a temporary problem: transcatheter valve-in-valve implantation for failed transcatheter aortic valve replacement, *JACC Cardiovasc Interv* 5(5):578–581, 2012 May.

24. Vasa-Nicotera M, Sinning JM, Chin D, et al: Impact of paravalvular leakage on outcome in patients after transcatheter aortic valve implantation, *JACC Cardiovasc Interv* 5(8):858–865, 2012 Aug.

25. Dumonteil N, Marcheix B, Lairez O, et al: Transcatheter aortic valve implantation for severe, noncalcified aortic regurgitation and narrow aortic root: description from a case report of a new approach to potentially avoid coronary artery obstruction, *Catheter Cardiovasc Interv* 82(2):E124–E127, 2013 Aug 1.

26. Lauten A, Zahn R, Horack M, et al: Transcatheter aortic valve implantation in patients with low-flow, low-gradient aortic stenosis, *JACC Cardiovasc Interv* 5(5):552–559, 2012 May.

27. Gotzmann M, Lindstaedt M, Bojara W, et al: Clinical outcome of transcatheter aortic valve implantation in patients with low-flow, low gradient aortic stenosis, *Catheter Cardiovasc Interv* 79(5):693–701, 2012 Apr 1.

28. D'Onofrio A, Gasparetto V, Napodano M, et al: Impact of preoperative mitral valve regurgitation on outcomes after transcatheter aortic valve implantation, *Eur J Cardiothorac Surg* 41(6):1271–1276, 2012 Jun.

29. Himbert D, Pontnau F, Messika-Zeitoun D, et al: Feasibility and outcomes of transcatheter aortic valve implantation in high-risk patients with stenotic bicuspid aortic valves, *Am J Cardiol* 110(6):877–883, 2012 Sep 15.

30. Genereux P, Head SJ, Van Mieghem NM, et al: Clinical outcomes after transcatheter aortic valve replacement using valve academic research consortium definitions: a weighted meta-analysis of 3519 patients from 16 studies, *J Am Coll Cardiol* 59(25):2317–2326, 2012 Jun 19.

31. Willson AB, Webb JG, Labounty TM, et al: Three-dimensional aortic annular assessment by multidetector computed tomography predicts moderate or severe paravalvular regurgitation after transcatheter aortic valve replacement: a multicenter retrospective analysis, *J Am Coll Cardiol* 59(14):1287–1294, 2012 Apr 3.

32. Jabbour A, Ismail TF, Moat N, et al: Multimodality imaging in transcatheter aortic valve implantation and postprocedural aortic regurgitation: comparison among cardiovascular magnetic resonance, cardiac computed tomography, and echocardiography, *J Am Coll Cardiol* 58(21):2165–2173, 2011 Nov 15.

33. Kempfert J, Van Linden A, Lehmkuhl L, et al: Aortic annulus sizing: echocardiographic versus computed tomography derived measurements in comparison with direct surgical sizing, *Eur J Cardiothorac Surg* 42(4):627–633, 2012 Oct.

34. Bloomfield GS, Gillam LD, Hahn RT, et al: A practical guide to multimodality imaging of transcatheter aortic valve replacement, *JACC Cardiovasc Imaging* 5(4):441–455, 2012 Apr.

35. Schultz CJ, Moelker A, Piazza N, et al: Three dimensional evaluation of the aortic annulus using multislice computer tomography: are manufacturer's guidelines for sizing for percutaneous aortic valve replacement helpful? *Eur Heart J* 31(7):849–856, 2010 Apr.

36. Jilaihawi H, Kashif M, Fontana G, et al: Cross-sectional computed tomographic assessment improves accuracy of aortic annular sizing for transcatheter aortic valve replacement and reduces the incidence of paravalvular aortic regurgitation, *J Am Coll Cardiol* 59(14):1275–1286, 2012 Apr 3.

37. Bapat VN, Attia RQ, Thomas M: Distribution of calcium in the ascending aorta in patients undergoing transcatheter aortic valve implantation and its relevance to the transaortic approach, *JACC Cardiovasc Interv* 5(5):470–476, 2012 May.

38. Pasic M, Unbehaun A, Dreysse S, et al: Rupture of the device landing zone during transcatheter aortic valve implantation: a life-threatening but treatable complication, *Circ Cardiovasc Interv* 5(3):424–432, 2012 Jun.

39. Tamborini G, Fusini L, Gripari P, et al: Feasibility and accuracy of 3DTEE versus CT for the evaluation of aortic valve annulus to left main ostium distance before transcatheter aortic valve implantation, *JACC Cardiovasc Imaging* 5(6):579–588, 2012 Jun.

40. Leipsic J, Wood D, Manders D, et al: The evolving role of MDCT in transcatheter aortic valve replacement: a radiologists' perspective, *AJR Am J Roentgenol* 193(3):W214–W219, 2009 Sep.

41. de Jaegere P, van Dijk L, Laborde J, et al: True percutaneous implantation of the CoreValve aortic valve prosthesis by the combined use of ultrasound guided vascular access, Prostar XL, and the TandemHeart, *EuroIntervention* 2:500–505, 2007.

42. Tchetche D, Modine T, Farah B, et al: Update on the need for a permanent pacemaker after transcatheter aortic valve implantation using the CoreValve(R) Accutrak system, *EuroIntervention* 8(5):556–562, 2012 Jun 15.

43. Nombela-Franco L, Rodes-Cabau J, DeLarochelliere R, et al: Predictive factors, efficacy, and safety of balloon post-dilation after transcatheter aortic valve implantation with a balloon-expandable valve, *JACC Cardiovasc Interv* 5(5):499–512, 2012 May.

44. Petronio AS, De Carlo M, Bedogni F, et al: Two-year results of CoreValve implantation through the subclavian access: a propensity-matched comparison with the femoral access, *J Am Coll Cardiol* 60(6):502–507, 2012 Aug 7.

45. Fraccaro C, Napodano M, Tarantini G, et al: Expanding the eligibility for transcatheter aortic valve implantation the trans-subclavian retrograde approach using: the III generation CoreValve revalving system, *JACC Cardiovasc Interv* 2(9):828–833, 2009 Sep.

46. Bojara W, Mumme A, Gerckens U, et al: Implantation of the CoreValve self-expanding valve prosthesis via a subclavian artery approach: a case report, *Clin Res Cardiol* 98(3):201–204, 2009 Mar.

47. Ruge H, Lange R, Bleiziffer S, et al: First successful aortic valve implantation with the CoreValve ReValving system via right subclavian artery access: a case report, *Heart Surg Forum* 11(5):E323–E324, 2008.

48. Alegria-Barrero E, Chan PH, Di Mario C, et al: Direct aortic transcatheter aortic valve implantation: a feasible approach for patients with severe peripheral vascular disease, *Cardiovasc Revasc Med* 13(3):201, 2012 May-Jun. e5–e7.

49. Bruschi G, De Marco F, Botta L, et al: Direct transaortic CoreValve implantation through right minithoracotomy in patients with patent coronary grafts, *Ann Thorac Surg* 93(4):1297–1299, 2012 Apr.

50. Bruschi G, de Marco F, Botta L, et al: Direct aortic access for transcatheter self-expanding aortic bioprosthetic valves implantation, *Ann Thorac Surg* 94(2):497–503, 2012 Aug.

51. Leon MB, Piazza N, Nikolsky E, et al: Standardized endpoint definitions for transcatheter aortic valve implantation clinical trials: a consensus report from the Valve Academic Research Consortium, *J Am Coll Cardiol* 57(3):253–269, 2011 Jan 18.

52. Leon MB, Piazza N, Nikolsky E, et al: Standardized endpoint definitions for transcatheter aortic valve implantation clinical trials: a consensus report from the Valve Academic Research Consortium, *Eur Heart J* 32(2):205–217, 2011 Jan.

53. Easton JD, Saver JL, Albers GW, et al: Definition and evaluation of transient ischemic attack: a scientific statement for healthcare professionals from the American Heart Association/American Stroke Association Stroke Council; Council on Cardiovascular Surgery and Anesthesia; Council on Cardiovascular Radiology and Intervention; Council on Cardiovascular Nursing; and the Interdisciplinary Council on Peripheral Vascular Disease. *Stroke* 40(6):2276–2293, 2009 Jun.

54. Iung B, Himbert D, Vahanian A: Atrial fibrillation following transcatheter aortic valve implantation: do we underestimate its frequency and impact? *J Am Coll Cardiol* 59(2):189–190, 2012 Jan 10.

55. Amat-Santos IJ, Rodes-Cabau J, Urena M, et al: Incidence, predictive factors, and prognostic value of new-onset atrial fibrillation following transcatheter aortic valve implantation, *J Am Coll Cardiol* 59(2):178–188, 2012 Jan 10.

56. Stortecky S, Windecker S, Pilgrim T, et al: Cerebrovascular accidents complicating transcatheter aortic valve implantation: frequency, timing and impact on outcomes, *EuroIntervention* 8(1):62–70, 2012 May 15.

57. Daneault B, Kirtane AJ, Kodali SK, et al: Stroke associated with surgical and transcatheter treatment of aortic stenosis: a comprehensive review, J Am Coll Cardiol 58(21):2143–2150, 2011 Nov 15.
58. Eggebrecht H, Schmermund A, Voigtlander T, et al: Risk of stroke after transcatheter aortic valve implantation (TAVI): a meta-analysis of 10,037 published patients, EuroIntervention 8(1):129–138, 2012 May 15.
59. Miller DC, Blackstone EH, Mack MJ, et al: Transcatheter (TAVR) versus surgical (AVR) aortic valve replacement: occurrence, hazard, risk factors, and consequences of neurologic events in the PARTNER trial, J Thorac Cardiovasc Surg 143(4):832–843, 2012 Apr. e13.
60. Fairbairn TA, Mather AN, Bijsterveld P, et al: Diffusion-weighted MRI determined cerebral embolic infarction following transcatheter aortic valve implantation: assessment of predictive risk factors and the relationship to subsequent health status, Heart 98(1):18–23, 2012 Jan.
61. Erdoes G, Basciani R, Huber C, et al: Transcranial Doppler-detected cerebral embolic load during transcatheter aortic valve implantation, Eur J Cardiothorac Surg 41(4):778–783, 2012 Apr. discussion 83–84.
62. Naber CK, Ghanem A, Abizaid AA, et al: First-in-man use of a novel embolic protection device for patients undergoing transcatheter aortic valve implantation, EuroIntervention 8(1):43–50, 2012 May 15.
63. Zahn R, Schiele R, Kilkowski C, et al: Correction of aortic regurgitation after transcatheter aortic valve implantation of the Medtronic CoreValve prosthesis due to a too-low implantation, using transcatheter repositioning, J Heart Valve Dis 20(1):64–69, 2011 Jan.
64. Yared K, Garcia-Camarero T, Fernandez-Friera L, et al: Impact of aortic regurgitation after transcatheter aortic valve implantation: results from the REVIVAL trial, JACC Cardiovasc Imaging 5(5):469–477, 2012 May.
65. Sinning JM, Hammerstingl C, Vasa-Nicotera M, et al: Aortic regurgitation index defines severity of periprosthetic regurgitation and predicts outcome in patients after transcatheter aortic valve implantation, J Am Coll Cardiol 59(13):1134–1141, 2012 Mar 27.
66. Haensig M, Lehmkuhl L, Rastan AJ, et al: Aortic valve calcium scoring is a predictor of significant paravalvular aortic insufficiency in transapical-aortic valve implantation, Eur J Cardiothorac Surg 41(6):1234–1240, 2012 Jan 12.
67. Piazza N, Onuma Y, Jesserun E, et al: Early and persistent intraventricular conduction abnormalities and requirements for pacemaking after percutaneous replacement of the aortic valve, JACC Cardiovasc Interv 1(3):310–316, 2008 Jun.
68. Houthuizen P, Van Garsse LA, Poels TT, et al: Left bundle-branch block induced by transcatheter aortic valve implantation increases risk of death, Circulation 126(6):720–728, 2012 Aug 7.
69. Buellesfeld L, Stortecky S, Heg D, et al: Impact of permanent pacemaker implantation on clinical outcome among patients undergoing transcatheter aortic valve implantation, J Am Coll Cardiol 60(6):493–501, 2012 Aug 7.
70. Bagur R, Rodes-Cabau J, Gurvitch R, et al: Need for permanent pacemaker as a complication of transcatheter aortic valve implantation and surgical aortic valve replacement in elderly patients with severe aortic stenosis and similar baseline electrocardiographic findings, JACC Cardiovasc Interv 5(5):540–551, 2012 May.
71. Chorianopoulos E, Krumsdorf U, Pleger ST, et al: Improved procedural results after CoreValve implantation with the new AccuTrak delivery system, J Interv Cardiol 25(2):174–179, 2012 Apr.
72. De Carlo M, Giannini C, Bedogni F, et al: Safety of a conservative strategy of permanent pacemaker implantation after transcatheter aortic CoreValve implantation, Am Heart J 163(3):492–499, 2012 Mar.
73. Roten L, Stortecky S, Scarcia F, et al: Atrioventricular conduction after transcatheter aortic valve implantation and surgical aortic valve replacement, J Cardiovasc Electrophysiol 23(10):1115–1122, 2012 Apr 16.
74. Stortecky S, Wenaweser P, Diehm N, et al: Percutaneous management of vascular complications in patients undergoing transcatheter aortic valve implantation, JACC Cardiovasc Interv 5(5):515–524, 2012 May.

Chapter 8

Percutaneous Pulmonary Valve Implantation

HARSIMRAN S. SINGH • LEE N. BENSON • MARK OSTEN • ERIC HORLICK

As the twenty-first century progresses, a new chapter in cardiac therapeutics is being written with the development of transcatheter valve technologies. Percutaneous pulmonary valve implantation (PPVI) has the distinction of being the first percutaneous valve replacement in humans and has allowed treatment of a growing patient population with congenital heart disease (CHD). These patients are at risk for traditional surgery because of multiple prior procedures or are often not surgical candidates. PPVI technologies minimize the number of lifetime sternotomies and can extend the life of previously implanted conduits.

This chapter reviews pulmonary valve pathology, including those conditions that require either surgical or percutaneous pulmonary valve replacement (PVR). The authors examine the experience to date for PPVI, highlighting indications, patient eligibility, currently available valve technologies, procedural considerations, potential complications and reported short- and long-term outcomes. Finally, future horizons for PPVI are discussed.

8.1 Pulmonary Valve Pathophysiology

The pulmonary valve (PV) is comprised of three semilunar cusps (anterior, right, and left) attached to the pulmonary trunk. The embryologic development of the PV begins at about 5 weeks' gestation arising from outpouching mesenchymal cushions and resulting in the septation of the common arterial trunk.[1] Unlike the cardiac valves in the left heart, the majority of PV clinical pathology is related to either a congenital anomaly or occurs secondary to a surgical intervention, including PV or right ventricular outflow tract (RVOT) obstruction and/or incompetence.

PULMONARY STENOSIS

Native PV or RVOT obstruction occurs in approximately 20% to 30% of patients with CHD, in isolation or in association with other congenital syndromes such as tetralogy of Fallot (TOF), Noonan syndrome, or congenital rubella. Up to 90% of isolated pulmonary stenosis (PS) is valvular, illustrated by systolic cusp doming caused by fusion of one or more of the valve commissures.[2] Occasionally, this may be in the setting of a bicuspid, quadricuspid, or dysplastic valve (e.g., Noonan syndrome) where there is little valve fusion but associated valve thickening, a small annulus, and short main pulmonary artery (PA). In addition to the valvular lesion, obstruction can occur in the subvalvular region in the RVOT, such as in a double-chambered right ventricle resulting from muscle bundles, or a supravalvular region, as seen in Williams syndrome. **Figure 8–1** illustrates the angiographic appearance of subvalvular, valvular, and supravalvular PS. TOF, the most common form of cyanotic heart disease, is represented by underdevelopment of the subpulmonary outflow caused by anterior deviation of the infundibular septum, resulting in the aorta overriding the ventricular septum and a malalignment ventricular septal defect (VSD).

Depending on the severity of the PS and adequacy of pulmonary blood flow, clinical symptoms may range from neonatal compromise with varying degrees of right ventricular (RV) hypoplasia requiring urgent neonatal intervention[3] to the gradual development of PS symptoms as the obstruction worsens with time.[4,5] Generally, PV gradients less than 20 mm Hg do not increase with the passage of time, whereas higher gradients may worsen. Increased RV systolic pressure leads to RV remodeling with either myocardial hyperplasia (when the exposure is during fetal or neonatal development) or hypertrophy outside the first months of life. This increase in RV mass decreases ventricular compliance and can progress to RV dilation and dysfunction in end stages. When PS manifests late, clinical manifestations include exertional intolerance, development of supraventricular or ventricular arrhythmias, endocarditis, cyanosis (in the presence of a concomitant interatrial shunt), and additional

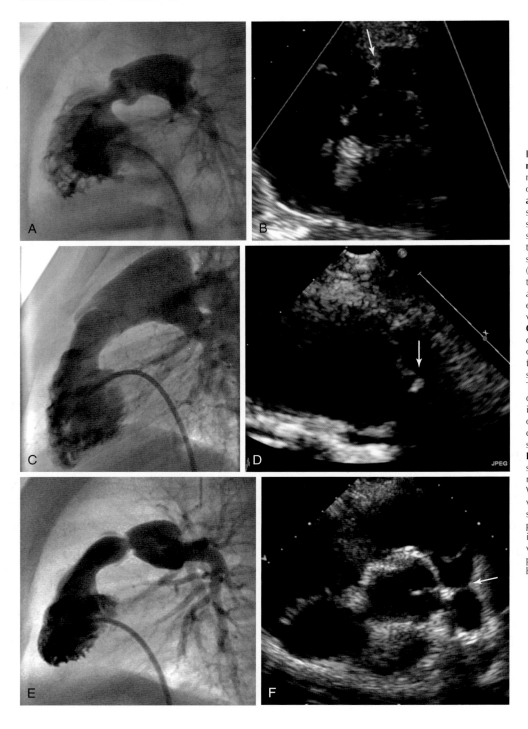

Figure 8–1 Imaging of Pulmonary Stenosis. These images document pulmonary stenosis and obstruction at the subvalvular (**A and B**), valvular (**C and D**), and supravalvular level (**E and F**). **A** shows evidence of infundibular stenosis of the RVOT in the setting of only mild-to-moderate stenosis of the pulmonary valve (20 mm Hg peak gradient across the valve vs. 30 mm Hg gradient across the RVOT). **B,** Transthoracic echo image demonstrates subvalvular pulmonary stenosis *(arrow)*. **C,** Valvular PS notable by the domed appearance of the valve cusps from commissural fusion on fluoroscopy. There is minimal visual obstruction across the RVOT. There is evidence of poststenotic dilation of the PA. **D,** Corresponding transthoracic echo image demonstrates doming of the pulmonary cusps *(arrow)* in a patient with severe valvular pulmonic stenosis. **E,** There is focal obstruction in the supravalvular lesion of the proximal main PA in this patient with Williams syndrome. On additional views, there are other levels of obstruction also present in the branch pulmonary arteries. **F,** Transthoracic echo image demonstrates supravalvular pulmonary stenosis in a patient with history of surgical PA banding *(arrow)*.

right-sided valvular disease (tricuspid or PR). Prognosis and symptoms are primarily determined by the severity of obstruction.[5]

Severe valvular PS, when isolated, can be treated by either surgical valvotomy or as in the past several decades, by percutaneous balloon valvuloplasty, both with excellent short- and long-term results in children and adults.[6,7] However, most patients with subvalvular, supravalvular, or multilevel obstruction require surgical correction. In children, surgical options for PVR have to

be balanced with future growth in addition to the individual anatomy. Bioprosthetic valves, homograft, and synthetic conduits (both valved and nonvalved) have been employed with varying frequency as valve replacements. Complete surgical repair of TOF typically includes reduction or elimination of the valvular and subvalvular RVOT obstruction, often a transannular patch reconstruction of the RVOT (particularly in the symptomatic infant), and closure of the malalignment VSD. As such, TOF repair often leads to significant pulmonary regurgitation (PR).

PULMONARY REGURGITATION

As noted, PR commonly occurs after surgical repair of TOF, especially with the use of a transannular patch. However, significant PR can also be found as an isolated condition, as a consequence of balloon or surgical pulmonary valvotomy, in the presence of bilateral PA or peripheral PA stenosis, or as a consequence of increased pulmonary vascular resistance.[8] Over time, nearly all surgical implants (bioprosthetic valves and conduits) in the pulmonary position become dysfunctional and develop some combination of PR and PS requiring additional management.

For many years, the contribution of PR to patient morbidity and ventricular dysfunction were overlooked, partly because PR can be well tolerated for a long time. However, approximately 30% of patients with chronic severe PR develop symptoms by the fourth decade of life.[9,10] In the repaired TOF population there is considerable variability in the anatomic dimension of the RVOT, pulmonary annulus, and branch PAs confounded by variations in TOF surgery that influence PR severity, the rate of RV dilation, and the development of symptoms.[11] The regurgitant volume back across the PV is driven by the diastolic pressure differential between the PA and right ventricle. This pressure differential is in turn determined by: 1) the RV compliance related to the degree of RV hypertrophy, stiffness, and fibrosis; 2) PA afterload consisting of the pulmonary vascular resistance and the presence of any PA stenosis; and 3) intrathoracic and airway pressure changes, typically contributing in the acute rather than chronic setting.[8,12,13]

Over time, significant PR results in RV dilation.[8,10] As a consequence, pressure–volume hemodynamic studies have shown RV volumes to increase while left ventricular (LV) volumes decrease.[14] In this setting, both ventricles have a diminished ability to augment ventricular output in response to inotropes. LV underfilling occurs as a consequence of RV dilation and secondary to septal bowing into the LV during diastole. The lack of mechanical–electrical synchrony between the ventricles also contributes to an overall reduction in biventricular function and efficiency.[15] Further dilation of the right ventricle can lead to RV dysfunction with symptomatic heart failure and secondary complications such as cardiac cirrhosis. Secondary tricuspid regurgitation can develop from annular dilation, further exacerbating the volume load on the right heart. Valvular regurgitation is associated with inhomogeneous electrical activation and slowed conduction velocities that are proarrhythmic and promote ventricular and supraventricular arrhythmias.[8,16]

The spectrum of clinical presentations secondary to chronic PR and RV dilation include dyspnea, fatigue, activity limiting palpitations, syncope, edema, diminished exercise capacity, and sudden cardiac death.[2,10,17,18] Several observational studies have suggested an association between PR and long-term outcomes including mortality.[19] In these studies, cardiac death was usually attributed to heart failure or sudden cardiac death.[8]

In the subset of patients who proscribe progressive and/or debilitating symptoms secondary to significant PR and RV dilation, the choice to offer a PVR is an easy one. The clinical decision making is less straightforward in those patients who deny symptoms or a change in functional status. Objective evidence of severe RV dilation or RV dysfunction attributable to PR is an indication for PVR in asymptomatic patients, though there remains diagnostic uncertainty as to the acceptable degree of RV dilation before proceeding with PVR. Small nonrandomized studies have looked at imaged-based parameters and suggested several cut-off points (i.e., an RV–end diastolic volume index [RVEDVI] of greater than 150 to 170 mL/m^2) to guide decision making for surgical intervention,[20,21] in addition to objective findings on formal exercise testing and Holter monitoring. Regardless of the exact timing for intervention, a majority of patients with severe PR require a PVR at some point.

8.2 Surgical Pulmonary Valve Replacement

For many years, surgical PVR had been the gold standard in the treatment of severe PR; mixed native PS or PR; or failure of a prior surgical bioprosthetic valve, homograft, monocusp, or conduit implants. Isolated surgical PVR is effective and can be performed with low perioperative mortality (reported 1% to 2%) and relatively minimal perioperative morbidity.[22] Surgical techniques for PVR depend on the choice of prosthesis, anatomy of the individual RVOT (e.g., replacing an RV-to-PA conduit vs. a bioprosthetic PVR with removal of transannular patch), and the need for any additional surgical repairs (e.g., tricuspid annuloplasty, PA enlargement, Maze procedure, and/or ventricular tachycardia ablation). Native valve surgical PVR is performed through a right ventriculotomy on cardiopulmonary bypass and most often using cardioplegia, though "beating heart" operations have been described. The valve is typically placed in the orthotopic position, although heterotopic RV-to-PA connections are constructed in certain instances. **Figure 8–2** provides an anatomic example of an RV-to-PA conduit in a patient with D-transposition of the great arteries (D-TGA). Valved surgical conduits can consist of cadaveric homografts (from the aortic or pulmonic position), manufactured bioprosthetic valves, or specialized bovine jugular valves that are sewn into synthetic conduit grafts **(Figure 8–3)**.

TYPES OF PROSTHESIS

The choice of prosthesis choice must take into account age, potential for growth, and the need for future reoperations or interventions. Mechanical valves are not implanted in the pulmonary position secondary to a high thrombosis risk observed during initial clinical experience.[23,24] although this has been contested in more recent retrospective series.[25] Homografts are commonly used in the primary correction of children with complex RVOT obstruction (e.g., TOF with pulmonary atresia or truncus

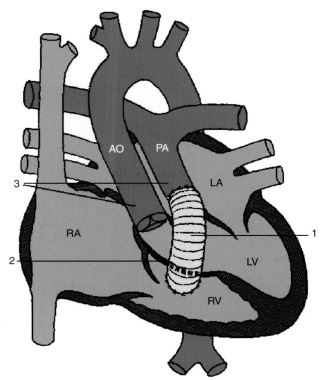

Figure 8–2 Schematic of a sample RV-to-PA conduit in a Rastelli repair for a patient with D-TGA. The RV-to-PA conduit *(1)* is placed in addition to construction of an intracardiac tunnel from LV to aorta *(2)* in patients with D-TGA, ventricular septal defect, and severe pulmonary stenosis or pulmonary atresia. *(Adapted from Mayer, Mullins, C. Congenital heart disease: a diagrammatic atlas. New York: Alan R. Liss, 1988, p. 5. Used with permission from Wiley-Liss, a subsidiary of John Wiley and Sons, Inc.)*

arteriosus) because of the availability of small diameters.[26] Retrospective surgical series of such implants suggest 75% to 85% 10-year freedom from reoperation, although significant implant dysfunction may be present in up to 50% at 10 years.[27]

Bioprosthetic implants are xenograft-based valves, constructed from either animal valves (porcine, bovine, or equine) or pericardial tissue. In the basic design, these valves are either "stented" when constructed within a sewing ring (usually three metal struts) or "stentless." There is no evidence that either bioprosthetic design is advantageous, although one retrospective series suggested that stentless valves pose an independent risk factor for redo PVR at 10 years.[22] In this study, other risk factors for bioprosthetic failure included younger age of valve implantation and a diagnosis of pulmonary atresia with VSD. Surgical series for bioprosthetic PVR show rates of 10-year valve dysfunction to be as high as 80%, with 10-year freedom from redo-PVR ranging from 52 to 86%.[22,28,29]

Monocusp valves are constructed individually by the surgeon to fit the patient's anatomy using pericardial tissue or polytetrafluoroethylene (PTFE).[30] Although they are described as having good short- to medium-term functional characteristics, their longevity has been questioned, due to variable surgical technique.[31,32] As they must be modeled in the operating room, monocusp

valve implantation may increase bypass and operative times. One published surgical series reported a 52% incidence of significant PR, although freedom from reoperation at 10 years was 82%.[31]

PROSTHESIS DURABILITY

Whereas some study cohorts have suggested improved longevity for homografts compared with bioprosthetic valves, there is little prospective evidence. Choice of valve is influenced by local availability and operator preference. The largest published pediatric surgical PVR series originates from Toronto and includes 945 valves, including homografts, bioprosthetic valves (porcine and pericardial), and bioprosthetic valved conduits.[33] Overall, there was an 81% freedom from reoperation at 5 years, 58% at 10 years, and 41% at 15 years. The risk factor associated with valve deterioration in the entire study group was a younger age at valve implantation (median age for surgery was 6.2 years). Risk factors in the 260-patient subgroup aged 13 to 65 years included smaller normalized valve prosthesis size for patient size, placement of endovascular stents, and increased number of previous valve placements. There was also a suggestion that homografts, conduits, and pericardial based bioprosthetic valves may be preferable to porcine bioprosthetic valves for long-term durability.

Valve degradation or homograft conduit dysfunction over time is theorized to be secondary to gradual calcification and fibrosis of the chemically or cryopreserved valve leaflets, in addition to an autoimmune response from the host. Alternate means of valve preservation, such as fresh decellularized pulmonary homografts may eventually result in increased freedom from explanation.[34] Although anti-calcification treatments and newer valve designs focus on improved valve durability, surgical valve replacements have limited durability, with the majority of patients requiring reoperation between 5 and 15 years.

8.3 Percutaneous Pulmonary Valve Implantation

RATIONALE FOR PERCUTANEOUS PULMONARY VALVE IMPLANTATION

With low morbidity and mortality rates, surgical PVR represents one of the medical success stories of cardiothoracic surgery. However, there are many instances when operative risks are high or surgery is prohibitive. Patients requiring RVOT reconstruction require multiple sternotomies and cardiac surgical procedures throughout their lives. A second, third, or even fourth reoperation is associated with increased surgical risk and perioperative mortality from adhesions, scar tissue, and anatomic disruption,[35] and each subsequent ventriculotomy increases the risk of developing scar-related ventricular arrhythmias. Redo sternotomies can be especially challenging when the RV-to-PA conduit or valve lies in an anterior position immediately behind the sternum. Other patients are simply not surgical candidates

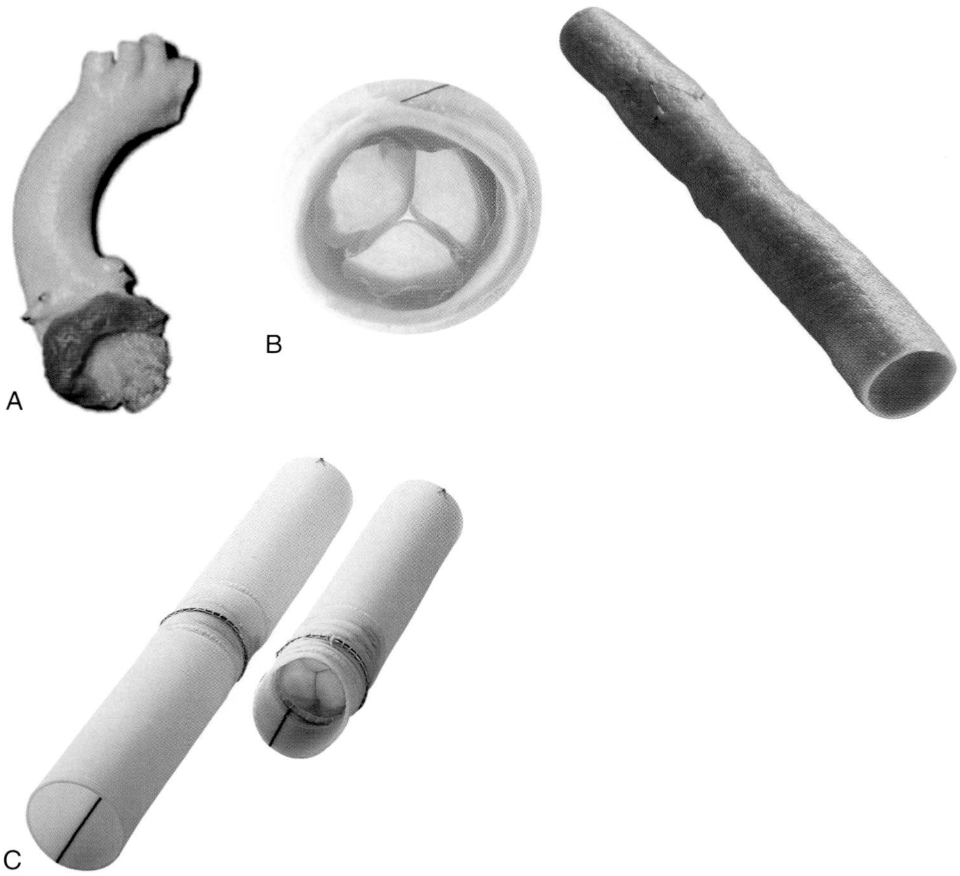

Figure 8–3 Different types of surgical conduits that are used for pulmonary valve replacement. A, Biologic homograft typically obtained from a cadaver (either aortic or pulmonic valve). **B,** The Contegra pulmonary valved conduit is an animal jugular vein that contains a valve with three leaflets that are similar to a human heart valve. The Contegra pulmonary valved conduit is approved for use in the United States as a humanitarian use device. Displayed images shows the interior and exterior of the Contegra conduit. **C,** The Hancock Bioprosthetic Valved Conduit consists of a porcine aortic valve sutured into the center of a woven fabric conduit. (*B* and *C published with permission from Medtronic.*)

because of comorbidities, and those with concomitant physical or mental challenges can make recovery after traditional surgery a daunting task.

The inspiration leading to the development of surgical alternatives arises from an innate human desire to minimize risk. Intuitively patients are looking for resolution and treatment of their medical problems but with minimal discomfort and recovery. There remain constraints to cardiac surgery, including incisional pain, wound healing, cosmetic appearance, length of rehabilitation, and the complications related to cardiopulmonary bypass.[36] These concerns are compounded by the reality that many patients requiring RVOT reconstruction are young and will need multiple reoperations in their lifetimes as they outgrow their implant or for prosthesis failure. A balance between the deleterious effects of RVOT dysfunction and the need to minimize the total number of lifetime surgeries for a given patient is a clinically challenging task prompting the need to develop minimally invasive valve therapies.

CURRENT TECHNOLOGIES FOR PERCUTANEOUS PULMUNARY VALVE IMPLANTATION

It has taken several decades of engineering innovation to develop fully compressible, competent valves and their corresponding transcatheter delivery systems for clinical application. The first-in-man PPVI was performed by Dr. Philipp Bonhoeffer and his colleagues in 2000 on a 12-year-old boy with a failing RV-to-PA conduit.[37] Since then, several thousand PVs have been implanted worldwide using primarily the Medtronic Melody valve (Minneapolis, Minn.). The Edwards SAPIEN valve (Edwards Lifesciences, Irvine, Calif.) was first implanted in 2005 and also remains an option for PVR.

The Melody valve and its corresponding Medtronic Ensemble delivery system **(Figure 8–4)** have been available in Canada and Europe since 2006 and were approved by the U.S. Food and Drug Administration (FDA) in 2010. It consists of a harvested valve from a bovine jugular vein that is sutured into a platinum-iridium stent frame that is 28 mm long and 18 mm in diameter. The valve is preserved in a proprietary mixture of glutaraldehyde and alcohol and must be manually crimped onto the Ensemble delivery balloon system at the time of implantation. The delivery system is 22F at its widest point (the crimped balloon valve assembly) with an integrated retractable covering sheath and a tapered tip to help the system traverse the acute angulations often found in the RVOT. The system uses a balloon-in-balloon catheter design (BIB; NuMED Hopkinton, N.Y.) for expansion of the valve, with outer balloon diameters of 18, 20, and 22 mm.

The Edwards SAPIEN valve and the Edwards RetroFlex III transfemoral delivery system **(Figure 8–5)** were initially designed and later FDA approved for

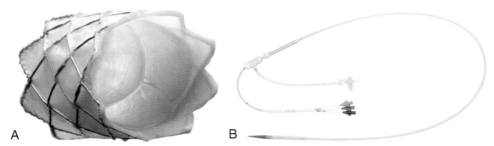

Figure 8–4 **Medtronic Melody transcatheter pulmonary valve and ensemble delivery system. A,** The Medtronic Melody valve is a harvested valve from a bovine jugular vein that is sewn onto a 28-mm long platinum/iridium frame. **B,** The Medtronic Ensemble delivery system is a 22F delivery system with an integrated sheath is designed for delivery of the Melody valve via the femoral or internal jugular veins. The Ensemble delivery system has catheters with balloon sizes of 18, 20, and 22 mm. The green port allows wire entry, and the orange port (outer balloon) and blue port (inner balloon) are part of the balloon-in-balloon design for expansion of the valve. *(Images published with permission of Medtronic.)*

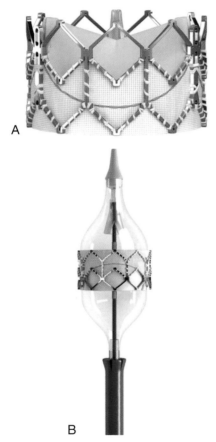

Figure 8–5 **Edwards SAPIEN transcatheter heart valve and transfemoral delivery. A.** The Edwards SAPIEN Valve consists of bovine pericardial leaflets sewn into a balloon-expandable cobalt chromium platform. It is available in 23-mm and 26-mm sizes **B,** The RetroFlex 3 delivery system is a transfemoral delivery catheter used for the Edwards SAPIEN valve. *(Image published with permission of Edwards Lifesciences LLC, Irvine, Calif. Edwards, Edwards Lifesciences, RetroFlex, RetroFlex II, RetroFlex 3, Retroplegia, RF3, SAPIEN, SAPIEN Therapeutics, SAPIEN XT, and SAPIEN 3 are trademarks of Edwards Lifesciences Corporation.)*

transcatheter aortic valve replacement in 2011;[38,39] however, the same valve and delivery system have been used for implantation in the pulmonary position. The SAPIEN valve consists of bovine pericardial leaflets sewn into a balloon-expandable stainless steel platform, currently available in 23-mm and 26-mm diameters (14-mm and 16-mm valve lengths, respectively), allowing for implantation in larger RVOTs than the Melody valve (see **Table 8–1** for schematic comparison of Melody and SAPIEN valves). The valve is preserved using the proprietary Carpentier Edwards ThermaFix process. The RetroFlex III delivery system is used for transfemoral delivery and has a tapered tip similar to the Ensemble system to ease valve delivery and requires a 22F or 24F hydrophilic sheath, depending on valve size. The SAPIEN valve must be crimped onto the 30-mm long Retroflex balloon using a proprietary Edwards Lifesciences crimper before implantation.

There are several noteworthy differences between the Melody and SAPIEN valves and delivery systems. The Melody valve remains sheathed until it is brought into position across the outflow tract at the landing zone, thereby minimizing potential damage and dislodgement of the stent valve during delivery. If needed, the Melody valve can be removed from the femoral vein (FV) before deployment. The availability of larger SAPIEN valve diameters allows for SAPIEN implantations into 23- to 26-mm conduits or bioprosthetic valves. However, once unsheathed in the inferior vena cava (IVC), a nonimplanted 26-mm SAPIEN valve cannot be removed from the body without a surgical cut-down.

INDICATIONS AND PATIENT SELECTION

Present indications for PPVI remain the same as those accepted for surgical PVR. In the setting of valvular PS, for the symptomatic patient, the RV pressure should be greater than 2/3 systemic; for the asymptomatic patient, a RV pressure of more than 3/4 systemic is generally accepted clinical criteria for intervention.[40,41] In the setting of moderate or severe PR progressive symptoms, exercise intolerance, arrhythmias, RV dilation, and RV dysfunction in various combinations are all considered reasonable criteria for replacement or implantation of a PV.[41] PR can be native, secondary to surgical intervention (e.g., as in transannular patch repair for TOF), or from failure of a previous outflow tract reconstruction or PVR (homograft, conduit, or bioprosthetic). With obstructive or mixed valvular lesions, patients typically experience earlier symptoms such as exercise intolerance.

TABLE 8–1

FDA-Approved Valves in North America that Are Used for Percutaneous Pulmonary Valve Implantation

	Medtronic Melody Valve	Edwards SAPIEN Valve
Available valve sizes	Initial length: 28 mm Initial diameter: 18 mm Crimped diameter: 6 mm Final diameter: 16 to 22 mm	Initial length: 16 mm Initial diameter: 14.6 or 16 mm Specialized crimper Final diameter: 21 to 23 mm, 24 to 26 mm
Valve type	Bovine jugular	Bovine pericardial
Balloon	BIB: 18, 20, 22 mm	Semicompliant 23 or 26 mm
Stent platform	Cheatham platinum	Stainless steel
Sheath size	22F	22F or 24F (outer diameter is 25F or 28F)
Delivery catheter shape	Ensemble delivery system Nose cone sheath	Retroflex 3 system Deflectable nose cone

BIB, Balloon-in-balloon (NuMED, Hopkinton, N.Y.)

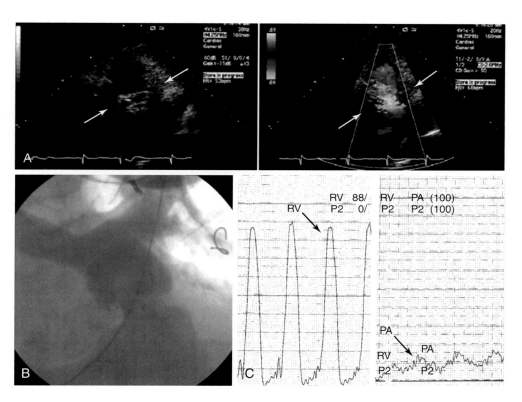

Figure 8–6 Diagnostic imaging performed before consideration of PPVI. A, Echocardiogram; two-dimensional image showing a 15-year old surgical bioprosthetic pulmonary valve *(arrows)* with color Doppler in the corresponding picture with free pulmonary regurgitation *(arrows)*. **B,** Angiography in the PA showing a dilated PA system with free pulmonary regurgitation. **C,** Catheter hemodynamics showing simultaneous right ventricular and PA pressure tracings in a patient with severe valvular pulmonic stenosis and approximately a 64-mm Hg valvular gradient.

Surgical PVR remains preferable to PPVI in cases where additional surgical lesions are necessary (e.g., television repair, cryoablation of ventricular arrhythmias, or atrial maze surgery. The presence of concomitant subvalvular and supravalvular PS may necessitate surgery, although on a case-by-case basis this may be treated percutaneously by stenting before PPVI.

Careful case selection for the procedure is crucial and should be performed by a multidisciplinary team. Although there are no universal screening protocols to determine eligibility, complete preprocedural diagnostics should confirm indications and determine whether the anatomy is suitable for the available percutaneous technologies **(Figure 8–6).** This typically includes: 1) echocardiography to assess outflow gradients and the presence of subvalvular, supravalvular, or branch PA stenosis; 2) cardiac magnetic resonance imaging (MRI) to quantify RV size and function in addition to calculating regurgitation fraction and three-dimensional reconstruction for the RVOT, PV annulus, and PA; 3) cardiopulmonary exercise testing as an objective measure of functional capacity, including parameters such as exercise time, peak oxygen uptake (peak $\dot{V}o_2$), anaerobic threshold, and minute ventilation/carbon dioxide production ratio ($V_E/\dot{V}co_2$); 4) a diagnostic catheterization to assess hemodynamics, confirming calibrated sizes across the RVOT for percutaneous suitability; and 5) coronary angiography, including an assessment for coronary impingement with balloon dilation of the RVOT.

With the current iterations of the Melody valve, the RVOT, PV annulus/ring, and proximal main PA must be 22 mm or less to prevent leaflet malcoaptation; typically it should be 16 mm or more. There is, however, limited experience with mounting the Melody valve on a 24-mm BIB balloon, with delivery through a 24F long sheath (Cook Medical Bloomington, Ind.). The Edwards SAPIEN valve allows for PV annulus sizes up to 25 mm. Balloon sizing should be performed during catheterization using a compliant sizing balloon to quantify the annulus or conduit size. Other considerations include patient size (minimum of 30 kg), adequate venous access (FV/IVC, jugular/superior vena cava) to allow for the large French-sized sheaths and that the coronary arteries are of an adequate distance away from the conduit to avoid compression when the conduit is expanded. The ideal anatomy for PPVI has a uniform diameter from RVOT to PA with adequate main PA length to avoid stenting into the PA bifurcation. Significant RVOT/subvalvular obstruction should be treated before valve implantation, or clinically significant gradients across the RVOT may remain after PPVI.

IMPLANTATION PROCEDURE

Whereas some operator variability is expected in any interventional procedure, there are certain axioms that are imperative during implantation. For an outline of the basic PPVI procedure, refer to **Box 8–1** and **Figure 8–7.** PPVI should be conducted under with the patient under general anesthesia to minimize patient discomfort and movement during valve delivery. Adequate angiography with multiple views (biplane if available) is crucial for visualization. Generally the lateral projection and the shallow right anterior oblique (RAO) projection provide the best views of the conduit. Both the FV and internal jugular (IJ) vein can be considered for valve delivery. On occasion, an IJ approach can lead to a more favorable anatomic curvature when positioning the valve compared to the FV. However, the FV approach is generally favored because of logistical considerations of fluoroscopy location, anesthesia presence at the head of the table, and operator preference.

A balloon-tipped catheter should be used to perform the right heart study and placement of the stiff exchange guidewire, thus avoiding entrapment in the tricuspid valve apparatus, which could be damaged by the large-caliber delivery systems. Given its vertical orientation, the left PA is often more preferable for achieving wire stability and traversing the RVOT with the delivery systems. It is imperative to use an extremely stiff 0.035-inch wire, because anatomic angulations, calcification, and fibrosis in the RVOT and PAs can challenge valve delivery. Stiff wires with distal PA wire position do increase the risk of periprocedural pulmonary hemorrhage, and thus great care is needed for maintaining wire stability during device delivery.

As noted above, it is crucial to test for potential coronary impingement. This can be done by simultaneous balloon dilation of the conduit and coronary angiography. Either coronary artery may be compromised, although the left main artery or proximal left anterior descending are the most often affected, running close to the outflow tract. A noncompliant balloon with inflations

to diameters close to the final diameter for the implant is performed across the pulmonary valve with simultaneous coronary angiography in multiple views. For very calcified conduits, slow serial dilation of the conduit with progressively larger balloons may mitigate some of the risk of conduit rupture. If coronary compression is documented in this testing phase **(Figure 8–8),** PPVI is contraindicated.

Prestenting of the RVOT is recommended to create a stable landing platform. This scaffolding is crucial when

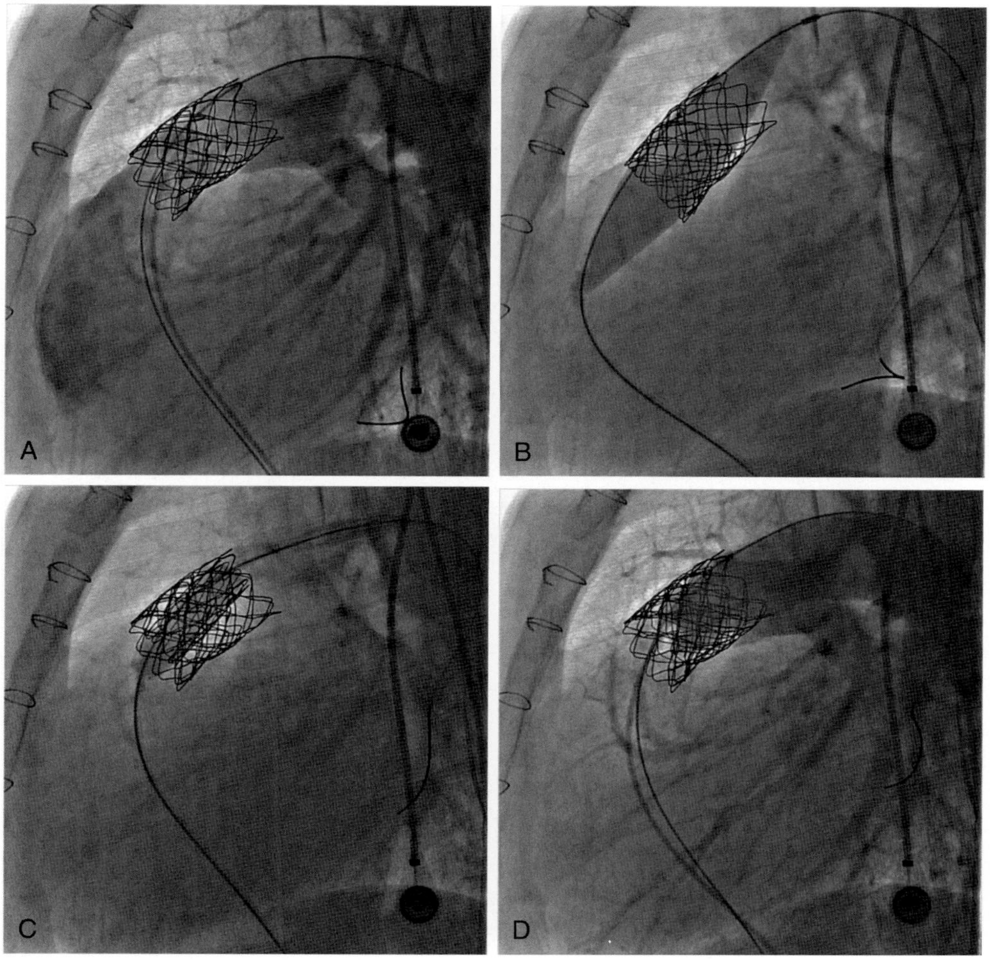

Figure 8–7 Fluoroscopic sequence for PPVI. A, Main PA angiogram; free pulmonary regurgitation (PR) is noted across the stented right ventricle-to-PA conduit. **B,** Balloon dilation of the older stent using a noncompliant balloon to diminish any conduit gradient. **C,** Implantation of Melody valve using a 22-mm balloon into the stented conduit. **D,** Final angiogram documenting a competent Melody valve without significant PR.

implantation is being attempted in a native RVOT and in conduits to reduce the incidence of stent fracture by decreasing the radial forces on the valve.[42] Stenting the area of greatest obstruction in the RVOT may also unmask additional regions of obstruction that should be treated before valve placement. Although a single stent may be adequate, several stent implants may be required until there is no conduit recoil upon balloon deflation.

A bare metal stent may be used, but there are advantages in using a covered stent to contain any conduit disruptions that may occur while preparing the outflow tract for implantation. The authors' institutional preference is to prestent using Cheatham platinum-covered (PC) stents (NuMED, Hopkinton, N.Y.) for homograft preparation. Palmaz XL series (Cordis Endovascular, Miami, Fla.) stents and Andrastent XL or XLL series stents (Andramed, Reutlingen, Germany) are used for prestenting when placing a covered stent is unfavorable. The stent(s) may require postimplant dilation (with a noncompliant balloon) to achieve the intended diameter. Full stent expansion at this stage helps prevent underexpansion during stent valve delivery. Hemodynamics after prestenting should document a minimal residual gradient across the outflow tract before the surgeon proceeds with valve implantation.

For both Melody and SAPIEN valves, proper balloon mounting and orientation should be confirmed before use. Valve positioning and catheter stability are the crucial tenets during implantation. Bringing the valve into position can be technically challenging and require multiple adjustments including wire repositioning, trialing sequentially stiffer wires, adding a second "buddy wire" (i.e., hydrophilic wire) to assist valve transit, and additional adjustments using stents to relieve any residual gradient/obstruction in the RVOT and PA. There have been published reports of using an RV subxiphoid hybrid approach for Melody valve implantation in cases where the valve is unable to be positioned through the venous system.[43] Once the Melody valve is unsheathed and in position, gradual sequential balloon inflations should be performed, the inner followed by the outer balloon. Slow inflation allows time to make microadjustments in the event of device slippage. The SAPIEN valve is inflated on a single balloon, but similarly careful and slow inflation minimize device slippage. Occasionally the implanted valves require postdilation with either the delivery balloon or a separate noncompliant balloon. After implantation, hemodynamics and repeat angiography should be performed to assess valve competence, the

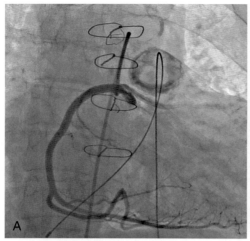
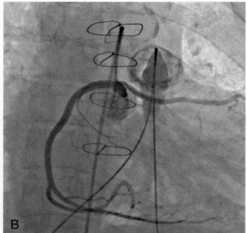
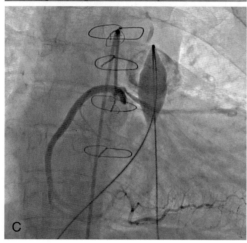

Figure 8–8 Coronary compression during balloon dilation. A. Baseline coronary angiogram. This angiogram documents an anomalous left main coronary system arising from the right coronary cusp with an interarterial course. The angiogram suggests baseline patency of left main and right coronary arteries. **B and C,** Inflation coronary angiograms performed during simultaneous balloon inflation across RV-to-PA conduit using a noncompliant balloon with increasing manual pressure. There is evidence of LM compression that worsens with increased balloon inflation. The balloon was deflated, and the decision was made to not proceed with PPVI given the risk of coronary compromise. The patient went to surgery for conduit replacement.

degree of residual outflow gradient, and the integrity of the outflow tract and PA.

POSTPROCEDURAL CARE

Uncomplicated cases are typically observed for 24 hours and discharged on the first postprocedure day. A transthoracic echocardiogram should be planned for the morning after the procedure to determine baseline hemodynamics. Antiplatelet therapy is not routinely prescribed, although some institutions use clopidogrel or aspirin empirically for 3 to 6 months and some prescribe it for life. There is little data supporting any particular antiplatelet regimen, and to date no definite reports of thromboembolism have been reported.

Given the large-vessel venous access, 4 to 5 hours of bed rest immediately after an uncomplicated procedure is routine regardless of whether closure devices or manual compression are used to achieve hemostasis. The patient is counseled for empiric low-level activity limitations for 72 hours after the procedure, and endocarditis prophylaxis before a dental procedures is reinforced. It is usually recommended that patients see their dentists before valve implantation. Routine cardiology follow-up care, including regular radiographic (e.g., chest x-ray) screening and fluoroscopic

evaluation (looking for stent fractures) if needed, is arranged. Postmarket surveillance conducted in certain countries requires specific follow-up and imaging protocols.

8.4 Outcomes for PPVI

PERIPROCEDURAL OUTCOMES

Melody Valve

Dr. Philipp Bonhoeffer's group, the originators of the valve, having begun in 2000, have the most experience, although an increasing number of institutions are also publishing their clinical experiences.[44-49] In appropriately screened patients, implantation can be performed with approximately 99% success with low rates of periprocedural complications that decrease as operators gain clinical experience. [47,50] The U.S. Melody Transcatheter Pulmonary Valve study is a prospective, nonrandomized trial with inclusion criteria designed to assess the safety, procedural success, and short-term efficacy of the valve in patients with dysfunctional RVOT conduits, and includes a 5-year follow-up study.[48,49] Implantation was performed in

124 of 136 enrolled subjects with an average age of 19 years old between 2007 and 2009. The majority of patients had a primary diagnosis of TOF, a prior Ross procedure, or transposition of the great arteries. In 12 patients, PPVI was not attempted because of procedural and study contraindications, including conduit morphology/size on balloon expansion, coronary location, or inadequate degree of conduit stenosis. PPVI resulted in an acute reduction in RV pressure to a median of 42 mm Hg and a reduction in peak gradients across the outflow tract to a median of 12 mm Hg. There was trace to no PR in 123 of 124 patients; 1 patient had moderate PR, and average procedure times were under 3 hours.

SAPIEN Valve

Although the Edwards SAPIEN valve and Retroflex III delivery system have been studied prospectively and FDA approved for aortic valve replacement,[38,39] their use in the pulmonary position has largely occurred on an off-label basis.[51] The first implantation of the CE-marked SAPIEN in the pulmonary position was performed in Europe in 2011.[52] A prospective, nonrandomized, multicenter study is currently ongoing to assess the efficacy and safety profile of the valve in the treatment of dysfunctional RV-to-PA conduits with moderate to severe PR, with or without stenosis. This trial, entitled COMPASSION (COngenital Multicenter trial of Pulmonic vAlve regurgitation Studying the SAPIEN interventIONal), published its FDA phase I clinical results, reporting on 36 patients with an average age of 30 years old who were enrolled between 2008 and 2010.[53] From this group, two patients were excluded for large conduit size, leaving 34 patients on whom PPVI was attempted with 97% implantation success. PPVI with the SAPIEN valve resulted in an acute reduction in RV pressure to a median of 42 mm Hg and a reduction in peak gradient across the RVOT to a median of 12 mm Hg. There was trace or no PR in 31 of 33 patients on postprocedural angiography with average procedure times just over 2 hours.

PROCEDURAL AND STENT COMPLICATIONS

Initial experience using the Melody valve from 2000 through 2007 reported a rate of 3% to 4% of acute complications requiring emergent surgery.[47,54] Three potential mechanisms of acute hemodynamic failure as a result of PPVI included: 1) valve dislodgement into the RVOT or PAs causing obstruction to pulmonary blood flow; 2) acute coronary compression with valve expansion leading to ischemia, hemodynamic collapse, and arrhythmias; and 3) hemorrhage from homograft rupture. The rate of serious complications in the U.S. prospective trial was reported at 6%, including death from coronary dissection (n = 1), conduit rupture (treated either with a covered stent or emergent surgery) (n = 2), unstable arrhythmias treated with cardioversion (n = 1), acute LV dysfunction caused by prolonged intubation (n = 1), wire perforation in to the distal PA (self-limited or treated with coil embolization; n = 2),

---

BOX 8–2 ▬▬▬▬▬▬

Reported Device and Procedural Complications after Percutaneous Pulmonary Valve Implantation

Death
Stent fracture
Device embolization
Coronary impingement
Hammock effect
Homograft rupture or hemorrhage
Perivalvular leak
Hemolysis
Venous occlusion
Infection/endocarditis
Thromboembolism
Valve failure (with stenosis or regurgitation)

---

and FV thrombosis (n = 1). With increased operator experience and refinement in patient selection and implantation techniques, more recent publications have suggested lower complication rates and a significantly decreased need for emergent surgery.[45,47]

Published data about use of the Edwards SAPIEN valve in the pulmonary position is significantly more limited.[51,53] Phase I of the COMPASSION trial reported 7 patients (21%) with adverse events, including migration or embolization of the stent valve (n = 4; three requiring surgical explantation and in one the valve was deployed into the IVC), unstable arrhythmias treated with cardioversion (n = 1), and wire perforation in to the distal PA (self-limited) (n = 2).[53]

Box 8–2 lists the more common complications that may be seen with the PPVI procedure; highlighted in the next paragraphs are several of the more prominent adverse events.

Coronary Impingement

Abrupt coronary closure after valve implantation can be a lethal complication that is mostly avoidable by careful patient screening using noninvasive and invasive imaging.[55] There is significant patient-to-patient variability in the precise anatomic location of the RVOT and conduit in relation to the coronary takeoff that depends on the atrioventricular and ventriculoarterial connection, the presence of anomalous coronaries, and prior surgical repair (e.g., thoracic location of RV to PA conduit; see **Figure 8–8**). The potential for coronary compromise most often involves the left main or proximal left anterior descending coronary artery, although the right coronary artery should also be assessed. Although noninvasive imaging may demonstrate significant anatomic distance between the RVOT and the coronary takeoffs, all patients should have simultaneous coronary angiography with balloon inflation across the outflow tract. The balloon should simulate the diameter anticipated by implant while assessing any decrease in coronary flow, transient stenosis, or "milking" of the vessel. If there is any suggestion of coronary involvement with test balloon inflation, then currently available technologies of PPVI are contraindicated.

Stent Fracture and Embolization

Stent fracture represents the most common and vexing early complication after Melody implantation. Nordmeyer et al. analyzed stent fracture data from the initial European experience and proposed a classification system[56] **(Figure 8–9):** Type I fractures (isolated fractures [one or more] but no effect on valve structural integrity) can be seen as often as in 40% of implantations; however, these are not linked with adverse clinical outcomes. Type II fractures (fractures plus loss of valve structural integrity) and type III fractures (type II fractures but with an embolized fragment) are less common. They may require treatment either by surgical replacement or repeat PPVI and are associated with early conduit restenosis and valve failure.[44] The majority of patients in the early PPVI experience did not receive prestenting of the RVOT.

Schievano et al. examined *in vitro* and *in vivo* mechanics of different stent platforms using MRI-constructed three-dimensional models from different RVOT morphologies.[57,58] Points of stent asymmetry after final valve deployment were at highest risk for stent fracture, typically caused by interaction of the valve with the individual RVOT anatomy. Although this type of modeling still requires clinical correlation, its use of anatomic parameters to help predict PPVI stent durability is promising. Previous experience with direct RVOT-to-PA conduit stents (using Palmaz stainless steel stents [Cordis Endovascular, Warren, N.J.] or Palmaz Genesis stents [Cordis Endovascular, Miami, Fla.]) found a fracture rate of 40% at 4 years, which may be an underestimate given the difficulty in diagnosing small stent fractures.[59] Over 90% of the fractures occurred when the conduit was in a substernal position; the type of stent used was also an independent risk factor in multivariate modeling. With PPVI, additional risk factors for stent fracture have included procedures performed in a native RVOT or a noncalcified RVOT and recoil of the PPVI during balloon deflation.[56]

Nordemeyer et al. found that prestenting the RVOT before valve stent implantation was associated with approximately a threefold relative risk reduction in developing stent fractures.[42] However, the study did not show differences in clinical outcomes between those patients who were prestented and those who had direct PPVI. Routine prestenting has been implemented as standard of care in most centers as an integral component of the PPVI procedure.[60] On follow-up study, it is recommended to use x-ray imaging and/or fluoroscopy at regular intervals to assess for stent fracture development. Early detection of fractures and subsequent reintervention may prolong conduit integrity.[61]

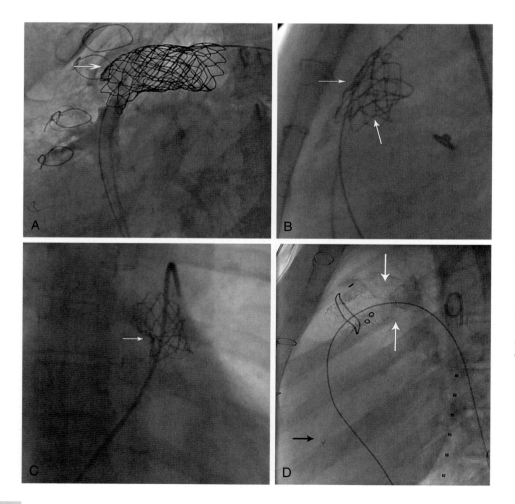

Figure 8–9 **Stent fracture classification system. A,** Type I: stent fracture of greater than or equal to 1 strut, without loss of stent integrity. The *arrows* delineate several Type I stent fractures. **B and C,** Type II: stent fracture of one or more struts with loss of stent integrity. Images show several fractures leading to stent compression; this patient had a clinically significant gradient across the stent. **D,** Type III: separation of stent segments or stent embolization. This image shows an RVOT stent (not a Melody valve) that had separated/broken to illustrate a Type III fracture. The classification system is described in Nordmeyer et al.[56]

Hammock Effect

This phenomenon was seen in the early Melody valve iterations when the stay sutures sewing the Contegra graft (Medtronic, Minneapolis, Mich.) to the stent were placed only on the stent distal ends.[62] Blood could freely traverse between valve tissue and the stent, creating the potential for pseudovalvular obstruction. In the most recent Melody valve, this design flaw has been corrected with additional sutures on the stent intersections, relegating this complication to historical significance only.

Undelivered Valve Explantation

Specific to the Edwards SAPIEN valve and corresponding Retroflex III delivery system, the valve is normally unsheathed in the IVC. If wire position is lost while attempting to bring the valve into place across the RVOT, the SAPIEN valve cannot be removed from the body percutaneously. At that point, if it is impossible to bring the valve into the appropriate delivery position, surgical removal of the valve from the venous system may be required (although a 23-mm SAPIEN valve can be removed through a 26F Retroflex III delivery sheath). Alternatively, the valve can be delivered in the IVC and then stented over to maintain IVC patency.[53]

HEMODYNAMIC AND CLINICAL OUTCOMES

In multiple prospective studies, PPVI has been found to be an effective therapy for decreasing RVOT gradients, decreasing RV pressures, and providing a competent PV without significant regurgitation. PPVI was compared to bare metal stenting (BMS) alone, across the RVOT by invasive hemodynamics and MRI.[63] Both therapies lead to a comparable initial decrease in RV pressures and RVOT gradients. However, BMS trades the physiology of a pressure loading with volume loading of the RV by induction of free PR. Effective right and LV stroke volume (RV stroke volume minus pulmonary regurgitant volume) improved with PPVI but was unchanged with BMS; this was further reflected by a heart rate decrease while maintaining steady cardiac output with the PPVI. Increases in LV end-diastolic volumes have been associated with improvement in early diastolic filling, decreased RV wall stress, and more balanced ventricular septal interaction.[64,65]

Two- to 3-year follow-up study after Melody PPVI has been reported in select patients. There is overall a low rate of periprocedural mortality (<1% across cohorts) or other serious complications. From Bonhoeffer's report of the initial 155 PPVI patients at approximately 28 months median follow-up study, freedom from reintervention or reoperation was 93% at 10 months and 86% at 30 months.[47] In the Melody Transcatheter Pulmonary Valve study, freedom from Melody valve dysfunction was 94% at 1 year and 86% at 2 years.[48] In the same study, freedom from RVOT reintervention was 95% at 1 year and 88% at 2 years. A smaller Toronto series examined PPVI performed in an adolescent population and found freedom from transcatheter reintervention

to be 91%, 80%, and 80%, at 12, 24, and 36 months, respectively.[46] Eicken et al. have published a two-institution clinical experience involving 102 patients who received a PPVI between 2006 and 2010.[45] Prestenting was routinely performed, and they reported one procedural death secondary to coronary compression. At a median 1-year clinical follow-up study, one valve (1%) was removed secondary to endocarditis; eight valves (8%) required repeat dilation for residual gradients, four of which led to repeat valve-in-valve procedures.

With regards to stent fractures, clinical series have reported 1-year rates ranging as low as 5% to as high as 40%, likely depending on case mix, incidence of prestenting, and the rigor of follow-up study.[45,48,56,62] At a mean of 13 months' follow-up study, Nordmeyer et al. report a 21% rate of stent fractures with fracture-free survival of 85.1% at 1 year, 74.5% at 2 years, and 69.2% at 3 years.[56] Most events were early in the first 400 days. The Melody Transcatheter Pulmonary Valve study has also reported stent fracture rates of approximately 22% at 14 months' follow-up study. There are considerably fewer PPVI patients who have received a SAPIEN valve compared with the Melody valve; however, there were no reported stent fractures at 6 months from the phase I COMPASSION trial.[53] Whether these findings will hold up over longer follow-up study and with increased patient numbers remains to be seen.

Published studies have consistently shown an improvement in New York Heart Association class after PPVI.[47] There are hemodynamic differences seen between lesions treated for predominantly RVOT obstruction versus significant PR.[65,66] Reduction of RV afterload leads to improvement in RV functional parameters and in functional capacity based on peak oxygen uptake during cardiopulmonary exercise testing, whereas this has not been found with resolution of PR alone.[66] The majority of the improvement in systolic RV function for obstructive lesions happens early and little additional improvement has been noted on sequential MRI evaluations 1 year later.[67]

In the cohort treated for severe PR, Plymen et al. found a statistically significant decrease in QRS duration and in QT_c dispersion, akin to observations after surgical PVR.[68] The decrease in QRS duration was not statistically significant for the cohort treated for RVOT obstruction. To date there is no evidence correlating improvement in electrocardiographic parameters after PPVI with reduction in clinical arrhythmia burden; however, it is hypothesized that increased homogeneity in repolarization is a sign of favorable electrical remodeling.

8.5 Future Horizons for PPVI

Whereas society-based appropriateness criteria for PPVI are lacking, there is debate as to whether patients should be offered PPVI at earlier stages of their disease (i.e., smaller overall RV end-diastolic volumes) than would be routinely done for surgical PVR. The argument for this is based on the relative periprocedural risks of a percutaneous procedure versus open-heart surgery.

There are no published or currently ongoing head-to-head trials comparing surgical PVR with PPVI. There are certain differences in case mix for PVR versus PPVI, including patient comorbidities, surgical risk, technological limitations, and need for additional surgeries that limit the generalizability of such comparisons. From a purely economic standpoint, cost models have suggested a PPVI-based strategy would add approximately $3000 to $7000 of health care expenses per patient over a 25-year period compared with surgical PVR strategy.[69]

One crucial question that remains to be answered is the long-term durability of the Melody and SAPIEN valves.[48] Over the next several years, longer follow-up studies can be expected both of previously published cohorts as well as of additional real-world experience. As a condition of the FDA's approval of the Melody valve, Medtronic is required to perform two postapproval studies to assess long-term risks and benefits in addition to the physician specialization needed to perform the procedure.[70] Medtronic must also maintain a clinical database of all Melody implants. The Melody Transcatheter Pulmonary Valve study will continue to report outcomes of its 150 participants through 5 years of follow-up study.[48,49] A second study of 100 new patients is underway to assess safety and adequacy of the training programs for PPVI. Similarly, the COMPASSION trial is moving forward with additional study participants and follow-up research using the Edwards SAPIEN PV.[53] There is considerable interest as to whether the SAPIEN valve can maintain low stent fracture rates with additional patients being enrolled and longer follow-up study. It also remains to be seen whether a decrease in stent fracture events will translate into differences in clinical outcomes. There are also several other percutaneous or hybrid PV systems that are at various stages of *in vitro*, animal, or preclinical investigation.[71-74]

The future "technologic burden" for PPVI rests with percutaneous valve delivery in native dilated outflow tracts, commonly found after TOF repair. Although initial experience with both Melody and SAPIEN valves examined valve implantation into RV-to-PA conduits, there has since been valve implantations into native RVOTs with transannular patches, when the annulus size was 22 mm or less for Melody and 26 mm or less for SAPIEN valves.[75,76] With a significantly dilated RVOT, hybrid surgical approaches have been reported using off-pump RVOT surgical reduction and ring placement coupled with PPVI. Also, a 29-mm SAPIEN valve is being used in the aortic position, which may allow the option of PPVI in patients with larger bioprosthetic rings.

Animal studies have proven the feasibility of valve implantation in the dilated native RVOT. The pulmonary trunk and infundibulum are downsized using modified hourglass-shaped stents that create a platform narrow enough for stent-valve deployment.[77,78] This concept of creating a stent based infundibular reducer is currently being studied with various different technologies. One such "native PV implant" produced by Medtronic is beginning human-research clinical trials. This self-expanding valved conduit is designed for placement in the main PA and native RVOT in patients with TOF, who have anatomy that precludes treatment with currently available transcatheter valve therapies.

With time there will likely be wider adoption of three-dimensional modeling to better assess patient suitability for PPVI and procedure planning. Patient heterogeneity will be countered by molding available valved stent platforms to better fit the contours of a particular patient.[79,80] Three-dimensional rapid prototyping systems recreated from MRI data have been used experimentally to create these models. These three-dimensional models also allow for the creation of patient-tailored percutaneous valves that are engineered to fit the individual anatomy.[81] Although this seems financially unfeasible at present, the authors believe that this is one of the end-goals of individualized medicine of the future.

REFERENCES

1. Xanthos T, Dalivigkas I, Ekmektzoglou KA: Anatomic variations of the cardiac valves and papillary muscles of the right heart, *Ital J Anat Embryol* 116:111–126, 2011.
2. Davlouros PA, Niwa K, Webb G, et al: The right ventricle in congenital heart disease, *Heart* 92(Suppl 1):i27–i38, 2006.
3. Freed MD, Rosenthal A, Bernhard WF, et al: Critical pulmonary stenosis with a diminutive right ventricle in neonates, *Circulation* 48:875–881, 1973.
4. Nugent EW, Freedom RM, Rowe RD, et al: Aneurysm of the membranous septum in ventricular septal defect, *Circulation* 56:182–184, 1977.
5. Hayes CJ, Gersony WM, Driscoll DJ, et al: Second natural history study of congenital heart defects: results of treatment of patients with pulmonary valvar stenosis, *Circulation* 87:128–137, 1993.
6. Chen CR, Cheng TO, Huang T, et al: Percutaneous balloon valvuloplasty for pulmonic stenosis in adolescents and adults, *N Engl J Med* 335:21–25, 1996.
7. Kan JS, White RI Jr, Mitchell SE, et al: Percutaneous balloon valvuloplasty: a new method for treating congenital pulmonary-valve stenosis, *N Engl J Med* 307:540–542, 1982.
8. Chaturvedi RR, Redington AN: Pulmonary regurgitation in congenital heart disease, *Heart* 93:880–889, 2007.
9. Oosterhof T, Hazekamp MG, Mulder BJ: Opportunities in pulmonary valve replacement, *Expert Rev Cardiovasc Ther* 7:1117–1122, 2009.
10. Shimazaki Y, Blackstone EH, Kirklin JW: The natural history of isolated congenital pulmonary valve incompetence: surgical implications, *Thorac Cardiovasc Surg* 32:257–259, 1984.
11. Shimazaki Y, Blackstone EH, Kirklin JW, et al: The dimensions of the right ventricular outflow tract and pulmonary arteries in tetralogy of Fallot and pulmonary stenosis, *J Thorac Cardiovasc Surg* 103:692–705, 1992.
12. Gatzoulis MA, Clark AL, Cullen S, et al: Right ventricular diastolic function 15 to 35 years after repair of tetralogy of Fallot: restrictive physiology predicts superior exercise performance, *Circulation* 91:1775–1781, 1995.
13. Chaturvedi RR, Kilner PJ, White PA, et al: Increased airway pressure and simulated branch pulmonary artery stenosis increase pulmonary regurgitation after repair of tetralogy of Fallot: real-time analysis with a conductance catheter technique, *Circulation* 95:643–649, 1997.
14. Kuehne T, Saeed M, Gleason K, et al: Effects of pulmonary insufficiency on biventricular function in the developing heart of growing swine, *Circulation* 108:2007–2013, 2003.
15. Davlouros PA, Kilner PJ, Hornung TS, et al: Right ventricular function in adults with repaired tetralogy of Fallot assessed with cardiovascular magnetic resonance imaging: detrimental role of right ventricular outflow aneurysms or akinesia and adverse right-to-left ventricular interaction, *J Am Coll Cardiol* 40:2044–2052, 2002.
16. Gray R, Greve G, Chen R, et al: Right ventricular myocardial responses to chronic pulmonary regurgitation in lambs: disturbances of activation and conduction, *Pediatr Res* 54:529–535, 2003.
17. Gatzoulis MA, Balaji S, Webber SA, et al: Risk factors for arrhythmia and sudden cardiac death late after repair of tetralogy of Fallot: a multicentre study, *Lancet* 356:975–981, 2000.

18. Therrien J, Siu SC, Harris L, et al: Impact of pulmonary valve replacement on arrhythmia propensity late after repair of tetralogy of Fallot, *Circulation* 103:2489–2494, 2001.
19. Nollert G, Fischlein T, Bouterwek S, et al: Long-term survival in patients with repair of tetralogy of Fallot: 36-year follow-up of 490 survivors of the first year after surgical repair, *J Am Coll Cardiol* 30:1374–1383, 1997.
20. Buechel ER, Dave HH, Kellenberger CJ, et al: Remodelling of the right ventricle after early pulmonary valve replacement in children with repaired tetralogy of Fallot: assessment by cardiovascular magnetic resonance, *Eur Heart J* 26:2721–2727, 2005.
21. Therrien J, Provost Y, Merchant N, et al: Optimal timing for pulmonary valve replacement in adults after tetralogy of Fallot repair, *Am J Cardiol* 95:779–782, 2005.
22. Lee C, Park CS, Lee CH, et al: Durability of bioprosthetic valves in the pulmonary position: long-term follow-up of 181 implants in patients with congenital heart disease: *J Thorac Cardiovasc Surg* 142:351–358, 2011.
23. Ilbawi MN, Lockhart CG, Idriss FS, et al: Experience with St. Jude Medical valve prosthesis in children: a word of caution regarding right-sided placement, *J Thorac Cardiovasc Surg* 93:73–79, 1987.
24. Miyamura H, Kanazawa H, Hayashi J, et al: Thrombosed St. Jude Medical valve prosthesis in the right side of the heart in patients with tetralogy of Fallot, *J Thorac Cardiovasc Surg* 94:148–150, 1987.
25. Waterbolk TW, Hoendermis ES, den Hamer IJ, et al: Pulmonary valve replacement with a mechanical prosthesis: promising results of 28 procedures in patients with congenital heart disease, *Eur J Cardiothorac Surg* 30:28–32, 2006.
26. Gulbins H, Kreuzer E, Reichart B: Homografts: a review, *Expert Rev Cardiovasc Ther* 1:533–539, 2003.
27. Oosterhof T, Meijboom FJ, Vliegen HW, et al: Long-term follow-up of homograft function after pulmonary valve replacement in patients with tetralogy of Fallot, *Eur Heart J* 27:1478–1484, 2006.
28. Discigil B, Dearani JA, Puga FJ, et al: Late pulmonary valve replacement after repair of tetralogy of Fallot, *J Thorac Cardiovasc Surg* 121:344–351, 2001.
29. Yemets IM, Williams WG, Webb GD, et al: Pulmonary valve replacement late after repair of tetralogy of Fallot, *Ann Thorac Surg* 64:526–530, 1997.
30. Turrentine MW, McCarthy RP, Vijay P, et al: Polytetrafluoroethylene monocusp valve technique for right ventricular outflow tract reconstruction, *Ann Thorac Surg* 74:2202–2205, 2002.
31. Brown JW, Ruzmetov M, Vijay P, et al: Right ventricular outflow tract reconstruction with a polytetrafluoroethylene monocusp valve: a twelve-year experience, *J Thorac Cardiovasc Surg* 133: 1336–1343, 2007.
32. Turrentine MW, McCarthy RP, Vijay P, et al: PTFE monocusp valve reconstruction of the right ventricular outflow tract, *Ann Thorac Surg* 73:871–879, 2002. discussion 9–80.
33. Caldarone CA, McCrindle BW, Van Arsdell GS, et al: Independent factors associated with longevity of prosthetic pulmonary valves and valved conduits, *J Thorac Cardiovasc Surg* 120:1022–1030, 2000. discussion 31.
34. Cebotari S, Tudorache I, Ciubotaru A, et al: Use of fresh decellularized allografts for pulmonary valve replacement may reduce the reoperation rate in children and young adults: early report, *Circulation* 124:S115–S123, 2011.
35. Holst KA, Dearani JA, Burkhart HM, et al: Risk factors and early outcomes of multiple reoperations in adults with congenital heart disease, *Ann Thorac Surg* 92:122–130, 2011.
36. Singh HS, Osten M, Horlick E: Future horizons for catheter-based interventions in adult congenital and structural heart disease, *Future Cardiol* 8:203–213, 2012.
37. Bonhoeffer P, Boudjemline Y, Saliba Z, et al: Percutaneous replacement of pulmonary valve in a right-ventricle to pulmonary-artery prosthetic conduit with valve dysfunction, *Lancet* 356:1403–1405, 2000.
38. Leon MB, Smith CR, Mack M, et al: Transcatheter aortic-valve implantation for aortic stenosis in patients who cannot undergo surgery, *N Engl J Med* 363:1597–1607, 2010.
39. Smith CR, Leon MB, Mack MJ, et al: Transcatheter versus surgical aortic-valve replacement in high-risk patients, *N Engl J Med* 364:2187–2198, 2011.
40. Feltes TF, Bacha E, Beekman RH 3rd, et al: Indications for cardiac catheterization and intervention in pediatric cardiac disease: a scientific statement from the American Heart Association: *Circulation*,123:2607–2652, 2011.
41. Warnes CA, Williams RG, Bashore TM, et al: ACC/AHA 2008 guidelines for the management of adults with congenital heart disease: a report of the American College of Cardiology/American Heart Association Task Force on Practice Guidelines (writing committee to develop guidelines on the management of adults with congenital heart disease), *Circulation* 118:e714–e833, 2008.
42. Nordmeyer J, Lurz P, Khambadkone S, et al: Pre-stenting with a bare metal stent before percutaneous pulmonary valve implantation: acute and 1-year outcomes, *Heart* 97:118–123, 2010.
43. Simpson KE, Huddleston CB, Foerster S, et al: Successful subxyphoid hybrid approach for placement of a Melody percutaneous pulmonary valve, *Catheter Cardiovasc Interv* 78:108–111, 2011.
44. Khambadkone S, Coats L, Taylor A, et al: Percutaneous pulmonary valve implantation in humans: results in 59 consecutive patients, *Circulation* 112:1189–1197, 2005.
45. Eicken A, Ewert P, Hager A, et al: Percutaneous pulmonary valve implantation: two-centre experience with more than 100 patients, *Eur Heart J* 32:1260–1265, 2011.
46. Vezmar M, Chaturvedi R, Lee KJ, et al: Percutaneous pulmonary valve implantation in the young 2-year follow-up, *J Am Coll Cardiol* 3:439–448, 2010.
47. Lurz P, Coats L, Khambadkone S, et al: Percutaneous pulmonary valve implantation: impact of evolving technology and learning curve on clinical outcome, *Circulation* 117:1964–1972, 2008.
48. McElhinney DB, Hellenbrand WE, Zahn EM, et al: Short- and medium-term outcomes after transcatheter pulmonary valve placement in the expanded multicenter US melody valve trial, *Circulation* 122:507–516, 2010.
49. Zahn EM, Hellenbrand WE, Lock JE, et al: Implantation of the melody transcatheter pulmonary valve in patients with a dysfunctional right ventricular outflow tract conduit early results from the U.S. clinical trial, *J Am Coll Cardiol* 54:1722–1729, 2009.
50. Neyt M, Vinck I, Gewillig M, et al: Percutaneous pulmonary and aortic valve insertion in Belgium: going for conditional reimbursement or waiting for further evidence? *Int J Technol Assess Health Care* 25:281–289, 2009.
51. Boone RH, Webb JG, Horlick E, et al: Transcatheter pulmonary valve implantation using the Edwards SAPIEN transcatheter heart valve, *Catheter Cardiovasc Interv* 75:286–294, 2010.
52. Ewert P, Horlick E, Berger F: First implantation of the CE-marked transcatheter SAPIEN pulmonic valve in Europe, *Clin Res Cardiol* 100:85–87, 2011.
53. Kenny D, Hijazi ZM, Kar S, et al: Percutaneous implantation of the Edwards SAPIEN transcatheter heart valve for conduit failure in the pulmonary position: early phase 1 results from an international multicenter clinical trial, *J Am Coll Cardiol* 58:2248–2256, 2011.
54. Kostolny M, Tsang V, Nordmeyer J, et al: Rescue surgery following percutaneous pulmonary valve implantation, *Eur J Cardiothorac Surg* 33:607–612, 2008.
55. Sridharan S, Coats L, Khambadkone S, et al: Images in cardiovascular medicine: transcatheter right ventricular outflow tract intervention: the risk to the coronary circulation, *Circulation* 113:e934–e935, 2006.
56. Nordmeyer J, Khambadkone S, Coats L, et al: Risk stratification, systematic classification, and anticipatory management strategies for stent fracture after percutaneous pulmonary valve implantation, *Circulation* 115:1392–1397, 2007.
57. Schievano S, Petrini L, Migliavacca F, et al: Finite element analysis of stent deployment: understanding stent fracture in percutaneous pulmonary valve implantation, *J Interv Cardiol* 20:546–554, 2007.
58. Schievano S, Taylor AM, Capelli C, et al: Patient specific finite element analysis results in more accurate prediction of stent fractures: application to percutaneous pulmonary valve implantation, *J Biomech* 43:687–693, 2010.
59. Peng LF, McElhinney DB, Nugent AW, et al: Endovascular stenting of obstructed right ventricle-to-pulmonary artery conduits: a 15-year experience, *Circulation* 113:2598–2605, 2006.
60. Demkow M, Biernacka EK, Spiewak M, et al: Percutaneous pulmonary valve implantation preceded by routine prestenting with a bare metal stent, *Catheter Cardiovasc Interv* 77:381–389, 2011.

61. Knirsch W, Haas NA, Lewin MA, et al: Longitudinal stent fracture 11 months after implantation in the left pulmonary artery and successful management by a stent-in-stent maneuver, *Catheter Cardiovasc Interv* 58:116–118, 2003.

62. Nordmeyer J, Coats L, Lurz P, et al: Percutaneous pulmonary valve-in-valve implantation: a successful treatment concept for early device failure, *Eur Heart J* 29:810–815, 2008.

63. Lurz P, Nordmeyer J, Muthurangu V, et al: Comparison of bare metal stenting and percutaneous pulmonary valve implantation for treatment of right ventricular outflow tract obstruction: use of an x-ray/magnetic resonance hybrid laboratory for acute physiological assessment, *Circulation* 119:2995–3001, 2009.

64. Lurz P, Puranik R, Nordmeyer J, et al: Improvement in left ventricular filling properties after relief of right ventricle to pulmonary artery conduit obstruction: contribution of septal motion and interventricular mechanical delay, *Eur Heart J* 30:2266–2274, 2009.

65. Coats L, Khambadkone S, Derrick G, et al: Physiological consequences of percutaneous pulmonary valve implantation: the different behaviour of volume- and pressure-overloaded ventricles, *Eur Heart J* 28:1886–1893, 2007.

66. Lurz P, Giardini A, Taylor AM, et al: Effect of altering pathologic right ventricular loading conditions by percutaneous pulmonary valve implantation on exercise capacity, *Am J Cardiol* 105:721–726, 2010.

67. Lurz P, Nordmeyer J, Giardini A, et al: Early versus late functional outcome after successful percutaneous pulmonary valve implantation: are the acute effects of altered right ventricular loading all we can expect? *J Am Coll Cardiol* 57:724–731, 2011.

68. Plymen CM, Bolger AP, Lurz P, et al: Electrical remodeling following percutaneous pulmonary valve implantation, *Am J Cardiol* 107:309–314, 2011.

69. Raikou M, McGuire A, Lurz P, et al: An assessment of the cost of percutaneous pulmonary valve implantation (PPVI) versus surgical pulmonary valve replacement (PVR) in patients with right ventricular outflow tract dysfunction, *J Med Econ* 14:47–52, 2011.

70. U.S. Food and Drug Administration (FDA): FDA *Approves First Percutaneous Heart Valve*, Jan. 25, 2010. Available at: http://www.fda.gov/NewsEvents/Newsroom/PressAnnouncements/ucm198597.htm. (Accessed March 15th, 2012., at http://www.fda.gov/NewsEvents/Newsroom/PressAnnouncements/ucm198597.htm.).

71. Attmann T, Jahnke T, Quaden R, et al: Advances in experimental percutaneous pulmonary valve replacement, *Ann Thorac Surg* 80:969–975, 2005.

72. Attmann T, Quaden R, Jahnke T, et al: Percutaneous pulmonary valve replacement: 3-month evaluation of self-expanding valved stents, *Ann Thorac Surg* 82:708–713, 2006.

73. Schreiber C, Horer J, Vogt M, et al: A new treatment option for pulmonary valvar insufficiency: first experiences with implantation of a self-expanding stented valve without use of cardiopulmonary bypass, *Eur J Cardiothorac Surg* 31:26–30, 2007.

74. Ruiz CE, Iemura M, Medie S, et al: Transcatheter placement of a low-profile biodegradable pulmonary valve made of small intestinal submucosa: a long-term study in a swine model, *J Thorac Cardiovasc Surg* 130:477–484, 2005.

75. Guccione P, Milanesi O, Hijazi ZM, et al: Transcatheter pulmonary valve implantation in native pulmonary outflow tract using the Edwards SAPIEN & trade; transcatheter heart valve, *Eur J Cardiothorac Surg* 41:1192–1194, 2012.

76. Thanopoulos BV, Giannakoulas G, Arampatzis CA: Percutaneous pulmonary valve implantation in the native right ventricular outflow tract, *Catheter Cardiovasc Interv* 79:427–429, 2012.

77. Mollet A, Basquin A, Stos B, et al: Off-pump replacement of the pulmonary valve in large right ventricular outflow tracts: a transcatheter approach using an intravascular infundibulum reducer, *Pediatr Res* 62:428–433, 2007.

78. Boudjemline Y, Agnoletti G, Bonnet D, et al: Percutaneous pulmonary valve replacement in a large right ventricular outflow tract: an experimental study, *J Am Coll Cardiol* 43:1082–1087, 2004.

79. Capelli C, Taylor AM, Migliavacca F, et al: Patient-specific reconstructed anatomies and computer simulations are fundamental for selecting medical device treatment: application to a new percutaneous pulmonary valve, *Philos Trans A Math Phys Eng Sci.* 368:3027–3038, 2010.

80. Schievano S, Taylor AM, Capelli C, et al: First-in-man implantation of a novel percutaneous valve: a new approach to medical device development, *EuroIntervention* 5:745–750, 2010.

81. Schievano S, Migliavacca F, Coats L, et al: Percutaneous pulmonary valve implantation based on rapid prototyping of right ventricular outflow tract and pulmonary trunk from MR data, *Radiology* 242:490–497, 2007.

Chapter 9

Percutaneous Balloon Valvuloplasty for Patients with Rheumatic Mitral and Tricuspid Stenosis

RONAN MARGEY • SAMMY ELMARIAH • IGOR F. PALACIOS

Before 1982, cardiac surgery was the conventional form of treatment for symptomatic stenotic valvular heart disease lesions.[1,2] Today, percutaneous balloon dilation of stenotic cardiac valves is being used in many centers for the treatment of patients with pulmonic, mitral, aortic, and tricuspid stenosis. Since its introduction in 1984 by Inoue et al.,[3] percutaneous mitral balloon commissurotomy or percutaneous mitral valvuloplasty (PMV) has been used successfully as an alternative to open or closed surgical mitral commissurotomy for the treatment of patients with symptomatic rheumatic mitral stenosis.[4-18] PMV produces good immediate hemodynamic outcome, low in-hospital complication rates, and clinical improvement in the majority of patients with rheumatic mitral stenosis. PMV is safe and effective, and it provides sustained clinical and hemodynamic improvement in patients with rheumatic mitral stenosis. The immediate and long-term results appear to be similar to those of surgical mitral commisssurotomy.[19-26] PMV is the preferred form of therapy for relief of mitral stenosis for a selected group of patients with symptomatic rheumatic mitral stenosis.

9.1 Patient Selection

Selection of patients for PMV should be based on symptoms, physical examination, and two-dimensional (2D) and Doppler echocardiographic findings.[4,17,27,28] PMV is usually performed electively. However, emergency PMV can be performed as a life-saving procedure in patients with mitral stenosis and severe pulmonary edema refractory to medical therapy and/or cardiogenic shock. Patients considered for PMV should be symptomatic (New York Heart Association [NYHA] ≥ II), should have no recent thromboembolic events, have less than two grades of mitral regurgitation (MR) by contrast ventriculography using the Sellers' classification,[29] and have no evidence of left atrial thrombus on 2D and transesophageal echocardiography **(Table 9–1).** Transthoracic and transesophageal echocardiography should be performed routinely before PMV. Patients in atrial fibrillation and patients with previous embolic episodes should have treatment with warfarin to achieve anticoagulation with a therapeutic international normalized ratio (INR) for at least 3 months before PMV. Patients with left-atrium thrombus on 2D-echocardiography should be excluded. However, PMV could be performed in these patients if left-atrium thrombus has resolved after warfarin therapy.

A multifactorial score derived from clinical, anatomic/echocardiographic, and hemodynamic variables can predict procedural success and clinical outcome **(Figure 9–1).**[28] Demographic data, echocardiographic parameters (including echocardiographic score, **Figure 9–2**), and procedure-related variables recorded from 1085 consecutive patients who underwent PMV at the Massachusetts General Hospital (MGH) and their long-term clinical follow-up data (i.e., death, mitral valve replacement, redo PMV) were used to derive this clinical score. Multivariate regression analysis of the first 800 procedures was performed to identify independent predictors of procedural success. Significant variables were formulated into a risk score and validated prospectively. Six independent predictors of PMV success were identified: (1) age younger than 55 years, (2) NYHA classes I and II, (3) pre-PMV mitral area of 1 cm^2 or greater, (4) pre-PMV MR grade less than 2, (5) echocardiographic score of 8 or less, and (6) male gender.[4,27,28] A score

TABLE 9–1

Recommendations for Percutaneous Mitral Valvuloplasty*

Current Indication	Class	Level of Evidence
Symptomatic patients (NYHA functional Class II, III, or IV), moderate or severe mitral stenosis (area <1.5 cm²), and valve morphology favorable for percutaneous balloon valvuloplasty in the absence of left atrial thrombus or moderate to severe mitral regurgitation (MR).	I	Grade A
Asymptomatic patients with moderate or severe mitral stenosis (area <1.5 cm²) and valve morphology favorable for percutaneous balloon valvuloplasty who have pulmonary hypertension (pulmonary artery systolic pressure >50 mmHg at rest or 60 mmHg with exercise) in the absence of left atrial thrombus or moderate to severe MR.	IIa	Grade C
Patients with NYHA functional Class III-IV, moderate or severe mitral stenosis (area <1.5 cm²), and a nonpliable calcified valve who are at high risk for surgery in the absence of left atrial thrombus or moderate to severe MR.	IIa	Grade B
Asymptomatic patients with moderate or severe mitral stenosis (area <1.5 cm²) and valve morphology favorable for percutaneous balloon valvuloplasty who have new onset of atrial fibrillation in the absence of left atrial thrombus or moderate to severe MR.	IIb	Grade B
Patients in NYHA functional Class III-IV who have moderate or severe mitral stenosis (area <1.5 cm²), and a nonpliable calcified valve who are low-risk candidates for surgery.	IIb	Grade C
Patients with mild mitral stenosis.	III	Grade C

NYHA, New York Heart Association.
*Adapted from currently American College of Cardiology/American Heart Association and European Guidelines for the management of patients with valvular heart disease.

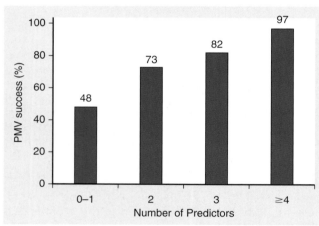

MULTIFACTORIAL DETERMINANTS OF PMV
PROCEDURAL SUCCESS

Figure 9–1 A multifactorial score derived from clinical, anatomic/echocardiographic, and hemodynamic variables would predict procedural success and clinical outcome. *PMV,* Percutaneous mitral balloon commissurotomy.

was constructed from the arithmetic sum of variables present per patient. Procedural success rates increased incrementally with increasing score (0% for a score of 0/6, 39.7% for 1/6, 54.4% for 2/6, 77.3% for 3/6, 85.7% for 4/6, 95% for 5/6, and 100% for 6/6; p < 0.001). In a validation cohort (n = 285 consecutive procedures), the multifactorial score remained a significant predictor of PMV success (p < 0.001). Comparison between the new score and the echocardiographic score confirmed that the new index is more sensitive and specific (p < 0.001). This new score also predicts long-term outcomes (p < 0.001). Clinical, anatomic, and hemodynamic variables predict PMV success and clinical outcome and may be formulated in a scoring system that would help to identify the best candidates for PMV.

9.2 Technique of Percutaneous Mitral Balloon Commissurotomy

PMV is performed when the patient is in the fasting state and under mild sedation. Antibiotics (500 mg dicloxacillin *per os* [po] q/6 hours for four doses started before the procedure or 1 g cefazolin intravenously [IV] at the time of the procedure) are used. Patients allergic to penicillin should receive 1 g vancomycin IV at the time of the procedure. All patients carefully chosen as candidates for mitral balloon valvuloplasty should undergo diagnostic right and transseptal left heart catheterization. After transseptal left heart catheterization, systemic anticoagulation is achieved by the intravenous administration of 100 units/kg of heparin. In patients older than 40 years, coronary arteriography is recommended and should also be performed.

Hemodynamic measurements, cardiac output, and cine left ventriculography are performed before and after PMV. Cardiac output is measured by thermodilution and Fick method techniques. Mitral valve calcification and angiographic severity of MR (Sellers' classification) are graded qualitatively from 0 to 4 as previously described.[29] An oxygen diagnostic run is performed before and after PMV to determine the presence of left-to-right shunt across the atrial septum after PMV.

There is not a unique technique of percutaneous mitral balloon valvuloplasty. Most of the techniques of PMV require transseptal left heart catheterization and use of the antegrade approach.[15-24,26,30-32] Antegrade PMV can be accomplished using double balloon technique **(Figure 9–3, A),** or the more commonly used single balloon technique **(Figure 9–3, B).** In this latter approach the two balloons could be placed through a single femoral vein and single transseptal puncture or through two femoral veins and two separate atrial septal puncture. In the retrograde technique of PMV the balloon dilating catheters are advanced percutaneously

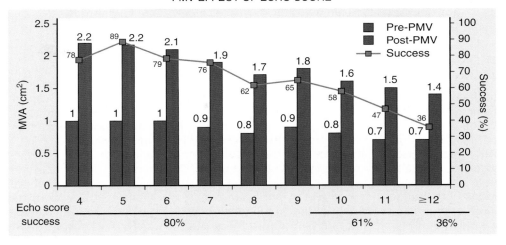

Figure 9–2 Relationship between the echo score, the pre- and post-PMV MVA, and immediate success after PMV. *MVA,* Mitral valve area; *PMV,* percutaneous mitral balloon commissurotomy.

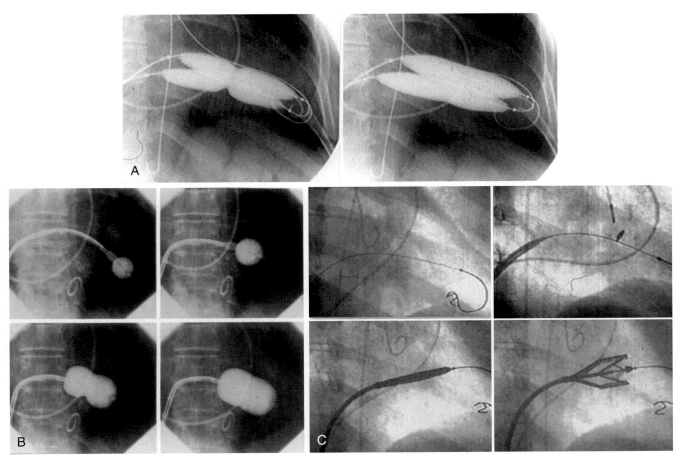

Figure 9–3 **Different percutaneous approaches of percutaneous mitral balloon commissurotomy. A,** The double balloon technique; **B,** the Inoue technique; and **C,** the metallic valvulotome.

through the right and left femoral arteries over guidewires that have been snared from the descending aorta. These guidewires have been advanced transseptally from the right femoral vein into the left atrium, the left ventricle, and the ascending aorta.[31] A retrograde non-transseptal technique of PMV has also been described.[15] A technique of PMV using a newly designed metallic

valvulotome has also been introduced.[16] The device consists of a detachable metallic cylinder with two articulated bars screwed onto the distal end of a disposable catheter, on which the proximal end is connected to activating pliers. Squeezing the pliers opens the bars up to a maximum of 40 mm **(see Figure 9–3, C).** The results with this device are at least comparable to those of the other balloon techniques of PMV.[16] However, multiple uses after sterilization should markedly decrease procedural costs.

THE ANTEGRADE DOUBLE BALLOON TECHNIQUE

In performing PMV using the antegrade double balloon technique (see Figure 9–3, A) two 0.0038-inch (260-cm) Teflon-coated exchange wires are placed across the mitral valve into the left ventricle, through the aortic valve into the ascending and then the descending aorta (see Double Balloon Antegrade PMV Technique).[4,18-19] Care should be taken to maintain large and smooth loops of the guidewires in the left ventricular cavity to allow appropriate placement of the dilating balloons. If a second guidewire cannot be placed into the ascending and descending aorta, a 0.038-inch Amplatz guidewire (Cook Inc., Bloomington, Ind.) with a preformed curl at its tip can be placed at the left ventricular apex. In patients with an aortic valve prosthesis, both guidewires with preformed curl tips should be placed at the left ventricular apex. When one or both guidewires are placed in the left ventricular apex, the balloons should be inflated sequentially. Care should be taken to avoid forward movement of the balloons and guidewires to prevent left ventricular perforation. Two balloon-dilating catheters are chosen according to the patient's body surface area such that the ratio of effective balloon-dilating area (EBDA) to body surface area is greater than 3.1 cm^2/m^2 and less than 4 cm^2/m^2 (Table 9–2). The balloon valvotomy catheters are then advanced over each one of the guidewires and positioned across the mitral valve parallel to the longitudinal axis of the left ventricle. The balloon valvotomy catheters are then inflated by hand until the indentation produced by the stenotic mitral valve is no longer seen. Generally one, but occasionally two or three, inflations are performed. After complete deflation, the balloons are removed sequentially.

THE INOUE TECHNIQUE

PMV can also be performed using the Inoue technique (see Figure 9–3, B).[3] The Inoue balloon is a 12F-shaft, coaxial, double-lumen catheter. The balloon is made of a double layer of rubber latex tubing with a layer of synthetic micromesh in between. After transseptal catheterization, a stainless steel guidewire is advanced through the transseptal catheter and placed with its tip coiled into the left atrium, and the transseptal catheter is removed. A 14F dilator is advanced over the guidewire and used to dilate the femoral vein and the atrial septum. A balloon catheter is chosen according to the patient's height using the formula:

Maximum balloon size (mm) = (height [cm] / 10)+10

The balloon catheter is advanced over the guidewire into the left atrium. The distal part of the balloon is partially inflated and advanced into the left ventricle with the help of the spring wire stylet, which has been inserted through the inner lumen of the catheter. The stylet is rotated in a counterclockwise fashion with gentle backward traction on the catheter. Once the catheter is in the left ventricle, the distal aspect of the balloon is inflated and moved back and forth inside the left ventricle to assure that it is free of the chordae tendineae. The catheter is then gently pulled against the mitral plane until resistance is felt. The balloon is then rapidly inflated to its full capacity and deflated quickly (Videos 9–1 and 9–2). During inflation of the balloon an indentation should be seen in its midportion. The catheter is withdrawn into the left atrium, and the mitral gradient and cardiac output are measured. If further dilations are required the stylet is introduced again and the sequence of steps described above is repeated at a larger balloon volume. After each dilation its effect should be assessed by pressure measurement, cardiac output, auscultation, and 2D echocardiography. If MR occurs, further dilation of the valve should not be performed.

MECHANISM OF PERCUTANEOUS MITRAL BALLOON COMMISSUROTOMY

The mechanism of successful PMV is splitting of the fused commissures toward the mitral annulus, resulting in commissural widening. This mechanism has been demonstrated by pathological, surgical, and echocardiographic studies.[27,33] In addition, in patients with calcific mitral stenosis the balloons could increase mitral valve flexibility by the fracture of the calcified deposits in the mitral valve leaflets.[33] Although rare, undesirable complications such as leaflet tears, left ventricular perforation, tear of the atrial septum, and rupture of chordae, mitral annulus, and papillary muscle could also occur.

IMMEDIATE OUTCOME

Figure 9–3 shows the hemodynamic changes produced by PMV in one patient. PMV resulted in a significant decrease in mitral gradient, mean left atrium pressure, and mean pulmonary artery pressure, and an increase in cardiac output and mitral valve area (MVA). Table 9–3 shows the changes in MVA reported by several investigators using different techniques of PMV. In most series, PMV is reported to increase MVA from less than 1.0 cm^2 to approximately 2.0 cm^2.[2,4,12-18,22,34]

Eight hundred and seventy nine consecutive patients with mitral stenosis underwent 939 consecutive PMVs at MGH between July 1986 and July 2000.[4] As shown in Figure 9–4, in this group of patients PMV resulted in a significant decrease in mitral gradient from 14 ± 6 to 6 ± 3 mmHg. The mean cardiac output significantly increased from 3.9 ± 1.1 to 4.5 ± 1.3 L/min, and the calculated MVA increased from 0.9 ± 0.3 to 1.9 ± 0.7 cm^2. In addition, mean pulmonary artery pressure significantly decreased from 36 ± 13 to 29 ± 11 mmHg, and the mean left atrial pressure decreased from 25 ± 7 to 17 ± 7 mmHg; consequently, the calculated pulmonary vascular resistances decreased significantly after PMV.

A successful hemodynamic outcome (defined as a post-PMV MVA ≥1.5 cm^2 and post-PMV MR <3 Sellers grade) was obtained in 72% of the patients. Although

TABLE 9–2
Effective Dilating Diameter (mm) for Double Balloon Technique

	5	**6**	**7**	**8**	**9**	**10**	**11**	**12**	**13**	**14**	**15**	**16**	**17**	**18**	**19**	**20**	**21**	**22**	**23**	**24**	**25**
5	8.2	9.0	9.9	10.7	11.6	12.5	13.5	14.4	15.3	16.2	17.2	18.1	19.1	20.0	21.0	21.9	22.9	23.9	24.8	25.8	26.8
6		9.8	10.7	11.5	12.4	13.3	14.1	15.1	16.0	16.9	17.8	18.7	19.7	20.6	21.6	22.5	23.5	24.4	25.4	26.3	27.3
7			11.5	12.3	13.1	14.0	14.9	15.8	16.7	17.6	18.5	19.4	20.3	21.2	22.2	23.1	24.1	25.0	25.9	26.9	27.8
8				13.1	13.9	14.8	15.8	16.5	17.4	18.3	19.2	20.1	21.0	21.9	22.8	23.7	24.7	25.6	26.5	27.5	28.4
9					14.7	15.6	16.4	17.3	18.1	19.0	19.9	20.8	21.7	22.6	23.5	24.4	25.3	26.2	27.2	28.1	29.0
10						16.4	17.2	18.0	18.9	19.7	20.6	21.5	22.4	23.3	24.2	25.1	26.0	26.9	27.8	28.8	29.7
11							18.0	18.8	19.7	20.5	21.4	22.2	23.1	24.0	24.9	25.8	26.7	27.6	28.5	29.4	30.3
12								19.8	20.5	21.3	22.1	23.0	23.9	24.7	25.6	26.5	27.4	28.3	29.2	30.1	31.0
13									21.3	22.1	22.9	23.8	24.6	25.5	26.4	27.2	28.1	29.0	29.9	30.8	31.7
14										22.9	23.7	24.8	25.4	26.3	27.1	28.0	28.9	29.7	30.6	31.5	32.4
15											24.5	25.4	26.2	27.0	27.9	28.8	29.6	30.5	31.4	32.2	33.1
16												26.2	27.0	27.8	28.7	29.5	30.4	31.2	32.1	33.0	33.9
17													27.8	28.6	29.5	30.3	31.2	32.0	32.9	33.7	34.1
18														29.5	30.3	31.1	32.0	32.8	33.6	34.5	35.4
19															31.1	31.9	32.7	33.6	34.4	35.3	36.1
20																32.7	33.6	34.4	35.2	36.1	36.9
21																	34.4	35.2	36.0	36.9	37.7
22																		36.0	36.8	37.7	38.5
23																			37.6	38.5	39.3
24																				39.3	40.1
25																					40.9

This chart can be used to determine the effective dilating diameter when two balloons are used simultaneously for mitral valvuloplasty. The bold numbers represent the diameters of the individual balloons; the intersection of these bold numbers reveals the effective dilating diameter.

TABLE 9–3

Immediate Changes in Mitral Valve Area after Percutaneous Mitral Valvuloplasty

Author	Institution	Number of Patients	Age	Pre-PMV	Post-PMV
Palacios et al.	MGH	879	55 ± 15	0.9 ± 0.3	1.9 ± 0.7
Vahanian et al.	Tenon	1514	45 ± 15	1.0 ± 0.2	1.9 ± 0.3
Hernández et al.	Clínico Madrid	561	53 ± 13	1.0 ± 0.2	1.8 ± 0.4
Stefanadis et al.	Athens University	438	44 ± 11	1.0 ± 0.3	2.1 ± 0.5
Chen et al.	Guangzhou	4832	37 ± 12	1.1 ± 0.3	2.1 ± 0.2
NHLBI	Multicenter	738	54 ± 12	1.0 ± 0.4	2.0 ± 0.2
Inoue et al.	Takeda	527	50 ± 10	1.1 ± 0.1	2.0 ± 0.1
Inoue Registry	Multicenter	1251	53 ± 15	1.0 ± 0.3	1.8 ± 0.6
Ben Farhat et al.	Fattouma	463	33 ± 12	1.0 ± 0.2	2.2 ± 0.4
Arora et al.	GB Pan	600	27 ± 8	0.8 ± 0.2	2.2 ± 0.4
Cribier et al.	Ruen	153	36 ± 15	1.0 ± 0.2	2.2 ± 0.4

MGH, Massachusetts General Hospital; *NHLBI,* National Heart, Lung, and Blood Institute; *PMV,* percutaneous mitral valvuloplasty.

MITRAL BALLOON VALVULOPLASTY
Immediate outcome

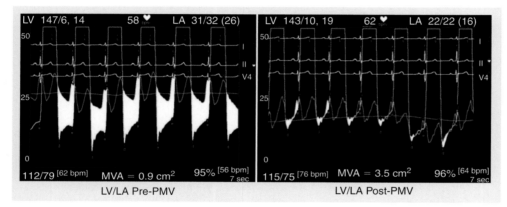

Figure 9–4 Hemodynamic changes produced by a successful PMV in one patient with severe mitral stenosis. Simultaneous left atrium and left ventricular pressures before *(left panel)* and after *(right panel)* PMV. The corresponding calculated MVAs are also displayed. *LA,* Left atrium; *LV,* left ventricle; *MVA,* mitral valve area; *PMV,* percutaneous mitral balloon valvuloplasty.

a suboptimal result occurred in 28% of the patients, a post-PMV MVA of 1.0 cm² or less (critical MVA) was present in only 8.7% of these patients.

9.3 Predictors of Increase in Mitral Valve Area and Procedural Success

Univariate analysis demonstrated that the increase in MVA with PMV is directly related to the balloon size employed because it reflects in the EBDA, and inversely related to the echocardiographic score **(see Figure 9–2),** the presence of atrial fibrillation, the presence of fluoroscopic calcium, the presence of previous surgical commissurotomy, older age, NYHA classification pre-PMV, and presence of MR before PMV. Multiple stepwise regression analysis identified balloon size (p < 0.02), the echocardiographic score (p < 0.0001), and the presence of atrial fibrillation (p < 0.009) and MR before PMV (p < 0.03) as independent predictors of the increase in MVA with PMV.[4]

Univariate predictors of procedural success included age, pre-PMV MVA, mean pre-PMV pulmonary artery pressure, male gender, echocardiographic score, pre-PMV MR of 2+ or greater, history of previous surgical

commissurotomy, presence of atrial fibrillation, and presence of mitral valve calcification under fluoroscopy.[4]

Multiple stepwise logistic regression analysis identified larger pre-PMV MVA (odds ratio [OR] 13.05; 95% confidence interval [CI] 7.74 to 22.51; p < 0.001), less degree of pre-PMV MR (OR 3.85; CI 2.27 to 6.66; p < 0.001), younger age (OR 3.33; CI 1.41 to 7.69; p = 0.006), absence of previous surgical commissurotomy (OR 1.85; CI 1.20 to 2.86; p = 0.004), male gender (OR 1.92; CI 1.19 to 3.13; p = 0.008), and echocardiographic score of 8 or lower (OR 1.69; CI 1.18 to 2.44; p = 0.004).[4]

THE ECHOCARDIOGRAPHIC SCORE

The echocardiographic examination of the mitral valve can accurately characterize the severity and extent of the pathologic process in patients with rheumatic mitral stenosis. The most utilized score to identify the anatomic abnormalities of the stenotic mitral valve is that described by Wilkins et al. **(see Figure 9–2 and Table 9–4).**[27,35,36] This echocardiographic score is an important predictor of the immediate and long-term outcome of PMV. In this morphologic score, leaflet rigidity, leaflet thickening, valvular calcification, and subvalvular disease are scored from 0 to 4. A higher score represents

TABLE 9–4

The Echocardiographic Score*

Echocardiographic Grading of the Severity and Extent of the Anatomic Abnormalities in Patients with Mitral Stenosis

Grade	Leaflet Mobility	Valvular Thickening	Valvular Calcification	Subvalvular Thickening
0	Normal	Normal	Normal	Normal
1	Highly mobile valve with restriction of only the leaflet tips	Leaflet near normal (4-5 mm)	A single area of increased echo brightness	Minimal thickening of chordal structures just below the valve
2	Middle portion and base of leaflets have reduced mobility	Midleaflet thickening, marked thickening of the margins	Scattered areas of brightness confined to leaflet margins	Thickening of chordae extending up to one third of chordal length
3	Valve leaflets move forward in diastole mainly at the base	Thickening extending through the entire leaflets (5-8 mm)	Brightness extending into the midportion of leaflets	Thickening extending to the distal third of the chordae
4	No or minimal forward movement of the leaflets in diastole	Marked thickening of all leaflet tissue (>8-10 mm)	Extensive brightness throughout most of the leaflet tissue	Extensive thickening and shortening of all chordae extending down to the papillary muscles

*The total score is the sum of each of these echocardiographic features (maximum 16).

a heavily calcified, thickened, and immobile valve with extensive thickening and calcification of the subvalvular apparatus. The increase in MVA with PMV is inversely related to the echocardiographic score. The best outcomes with PMV occur in those patients with echocardiographic scores of 8 or lower. The increase in MVA is significantly greater in patients with echocardiographic scores of 8 or higher than in those with echocardiographic scores higher than 8 (Videos 9–3 and 9–4). Among the four components of the echocardiographic score, valve leaflets thickening and subvalvular disease correlate the best with the increase in MVA produced by PMV.[37] Therefore suboptimal results with PMV are more likely to occur in patients with valves that are more rigid and more thickened and in those patients with more subvalvular fibrosis and calcification.

BALLOON SIZE AND EFFECTIVE BALLOON DILATING AREA

The increase in MVA with PMV is directly related to balloon size. This effect was first demonstrated in a subgroup of patients who underwent repeat PMV. They initially underwent PMV with a single balloon, resulting in a mean MVA of 1.2 ± 0.2 cm^2. They underwent repeat PMV using the double balloon technique, which increased the EBDA normalized by body surface area from 3.41 ± 0.2 to 4.51 ± 0.2 cm^2/m^2. The mean MVA in this group after repeat PMV was 1.8 ± 0.7 cm^2. The increase in MVA in patients who underwent PMV at MGH using the double balloon technique (EBDA of 6.4 ± 0.03 cm^2) was significantly greater than the increase in MVA achieved in patients who underwent PMV using the single balloon technique (EBDA of 4.3 ± 0.02 cm^2).[38] The mean MVAs were 1.9 ± 0.7 and 1.4 ± 0.1 cm^2 for patients who underwent PMV with the double balloon and the single balloon techniques, respectively. However, as previously mentioned, care should be taken

in the selection of dilating balloon catheters so as to obtain an adequate final MVA and no change or a minimal increase in MR.

MITRAL VALVE CALCIFICATION

The immediate outcome of patients undergoing PMV is inversely related to the severity of valvular calcification seen by fluoroscopy. Patients without fluoroscopic calcium have a greater increase in MVA after PMV than patients with calcified valves. Patients with either no or 1+ fluoroscopic calcium have a greater increase in MVA after PMV (1.1 ± 0.6 and 0.9 ± 0.5 cm^2, respectively) than those patients with 2+, 3+, or 4+ fluoroscopic calcium (0.8 ± 0.6, 0.8 ± 0.5, and 0.6 ± 0.4 cm^2, respectively).[39]

PREVIOUS SURGICAL COMMISSUROTOMY

Although the increase in MVA with PMV is inversely related to the presence of previous surgical mitral commissurotomy, PMV can produce a good outcome in this group of patients. The post-PMV mean MVA in 154 patients with previous surgical commissurotomy was 1.8 ± 0.7 cm^2, compared with a valve area of 1.9 ± 0.6 cm^2 in patients without previous surgical commissurotomy ($p < 0.05$). In this group of patients an echocardiographic score of 8 or lower was an important predictor of a successful hemodynamic immediate outcome.[40]

AGE

The immediate outcome of PMV is directly related to the age of the patient. The percentage of patients obtaining a good result with this technique decreases as age increases. A successful hemodynamic outcome from PMV was obtained in fewer than 50% of patients 65 years or older.[30,41] This inverse relationship between age and the immediate outcome from PMV is the result of the

TABLE 9–5

Complications after Percutaneous Mitral Valvuloplasty

Author	Number of Patients	Mortality	Tamponade	Severe MR	Embolism
Palacios et al.	879	0.6%	1.0%	3.4%	1.8%
Vahanian et al.	1514	0.4%	0.3%	3.4%	0.3%
Hernández et al.	561	0.4%	0.6%	4.5%	N/A
Stefanadis et al.	438	0.2%	0%	3.4%	0%
Chen et al.	4832	0.1%	0.8%	1.4%	0.5%
NHLBI	738	3.0%	4.0%	3.0%	3.0%
Inoue et al.	527	0%	1.6%	1.9%	0.6%
Inoue Registry	1251	0.6%	1.4%	3.8%	0.9%
Ben Farhat et al.	463	0.4%	0.7%	4.6%	2.0%
Arora et al.	600	1.0%	1.3%	1.0%	0.5%
Cribier et al.	153	0%	0.7%	1.4%	0.7%

MR, Mitral regurgitation; *NHLBI,* National Heart, Lung, and Blood Institute.

higher frequency of atrial fibrillation, calcified valves, and higher echocardiographic scores in elderly patients.

ATRIAL FIBRILLATION

The increase in MVA with PMV is inversely related to the presence of atrial fibrillation; the post-PMV MVA of patients in normal sinus rhythm was 2.0 ± 0.7 cm^2, compared with a valve area of 1.7 ± 0.6 cm^2 of those patients in atrial fibrillation. The inferior immediate outcome of PMV in patients with mitral stenosis who are in atrial fibrillation is more likely related to the presence of clinical and morphological characteristics such as advanced age, echocardiographic scores greater than 8, NYHA functional class IV, calcified mitral valves under fluoroscopy, and a previous history of surgical mitral commissurotomy.[42]

MITRAL REGURGITATION BEFORE PERCUTANEOUS MITRAL BALLOON COMMISSUROTOMY

The presence and severity of MR before PMV is an independent predictor of unfavorable outcome of PMV. The increase in MVA after PMV is inversely related to the severity of MR determined by angiography before the procedure. This inverse relationship between the presence of MR and immediate outcome of PMV is in part caused by the higher frequency of atrial fibrillation, higher echocardiographic scores, calcified mitral valves under fluoroscopy, and older age in patients with MR before PMV.[28,42]

9.4 Complications

Table 9–5 shows the complications reported by several investigators after PMV.[4,12-18,22,34] Mortality and morbidity with PMV are low and similar to surgical commissurotomy. Overall, there is a less than 1% procedural mortality. Severe MR (4 grades by angiography) has been reported in 1% to 5.2% of patients, with some of these patients requiring in-hospital mitral valve replacement.

Thromboembolic episodes and stroke have been reported in 0% to 3.1% and pericardial tamponade in 0.2% to 4.6% of cases in these series. Pericardial tamponade can occur from transseptal catheterization and more rarely from ventricular perforation. PMV is associated with a 3% to 16% incidence of left-to-right shunt documented by oxymetry immediately after the procedure. However, the pulmonary-to-systemic flow ratio is greater than or equal to 2:1 in only a minimum number of patients.

Severe MR (4 grades by angiography) occurs in about 3% of patients undergoing PMV.[28,42] An undesirable increase in MR (≥2 grades by angiography) occurred in 10.1% of patients. This undesirable increase in MR is well tolerated in most patients. Furthermore, more than half of them have less MR at follow-up cardiac catheterization. The ratio of the EBDA to body surface area is a predictor of increased MR after PMV.[28,42,43] The EBDA is calculated using standard geometric formulas **(see Table 9–2).** The incidence of MR is lower if balloon sizes are chosen so that EBDA/body surface area is less than or equal to 4.0 cm^2/m^2. The single balloon technique results in a lower incidence of MR but provides less relief of mitral stenosis than the double balloon technique. Thus there is an optimal EBDA between 3.1 and 4.0 cm^2/m^2 that achieves a maximal MVA with a minimal increase in MR. An echocardiographic score for the mitral valve that can predict the development of severe MR after PMV has also been described.[35] This score takes into account the distribution (even or uneven) of leaflet thickening and calcification, the degree and symmetry of commissural disease, and the severity of subvalvular disease **(Table 9–6).**

Left-to-right shunt through the created atrial communication determined by oximetry occurred in 3% to 16% of patients undergoing PMV. The size of the defect is small as reflected in the pulmonary-to-systemic flow ratio of less than 2:1 in the majority of patients. Older age, fluoroscopic evidence of mitral valve calcification, higher echocardiographic score, pre-PMV lower cardiac output, and higher pre-PMV NYHA functional class are the factors that predispose patients to develop left-to-right shunt post-PMV.[44] Clinical, echocardiographic, surgical, and hemodynamic follow-up study of patients with post-PMV left-to-right shunt demonstrated that the defect closed

TABLE 9–6
The Echocardiographic Score* for Severe Mitral Regurgitation after Percutaneous Mitral Commissurotomy

I-II	Valvular thickening (score each leaflet separately)
	Leaflet near normal (4-5 mm) or with only a thick segment
	Leaflet fibrotic and/or calcified evenly; no thin areas
	Leaflet fibrotic and/or calcified with uneven distribution; thinner segments are mildly thickened (5-8 mm)
	Leaflet fibrotic and/or calcified with uneven distribution; thinner segments are near normal (4-5 mm)
III	Commissural calcification
	Fibrosis and/or calcium in only one commissure
	Both commissures mildly affected
	Calcium in both commissures, one markedly affected
	Calcium in both commissures, both markedly affected
IV	Subvalvular disease
	Minimal thickening of chordal structures just below the valve
	Thickening of chordae extending to one third of chordal length
	Thickening to the distal third of the chordae
	Extensive thickening and shortening of all chordae extending down to papillary muscle

*The total score is the sum of each of these echocardiographic features (maximum 16).

TABLE 9–7
Clinical Long-Term Follow-Up after Percutaneous Mitral Valvuloplasty

Author	Number of Patients	Age	Follow-Up Study (Years)	Survival	Event-Free Survival
Palacios et al.	879	55	12	74%	33%
Iung et al.	1024	49	10	85%	56%
Hernández et al.	561	53	7	95%	69%
Orrange et al.	132	44	7	83%	65%
Ben Farhat et al.	30	29	7	100%	90%
Stefanadis et al.	441	44	9	98%	75%

in approximately 60% of patients. Persistent left-to-right shunt at follow-up study is small ($\dot{Q}P/\dot{Q}S < 2:1$) and clinically well tolerated. In the series from MGH there is one patient in whom the atrial shunt remained hemodynamically significant at follow-up study. This patient underwent percutaneous transcatheter closure of her iatrogenic residual atrial defect with a clamshell device. Desideri et al.[45] reported atrial shunting determined by color flow transthoracic echocardiography in 61% of 57 patients immediately after PMV. The shunt persisted in 30% of patients at 19 ± 6 (range 9 to 33) months' follow-up examination. They identified the magnitude of the post-PMV atrial shunt ($\dot{Q}P/\dot{Q}S > 1.5:1$), use of bifoil balloon (2 balloons on 1 shaft), and smaller post-PMV MVA as independent predictors of the persistence of atrial shunt at long-term follow-up study. Together with the authors' results, these findings suggest that those patients with persistently elevated left atrial pressures resulting from either suboptimal PMV or poor diastolic compliance after PMV are more likely to experience persistent left-to-right shunting.

9.5 Clinical Follow-Up Studies

Long-term follow-up studies after PMV are encouraging.[4,22-26,30,46-60] After PMV, the majority of patients have marked clinical improvement and are scored at NYHA Class I or II. The symptomatic, echocardiographic, and hemodynamic improvement produced by PMV persists in intermediate and long-term follow-up study. The best long-term results are seen in patients with echocardiographic scores of 8 or less. When PMV produces a good immediate outcome in this group of patients, restenosis is unlikely to occur at follow-up study. Although PMV can result in a good outcome in patients with echocardiographic scores higher than 8, hemodynamic and echocardiographic restenosis is often demonstrated at follow-up study despite ongoing clinical improvement. **Table 9–7** shows long-term follow-up results of patients undergoing PMV at different institutes. An estimated 12-year survival rate of 74% in a cohort of 879 patients undergoing PMV at the MGH was reported **(Figure 9–5).**[4] Death at follow-up study was directly related to age, post-PMV pulmonary artery pressure, and pre-PMV NYHA functional class IV. In the same group of patients, the 12-year event-free survival rate (alive and free of mitral valve replacement or repair and redo PMV) was 33% **(Figure 9–6).** Cox regression analysis identified age (risk ratio [RR] 1.02; CI 1.01 to 1.03; p < 0.0001), pre-PMV NYHA functional class IV (RR 1.35; CI 1.00 to 1.81; p = 0.05), prior commissurotomy (RR 1.50; CI 1.16 to 1.92; p = 0.002), the echocardiographic score (RR 1.31; CI 1.02 to 1.67; p = 0.003), pre-PMV MR greater than or equal to 2+ (RR 1.56; CI 1.09 to 2.22; p = 0.02), post-PMV MR greater than or equal to 3+ (RR 3.54; CI 2.61 to 4.72; p < 0.0001), and post-PMV mean pulmonary artery pressure (RR 1.02; CI 1.01 to 1.03; p < 0.0001) as independent predictors of combined events at long-term follow-up study.

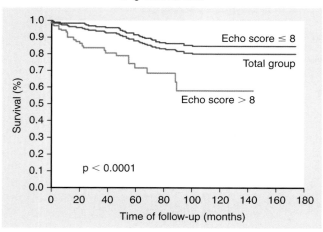

Figure 9–5 Fifteen-year survival rates for all patients and for patients with echocardiographic scores of 8 or lower and greater than 8 undergoing percutaneous mitral balloon valvuloplasty at MGH.

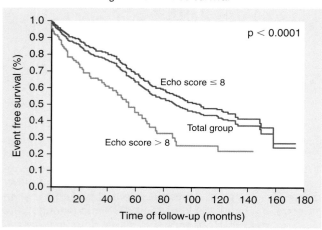

Figure 9–6 Fifteen-year event-free survival rates for all patients and for patients with echocardiographic scores of less than or equal to 8 and greater than 8 undergoing percutaneous mitral balloon valvuloplasty at MGH.

Actuarial survival and event-free survival rates throughout the follow-up period were significantly better in patients with echocardiographic scores of 8 or lower. Survival rates were 82% for patients with echocardiographic score of 8 or lower and 57% for patients with score higher than 8 at a follow-up time of 15 years (p < 0.0001). Event-free survival (38% vs 22%; p < 0.0001) at 15 years follow-up study were also significantly higher for patients with echocardiographic score of 8 or less. Similar follow-up studies have been reported in other series with the double balloon technique and with the Inoue technique of PMV.[4] Over 90% of young patients with pliable valves, in sinus rhythm, and with no evidence of calcium under fluoroscopy remain free of cardiovascular events at an approximate follow-up time of 5 years.[4]

Functional deterioration at follow-up study is late and related primarily to mitral restenosis.[36] The incidence of restenosis, as assessed by sequential echocardiography, is approximately 40% after 7 years.[36] Repeat PMV can be proposed if recurrent stenosis leads to symptoms. At the moment, there are only a small number of series available on redo PMV. They show encouraging results in selected patients with favorable characteristics when restenosis occurs several years after an initially successful procedure and if the predominant mechanism of restenosis is commissural refusion.

THE ELDERLY

Tuzcu et al.[30] reported the outcome of PMV in 99 elderly patients (≥ 65 years). A successful outcome (valve area ≥ 1.5 cm² without ≥ 2+ increase in MR and without left-to-right shunt of ≥ 1.5:1) was achieved in 46 patients. The best multivariate predictor of success was the combination of echocardiographic score, NYHA functional class, and inverse of MVA. Patients who had an unsuccessful outcome from PMV were in a higher NYHA functional class, had higher echocardiographic scores, and smaller MVAs pre-PMV compared with those patients who had a successful outcome. Low echocardiographic score was the only independent predictor of survival, and lack of mitral valve calcification was the strongest predictor of event free survival.

Recent data have shown that patients aged 75 years and older present a lower pre-PMV MVA (0.8 ± 0.3 vs. 0.9 ± 0.3; p = 0.005) and that PMV is less often successful (51% versus 71.4%; p < 0.0001) compared with patients younger than 75 years.[41] Older patients also exhibited a higher in-hospital mortality (3.1% vs. 0.3%) with no significant differences in the other procedure-related complications (cardiac tamponade, severe MR, significant left-to-right shunt and embolism). The echo score appears to be an imperfect predictor of hemodynamic improvement in elderly patients.[30,41]

Unfortunately, no randomized study is available for elderly patients, and a comparison of the results of PMV with those of surgical series is difficult because of the differences in the patients and surgical techniques involved.

PATIENTS WITH CALCIFIED MITRAL VALVES

The presence of fluoroscopically visible calcification on the mitral valve influences the success of PMV. Patients with heavily calcified valves (≥3 grades) under fluoroscopy have a poorer immediate outcome as reflected in a smaller post-PMV MVA and greater post-PMV mitral valve gradient. The long-term results of PMV are significantly different in calcified and uncalcified groups and in subgroups of the calcified group.[39] Estimated 2-year survival is significantly lower for patients with calcified mitral valves than for those with noncalcified valves (80% vs. 99%, p < 0.0001), and survival becomes worse as the severity of valvular calcification becomes more severe. Freedom from mitral valve replacement at 2 years was significantly lower for patients with calcified valves than for those with noncalcified valves (67% vs. 93%, p < 0.00005). These findings are in agreement with several follow-up studies of surgical commissurotomy that previously demonstrated that patients with calcified mitral valves had poorer survival rates compared with those patients with noncalcified valves.[1,2,39]

PATIENTS WITH PREVIOUS SURGICAL COMMISSUROTOMY

PMV also has been shown to be a safe procedure in patients with previous surgical mitral commissurotomy.[40] Although a good immediate outcome is often achieved in these patients, follow-up results are not as favorable as those obtained in patients without previous surgical commissurotomy. Although there is no difference in mortality between patients with or without a history of previous surgical commissurotomy at 4-year follow-up study, the number of patients who required mitral valve replacement (26% vs. 8%) and/or were in NYHA class III or IV (35% vs. 13%) was significantly higher among those patients with previous commissurotomy. However, when the patients are carefully selected according to the echocardiographic score (≤8), the immediate outcome and the 4-year follow-up results are excellent and similar to those seen in patients without previous surgical commissurotomy.

PATIENTS WITH ATRIAL FIBRILLATION

It has been reported that the presence of atrial fibrillation is associated with inferior immediate and long-term outcome after PMV as reflected in a smaller post-PMV MVA and a lower event-free survival rate (freedom of death, redo-PMV, and mitral valve surgery) at a median follow-up time of 61 months (32% vs. 61%; p < 0.0001).[41] Analysis of preprocedural and procedural characteristics revealed that this association is most likely explained by the presence of multiple factors in the atrial fibrillation group that adversely affect the immediate and long-term outcome of PMV. Patients in atrial fibrillation are older and more often were rated at NYHA class IV, had an echocardiographic score of greater than 8, showed evidence of calcified valves under fluoroscopy, and had a history of previous surgical commissurotomy. In the group of patients in atrial fibrillation, severe post-PMV MR (≥3+; p = 0.0001), echocardiographic score greater than 8 (p = 0.004), and pre-PMV NYHA class IV (p = 0.046) were identified as independent predictors of combined events at follow-up study. The presence of atrial fibrillation per se should not be the only determinant in the decision process regarding treatment options in a patient with rheumatic mitral stenosis. The presence of an echocardiographic score of 8 or less primarily identifies a subgroup of patients in atrial fibrillation in whom percutaneous balloon valvotomy is very likely to be successful and provide good long-term results. Therefore in this group of patients, PMV should be the procedure of choice.

PATIENTS WITH PULMONARY ARTERY HYPERTENSION

The degree of pulmonary artery hypertension before PMV is inversely related to the immediate and long-term outcome of PMV. Chen et al.[46] divided 564 patients undergoing PMV at MGH into three groups on the basis of the pulmonary vascular resistance (PVR) obtained at cardiac catheterization immediately before PMV: group I had a PVR less than or equal to 250 dyne · sec/cm^{-5} (normal/mildly elevated resistance) and comprised 332 patients (59%); group II had a PVR between 251 and 400 dyne · sec/cm^{-5} (moderately elevated resistance) and comprised 110 patients (19.5%); group III had a PVR greater than or equal to 400 dyne · sec/cm^{-5} and comprised of 122 patients (21.5%). Patients in Group I and II were younger, had less severe heart failure symptoms measured by NYHA class and a lower incidence of echocardiographic scores higher than 8, atrial fibrillation, and calcium noted on fluoroscopy than patients in group III. Before and after PMV, patients with higher PVR had a smaller MVA, lower cardiac output, and higher mean pulmonary artery pressure. For Group I, II, and III patients, the immediate success rates for PMV were 68%, 56%, and 45%, respectively. Therefore patients in the group with severely elevated pulmonary artery resistance before the procedure had lower immediate success rates of PMV. At long-term follow-up study, patients with severely elevated pulmonary vascular resistance had significantly lower rates of survival and event-free survival (survival with freedom from mitral valve surgery or NYHA Class III or IV heart failure).

PATIENTS WITH TRICUSPID REGURGITATION

The degree of tricuspid regurgitation before PMV is inversely related to the immediate and long-term outcome of PMV. Sagie et al.[47] divided patients undergoing PMV at MGH into three groups on the basis of the degree of tricuspid regurgitation determined by 2D and color-flow Doppler echocardiography before PMV. Patients with severe tricuspid regurgitation before PMV were older, had more severe heart failure symptoms measured by NYHA class, and a higher incidence of echocardiographic scores greater than 8, atrial fibrillation, and calcified mitral valves on fluoroscopy than patients with mild or moderate tricuspid regurgitation. Patients with severe tricuspid regurgitation had a smaller MVAs before and after PMV than the patients with mild or moderate tricuspid regurgitation. At long-term follow-up study, patients with severe tricuspid regurgitation had significant lower rates of survival and event-free survival (survival with freedom from mitral valve surgery or NYHA Class III or IV heart failure). The degree of tricuspid regurgitation can be diminished when the transmitral pressure gradient is sufficiently relieved with PMV.[61]

THE BEST PATIENTS FOR PMV

In patients identified as optimal candidates for PMV, this technique results in excellent immediate and long-term outcomes. Optimal candidates for PMV are those patients meeting the following characteristics: (1) age 45 years old or younger; (2) normal sinus rhythm; (3) echocardiographic score less than or equal to 8; (4) no history of previous surgical commissurotomy; and (5) pre-PMV MR less than or equal to 1+ Sellers grade. From 879 consecutive patients undergoing percutaneous mitral balloon valvuloplasty (PMV) 136 patients with optimal preprocedure characteristics were identified. In these patients PMV results in an 81% success rate and a 3.4% incidence of major in-hospital combined events (death and/or MVR). In these patients, PMV results in a 95% survival and 61% event-free survival at a 12-year follow-up study.[4]

THE DOUBLE BALLOON VS. THE INOUE BALLOON TECHNIQUES

Today the Inoue approach of PMV is the technique more widely used. There was controversy as to whether the double balloon or the Inoue technique provided superior immediate and long-term results. The authors compared the immediate procedural and the long-term clinical outcomes after PMV using the double balloon technique (n = 659) and Inoue technique (n = 233).[48] There were no statistically significant differences in baseline clinical and morphologic characteristics between patients undergoing either the double balloon or Inoue procedure. Although the post-PMV MVA was larger with the double-balloon technique (1.94 ± 0.72 vs. 1.81 ± 0.58; p = 0.01), the success rate (71.3% vs. 69.1%; p = NS), incidence of 3+ or greater MR (9% vs 9%), in-hospital complications, and long-term and event-free survival rates were similar with both techniques. In conclusion, both the Inoue and the double-balloon techniques are equally effective techniques of PMV, and the procedure of choice should be performed based on the interventionist's experience in the technique.

ECHOCARDIOGRAPHIC AND HEMODYNAMIC FOLLOW-UP STUDY

Follow-up studies have shown that the incidence of hemodynamic and echocardiographic restenosis is low after PMV.[4,30,49] A study of patients undergoing simultaneous clinical evaluation, 2D-Doppler echocardiography, and transseptal catheterization 2 years after PMV found 90% of patients to be in NYHA classes I and II.[48] Although a discrepancy between hemodynamic and echocardiographic MVA is often observed immediately after PMV because of the contribution of left-to-right shunting (undetected by oximetry) across the created interatrial communication,[50] Desideri et al. showed no significant differences in MVA (measured by Doppler echocardiography) at 19 ± 6 (range 9 to 33) months' follow-up examination between the post-PMV and follow-up MVAs.[45] Echocardiographic restenosis (MVA ≤ 1.5 cm^2 with >50% reduction of the gain) was estimated to occur in 39% of patients at 7 years after the Inoue technique. A mitral area loss of 0.3 cm^2 or more was seen in 12%, 22%, and 27% of patients at 3, 5, and 7 years, respectively.

Predictors of restenosis included a post-MVA less than 1.8 cm^2 and an echo score higher than 8.[45]

PERCUTANEOUS MITRAL BALLOON COMMISSUROTOMY VS. SURGICAL MITRAL COMMISSUROTOMY

Restenosis after both closed and open surgical mitral commissurotomy has been well documented.[52-56] Although surgical closed mitral commissurotomy is uncommonly performed in the United States, it is still used often in other countries. Long-term follow-up study of 267 patients who underwent surgical transventricular mitral commissurotomy at the Mayo Clinic showed 79%, 67%, and 55% survival rates at 10, 15, and 20 years, respectively. Survival with freedom from mitral valve replacement were 57%, 36%, and 24%, respectively.[56] Age, atrial fibrillation, and male gender were independent predictors of death, whereas mitral valve calcification, cardiomegaly, and MR were independent predictors of repeat mitral valve surgery.

Interpretation of long-term clinical follow-up study of patients undergoing percutaneous mitral balloon valvuloplasty as well as their comparison with surgical commissurotomy series are confounded by heterogeneity in the patient's population. Most surgical series have included a younger population with optimal mitral valve morphology. Differences in age and valve morphology may also account for the lower and event-free survival rates of PMV series from United States and Europe.[26]

Several studies have compared the immediate and early follow-up results of PMV versus closed surgical commissurotomy in patients with optimal valve morphology. The results of these studies have been controversial, showing either superior outcome from PMV or no significant differences between both techniques.[20-25] Patel et al.[20] randomized 45 patients with mitral stenosis to closed surgical commissurotomy or PMV. They demonstrated a larger increase in MVA with PMV than with surgery (2.1 ± 0.7 cm^2 vs. 1.3 ± 0.3 cm^2). Shrivastava et al.[21] compared the results of single balloon PMV, double balloon PMV, and closed surgical commissurotomy in three groups of 20 patients each. The MVA after intervention was larger for the double balloon technique of PMV. Postintervention valve areas were 1.9 ± 0.8, 1.5 ± 0.4 and 1.5 ± 0.5 for the double balloon, the single balloon, and the closed surgical commissurotomy techniques, respectively. On the other hand, several randomized studies have found similar postintervention MVAs.[21-25] Arora and colleagues also reported identical event-free survival at a mean follow-up period of 22 ± 6 months.[22] Ben Farhat et al.[25] reported the results of a randomized trial designed to compare the immediate and long-term results of double balloon PMV versus those of open and closed surgical mitral commissurotomy. Their results demonstrate that the immediate and long-term results of PMV are comparable to those of open mitral commissurotomy and superior to those of closed commissurotomy. Since open commissurotomy is associated with a thoracotomy, need for cardiopulmonary bypass, higher cost, longer length of hospital stay, and a longer period of convalescence, PMV should be the procedure of choice for the treatment of patients with rheumatic mitral stenosis who are, from the clinical and morphological point of view, optimal candidates for PMV.[28]

PERCUTANEOUS MITRAL BALLOON COMMISSUROTOMY IN PREGNANT WOMEN

Surgical mitral commissurotomy has been performed in pregnant women with severe mitral stenosis. Because the risk of anesthesia and surgery for the mother and the fetus are increased, this operation is reserved for those patients with incapacitating symptoms refractory to medical therapy.[57-59] Under this condition PMV can be performed safely after the twentieth week of pregnancy with minimal radiation to the fetus. Because of the definite risk in women with severe mitral stenosis of developing symptoms during pregnancy, PMV should be considered when the patient is considering becoming pregnant.

DIFFERENCE IN OUTCOME AMONG WOMEN AND MEN AFTER PERCUTANEOUS MITRAL VALVULOPLASTY

The authors evaluated measures of procedural success and clinical outcome in 1015 consecutive patients (839 women and 176 men) who underwent PMV. Despite a lower baseline echocardiographic score (7.47 ± 2.15 vs. 8.02 ± 2.18, p = 0.002), women were less likely to achieve PMV success (69% vs. 83%, adjusted OR 0.44; 95% CI 0.27 to 0.74; p = 0.002), and had a smaller postprocedural MV area (1.86 ± 0.7 vs. 2.07 ± 0.7 cm^2, p < 0.001). Overall procedural and in-hospital complication rates did not differ significantly between women and men. However, women were significantly more likely to develop severe MR immediately after PMV (adjusted OR 2.41; 95% CI 1.0 to 5.83; p = 0.05) or to undergo MV surgery (adjusted HR 1.54; 95% CI 1.03 to 2.3; p = 0.037) after a median follow-up of 3.1 years. Thus compared to men, women with rheumatic mitral stenosis who undergo PMV are less likely to have a successful outcome and more likely to require MV surgery on long-term follow-up despite more favorable baseline mitral valve anatomy.[60]

9.6 Summary

PMV should be the procedure of choice for the treatment of patients with rheumatic mitral stenosis who are, from the clinical and morphological points of view, optimal candidates for PMV.[62] Patients with echocardiographic scores of 8 or lower have the best results, particularly if they are young, are in sinus rhythm, have no pulmonary hypertension, and show no evidence of calcification of the mitral valve under fluoroscopy. The immediate and long-term results of PMV in this group of patients are similar to those reported after surgical mitral commissurotomy. Patients with echocardiographic scores higher than 8 have only a 50% chance to obtain a successful

hemodynamic result with PMV, and long-term follow-up results are not as good as those from patients with echocardiographic scores less than or equal to 8. In patients with echocardiographic scores of 12 or higher, it is unlikely that PMV could produce good immediate or long-term results. They preferably should undergo open heart surgery. PMV could be performed in these patients if they are not high-risk candidates for surgery. Finally, much remains to be done in refining indications for patients with few or no symptoms and those with unfavorable anatomy. However, surgical therapy for mitral stenosis should actually be reserved for patients who have Sellers' grades of 2 or higher for MR by angiography, which can be better treated by mitral valve repair, and for those patients with severe mitral valve thickening and calcification or with significant subvalvular scarring to warrant valve replacement.

9.7 Percutaneous Tricuspid Balloon Valvuloplasty

Tricuspid stenosis is an uncommon valvular abnormality that most commonly occurs in association with other valvular lesions.[62] For many years, surgical commissurotomy and valvuloplasty were the only available methods to correct tricuspid stenosis.[63,64] The development of percutaneous balloon valvuloplasty techniques has revolutionized the management of mitral stenosis.[61,65,66] Similar techniques can be used to treat tricuspid stenosis.[61,66-74] Tricuspid stenosis is most commonly of rheumatic etiology; the majority of cases present with tricuspid regurgitation or a combination of regurgitation and stenosis. Other causes of flow obstruction at the level of the tricuspid valve include: (1) congenital atresia or stenosis of the valve; (2) right atrial or metastatic tumors; (3) the carcinoid syndrome, which may cause stenosis, although tricuspid regurgitation is more common; and (4) bacterial endocarditis, particularly in association with a permanent pacemaker lead or a prosthetic valve.[62,70,75-77]

Echocardiographic features of tricuspid stenosis include limited mobility of the leaflets, reduced separation of the leaflet tips, a reduction in the diameter of the tricuspid annulus, and diastolic doming of the valve.[62] Although leaflet thickening is seen, the degree of thickening and calcification is generally less pronounced than in rheumatic mitral stenosis. Doppler echocardiography reveals high velocity turbulent diastolic flow across the stenotic orifice and prolonged pressure half-time. A tricuspid valve area less than 1.0 cm^2 indicates severe tricuspid stenosis. It is important to assess the presence and severity of tricuspid regurgitation because this can influence the decision to proceed with balloon valvuloplasty.[62]

Patients with signs and symptoms of systemic venous hypertension and congestion should be considered for balloon valvuloplasty. Transvalvular pressure gradients as low as 3 mmHg and valve areas less than 1.5 cm^2 can indicate serious, but treatable, stenosis. Tricuspid regurgitation that is greater than mild is generally thought to be a contraindication to valvuloplasty, but a few patients with moderate regurgitation have been successfully treated with this technique. Tumor masses, vegetations, and thrombi are contraindications to valvuloplasty.[62,70,73,74,78]

There is far less experience with tricuspid valvuloplasty than with mitral valvuloplasty. Valve areas generally increase from less than 1 to almost 2 cm². Although some stenosis persists, this change in area is sufficient to produce a significant reduction in the transvalvular pressure gradient and a decrease in right atrial pressure.[66,73,74]

Percutaneous balloon tricuspid valvuloplasty for tricuspid stenosis seems to be effective and associated with a low morbidity. Thus if symptoms of systemic venous hypertension and congestion are not adequately controlled with diuretics and angiotensin-converting enzyme (ACE) inhibitors or angiotensin receptor antagonists, balloon valvuloplasty of the stenotic tricuspid valve should be performed.[73,74] Surgical correction of the stenotic lesion should be reserved for those patients whose valve is not treatable with balloon techniques.[62]

9.8 Technique of Percutaneous Mitral Valvuloplasty

GENERAL CONSIDERATIONS

- PMV is usually performed on fasting patients with mild to moderate levels of conscious sedation.
- It is guided by the use of intraprocedural transthoracic echocardiography to assess the baseline valve characteristics and the degree of MR after each balloon inflation.
- It is the authors' practice to obtain a transesophageal echocardiogram within 24 hours of the proposed PMV to confirm the pre-PMV Wilkins valve score, quantify the baseline degree of MR, and primarily to rule out the presence of intracardiac thrombus, in particular left atrial appendage thrombus.
- If left atrial appendage thrombus is present, the authors generally anticoagulate patients with strict supervision of their INR for 4 to 8 weeks before reattempting PMV.
- Antibiotic prophylaxis is given before obtaining access, with a 1 to 2 g dose of cephazolin administered IV. In patients with a penicillin allergy, 1g vancomycin IV is administered over 1 hour.
- All patients carefully chosen to undergo mitral balloon valvuloplasty should undergo diagnostic right and transseptal left heart catheterization.
- The authors typically obtain 5F right femoral arterial access, 8F right femoral venous access for transseptal sheath placement, and a further 7F femoral venous access for right heart catheterization, which can be placed in either groin.
- Transseptal catheterization, which allows access to the left atrium, is the first step of the PMV procedure and one of the most crucial steps.

- After transseptal left heart catheterization, systemic anticoagulation is achieved by the IV administration of 100 units/kg of heparin.
- In patients older than 40 years, coronary arteriography should also be performed.
- Hemodynamic measurements, cardiac output, and cine left ventriculography are performed before and after PMV.
- Cardiac output is measured by thermodilution and Fick method techniques. Mitral valve calcification and angiographic severity of MR (Sellers' classification) are graded qualitatively from 0 to 4. An oxygen diagnostic run is performed before and after PMV to determine the presence of left-to-right shunt after PMV.

TRANSSEPTAL PUNCTURE TECHNIQUE

- Transseptal catheterization is performed using the percutaneous technique only from the right femoral vein.
- However, it is technically possible to perform transseptal access from the right jugular, right subclavian, or left femoral vein, albeit with higher degrees of technical difficulty and procedural complications.
- Biplane fluoroscopy, if available, is the ideal imaging system. However, a single plane C-arm fluoroscope, which can be rotated from the anteroposterior to lateral position, may also be used.
- The authors use an 8F Mullins sheath and dilator (Medtronic, Minneapolis, Minn., and Cook Medical, Bloomington, Ind.) and a standard Brockenbrough needle and stylet (Cook Medical, Bloomington, Ind.) to perform transseptal puncture.
- Before attempted puncture of the interatrial septum, full familiarity with the transseptal apparatus (Mullins sheath and dilator, Brockenbrough needle and stylet) is essential.
- The Mullins transseptal introducer is composed of a 59-cm sheath and a 67-cm dilator. The distance the dilator protrudes from the sheath should be noted before the procedure **(Figure 9–7, A)**.
- The Brockenbrough needle is 71 cm in length. The flange of the needle has an arrow that points to the position of the tip of the needle **(see Figure 9–7, B)**. Before use, the operator should be sure that the needle is straight and that the arrow of the flange is perfectly aligned with the needle tip.
- This arrow will allow the operator to know exactly where the distal tip of the needle is pointing. When the needle tip lies just within the dilator there is approximately 1.5 to 2 cm distance between the dilator hub and the needle flange. This measurement also should be noted.
- Via the preexisting 8F venous access, a standard J-tipped 0.035-inch guidewire is advanced from the femoral vein through the inferior vena cava and right atrium into the superior vena cava and placed at the junction of the superior vena cava and the left innominate vein.

• A 5F straight pigtail catheter is advanced into the aortic root and placed into the right coronary sinus. This catheter should be connected to continuous arterial monitoring and flushed every 3 minutes with heparinized saline to prevent thrombosis and embolic complications.
• Under fluoroscopic guidance, the Mullins sheath and dilator are advanced over the J-wire into the superior

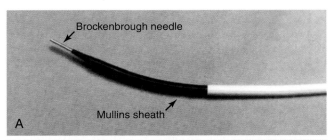

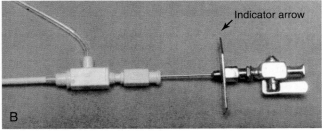

Figure 9–7 **Mullins sheath with Brockenbrough needle. A,** The tip of a Mullins sheath is shown with the dilator and Brockenbrough needle protruding through it. The relationship of the three is important to note before use. **B,** The indicator arrow on the Brockenbrough needle points in the direction of the curve on the distal end of the needle. This arrow allows the operator to know the direction in which the needle is pointing and allows for accurate rotation of the needle during transseptal puncture.

vena cava/left innominate vein junction. The sheath must never be advanced without the wire, because the stiff dilator can readily perforate the inferior vena cava, superior vena cava, or right atrium. Once the Mullins sheath is properly placed, the wire is removed. The sheath is allowed to bleed back and then flushed with heparinized saline to prevent clot formation.
• The Brockenbrough needle is then advanced to lie just inside the dilator, using the predetermined distance between the needle flange and dilator as a guide. When advancing the needle to this position, it must rotate freely within the dilator and not be forcibly turned to prevent damage to the needle tip or dilator. Occasionally there is some resistance as the transseptal needle is advanced through the iliac vein or the inferior vena cava, particularly at the pelvic brim. Under this circumstance the needle should not be forcibly advanced; instead the needle with its stylet inside and the Mullins sheath should be advanced as a unit through the areas of resistance.
• The Brockenbrough needle stylet is then removed, and the needle is allowed to bleed back again before being flushed with heparinized saline and connected to a pressure recording line. At this point, the authors display a single pressure tracing on 40 to 50 mmHg scale only, demonstrating pressure at the needle tip in order to avoid confusion.
• At this point, proper orientation of the assembly is critical. The side arm of the sheath and needle flange should always have the same orientation. Initially, they point horizontally and to the patient's left. This directs the tip of the apparatus medially in the anteroposterior fluoroscopic view **(Figure 9–8, A).** The entire system is then rotated clockwise until

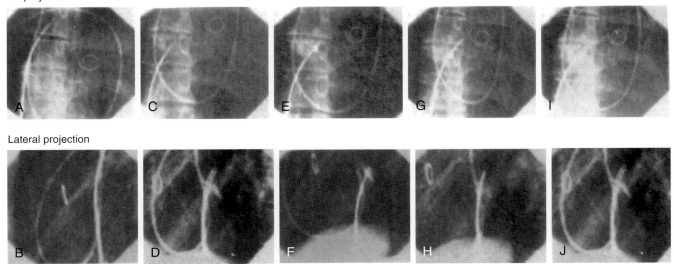

Figure 9–8 Fluoroscopic images depicting steps of transseptal puncture in the anteroposterior *(AP)* and lateral fluoroscopic projections. A Swan-Ganz catheter is in place throughout the procedure. A pigtail catheter is seen in the right aortic cusp throughout the series of images. The transseptal catheter system is withdrawn across three sequential landmark "bumps." On a lateral view, the correct position for puncture of the apparatus is posterior and inferior to the aorta (marked by the pigtail catheter), usually midway between an imaginary line from the pigtail tip to the right border of the spine. Contrast can be injected with the needle against or within the septum to confirm its position ("tattooing the septum") as shown here. *(Reproduced with permission from Roelke M, Smith AJ, Palacios IF. The technique and safety of transseptal left heart catheterization: the Massachusetts General Hospital experience with 1279 procedures. Catheter Cardiovasc Diagn 1994;32[4]:332-9.)*

the needle flange arrow and sheath side arm are positioned at 4 o'clock (with the patient's forehead representing 12 o'clock and the patient's occipital 6 o'clock). This directs the assembly to the left and slightly posterior.

- Under anteroposterior fluoroscopy, the entire system is then withdrawn across three sequential landmark "bumps," or leftward movements of the needle **(see Figure 9–8, A, C, and D)**. These landmark bumps represent movement of the apparatus: (1) as it enters the right atrium/superior vena cava junction, (2) as it moves over the ascending aorta where the tactile sensation of aortic pulsations aids in localization, and (3) as it passes over the limbus to intrude into the fossa ovalis. On a lateral view, the correct position for puncture of the apparatus is posterior and inferior to the aorta (marked by the pigtail catheter), usually midway between an imaginary line from the pigtail tip to the right border of the spine **(see Figure 9–8, F)**.[79]

- The system is advanced (needle within the dilator) until further movement is limited by the limbus. In approximately 10% of cases, the foramen ovale is patent and the apparatus directly enters the left atrium. In the remainder, the tip of the Brockenbrough needle is advanced into the left atrium under continuous fluoroscopic and pressure monitoring.

- Successful penetration of the septum is confirmed by a change in the pressure tracing from right atrial to left atrial pressure morphology. Furthermore, successful left atrial access can be confirmed by sampling a direct left atrial saturation.

- If the pressure tracing is damped, injection of contrast will aid in localizing the puncture site. If there is staining of the interatrial septum, the needle must be advanced further **(see Figure 9–8, E and F)**. A stained septum may indeed be used as a guide for future attempts.

- At this point after successful interatrial puncture, the entire system is rotated counterclockwise to 3 o'clock and carefully advanced under fluoroscopic and hemodynamic guidance until it is certain the dilator lies within the left atrium **(see Figure 9–8, G and H)**. The needle is withdrawn into the dilator.

- The sheath is then advanced into the left atrium, keeping the needle within the sheath to avoid puncturing the left atrium **(see Figure 9–8, I and J)**. The needle and dilator are then removed, and the sheath is double flushed before it is connected to pressure tubing. If the sheath has entered an inferior pulmonary vein, it must be withdrawn slightly with counterclockwise rotation to position it in the left atrium.

- Care should be taken after entering the left atrium with the needle. Perforation of the left atrial wall could occur if the system is advanced without careful pressure and fluoroscopic monitoring. If the left atrial pressure becomes damped, the apparatus may be against the left atrial wall and further advancement of the system could result in perforation and tamponade.

- Immediately after completion of transseptal left heart catheterization, 5000 units of IV heparin is administered.

INOUE TECHNIQUE OF ANTEGRADE BALLOON MITRAL VALVULOPLASTY

- The Inoue balloon is a 12F shaft, coaxial, double-lumen catheter. The balloon is made of a double layer of rubber tubing with a layer of synthetic micromesh in between. It is essential that the operator is experienced with the preparation and selection of an appropriately-sized Inoue balloon catheter.

- After transseptal catheterization, a stainless steel guidewire is advanced through the transseptal catheter and placed with its tip coiled into the left atrium and the transseptal catheter is removed **(Figure 9–9).**

- A 14F dilator is advanced over the guidewire and used to dilate the skin tract, femoral vein, and atrial septum **(see Figure 9–9)**. The authors typically perform two passes of the dilator across the septum with rotation in addition to forward traction on the dilator to ensure adequate dilation.

- A balloon catheter is chosen according to the patient's height, using a simple calculation of the patient's height in centimeters divided by 10, plus 10. For example, a 180-cm patient would have an optimal balloon diameter of 180/10 + 10, or 28 mm. Typically, the authors start at 2 mm below the optimal balloon size and increase with 1cc of extra saline/contrast mix until the optimal balloon size is reached or an increase of more than 1+ MR is achieved on echocardiography.

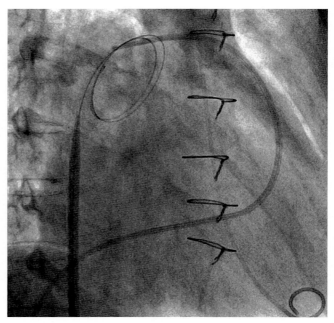

Figure 9–9 Fluoroscopic image demonstrating an Inoue wire coiled in the left atrium. A 14F dilator is advanced over the wire in order to dilate the skin tract, the femoral venous access site, and the intraatrial septum.

- After selecting the correct balloon, the central metal lumen is flushed with heparinized saline and the metal dilator is flushed with heparinized saline. Next, the vent port on the balloon catheter is flushed with a 70:30 saline/contrast mix until no further air is expelled from the balloon port. At this point, the stopcock on the vent port is closed and the balloon inflation syringe, containing the predetermined inflation column of saline/contrast mix, is attached. The balloon is then inflated under saline twice to ensure any residual air is expelled, and finally the maximum inflated balloon waist diameter is measured to confirm it is adequate. At this point, the balloon is deflated.
- The central metal dilator is advanced through the balloon catheter and locked in place. The metal shaft of the balloon catheter is then advanced forward into the plastic balloon catheter hub and locked in place. (Hence, the saying "metal to metal, metal to plastic.") The catheter is now ready for insertion into the body.
- The balloon catheter is then advanced over the stiffened guidewire into the right atrium until its tip engages the septum.
- With a single forward motion, the balloon tip is used to stab the septum. At this point, with the distal tip across the septum the rigid metal dilator is withdrawn, the metal-to-plastic lock is undone, and the balloon is allowed to advance into the left atrium over the central metal lumen, which acts as a railroad.
- The distal part of the balloon is inflated and advanced into the left ventricle with the help of a spring-wire stylet, which has been inserted through the inner lumen of the catheter.
- After insertion of the stylet the catheter is advanced toward the mitral valve plane and, by using counterclockwise rotation of the stylet and gentle backward traction on the catheter, facilitates entry into the left ventricle **(Video 9–5).**
- Occasionally and particularly in patients with a large left atrium or suboptimal transseptal puncture site, the previous maneuver does not allow entry into the left ventricle.
- In this circumstance, the authors rotate the stylet clockwise, allowing the catheter to initially rotate posteriorly in front of the pulmonary veins and then by advancing further the partially inflated balloon to the mitral plane; gentle movements of the stylet back and forth allow the balloon to enter the left ventricle.
- Once the catheter is in the left ventricle, the partially inflated balloon is moved back and forth inside the left ventricle to assure that it is free of the chordae tendineae **(see Figure 9–9, B).**
- The catheter is then gently pulled against the mitral plane until resistance is felt. The balloon is then rapidly inflated to its full capacity and then deflated quickly. During inflation of the balloon an indentation should be seen in its midportion **(see Video 9–2).**

- The catheter is withdrawn into the left atrium, and the mitral gradient and cardiac output are measured. If further dilations are required, the stylet is introduced again and the sequence of steps is repeated at a larger balloon volume.
- The criteria for stopping the procedure are complete opening of at least one of the commissures with a valve area greater than 1 cm²/m² body surface area or greater than 1.5 cm², or the appearance of regurgitation or its increase by 25%.
- To remove the balloon catheter, the balloon is deflated, the central dilator is readvanced partially, and the Inoue guidewire is readvanced such that the floppy tip of the guidewire is within the left atrium. The catheter is withdrawn back to rest against the septum.
- The central plastic portion of the balloon catheter is withdrawn back to meet the central metal lumen and locked in place. The central metal lumen is then withdrawn back to lock with the central dilator. The guidewire is then withdrawn into the right atrium, and the balloon catheter is removed and a 12F or 14F sheath is placed into the femoral vein.

DOUBLE BALLOON ANTEGRADE PERCUTANEOUS MITRAL BALLOON COMMISSUROTOMY TECHNIQUE

- This technique involves placing two balloons across the mitral valve from either a single femoral venous access and transseptal puncture or from two separate femoral venous punctures and atrial septal punctures.
- A 7F flow-directed balloon catheter is advanced through the transseptal sheath across the mitral valve into the left ventricle.
- The catheter is then advanced through the aortic valve into the ascending and then the descending aorta. A 0.035- or 0.038-inch, 260-cm long Teflon-coated exchange wire is then passed through the catheter. The sheath and the catheter are removed, leaving the wire behind.
- A 5-mm balloon dilating catheter is used to dilate the atrial septum. A second exchange guidewire is passed parallel to the first guidewire through the same femoral vein and atrial septum punctures using a double lumen catheter. The double lumen catheter is then removed, leaving the two guidewires across the mitral valve in the ascending and descending aorta.
- During these maneuvers, care should be taken to maintain large and smooth loops of the guidewires in the left ventricular cavity to allow appropriate placement of the dilating balloons.
- Two balloon dilating catheters, chosen according to the patient's body surface area **(see Table 9–5),** are then advanced over each one of the guidewires and positioned across the mitral valve, parallel to the longitudinal axis of the left ventricle.
- The balloon valvuloplasty catheters are then inflated by hand until the indentation produced by the stenotic mitral valve is no longer seen.

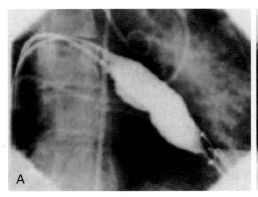
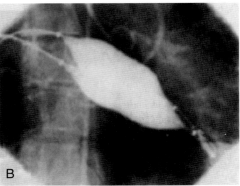

Figure 9–10 Fluoroscopic images in the anteroposterior projection demonstrating the double balloon technique of percutaneous tricuspid valvuloplasty. Images depict early **(A)** and late **(B)** stages of balloon inflation with disappearance of the "waste" after full balloon inflation. *(Reproduced with permission from Konugres GS, Lau FY, Ruiz CE. Successful percutaneous double-balloon mitral, aortic, and tricuspid valvotomy in rheumatic trivalvular stenosis. Am Heart J1990;119(3 Pt 1):663-6.)*

- Generally one, but occasionally two or three, inflations are performed. After complete deflation, the balloons are removed sequentially.
- The double balloon technique of PMV is effective but demanding and carries the risk of left ventricular perforation by the guidewires or the tip of the balloons.

9.9 Technique of Percutaneous Tricuspid Valvuloplasty

DOUBLE BALLOON PERCUTANEOUS TRICUSPID VALVULOPLASTY TECHNIQUE

- This technique involves placing two balloons across the tricuspid valve from a single femoral venous access, although bilateral access can be used as well.
- A 7F flow-directed balloon catheter is advanced through the right heart to the pulmonary artery.
- A 0.035- or 0.038-inch, 260-cm long Teflon-coated exchange wire, the tip of which has been formed into a curve, is then passed through the catheter. The sheath and the catheter are removed, leaving the wires behind. The wires can be left in the pulmonary artery or the apex of the right ventricle.
- A second exchange guidewire is passed parallel to the first guidewire through the same femoral vein using a double lumen catheter. The double lumen catheter is then removed, leaving the two guidewires across the tricuspid valve. Alternatively, a second balloon catheter can be advanced from the contralateral femoral vein to the pulmonary artery and the second guidewire placed.
- Two balloon dilating catheters, chosen in order to obtain an EBDA/BSA ratio between 3.41 ± 0.2 and 4.51 ± 0.2 cm²/m², as with PMV **(see Table 9–2).**
- The balloon valvuloplasty catheters are then inflated by hand until the indentation produced by the stenotic tricuspid valve is no longer seen **(Figure 9–10).**[80]
- Generally one inflation is performed. After complete deflation, the balloons are removed sequentially.

REFERENCES

1. Williams JA, Littmann D, Warren R: Experience with the surgical treatment of mitral stenosis, N Engl J Med 258:623–630, 1958.
2. Scannell JG, Burke JF, Saidi F, et al: Five-year follow-up study of closed mitral valvotomy, J Thorac Cardiovasc Surg 40:723–730, 1960.
3. Inoue K, Owaki T, Nakamura T, et al: Clinical application of transvenous mitral commissurotomy by a new balloon catheter, J Thorac Cardiovasc Surg 87:394–402, 1984.
4. Palacios IF, Sanchez PL, Harrell LC, et al: Which patients benefit from percutaneous mitral balloon valvuloplasty? Prevalvuloplasty and postvalvuloplasty variables that predict long-term outcome, Circulation 105:1465–1471, 2002.
5. Lock JE, Kalilullah M, Shrivastava S, et al: Percutaneous catheter commissurotomy in rheumatic mitral stenosis, N Engl J Med 313:1515–1518, 1985.
6. Al Zaibag M, Ribeiro PA, Al Kassab SA, et al: Percutaneous double balloon mitral valvotomy for rheumatic mitral stenosis, Lancet 1:757–761, 1986.
7. Palacios I, Block PC, Brandi S, et al: Percutaneous balloon valvotomy for patients with severe mitral stenosis, Circulation 75:778–784, 1987.
8. Mc Kay CR, Kawanishi DT, Rahimtoola SH: Catheter balloon valvuloplasty of the mitral valve in adults using a double balloon technique: early hemodynamic results, JAMA 257:1753–1761, 1987.
9. Cohen DJ, Kuntz RE, Gordon SPF, et al: Predictors of long-term outcome after percutaneous mitral valvuloplasty, N Engl J Med 327:1329–1335, 1991.
10. Arora R, Kalra GS, Murty GS, et al: Percutaneous transatrial mitral commissurotomy: immediate and intermediate results, J Am Coll Cardiol 23:1327–1332, 1994.
11. Chen CR, Cheng TO: Percutaneous balloon mitral valvuloplasty by the Inoue technique: a multicenter study of 4832 patients in China, Am Heart J 129:1197–1203, 1995.
12. Dean LS, Mickel M, Bonan R, et al: Four-year follow-up of patients undergoing percutaneous balloon mitral commissurotomy: a report from the National Heart, Lung, and Blood Institute Balloon Valvuloplasty Registry, J Am Coll Cardiol 28:1452–1457, 1996.
13. Orrange SE, Kawanishi DT, Lopez BM, et al: Actuarial outcome after catheter balloon commissurotomy in patients with mitral stenosis, Circulation 97:245–250, 1997.
14. Chen CR, Cheng TO, Chen JY, et al: Long-term results of percutaneous balloon mitral valvuloplasty for mitral stenosis: a follow-up study to 11 years in 202 patients, Catheter Cardiovasc Diagn 43:132–139, 1998.
15. Stefanadis CI, Stratos CG, Lambrou SG, et al: Retrograde nontransseptal balloon mitral valvuloplasty: immediate results and intermediate long-term outcome in 441 cases—a multicenter experience, J Am Coll Cardiol 32:1009–1016, 1998.
16. Cribier A, Eltchaninoff H, Koning R, et al: Percutaneous mechanical mitral commissurotomy with a newly designed metallic valvulotome: immediate results of the initial experience in 153 patients, Circulation 99:793–799, 1999.
17. Hernandez R, Banuelos C, Alfonso F, et al: Long-term clinical and echocardiographic follow-up after percutaneous mitral valvuloplasty with the Inoue balloon, Circulation 99:1580–1586, 1999.

18. Iung B, Garbarz E, Michaud P, et al: Late results of percutaneous mitral commissurotomy in a series of 1024 patients: analysis of late clinical deterioration: frequency, anatomic findings and predictive factors, *Circulation* 99:3272–3278, 1999.
19. Cribier A, Eltchaninoff H, Carlot R, et al: Percutaneous mechanical mitral commissurotomy with the metallic valvulotome: detailed technical aspects and overview of the results of the multicenter registry in 882 patients, *J Interv Cardiol* 13:255–262, 2000.
20. Patel JJ, Shama D, Mitha AS, et al: Balloon valvuloplasty versus closed commissurotomy for pliable mitral stenosis: a prospective hemodynamic study, *J Am Coll Cardiol* 18:1318–1322, 1991.
21. Shrivastava S, Mathur A, Dev V, et al: A comparison of immediate hemodynamic response of closed mitral commissurotomy, single-balloon, and double-balloon mitral valvuloplasty in rheumatic mitral stenosis, *J Thorac Cardiovasc Surg* 104:1264–1267, 1992.
22. Arora R, Nair M, Kalra GS, et al: Immediate and long-term results of balloon and surgical closed mitral valvotomy: a randomized comparative study, *Am Heart J* 125:1091–1094, 1993.
23. Turi ZG, Reyes VP, Raju BS, et al: Percutaneous balloon versus surgical closed commissurotomy for mitral stenosis: a prospective, randomized trial, *Circulation* 83:1179–1185, 1991.
24. Reyes VP, Raju BS, Wynne J, et al: Percutaneous balloon valvuloplasty compared with open surgical commissurotomy for mitral stenosis, *N Engl J Med* 331:961–967, 1994.
25. Ben Farhat M, Ayari M, Maatouk F, et al: Percutaneous balloon versus surgical closed and open mitral commissurotomy: seven-year follow-up results of a randomized trial, *Circulation* 97:245–250, 1998.
26. Vahanian A, Palacios IF: Percutaneous approaches to valvular disease, *Circulation* 109:1572–1579, 2004.
27. Wilkins GT, Weyman AE, Abascal VM, et al: Percutaneous balloon dilation of the mitral valve: an analysis of echocardiographic variables related to outcome and the mechanism of dilation, *Br Heart J* 60:229–308, 1988.
28. Cruz-Gonzalez I, Sanchez-Ledesma M, Sanchez PL, et al: Predicting success and long-term outcomes of percutaneous mitral valvuloplasty; a multifactorial score, *Am J Med* 122:581–589, 2009.
29. Sellers RD, Levy MJ, Amplatz K, et al: Left retrograde cardioangiography in acquired cardiac disease, *Am J Cardiol* 14:437–447, 1964.
30. Tuzcu EM, Block PC, Griffin BP, et al: Immediate and long-term outcome of percutaneous mitral valvotomy in patients 65 years and older, *Circulation* 85:963–971, 1992.
31. Babic UU, Pejcic P, Djurisic Z, et al: Percutaneous transarterial balloon valvuloplasty for mitral valve stenosis, *Am J Cardiol* 57:1101–1104, 1986.
32. Stefanadis C, Stratos C, Pitsavos C, et al: Retrograde nontransseptal balloon mitral valvuloplasty: immediate results and long term follow-up, *Circulation* 85:1760–1767, 1992.
33. Mc Kay RG, Lock JE, Safian RD, et al: Balloon dilation of mitral stenosis in adults patients: postmortem and percutaneous mitral valvuloplasty studies, *J Am Coll Cardiol* 9:723–731, 1987.
34. Herrmann HC, Lima JA, Feldman T, et al: Mechanisms and outcome of severe mitral regurgitation after Inoue balloon valvuloplasty, *J Am Coll Cardiol* 27:783–789, 1993.
35. Padial LR, Freitas N, Sagie A, et al: Echocardiography can predict which patients will develop severe mitral regurgitation after percutaneous mitral valvulotomy, *J Am Coll Cardiol* 27:1225–1231, 1996.
36. Abascal VM, O'Shea JP, Wilkins GT, et al: Prediction of successful outcome in 130 patients undergoing percutaneous balloon mitral valvotomy, *Circulation* 82:448–456, 1990.
37. Abascal VM, Wilkins GT, Choong CY, et al: Mitral regurgitation after percutaneous mitral valvuloplasty in adults: evaluation by pulsed Doppler echocardiography, *J Am Coll Cardiol* 2:257–263, 1988.
38. Herrman HC, Wilkins GT, Abascal VM, et al: Percutaneous balloon mitral valvotomy for patients with mitral stenosis: analysis of factors influencing early results, *J Thorac Cardiovasc Surg* 96:33–38, 1988.
39. Tuzcu EM, Block PC, Griffin B, et al: Percutaneous mitral balloon valvotomy in patients with calcific mitral stenosis: immediate and long term outcome, *J Am Coll Cardiol* 23:1604–1609, 1994.
40. Jang IK, Block PC, Newell JB, et al: Percutaneous mitral balloon valvotomy for recurrent mitral stenosis after surgical commissurotomy, *Am J Cardiol* 75:601–605, 1995.
41. Sanchez PL, Rodríguez-Alemparte M, Inglessis I, et al: The impact of age in the immediate and long-term outcomes of percutaneous mitral balloon valvuloplasty, *J Invasive Cardiol* 18:217–225, 2005.
42. Leon MN, Harrell LC, Simosa HF, et al: Mitral balloon valvotomy for patients with mitral stenosis in atrial fibrillation: immediate and long-term results, *J Am Coll Cardiol* 34:1145–1152, 1999.
43. Roth RB, Block PC, Palacios IF: Predictors of increased mitral regurgitation after percutaneous mitral balloon valvotomy, *Catheter Cardiovasc Diagn* 20:17–21, 1990.
44. Casale P, Block PC, O'Shea JP, et al: Atrial septal defect after percutaneous mitral balloon valvuloplasty: immediate results and follow-up, *J Am Coll Cardiol* 15:1300–1304, 1990.
45. Desideri A, Vanderperren O, Serra A, et al: Long term (9 to 33 months) echocardiographic follow-up after successful percutaneous mitral commissurotomy, *Am J Cardiol* 69:1602–1606, 1992.
46. Chen MH, Semigran M, Schwammenthal E, et al: Impact of pulmonary resistance on short and long term outcome after percutaneous mitral valvuloplasty, *Circulation*(Suppl I):1825, 1993.
47. Sagie A, Schwammenthal E, Newell JB, et al: Significant tricuspid regurgitation is a marker for adverse outcome in patients undergoing mitral balloon valvotomy, *J Am Coll Cardiol* 24:696–702, 1994.
48. Sanchez PL, Harrell LC, Salas RE, et al: Learning curve of the Inoue technique of percutaneous mitral balloon valvuloplasty, *Am J Cardiol* 88:662–667, 2001.
49. Block PC, Palacios IF, Block EH, et al: Late (two year) follow-up after percutaneous mitral balloon valvotomy, *Am J Cardiol* 69:537–541, 1992.
50. Petrossian GA, Tuzcu EM, Ziskind AA, et al: Atrial septal occlusion improves the accuracy of mitral valve area determination following percutaneous mitral balloon valvotomy, *Catheter Cardiovasc Diagn* 22:21–24, 1991.
51. John S, Bashi VV, Jairaj PS, et al: Closed mitral valvotomy: early results and long term follow up of 3724 patients, *Circulation* 68:891–896, 1983.
52. Kirklin JW: Percutaneous balloon versus surgical closed commissurotomy for mitral stenosis, *Circulation* 83:1450–1451, 1991.
53. Higgs LM, Glancy DL, O'Brien KP, et al: Mitral restenosis: an uncommon cause of recurrent symptoms following mitral commissurotomy, *Am J Cardiol* 26:34–37, 1970.
54. Glover RP, Davila JC, O'Neil TJE, et al: Does mitral stenosis recur after commissurotomy? *Circulation* 11:14–28, 1955.
55. Hickey MSJ, Blackstone EH, Kirklin JW, et al: Outcome probabilities and life history after surgical mitral commissurotomy: implications for balloon commissurotomy, *J Am Coll Cardiol* 17:29–42, 1991.
56. Rihal CS, Schaff HV, Frye RL, et al: Long-term follow-up of patients undergoing closed transventricular mitral commissurotomy: a useful surrogate for percutaneous balloon mitral valvuloplasty, *J Am Coll Cardiol* 20:781–786, 1992.
57. Palacios IF, Block PC, Wilkins GT, et al: Percutaneous mitral balloon valvotomy during pregnancy in patients with severe mitral stenosis, *Catheter Cardiovasc Diagn* 15:109–111, 1988.
58. Mangione JA, Zuliani MF, Del Castillo JM, et al: Percutaneous double balloon mitral valvuloplasty in pregnant women, *Am J Cardiol* 64:99–102, 1989.
59. Esteves CA, Munoz JS, Braga S, et al: Immediate and long-term follow-up of percutaneous balloon mitral valvuloplasty in pregnant patients with rheumatic mitral stenosis, *Am J Cardiol* 98:812–816, 2006.
60. Cruz-Gonzalez I, Jneid H, Sanchez-Ledesma M, et al: Difference in outcome among women and men after percutaneous mitral valvuloplasty, *Catheter Cardiovasc Interv* 77(1):115–120, 2011, Jan 1.
61. Bahl VK, Chandra S, Mishra S: Concurrent balloon dilation of mitral and tricuspid stenosis during pregnancy using an Inoue balloon, *Int J Cardiol* 59(2):199–202, 1997.
62. Bonow RO, Carabello BA, Chatterjee K, et al: 2008 focused update incorporated into the ACC/AHA 2006 guidelines for the management of patients with valvular heart disease: a report of the American College of Cardiology/American Heart Association task force on practice guidelines (writing committee to revise the 1998 guidelines for the management of patients with valvular heart disease). Endorsed by the society of cardiovascular anesthesiologists, society for cardiovascular angiography and interventions, and society of thoracic surgeons, *Circulation* 118:e523–e661, 2008.
63. Rizzoli G, De Perini L, Bottio T, et al: Prosthetic replacement of the tricuspid valve: Biological or mechanical? *Ann Thorac Surg* 66(6 Suppl):S62–S67, 1998.
64. Juarez Hernandez A: Is the tricuspid valve an enigma? Surgical treatment: valvuloplasty or valve change? Which prosthesis? *Arch Cardiol Mex* 71(1):73–77, 2001.

65. Cubeddu RJ, Palacios IF: Percutaneous techniques for mitral valve disease, *Cardiol Clin* 28(1):139–153, 2010, doi: 10.1016/j.ccl.2009.09.006.

66. Ashraf T, Pathan A, Kundi A: Percutaneous balloon valvuloplasty of coexisting mitral and tricuspid stenosis: single-wire, double-balloon technique, *J Invasive Cardiol* 20(4):E126–E128, 2008.

67. Boccuzzi G, Gigli N, Cian D, et al: Percutaneous transcatheter balloon valvuloplasty for severe tricuspid valve stenosis in Ebstein's anomaly, *J Cardiovasc Med (Hagerstown)* 10(6):510–515, 2009.

68. Cheng TO: Concurrent balloon valvuloplasty for combined mitral and tricuspid stenoses, *Int J Cardiol* 61(2):197, 1997.

69. Gamra H, Betbout F, Ayari M, et al: Recurrent miscarriages as an indication for percutaneous tricuspid valvuloplasty during pregnancy, *Catheter Cardiovasc Diagn* 40(3):283–286, 1997.

70. Hussain T, Knight WB, McLeod KA: Lead-induced tricuspid stenosis: successful management by balloon angioplasty, *Pacing Clin Electrophysiol* 32(1):140–142, 2009, doi: 10.1111/j.1540-8159.2009.02189.x.

71. Harle T, Kronberg K, Motz R, et al: Balloon valvuloplasty of a tricuspid valve stenosis in double balloon technique, *Clin Res Cardiol* 99(3):203–205, 2010, doi: 10.1007/s00392-009-0107-0.

72. Joseph G, Rajendiran G, Rajpal KA: Transjugular approach to concurrent mitral-aortic and mitral-tricuspid balloon valvuloplasty, *Catheter Cardiovasc Interv* 49(3):335–341, 2000.

73. Pfitzner R, Traczynski K: Early and late results of tricuspid valvuloplasty, *Acta Cardiol* 59(2):224–225, 2004.

74. Sancaktar O, Kumbasar SD, Semiz E, et al: Late results of combined percutaneous balloon valvuloplasty of mitral and tricuspid valves, *Catheter Cardiovasc Diagn* 45(3):246–250, 1998.

75. Robiolio PA, Rigolin VH, Harrison JK, et al: Predictors of outcome of tricuspid valve replacement in carcinoid heart disease, *Am J Cardiol* 75(7):485–488, 1995.

76. Moyssakis IE, Rallidis LS, Guida GF, et al: Incidence and evolution of carcinoid syndrome in the heart, *J Heart Valve Dis* 6(6):625–630, 1997.

77. Egred M, Albouaini K, Morrison WL: Images in cardiovascular medicine. Balloon valvuloplasty of a stenosed bioprosthetic tricuspid valve, *Circulation* 113(18):e745–e747, 2006, doi: 10.1161/CIRCULATIONAHA.105.568238.

78. Patel TM, Dani SI, Shah SC, et al: Tricuspid balloon valvuloplasty: a more simplified approach using Inouye balloon, *Catheter Cardiovasc Diagn* 37(1):86–88, 1996.

79. Roelke M, Smith AJ, Palacios IF: The technique and safety of transseptal left heart catheterization: the Massachusetts General Hospital experience with 1279 procedures, *Catheter Cardiovasc Diagn* 32(4):332–339, 1994.

80. Konugres GS, Lau FY, Ruiz CE: Successful percutaneous double-balloon mitral, aortic, and tricuspid valvotomy in rheumatic trivalvular stenosis, *Am Heart J* 119(3 Pt 1):663–666, 1990.

Chapter 10

Percutaneous Approaches for Treating Mitral Regurgitation

JASON H. ROGERS • EHRIN J. ARMSTRONG • STEVEN F. BOLLING

Percutaneous treatment of mitral regurgitation (MR) remains one of the most important areas of innovation and unmet clinical need in the field of adult structural heart disease. It is also one of the most challenging areas for device development because of the complexity of mitral valve (MV) function and the numerous pathologies that have traditionally required highly individualized surgical corrective therapy. Mitral leaflet mobility and coaptation rely on integrated function of the mitral annulus, chordae tendineae, papillary muscles, left ventricle, and left atrium. Together these structures are referred to as the *mitral apparatus* **(Figure 10–1)**. MR is an important and often underrecognized entity in which blood regurgitates into the left atrium from the left ventricle during systole. Published guidelines have established indications for surgical MV correction, generally for patients with symptoms, evidence of left ventricular (LV) enlargement or systolic dysfunction, or atrial fibrillation.[1,2] These guidelines have resulted in approximately 40,000 MV operations annually in the United States and a comparable number in Europe.[3] However, an unmet clinical need exists for a large population of patients with congestive heart failure–associated MR, with comorbidities, or at high surgical risk.[4,5] Because MR reduction in these patients can improve quality of life and result in favorable LV remodeling, numerous percutaneous approaches for treating MR have been developed in the last decade. This chapter describes existing and emerging therapies that are rapidly assuming importance as therapeutic options for patients with MR.

10.1 Mitral Regurgitation: Etiology, Prevalence, and Clinical Background

MR is a heterogeneous disease reflecting multiple underlying etiologies that converge on systolic regurgitation of the MV. Carpentier, Barlow, and others have described three general categories of MR with associated subclassifications **(Figure 10–2)**.[6-8] Degenerative MR (DMR; Carpentier Type II dysfunction) results from structurally abnormal leaflets or chordae and occurs in fibroelastic deficiency with leaflet prolapse, myxomatous leaflet degeneration, or Barlow disease with diffuse excess tissue and chordal elongation. Over the course of 10 years, 90% of patients with severe MR caused by a flail posterior leaflet will either die or require MV surgery.[9] Surgical MV repair is the preferred treatment for degenerative MR because it is associated with improved postoperative outcomes and survival when compared to MV replacement.[10] Multiple surgical repair techniques exist, including leaflet repair with resection, chordal transfer, use of polytetrafluoroethylene neochordae, and prosthetic ring or band annuloplasty.[11] Novel therapies addressed later in this chapter include percutaneous approaches to these leaflet and chordal repair strategies.

Functional MR (FMR; Carpentier Type I or IIIb) results from underlying LV dysfunction and annular dilation, leading to impaired coaptation of otherwise structurally normal leaflets. Surgical correction of FMR improves functional class and LV remodeling,[12] but it is uncertain whether this is associated with reduced mortality.[13] Even with modern surgical annuloplasty techniques, up to one third of patients with FMR develop recurrent moderate or greater MR within 1 year of surgery.[14-16] A number of predictors for recurrent MR after restrictive annuloplasty have been identified, including LV end-diastolic diameter greater than 65 mm,[17] posterior leaflet angle of 45 degrees or greater,[18] and MV coaptation depth of 11 mm or more.[19] As many as 500,000 people in North America have clinically significant congestive heart failure–associated MR, but the majority of those patients are not offered any MV intervention. Given that even asymptomatic patients with severe MR have higher 5-year rates of death, heart failure, and atrial fibrillation, a significant need exists for improved FMR therapies.

Many of the devices discussed in this chapter attempt to address percutaneous approaches for treatment of FMR, primarily through percutaneous annuloplasty.

From an anatomic and interventional perspective, technologies for addressing MR can be categorized into treatments focused on leaflet repair, annuloplasty, chordal implants, LV remodeling techniques, and percutaneous MV replacement **(Table 10–1).**[20] The following discussion examines interventional techniques in development for each of these approaches.

10.2 Leaflet Repair

MITRACLIP THERAPY

MitraClip (Abbott Vascular Structural Heart, Menlo Park, Calif.) therapy has become an important therapeutic option for patients with MR, and important investigations centered on this therapy have given credence and momentum to the entire field of percutaneous MV

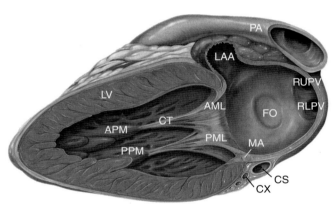

Figure 10–1 The mitral valve apparatus. Anatomy as seen from a section though the left ventricle and left atrium. *AML,* Anterior mitral leaflet; *APM,* anterior papillary muscle; *CS,* coronary sinus; *CT,* chordae tendineae; *CX,* circumflex coronary artery; *FO,* fossa ovalis; *LAA,* left atrial appendage; *LV,* left ventricle; *MA,* mitral annulus; *PA,* pulmonary artery; *PML,* posterior mitral leaflet; *PPM,* posterior papillary muscle; *RLPV,* right lower pulmonary vein; *RUPV,* right upper pulmonary vein.

repair.[21] MitraClip therapy is based on the surgical edge-to-edge repair first described by Alfieri.[22] Because of the wealth of data and clinical experience related to Mitra-Clip therapy, this technique is the subject of a separate chapter in this volume (Chapter 11).

OTHER LEAFLET REPAIR TECHNOLOGIES

The Cardiosolutions Percu-Pro system (Cardiosolutions Inc., Stoughton, Mass.) is a percutaneously delivered polyurethane-silicone polymer "Mitra-Spacer." The spacer is balloon-shaped, occupies the regurgitant mitral orifice, and is anchored to the LV apex **(Figure 10–3).** The spacer has the ability to "self-center" within the regurgitant orifice. Animal studies have shown that the device is not associated with any significant inflammatory response, and early clinical trials are underway.

Middle Peak Medical (Palo Alto, Calif.) is developing a unique solution that involves minimally invasive or transcatheter implantation of a posterior "neoleaflet." The potential advantage of this approach is that the neoleaflet can restore coaptation with the anterior leaflet despite a variety of underlying degenerative or functional etiologies. Because the device consists only of this thin neoleaflet, the delivery profile is much smaller than a complete transcatheter mitral replacement. Since native posterior leaflet function is rendered inactive by the neoleaflet, no complex repair strategies are required. The implant does not interfere with the mitral support apparatus, so that ventricular–annular mechanical coupling is preserved. At publication, the device is undergoing preclinical development; a schematic of the technology is shown in **Figure 10–4.**

The MOBIUS device (Edwards Lifesciences, Irvine, Calif.) utilized an innovative transseptal catheter that possessed suction capability in order to grasp the leaflets. Once the leaflets were grasped, a suture was delivered to the leaflets to create a double-orifice valve. In the initial in-human experience, the procedure was performed successfully on 15 patients. Nine of the patients had acute reduction of MR by 1 grade or more, and 6 patients had sustained improvement at 30 days.

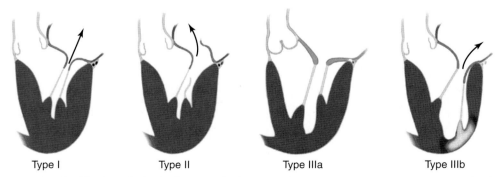

| Type I | Type II | Type IIIa | Type IIIb |

Figure 10–2   The Carpentier classification of mitral valve regurgitation. More than one type can coexist in a given individual. *Type I:* Normal leaflet motion with annular dilation and centrally directed jet of mitral regurgitation (MR). *Type II:* Increased leaflet motion (leaflet prolapse or flail) with eccentric jet of MR. *Type IIIa:* Restricted leaflet motion in systole and diastole, usually associated with leaflet and subvalvular thickening/scarring (rheumatic). *Type IIIb:* Restricted leaflet motion in systole, as seen in ischemic cardiomyopathy with history of infarct (light region in left ventricle). One or more leaflets may be "tethered" below the coaptation plane, resulting in MR.

This device is no longer in further development because of the lack of apparent durability in the initial studies.[23]

10.3 Chordal Implantation

NEOCHORD

The NeoChord device (NeoChord, Inc., Eden Prairie, Minn.) utilizes a transapical approach for implantation of artificial chordae tendineae in patients with leaflet prolapse or flail **(Figure 10–5).** The LV apex is exposed via a left lateral minithoracotomy, and a sheath is advanced via the apex towards the MV leaflets. With the guidance of transesophageal echocardiography (TEE), a catheter is used to grasp the leaflets and attach artificial chordae, which are then anchored to the LV apex. The system utilizes a unique fiber optic feedback system to ensure that the target leaflet is appropriately centered in the jaws of the device. Once the NeoChord is attached, the operator

TABLE 10–1

Past and Present Percutaneous Therapies for Mitral Valve Regurgitation

Target of Therapy	Device Name (Manufacturer)	Mechanism of Action
Leaflet repair	MitraClip (Abbott)	Clip-based edge-to-edge repair
	Percu-Pro (Cardiosolutions)	Space-occupying in regurgitant orifice
	MOBIUS (Edwards)	Suture-based edge-to-edge repair
Chordal implant	NeoChord (NeoChord)	Synthetic chordae tendineae
Neoleaflet implant	Middle Peak Medical	Synthetic neoleaflet
Indirect annuloplasty	CARILLON (Cardiac Dimensions)	Coronary sinus reshaping
	MONARC (Edwards)	Coronary sinus reshaping
	PTMA device (Viacor)	Coronary sinus reshaping
	Mitral cerclage (NIH)	Coronary sinus-right atrial encircling
	PS³ System (MVRx)	Transatrial coronary sinoatrial septal shortening
Direct annuloplasty	Mitralign (Mitralign)	2 × 2 Plicating anchors through posterior annulus
	Accucinch (Guided Delivery Systems)	Plicating anchors on ventricular side of mitral annulus
	Cardioband (Valtech)	Plicating anchors on atrial side of mitral annulus
	QuantumCor (QuantumCor)	Radiofrequency energy shrinking annular collagen
	Millipede (Millipede)	Semirigid circumferential annular ring
Left ventricular reshaping	iCoapsys (Edwards)	Transventricular reshaping
	BACE (Mardil)	External basal myocardial reshaping
Mitral annular anchor	M-Valve	Percutaneous anchor to allow fixation of transcatheter valve
Mitral valve replacement	Endovalve-Herrmann (Endovalve)	Valve replacement
	CardiAQ (CardiAQ)	Valve replacement
	Tiara (Neovasc)	Valve replacement

PTMA, Percutaneous transvenous mitral annuloplasty.

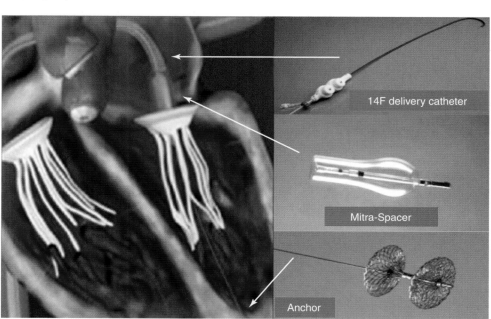

Figure 10–3 The Percu-Pro system. The space occupying Mitra-Spacer balloon acts as a "buoy," filling the mitral regurgitant orifice, and is anchored by a tether to the left ventricular apex. *Arrows* correspond to the positions of the delivery catheter, Mitra-Spacer, and anchor.

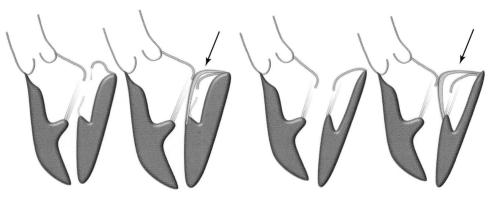

Figure 10–4 Middle Peak medical neoleaflet. The concept is shown by the arrows. A posterior neoleaflet *(blue)* is implanted and restores leaflet coaptation in either DMR or FMR.

Degenerative mitral regurgitation (DMR)

Functional mitral regurgitation (FMR)

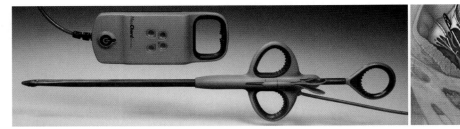

Figure 10–5   NeoChord device (NeoChord, Inc., Eden Prairie, Minn.). The NeoChord device is shown in the left panel and consists of a catheter to grasp the leaflet, an exchangeable cartridge containing expanded polytetrafluoroethylene (ePTFE) suture, and an integrated fiber optic display to verify leaflet capture. The device is delivered from the transapical approach as shown in the right panel.

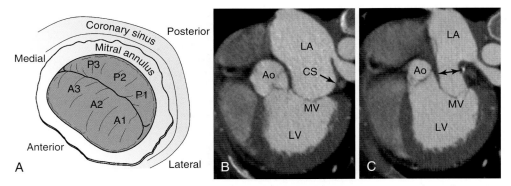

Figure 10–6   Indirect mitral annuloplasty using the coronary sinus. A, The CS encircles the posterior mitral annulus. **B,** Computed tomography scan of subject with FMR showing relationship of CS *(arrow)* to the MV. Note that they are not coplanar. **C,** Movement of the CS with device results in narrowing of the left atrial lumen above the MV *(double-headed arrow)*, with secondary indirect decrease in the mitral annulus diameter. *Ao,* Aorta; *CS,* coronary sinus; *LA,* left atrium; *LV,* left ventricle; *MV,* mitral valve.

can optimize real-time reduction in MR by varying chord tension and the extent of MV prolapse. The European Transapical Artificial Chordae Tendineae (TACT) trial is still underway at publication of this chapter and will target subjects with severe DMR.

ANNULAR SHAPE-CHANGE APPROACHES

Surgical annuloplasty is often a stand-alone treatment for FMR and is an important adjunct to leaflet repair procedures for DMR. The importance of annuloplasty to durable long-term results has led to the concept that multiple transcatheter interventions (e.g., both Mitra-Clip and annuloplasty) may be necessary to treat MR in a given patient.

Most percutaneous approaches for annuloplasty have attempted to reshape the annulus "indirectly" by reshaping the coronary sinus (CS). The CS travels in close proximity to the mitral annulus **(Figure 10–6).** Importantly, however, the CS does not directly lie in the annulus, but rather travels 5 to 10 mm superior and diagonally to the plane of the mitral annulus.[24] Any conformational change in the CS must be transmitted through sinoannular tissue, which attenuates any applied force. Additionally, the sinoannular tissue may remodel and redilate over time, thereby compromising durability of MR reduction. Several devices have been developed for placement within the CS. Each of these systems creates focal tension to reduce the circumference of the mitral annulus and the septal–lateral (SL) dimensions, with resulting reduction in MR. Although these devices are relatively easy to deploy, reproducible efficacy is a limitation because of the variable relationship of the CS to the annulus, and these devices all harbor the risk of circumflex coronary artery compression.[25]

Other techniques employ more "direct" annuloplasty by attaching a series of anchors near or on the annulus that can be drawn together (plicated) with suture, with the goal of reducing the mitral annular circumference and the SL dimension. This approach may have the advantage of more closely approximating the annulus but is also more technically challenging from an engineering and procedural standpoint. Technologies are also under development to completely replicate a surgical annuloplasty with a semirigid implantable circumferential annular ring.

CARDIAC DIMENSIONS CARILLON DEVICE

The CARILLON Mitral Contour System (Cardiac Dimensions, Kirkland, Wash.) consists of a pair of helical self-expanding nitinol distal and proximal anchors connected by a nitinol bridge. The device is placed percutaneously in the CS from a right internal jugular vein approach and can be retrieved acutely if positioning or MR reduction is not favorable. The bridge can be shortened after the anchors are deployed in order to plicate posterior annular tissue and create movement of the posterior annulus anteriorly, thereby reducing the SL dimension **(Figure 10–7)**. The device has undergone several design iterations (additional "twists" to the anchor portions to prevent slippage and reinforcement of the device at its ends to prevent fracture) and on publication exists as the modified XE2 (mXE2) device.

The AMADEUS trial was the first investigation of a percutaneous CS-based intervention to reduce FMR in patients with heart failure.[26] The AMADEUS trial enrolled 48 symptomatic patients with dilated cardiomyopathy, at least moderate FMR, and an ejection fraction of less than 40%. Thirty patients had successful device implantation with the primary safety endpoint—a composite of death, myocardial infarction, or device-related complication—evaluated at 30 days. Echocardiographic FMR grade and functional indices (New York Heart Association functional class, Kansas City Cardiomyopathy Questionnaire, and 6-minute walk test) were assessed at baseline, 1 month, and 6 months. Of the 48 patients in the trial, 6 (13%) experienced a major adverse event within 30 days; 1 of these 6 patients died, with the remaining events consisting of either clinically silent myocardial infarction or CS dissection and/or perforation. The early findings of CS injury led to changes in procedural technique that dramatically reduced the occurrence of this adverse event. Coronary arteries were crossed in 36 of 43 (84%) implant attempts. When coronary compromise was identified, the CARILLON device could be safely removed before implantation. There was a 22% to 32% reduction in MR grade at 6 months by a composite of four echocardiographic parameters used, with no significant worsening of the 30-day MR values at 6 months. Although quality of life and functional indices

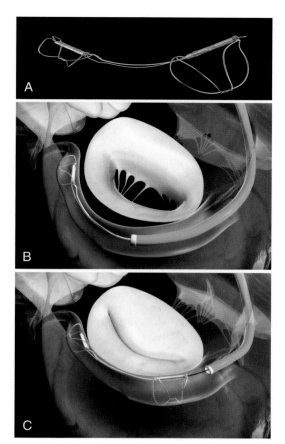

Figure 10–7 Cardiac Dimensions CARILLON device. The mXE2 CARILLON device **(A).** The distal anchor is smaller and deployed first **(B),** and traction is applied, followed by proximal anchor deployment **(C).** The device is delivered from the internal jugular vein (shown as green delivery catheter).

all improved in follow-up studies, there was no significant change in LV size or LV ejection fraction at 6 months. Additionally, the anteroposterior mitral annular diameter decreased from an average of 42 mm at baseline to 37.8 mm at 6-month follow-up study—representing a relatively small 10% diameter reduction—and never attained a correction back to normal. Despite these limitations, the AMADEUS trial provided important evidence that a CS-based device could be used safely to reduce MR and improve quality of life in patients with FMR. On the basis of the findings, the CARILLON device was granted CE-mark approval in 2009.

The TITAN trial was a prospective nonrandomized trial in which 53 patients with symptomatic FMR were enrolled for CARILLON device therapy.[27] Thirty-six patients (68%) underwent successful device implantation, whereas 17 devices were not implanted because of insufficient MR reduction (n = 9) or transient coronary compromise (n = 8) in patients. Successful device therapy showed significant reduction in MR grade, favorable LV remodeling, and improved quality of life when compared with the control group of subjects who did not receive implants. There were nine wireform device fractures seen in this trial, with no advents attributable to this finding. In only one of the patients with device fracture was a reduction in FMR observed. A newer CARILLON mXE2 device has been introduced and will be used in future trials. Preprocedure computed tomography scanning has also been used in the CARILLON studies and can provide some useful anatomic information for planning the procedure, but has not reliably been able to predict efficacy or coronary artery compression.

EDWARDS MONARC DEVICE

The MONARC device (Edwards Lifesciences, Irvine, Calif.) is an annular device with a distal self-expanding anchor, a middle springlike "bridge," and a proximal self-expanding anchor. The distal anchor is placed near the anterior interventricular vein, and the proximal anchor is placed near the ostium of the CS. The bridge has shape-memory properties that result in shortening forces at body temperature after dissipation of a dissolvable element in the center of the device. After device placement, there is no acute reduction in MR. Instead, MR reduction occurs over a 3- to 6-week period as the spacer material dissolves and results in device shortening. This delayed-shortening property has raised concerns for late coronary artery compression. A pilot study in humans with the first-generation Viking device (Edwards Lifesciences, Irvine, Calif.) showed some improvement in chronic MR, but 1 out of the 5 patients could not have the device successfully implanted, and 3 of the 4 who did had evidence of bridge separation or fracture during follow-up study.[28] A second-generation device (MONARC device) correcting these problems was then studied in the prospective nonrandomized Clinical Evaluation of the Edwards Lifesciences Percutaneous Mitral Annuloplasty System for The Treatment of Mitral Regurgitation (EVOLUTION I and II) trials. The EVOLUTION I trial of FMR demonstrated implantation success in 82% (59 of 72 patients), with 13 failures (18%) because of tortuous anatomy or inappropriate CS dimensions. Two myocardial infarctions occurred as a result of coronary artery compression. Event-free survival was 91% at 30 days and 82% at 1 year. MR reduction of 1 grade or more was seen in 50% of subjects at 12 months.[29] Despite encouraging initial clinical results, the MONARC device is not undergoing further clinical development.

VIACOR PERCUTANEOUS TRANSVENOUS MITRAL ANNULOPLASTY DEVICE

The Viacor percutaneous transvenous mitral annuloplasty device (Viacor, Wilmington, Mass.) uses a CS catheter containing up to three nitinol rods of varying length and stiffness that exert an anterior displacement force. The safety and feasibility of this device was reported for 19 subjects who underwent temporary "diagnostic device" implantation to assess acute MR reduction. The device was successfully implanted in nine subjects. Four of the implants were subsequently removed because of device migration and/or diminished efficacy. There were no procedure or device-related major adverse events with permanent effects in any of the patients who had diagnostic studies or implants.

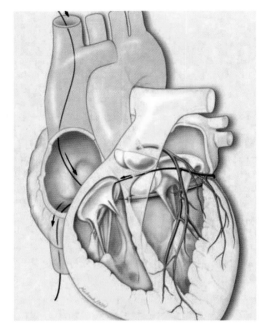

Figure 10–8 Cerclage annuloplasty. The mitral valve is encircled by a guidewire *(black arrows)* that can be tensioned to reduce the mitral annular circumference and diameter.

Further device development has been abandoned because of limited MR reduction and technical issues.[30]

OTHER CORONARY SINUS–BASED DEVICES

Cerclage annuloplasty **(Figure 10–8)** is an investigational technique that uses magnetic resonance imaging merged with fluoroscopic guidance to pass a wire from the right atrium, through the CS, and back into the right atrium by traversing a short segment of the basal septal myocardium. In this way it encircles the annulus. By tensioning the guidewire in a porcine model of ischemic cardiomyopathy, mitral annular size and MR grade can be decreased. A small nitinol tube has also been developed to prevent guidewire coronary artery compression by acting as a miniature arch over the artery.[31] This device remains in the preclinical development phase.

The Percutaneous Septal Sinus Shortening system (PS[3] system; MVRx, Belmont, Calif.) uses magnetic catheters in order to allow accurate placement of a "bridge" that connects anchors in the CS and the interatrial septum **(Figure 10–9)**. Once this connection is made between the CS and the interatrial septum, tension can be applied to the bridge element, effectively shortening the SL dimension. Using an ovine model, investigators found that device implantation with an average 24% SL diameter reduction resulted in acute and chronic MR reduction.[32] Because this approach had shown early promise, temporary devices were implanted in patients in a first-in-human study, confirming efficacy and significantly reducing MR.[33] Permanent implants in humans have also been performed demonstrating safety and moderate efficacy. However, additional studies have not been performed and the technology is currently undergoing device refinement.

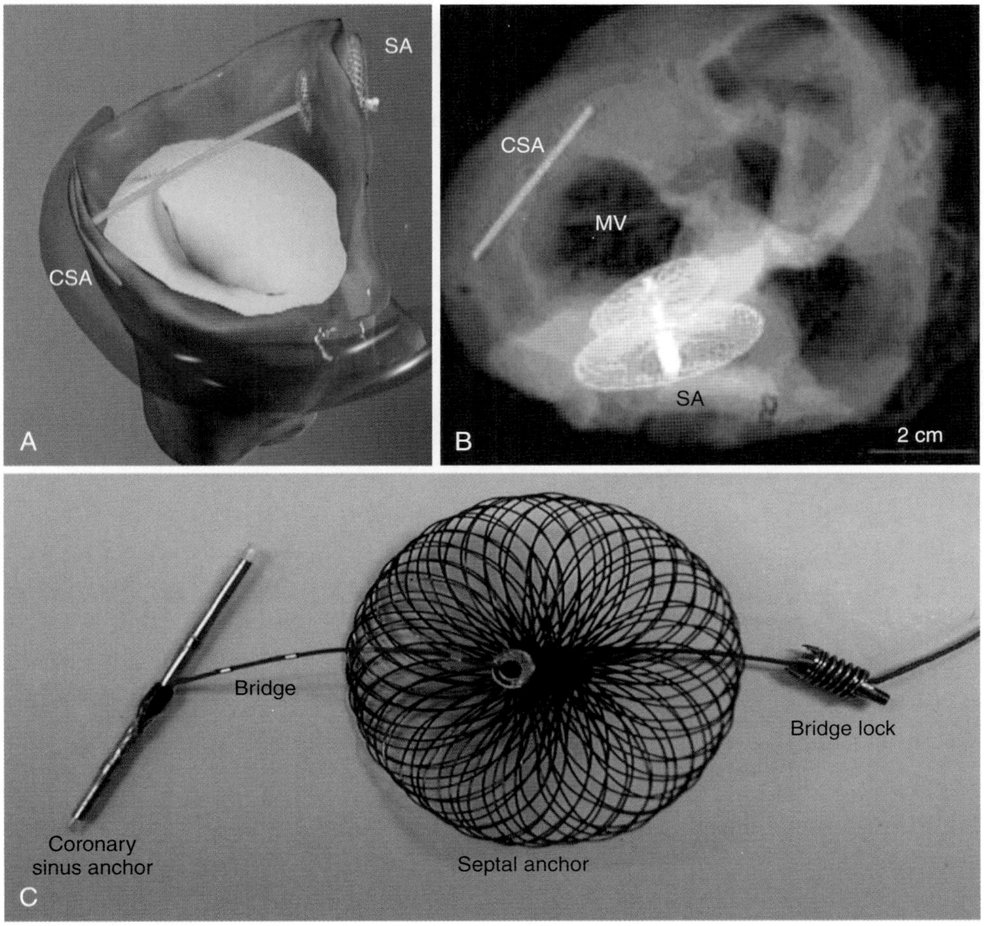

Figure 10–9 **Percutaneous septal-sinus shortening (PS³) procedure.** The PS³ system is placed using magnetically tipped catheters with simultaneous coronary sinus (CS) and transseptal left atrial access. **A,** Schematic of the PS³ system showing the CS anchor *(CSA)* and septal anchor *(SA)*. These are connected using a suture bridge *(light blue)* that can be tensioned, reducing the septal-lateral dimension. **B,** X-ray image of the PS³ System in an animal model demonstrating the relationship between the CS and septal anchors in relation to the mitral valve. **C,** Components of the PS³ system.

10.4 Direct Annuloplasty

Surgical closed-ring mitral annuloplasty is currently considered the gold standard for the treatment of functional MR, with predictable and durable reductions in mitral annular circumference and the SL diameter. Before the advent of open and closed rigid rings, suture-based annuloplasty based on prior work by Paneth and Burr had been used.[34] This technique has been shown to reduce the SL diameter in patients undergoing adjunctive annuloplasty in the setting of degenerative leaflet repair, or for repair of functional MR.[35,36] However, the durability of suture-based or nonrigid annuloplasty is inferior to rigid mitral annular rings, with progression in mitral annular dimensions over time.[16,35] Nonetheless, several percutaneous approaches have been developed. Other novel approaches include the application of radiofrequency energy and the development of a percutaneously delivered semirigid circumferential mitral annuloplasty ring.

MITRALIGN PERCUTANEOUS ANNULOPLASTY SYSTEM

The Mitralign percutaneous annuloplasty system (Mitralign, Tewksbury, Mass.) is based on surgical suture annuloplasty of the MV. The Mitralign procedure involves an LV approach through retrograde femoral arterial access. A deflectable catheter is placed under the posterior mitral leaflet and adjacent to the annular tissue beneath the valve. A specially designed catheter carries two crossing wires (the "bident") that are passed from the ventricular aspect of the annulus into the left atrium using brief application of radiofrequency energy. These wires serve as the guides over which two sets of paired anchors are placed through the posterior annulus of the MV. These anchors are plicated, resulting in a segmental posterior annuloplasty and reduction in MR **(Figure 10–10).** This technology is undergoing safety and feasibility testing in Europe and South America.

GUIDED DELIVERY SYSTEMS ACCUCINCH SYSTEM

The Accucinch system (Guided Delivery Systems, Santa Clara, Calif.) is also based on suture annuloplasty. The procedure uses a retrograde femoral arterial approach to gain access to the ventricular aspect of the mitral annulus. A proprietary catheter is placed under the posterior mitral leaflet, adjacent to the annular tissue beneath the valve. Using this catheter, 9 to 12 anchors can be placed from the anterior to posterior commissures along the posterior mitral annulus. The anchors

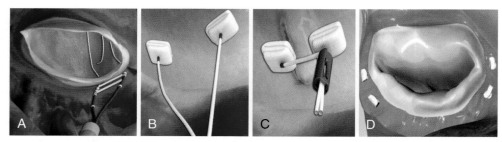

Figure 10–10 **Mitralign annuloplasty system. A,** A retrograde aortic deflectable catheter *(blue)* allows passage of the "bident" crossing wires through the mitral annulus from the left ventricle to the left atrium. **B,** Paired pledgeted sutures are placed along the posterior annulus. **C,** The pledgeted sutures are tensioned and locked, and the suture is cut. The procedure is repeated to place an additional set of anchors. **D,** Final appearance of 2 × 2 annular plication.

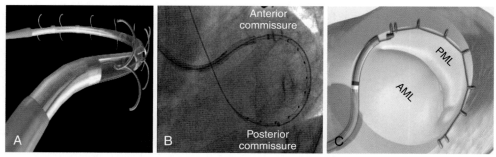

Figure 10–11 **Accucinch annuloplasty system. A,** Schematic of Accucinch system showing delivery catheter *(green)* and anchors that are placed in the left ventricular myocardium directly below the posterior mitral annulus. **B,** Fluoroscopic view of Accucinch delivery system encircling the mitral valve. **C,** Illustration demonstrating placement of anchors in the ventricular tissue under the mitral leaflets. *AML,* Anterior mitral leaflet; *PML,* posterior mitral leaflet.

are then connected by a suture element and plicated to reduce the mitral annular circumference and MR **(Figure 10–11).** This technique could be used to plicate the posterior wall of the left ventricle to improve ventricular geometry and potentially reduce FMR. Chronic surgical implants in humans have been completed, and percutaneous human implants are under development.

THE QUANTUMCOR SYSTEM

The QuantumCor system (QuantumCor, Bothell, Wash.) is based on the concept of thermal remodeling of collagen. Since the MV annulus has significant collagen content, catheter-based application of radiofrequency (RF) energy at subablative temperatures to the mitral annulus can heat and contract the collagen fibers, thereby reducing mitral annular circumference. Animal models have confirmed reduction in mitral annular dimensions and MR after treatment.[37] Histologic follow-up study showed that the annular lesions did not compromise the structural integrity of the atrium or mitral leaflets. The energy is applied circumferentially to the mitral annulus using a proprietary RF catheter. Favorable aspects of this technology are that no material is left behind and that repeat applications can be applied. Therapy in humans has not yet been reported.

SUPRAANNULAR RINGS

The Millipede system (Millipede, Austin, Tex.) is a device in preclinical development that mimics a surgical circumferential and rigid annuloplasty. This technique consists of placement of a novel expandable annular ring with an innovative attachment system via either minimally invasive surgical or percutaneous methods to restore the native mitral annular shape and diameter. The device can be used to treat FMR or as an adjunct to leaflet repair technologies.

The Cardioband (Valtech, Or Yehuda, Israel), in early clinical development, allows percutaneous placement of a series of small corkscrew anchors under TEE guidance into the left atrial aspect of the mitral annulus. These anchors are connected by a sleeve that can be tensioned, resulting in reduction of the mitral annular circumference. The system is delivered by means of a nested catheter system that allows the operator to achieve multiple degrees of movement within the left atrium **(Figure 10–12).**

10.5 Ventricular Reshaping Technologies

The iCoapsys system (Edwards Lifesciences, Irvine, Calif.) is a novel method of reshaping the left ventricle by means of a percutaneously placed system. The procedure is based on the surgically placed Coapsys system, which has demonstrated sustained reduction in MR at 1 year.[38] Under fluoroscopic and echocardiographic guidance, intrapericardial anchoring devices are placed on the epicardial ventricular surface in an anteroposterior configuration and are connected by a tethering or anchoring suture that

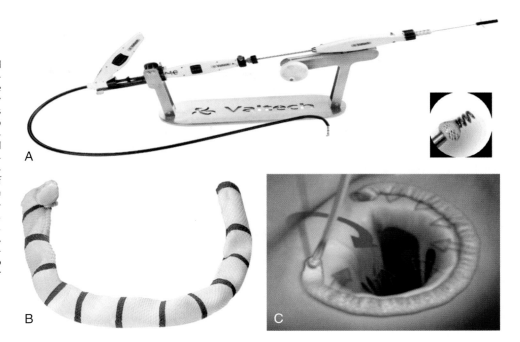

Figure 10–12 Valtech Cardioband system. The Cardioband is a percutaneous sutureless and adjustable annuloplasty system. **A,** The delivery system rests on a stand and allows control of a transseptal catheter tip in the left atrium. A series of corkscrew anchors *(inset)* are placed under fluoroscopic and echocardiographic guidance into the mitral annulus. **B,** Detailed image of the Cardioband device. The design is similar to a sleeve, and the anchors are delivered from the inside, through the Cardioband material, and then into the mitral annulus. **C,** After delivery of all anchors, the annuloplasty band can be tightened to achieve the desired mitral annular reduction.

passes horizontally through the left ventricle. By applying tension to the anchoring suture, the geometry of the ventricle is changed. Likewise, the mitral annular diameter is decreased, resulting in improved leaflet coaptation. After several human implants, further development of the device was terminated because of device complexity and other technical issues. Nonetheless, the device was important in validating the concept that FMR is a ventricular disease and that remodeling of the LV can effect significant MR reduction.

The Basal Annuloplasty of the Cardia Externally (BACE) device (Mardil, Morrisville, N.C.) requires a minithoracotomy and is implanted on a beating heart. A silicone band with an inflatable chamber is placed around the left ventricle by means of a transapical approach. By inflating the device, the ventricular shape is changed, improving ventricular–mitral dynamics and reducing FMR.

10.6 Percutaneous Mitral Valve Replacement

Although surgical MV repair is generally preferable to replacement for degenerative MR, transcatheter MV replacement therapies are important for several reasons. First, some complex MV pathologies are not amenable to percutaneous repair or require combinations of percutaneous technologies that may not be feasible. Percutaneous valve replacement may result in superior reduction of MR compared to repair, and this may be of particular importance if the goal of a procedure is to attain "zero MR." For patients with FMR, replacement may also be an attractive option, because there is no mortality difference between repair versus replacement in patients with ischemic MR up to 6 years after surgery.[39] However, multiple challenges remain. Secure anchoring and attachment of percutaneous valves is crucial, because

paravalvular leaks are likely not well tolerated. Patients with FMR treated with a transcatheter valve generally have large mitral annular diameters, and developing devices that expand to fill these large diameters will also be necessary.

The Endovalve-Herrmann Mitral Valve (Micro-Interventional Devices, Bethlehem, Pa.) is a foldable nitinol valve with a sealing skirt that attaches to the MV apparatus. It is fully valve-sparing and repositionable before release. The CardiAQ prosthesis (CardiAQ Valve Technologies, Irvine, Calif.) is a transcatheter valve delivered by a transseptal approach. The valve is attached to a self-expanding nitinol frame that self-centers on the mitral annulus **(Figure 10–13).** A first-in-man implant of the CardiAQ valve was performed in Europe in 2012. The Tiara valve (Neovasc, Richmond, British Columbia, Canada) is a catheter-based self-expanding mitral bioprosthesis. The Tiara valve has a unique **D**-shape to match the shape of the mitral orifice, with the flat side of the **D** positioned anteriorly to prevent impingement of the LV outflow tract. Preclinical work in domestic swine has shown safety and feasibility.[40]

In addition to transcatheter MV replacement for MR, transcatheter valve-in-valve implantation inside of a degenerated MV bioprosthesis is increasingly performed and is described in Chapter 13. The majority of these procedures have been performed via the transapical approach because of the favorable anatomic alignment of the catheter from the LV apex to the MV. Although mitral valve-in-valve procedures will remain limited to those with prior valve implantation, the success of this approach demonstrates the feasibility of transcatheter MV replacement. Others are developing a percutaneously delivered anchoring system, which is placed on the mitral annulus (M-Valve, La Jolla, Calif.). The theory is that once this implant is securely positioned, it may serve as an anchor to allow deployment of any one of a variety of

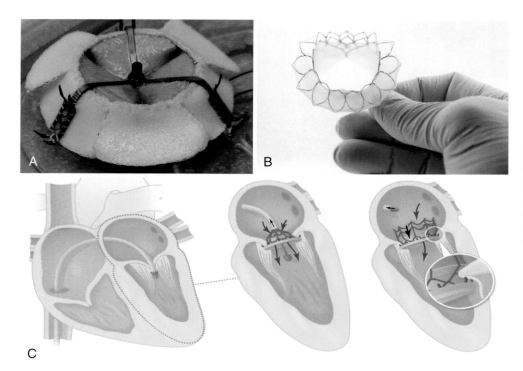

Figure 10–13 Percutaneous mitral valve replacements. A, Prototype of the Endovalve-Herrmann prosthesis. **B,** The Tiara valve. Note unique D-shape to avoid impingement on the left ventricular outflow tract. **C,** Schematic of delivery of CardiAQ prosthesis via transseptal route with self-expanding frame.

commercially available transcatheter valves. Percutaneous closure of mitral paravalvular leaks is also increasingly performed, and this topic is covered in Chapter 12.

10.7 Summary

Interventional cardiology has seen the advent of a new era in the transcatheter management of MV disease. The challenges for all these devices are to demonstrate safety and either equivalent or superior efficacy in comparison to traditional management strategies, whether medical or surgical. Interventionists must strive to properly select patients for these new therapies and to develop effective technologies to treat populations at high risk for surgery. Patience, collaboration, and vision are needed to fully develop these strategies.

REFERENCES

1. Bonow RO, Carabello BA, Chatterjee K, et al: 2008 Focused update incorporated into the ACC/AHA 2006 guidelines for the management of patients with valvular heart disease: a report of the American College of Cardiology/American Heart Association Task Force on Practice Guidelines (Writing Committee to Revise the 1998 Guidelines for the Management of Patients With Valvular Heart Disease): endorsed by the Society of Cardiovascular Anesthesiologists, Society for Cardiovascular Angiography and Interventions, and Society of Thoracic Surgeons, *Circulation* 118(15):e523–e661, Oct 7 2008.
2. Vahanian A, Baumgartner H, Bax J, et al: Guidelines on the management of valvular heart disease: The Task Force on the Management of Valvular Heart Disease of the European Society of Cardiology, *Eur Heart J* 28(2):230–268, Jan 2007.
3. Gammie JS, O'Brien SM, Griffith BP, et al: Influence of hospital procedural volume on care process and mortality for patients undergoing elective surgery for mitral regurgitation, *Circulation* 115(7):881–887, Feb 20 2007.
4. Mirabel M, Iung B, Baron G, et al: What are the characteristics of patients with severe, symptomatic, mitral regurgitation who are denied surgery? *Eur Heart J* 28(11):1358–1365, Jun 2007.
5. O'Brien SM, Shahian DM, Filardo G, et al: The Society of Thoracic Surgeons 2008 cardiac surgery risk models. Part 2. Isolated valve surgery, *Ann Thorac Surg* 88(1 Suppl):S23–S42, Jul 2009.
6. Carpentier A: Cardiac valve surgery: the "French correction." *J Thorac Cardiovasc Surg* 86(3):323–337, Sep 1983.
7. Adams DH, Rosenhek R, Falk V: Degenerative mitral valve regurgitation: best practice revolution, *Eur Heart J* 31(16):1958–1966, Aug 2010.
8. Barlow JB, Pocock WA: The significance of late systolic murmurs and mid-late systolic clicks, *Md State Med J* 12:76–77, Feb 1963.
9. Ling LH, Enriquez-Sarano M, Seward JB, et al: Clinical outcome of mitral regurgitation due to flail leaflet, *N Engl J Med* 335(19):1417–1423, Nov 7 1996.
10. Enriquez-Sarano M, Schaff HV, Orszulak TA, et al: Valve repair improves the outcome of surgery for mitral regurgitation: a multivariate analysis, *Circulation* 91(4):1022–1028, Feb 15 1995.
11. Seeburger J, Falk V, Borger MA, et al: Chordae replacement versus resection for repair of isolated posterior mitral leaflet prolapse: à égalité, *Ann Thorac Surg* 87(6):1715–1720, Jun 2009.
12. Bax JJ, Braun J, Somer ST, et al: Restrictive annuloplasty and coronary revascularization in ischemic mitral regurgitation results in reverse left ventricular remodeling, *Circulation* 110(11 Suppl 1):II103–II108, Sep 14 2004.
13. Wu AH, Aaronson KD, Bolling SF, et al: Impact of mitral valve annuloplasty on mortality risk in patients with mitral regurgitation and left ventricular systolic dysfunction, *J Am Coll Cardiol* 45(3):381–387, Feb 1 2005.
14. Hung J, Papakostas L, Tahta SA, et al: Mechanism of recurrent ischemic mitral regurgitation after annuloplasty: continued LV remodeling as a moving target, *Circulation* 110(11 Suppl 1):II85–II90, Sep 14 2004.
15. Marwick TH: Restrictive annuloplasty for ischemic mitral regurgitation: too little or too much? *J Am Coll Cardiol* 51(17):1702–1703, Apr 29 2008.
16. McGee EC, Gillinov AM, Blackstone EH, et al: Recurrent mitral regurgitation after annuloplasty for functional ischemic mitral regurgitation, *J Thorac Cardiovasc Surg* 128(6):916–924, Dec 2004.
17. Braun J, van de Veire NR, Klautz RJ, et al: Restrictive mitral annuloplasty cures ischemic mitral regurgitation and heart failure, *Ann Thorac Surg* 85(2):430–436, Feb 2008, discussion 436–437.
18. Magne J, Pibarot P, Dagenais F, et al: Preoperative posterior leaflet angle accurately predicts outcome after restrictive mitral valve annuloplasty for ischemic mitral regurgitation, *Circulation* 115(6):782–791, Feb 13 2007.

19. Calafiore AM, Gallina S, Di Mauro M, et al: Mitral valve procedure in dilated cardiomyopathy: repair or replacement? *Ann Thorac Surg* 71(4):1146–1152, Apr 2001, discussion 1152–1143.

20. Chiam PT, Ruiz CE: Percutaneous transcatheter mitral valve repair: a classification of the technology, *JACC Cardiovasc Interv* 4(1):1–13, Jan 2011.

21. Rogers JH, Franzen O: Percutaneous edge-to-edge MitraClip therapy in the management of mitral regurgitation, *Eur Heart J* 32(19):2350–2357, 2011.

22. Alfieri O, Maisano F, De Bonis M, et al: The double-orifice technique in mitral valve repair: a simple solution for complex problems, *J Thorac Cardiovasc Surg* 122(4):674–681, Oct 2001.

23. Webb JG, Maisano F, Vahanian A, et al: Percutaneous suture edge-to-edge repair of the mitral valve, *EuroIntervention* 5(1):86–89, May 2009.

24. Maselli D, Guarracino F, Chiaramonti F, et al: Percutaneous mitral annuloplasty: an anatomic study of human coronary sinus and its relation with mitral valve annulus and coronary arteries, *Circulation* 114(5):377–380, Aug 1 2006.

25. Tops LF, Van de Veire NR, Schuijf JD, et al: Noninvasive evaluation of coronary sinus anatomy and its relation to the mitral valve annulus: implications for percutaneous mitral annuloplasty, *Circulation* 115(11):1426–1432, Mar 20 2007.

26. Schofer J, Siminiak T, Haude M, et al: Percutaneous mitral annuloplasty for functional mitral regurgitation: results of the CARILLON Mitral Annuloplasty Device European Union Study, *Circulation* 120(4):326–333, Jul 28 2009.

27. Siminiak T, Wu JC, Haude M, et al: Treatment of functional mitral regurgitation by percutaneous annuloplasty: results of the TITAN Trial, *Eur J Heart Fail* 14(8):931–938, Aug 2012.

28. Webb JG, Harnek J, Munt BI, et al: Percutaneous transvenous mitral annuloplasty: initial human experience with device implantation in the coronary sinus, *Circulation* 113(6):851–855, Feb 14 2006.

29. Harnek J, Webb JG, Kuck KH, et al: Transcatheter implantation of the MONARC coronary sinus device for mitral regurgitation: 1-year results from the EVOLUTION phase I study (clinical evaluation of the Edwards Lifesciences percutaneous mitral annuloplasty system for the treatment of mitral regurgitation), *JACC Cardiovasc Interv* 4(1):115–122, Jan 2011.

30. Sack S, Kahlert P, Bilodeau L, et al: Percutaneous transvenous mitral annuloplasty: initial human experience with a novel coronary sinus implant device, *Circ Cardiovasc Interv* 2(4):277–284, Aug 2009.

31. Kim JH, Kocaturk O, Ozturk C, et al: Mitral cerclage annuloplasty, a novel transcatheter treatment for secondary mitral valve regurgitation: initial results in swine, *J Am Coll Cardiol* 54(7):638–651, Aug 11 2009.

32. Rogers JH, Macoviak JA, Rahdert DA, et al: Percutaneous septal sinus shortening. a novel procedure for the treatment of functional mitral regurgitation, *Circulation* 113(19):2329–2334, May 16 2006.

33. Palacios IF, Condado JA, Brandi S, et al: Safety and feasibility of acute percutaneous septal sinus shortening: first-in-human experience, *Catheter Cardiovasc Interv* 69(4):513–518, Mar 1 2007.

34. Burr LH, Krayenbuhl C, Sutton MS: The mitral plication suture: a new technique of mitral valve repair, *J Thorac Cardiovasc Surg* 73(4):589–595, Apr 1977.

35. Aybek T, Risteski P, Miskovic A, et al: Seven years' experience with suture annuloplasty for mitral valve repair, *J Thorac Cardiovasc Surg* 131(1):99–106, Jan 2006.

36. Nagy ZL, Bodi A, Vaszily M, et al: Five-year experience with a suture annuloplasty for mitral valve repair, *Scand Cardiovasc J* 34(5):528–532, Oct 2000.

37. Heuser RR, Witzel T, Dickens D, et al: Percutaneous treatment for mitral regurgitation: the QuantumCor system, *J Interv Cardiol* 21(2):178–182, Apr 2008.

38. Mishra YK, Mittal S, Jaguri P, et al: Coapsys mitral annuloplasty for chronic functional ischemic MR: 1-year results, *Ann Thorac Surg* 81(1):42–46, Jan 2006.

39. Magne J, Girerd N, Senechal M, et al: Mitral repair versus replacement for ischemic MR: comparison of short-term and long-term survival, *Circulation* 120(Suppl 11):S104–S111, Sep 15 2009.

40. Banai S, Jolicoeur EM, Schwartz M, et al: Tiara: a novel catheter-based mitral valve bioprosthesis: initial experiments and short-term pre-clinical results, *J Am Coll Cardiol* 60(15):1430–1431, Oct 9 2012.

Chapter 11

The MitraClip Device and Procedural Overview

D. SCOTT LIM

11.1 Key Points

- Percutaneous transcatheter therapies for mitral regurgitation (MR) have found a role for patients at high operative risk with both degenerative and functional pathologies.
- The MitraClip (Abbott Vascular Structural Heart, Menlo Park, Calif.) therapy utilizes a catheter-based system to deliver a clip-type implant to provide apposition between anterior and posterior mitral leaflets.
- Careful patient selection with a thoughtful eye to appropriate mitral pathology remains paramount for success with the MitraClip.
- Technical success is dependent on skill with echocardiographic imaging, with three-dimensional transesophageal echocardiography (TEE) being particularly valuable.

11.2 Background

MR from nonrheumatic etiology may be the result of either degenerative valve disease, such as prolapse, chordal rupture, or myxomatous degeneration, or of functional etiologies such as ischemic cardiomyopathy and secondary MR. Additionally, as surgical or transcatheter therapies focus on functional etiologies of MR, the knowledge base of how the disease of the ventricle affects the mitral apparatus will increase. Significant MR (3+ or 4+) occurs in 0.5% of the population,[1] with approximately 250,000 new cases annually in the United States. For patients with significant organic MR, medical therapy has been shown to be ineffective in treating the underlying pathophysiology and is unable to retard disease progression. Surgical repair or replacement is the standard of care, because it is efficacious and low risk.[2] However, it has been estimated that only about 20% of patients with significant MR undergo surgery. Therefore there is a significant unmet therapeutic need for patients with mitral valve regurgitation, and particularly for patients at high surgical risk, a significant opportunity for novel catheter-based therapies.

11.3 Adapted from a Surgical Approach to Mitral Regurgitation

Currently, surgery for MR has become a mature therapy, with a wide range of different techniques involving leaflet, chordal, and annular approaches. Concepts behind each of these approaches have been used by novel transcatheter approaches to repair of MR. Additionally, work continues to create a transcatheter replacement option for mitral valve disease.

11.4 MitraClip System

This novel percutaneous approach was the first to achieve success in prehuman and clinical trials for treatment of patients with nonrheumatic MR. The concept of grasping a leaflet with a clip mechanism on the regurgitant portions of the mitral valve became the hallmark of the final design iteration of the MitraClip (Figure 11–1).[3,4] The MitraClip is introduced from a percutaneous, transvenous, transseptal approach to the mitral valve (Figure 11–2). The traditional imaging modality in the catheterization lab of fluoroscopy is of limited utility in this procedure, because it cannot visualize the mitral leaflets. Therefore the procedure is guided by simultaneous transesophageal imaging, ideally using both two- and three-dimensional echocardiography (Figures 11–3 and 11–4). Combined with the reality that the MitraClip delivery system is manipulated by a mechanical-based device, it is more important that the valve interventionalist be skilled in transesophageal imaging than in the standard catheter and wire skills.

When the MitraClip is placed on the central portions of the anterior and posterior leaflets, it acts to anchor prolapsing or flail segments, as well as coapt tethered

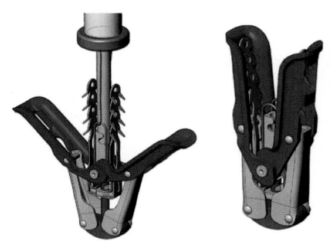

Figure 11–1 A schematic view of the MitraClip, used for percutaneous repair of MR, is shown. The blue arms are mechanically hinged and allow the operator to change the angle between them. These arms are designed to be pulled up from the ventricular side of the mitral leaflets to bring them together. The reddish spiked frictional elements may be lowered onto the atrial side of the leaflets, thereby sandwiching each leaflet between the blue arm and the red frictional element. *(Image provided courtesy of Abbott Vascular Structural Heart, Menlo Park, Calif.)*

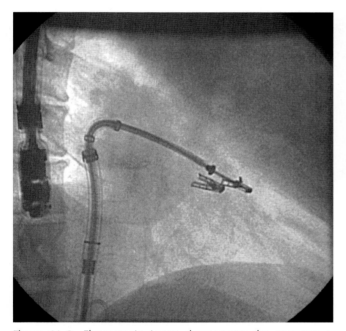

Figure 11–2 Fluoroscopic image demonstrates the transvenous, transseptal approach to introduce the MitraClip to the mitral valve.

leaflets so that it reduces the time and force required to close the valve. By decreasing MR, the left ventricular (LV) volumes are in turn reduced, leading to beneficial left ventricular remodeling.[5] Anatomically, the MitraClip creates a tissue bridge between the two leaflets that limits dilation of the mitral annulus in the septal–lateral dimension, which supports the durability of this repair.[4]

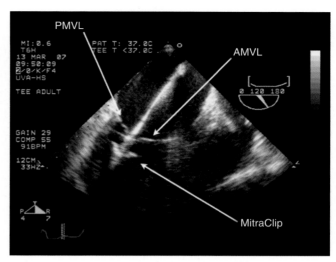

Figure 11–3 Two-dimensional TEE image of the MitraClip and its orientation to the anterior *(AMVL)* and posterior mitral valve leaflets *(PMVL)* is shown. This three-chamber view of the mitral valve is used to orient the MitraClip in an anteroposterior direction on the valve.

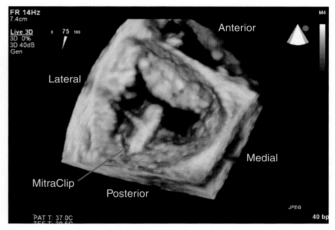

Figure 11–4 Three-dimensional TEE image of the MitraClip and its orientation to the mitral valve is shown. The arms of the MitraClip are oriented perpendicular to the line of coaptation of the valve and over the point of pathology. To maintain operator orientation, the atrial septum is on the right side of the screen, with the aortic valve at approximately the 12 o'clock position.

11.5 EVEREST I and II Trials

This MitraClip approach to percutaneous mitral valve repair was evaluated in the EVEREST trials. EVEREST I was the safety and feasibility registry and enrolled 55 patients in a nonrandomized clinical trial.[6] EVEREST II was the pivotal clinical trial in which 279 patients with 3+ or 4+ MR were randomized to either MitraClip therapy or standard surgical therapy (either mitral valve repair or replacement).[7,8] It is important to note that this involved patients at low and moderate risk, in contrast to the EVEREST High Risk Registry, which enrolled 79 patients who were nonoperative candidates to the MitraClip therapy. In the early nonrandomized experience with the MitraClip, procedural success (reduction of MR to 2+ or less) was achieved in 74%, and 66% were free from death, mitral valve surgery, or MR greater than 2+ at 12 months.[8] These outcomes were similar for those with either degenerative (79%) or functional (21%) etiology of MR. It is also important to note that this represents the initial experience with this novel technology that has a steep learning curve.

The randomized EVEREST II trial included patients who were operative candidates for either moderately severe or severe MR. Patients were either symptomatic, with a left ventricular ejection fraction (LVEF) greater than 25% and left ventricular end-systolic dimension (LVESD) of less than 55 mm, or they were asymptomatic with ventricular dysfunction (defined as LVEF of 25% to 60% or LVESD greater than 40 mm) or pulmonary hypertension. Patients were excluded if they had need for other cardiac surgery, recent acute myocardial infarction (within 12 weeks), severe renal insufficiency (creatinine greater than 2.5 mg/dL), endocarditis, or rheumatic etiology of valvar dysfunction. Additionally, patients were excluded for certain anatomic issues of the mitral valve: stenosis with mitral valve area of less than 4.0 cm^2, a severely broad flail width (>15 mm) and flail gap (>10 mm), or deficient coaptation length (<2 mm).

Compared with patients from either the Society of Thoracic Surgery database[9] or those undergoing first time elective mitral valve surgery,[10] those enrolling in the EVEREST II trial were significantly older with more comorbidities. This likely is because of the preference for the initial experience with novel percutaneous therapies to be reserved for patients who are less ideal surgical candidates. This randomized trial was designed to have a primary safety endpoint powered for a superiority hypothesis—for major adverse events at 30 days. The primary effectiveness endpoint was powered for a noninferiority hypothesis—for the 12-month composite of freedom from death, mitral valve surgery, reoperation, or MR greater than 2+. Additional endpoints included echocardiographic-assessed MR severity, left ventricular function, New York Heart Association (NYHA) functional class, and quality of life indices.

From the primary safety endpoint, with an intention to treat statistical analysis, those randomized to the MitraClip arm had a major adverse event rate of 15% at 30 days, versus those in the surgical arm who had an event rate of 48% (psup < 0.0001).[7] Further detailed analyses of the major adverse events such as death, stroke, reoperation, or emergent surgery demonstrated no such events occurring in patients receiving the MitraClip alone, but adverse events occurred in those crossing over to surgical therapy after unsuccessful MitraClip therapy. Therefore in a per-protocol analysis, which evaluates just the performance of the device alone rather than a strategy approach, the major adverse event rate was under 10% at 30 days.

From the primary effectiveness endpoint, in terms of the clinical composite of freedom from death, mitral valve surgery/reoperation, or MR greater than 2+ at 12 months with an intention to treat analysis, the MitraClip arm had a success rate of 55% versus the surgical arm,

which had a success rate of 73% (pNI < 0.0012). At 24 months, the primary effectiveness rate dropped in both groups to 52% and 66%.[7] Further analysis of the events driving the composite endpoint demonstrates that there was no significant difference between the MitraClip arm and the surgical control arm with respect to death or freedom from severe MR, but that the difference in composite endpoints was the result of a difference in subsequent surgery for mitral valve dysfunction (p < 0.001). MR reduction to the goal and maintenance at 12 and 24 months of 2+ or less was achieved in 81% of the patients receiving the MitraClip, versus 97% of patients who had surgery, although this was achieved by mitral valve replacement in 12% of surgical patients. Despite this difference in echocardiographic-measured MR reduction, there were similar reductions in left ventricular dimensions and volumes achieved at up to 24 months. Interestingly, the left ventricular volumes continued to remodel beneficially between 1 and 2 years. Additionally and paradoxically, despite the differences in apparent MR reduction, there were a greater percentage of patients from the MitraClip arm who were asymptomatic or minimally symptomatic at 24 months (98%), versus those in the surgical arm (88%). Some of these apparent inconsistencies may be because of the difficulties in quantifying the degree of residual MR after a MitraClip has been placed in the center of the valve.

Quality of life indices, as measured by a Short Form (SF)-36 survey, demonstrated improved scores on both physical and mental evaluations in the MitraClip arm at 30 days, versus impaired physical and indeterminate mental scores at 30 days in the surgical arm. At 12 months, there were improvements in all study arms.

11.6 EVEREST High-Risk Registry

A separate United States registry was created for patients who were nonoperative candidates with severe MR that was of either degenerative (prolapse or flail) or functional etiologies (MR secondary to ischemic or nonischemic cardiomyopathy), the EVEREST High Risk Registry. This registry enrolled 79 patients rapidly, because there was significant support for it from surgical colleagues. The majority of patients in the EVEREST High Risk Registry had functional etiology of their MR, as would be expected from finding more patients with ischemic etiologies in a higher risk subgroup. Additionally, patients were older (average age of 76 years, with 68% over age 75 years) and more symptomatic (New York Heart Association functional class III or IV in 89%) than the randomized EVEREST population.

Data presented showed that whereas at 30 days the predicted mortality for the group was 18%, the actual mortality was under 8%, with 76% surviving at 1 year and 79% of the survivors in New York Heart Association symptom class I or II.[11] In a nonrandomized comparison to similar high-risk patients treated medically, there was a survival advantage at 1 year, with 76% alive in the MitraClip group, versus 55% in the medically treated group (p = 0.037). This data gives support to the concept that

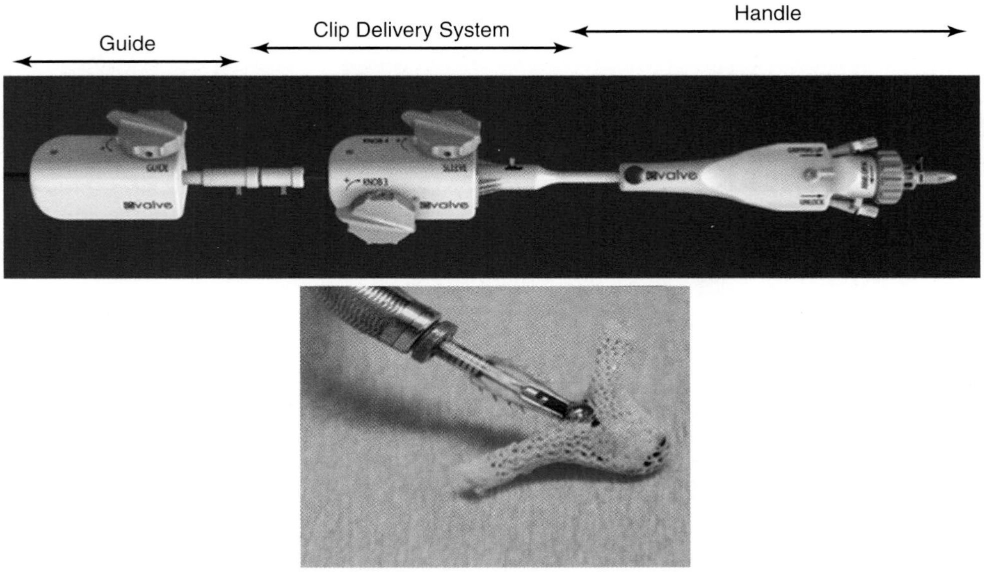

Figure 11–5 The mechanical MitraClip system is controlled by knobs and levers on a complex handle system that in turn actuates wires running the length of the catheter. The proximal part contains the controls to the steerable and deflectable guide, which essentially is a 24F system to deliver the MitraClip-containing catheter to the left atrium. The middle section is the Clip Delivery System, and the distal part is the control handle.

particularly for those patients who are not candidates for surgery, novel percutaneous options are attractive.

In Europe, along with the MitraClip having become a commercially available therapy, there is an ongoing nonrandomized registry collecting clinical and health economic data on treatment options for MR. Based on physician and patient choice, patients either receive MitraClip therapy, medical management, or standard surgical therapy. The patients undergoing MitraClip therapy continue to be older (41% older than age 75 years), with more comorbidities (49% with cardiomyopathy, 45% with renal disease, and 19% with lung disease), and at high risk (average logistic EuroSCORE predicting mortality in 20%). Interestingly, unlike the U.S. experience, 87% had functional etiology (either underlying ischemic or nonischemic cardiomyopathy as causes of MR) and 41% had LVEFs between 10% and 30%. It is evident that the "sweet spot" for patient selection for this therapy is those patients who are not ideal operative candidates.

Not all patients who have undergone percutaneous mitral valve repair with the MitraClip will have adequate reduction of MR or perfect durability of that repair. Clearly the time and energy spent up front with appropriate patient selection will pay dividends in terms of outcomes. However, for those patients who have inadequate or nonsustained MR reduction after MitraClip implantation, subsequent surgical repair has been performed. The rate of surgical repair of MR after MitraClip implantation was 89% (n = 20), which compares favorably to the repair rate in those randomized to the surgical control arm of EVEREST II (86%, n = 69), or as found in the 2007 Society of Thoracic Surgery database (59%). Anterior or bileaflet disease was an independent predictor of mitral valve replacement after MitraClip therapy, but age, etiology, or surgeon experience was not. Additionally, successful mitral valve surgery has been performed up to 5 years after MitraClip implantation, and in these small numbers of patients, it does not appear that increasing time decreases the repair rate.[12]

TECHNICAL AND EQUIPMENT ISSUES

The MitraClip system is designed to deliver the MitraClip to the mitral leaflets and is comprised of a steerable and deflectable guide, a Clip Delivery System, and a control handle **(Figure 11–5).** The steerable guide has a diameter of 24F at the skin entrance and tapers to 22F diameter as it crosses the atrial septum. The control knob on its handle allows the distal tip of the steerable guide to be either deflected or straightened. The steerable guide is placed within a stabilizer unit, which allows the guide to be iteratively advanced or retracted, as well as rotated. After a transseptal puncture, a stiff 0.035-inch guidewire is placed into the left atrium. Over this guidewire the steerable guide is advanced with a dilator in place. The distal tip of the dilator has a spiral groove cut into it, facilitating echocardiographic visualization. After identification of the guide into the left atrium, the dilator is removed and the guide is secured using the stabilizer unit. The MitraClip and Clip Delivery System are then inserted into the steerable guide and keyed into the precut channels within the guide, ensuring proper orientation **(Figure 11–6).** The Clip Delivery System is advanced until the radiopaque double markers are aligned with the distal thicker radiopaque band of the steerable guide. During this advancement, care must be taken to visualize the distal tip of the MitraClip by echocardiography to make sure that it is not inadvertently advanced out the back wall of the left atrium.

The two knobs on the handle of the Clip Delivery System allow deflection of the catheter in medial and lateral directions, as well as anterior and posterior directions. These deflection mechanisms are used to orient the MitraClip coaxial to the mitral valve and positioned over the point of leaflet pathology.

The MitraClip control handle adjusts the mechanism within the MitraClip **(Figure 11–7)**. The handle itself may be advanced or retracted in order to advance or retract the catheter on which the MitraClip is mounted. The

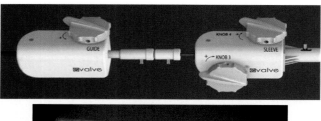

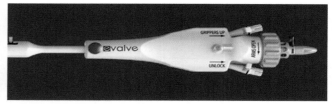

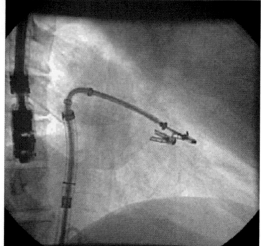

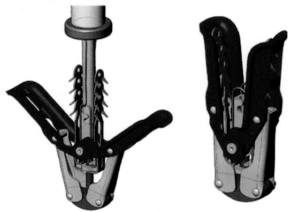

Figure 11–6 The Clip Delivery System fits in a keyed groove in the steerable guide, and the top and side knobs then control anterior/posterior and medial/lateral defections of the catheter.

Figure 11–7 The handle controls actuate the MitraClip's functions, with the rotary knob in *light blue (top)* controlling the angle of the clip arms *(dark blue)* and the gripper lever raising and lowering the frictional gripper elements *(brown)* on the MitraClip.

handle may also be rotated to change the angle of the MitraClip's arms relative to the line of coaptation of the mitral valve. In order to change the angle of the arms of the MitraClip, the lock lever is opened, and then the rotary knob is rotated counterclockwise **(Figure 11–7, blue)**. The MitraClip arms are opened to 180 degrees for optimal visualization of their position relative to the valve leaflets, closed to 120 degrees for performing a grab of the leaflets, and closed to approximately 60 degrees after the grab. Once adequate leaflet insertion has been confirmed, they may be closed fully. Additionally, the arms may be inverted to allow retraction of the clip back into the atrium without interfering with the mitral leaflet tissue. The other lever on the handle controls the frictional gripper elements **(Figure 11–7, brown)**. After grabbing the mitral leaflets, these are rapidly lowered into place, sandwiching the mitral leaflets between the frictional gripper elements and the MitraClip arms.

After a successful grab with adequate leaflet insertion between the MitraClip arm and gripper, the entire system may be detached from the MitraClip by successive removal of the lock line, control shaft, and gripper line.

PROPER PATIENT SELECTION

Many of the aspects of percutaneous mitral valve therapies rely on skills and technology not usually available to the standard cardiac interventionalist. Therefore collaboration for both patient selection as well as procedural success is required between interventionalists, echocardiologists, and cardiac surgeons.

Key in patient selection is understanding the different pathologic subtypes of MR, both degenerative and functional. In degenerative MR, open surgical mitral valve repair by skilled mitral surgeons has proven to be of high success and low risk in most patients. Therefore it is important to delineate which mitral pathology may not be amenable to repair and thus in need of mitral valve replacement. Additionally, it is important to define the type of degenerative pathology likely to have success with the MitraClip: central, relatively narrow prolapse, or flail segments. Unlike surgical approaches that have had demonstrably better success with posterior pathology, the MitraClip has had success with both anterior and posterior leaflet disease. Less experience is available for commissural pathology (such as a flail P1 segment) with the MitraClip, although it is the author's personal experience that it can be successfully treated.

For functional MR, it is important to determine whether the patient with ischemic cardiomyopathy has a need for concomitant revascularization. It is also important, although difficult, to determine whether the patient's primary issue is pump failure versus MR, because that will have bearing on whether the patient's needs are able to be met by the MitraClip.

Imaging with both transthoracic and TEE is paramount for proper patient selection. The screening transthoracic echocardiogram is used to determine severity of MR, presence of mitral stenosis, and left ventricular function. Patients with a mitral valve area of less than 4 cm^2 are at risk of developing significant mitral stenosis after the MitraClip procedure.

The screening TEE is used to determine the mechanism of MR. Patients with complex degenerative pathology including particularly wide flails or mixed disease (i.e., restrictive posterior leaflet with commissural flail segment) are unlikely to experience success with the MitraClip. Three-dimensional TEE is helpful for understanding the complex pathology in its entirety.

Lastly, the MitraClip therapy has not been found to be ideal for emergency use nor as a bastion of last hope. Patients with hemodynamic instability are unlikely to benefit solely from correction of their MR, nor would patients who are truly end-stage.

PRACTICAL PROCEDURAL ISSUES

The MitraClip procedure, with its current dependence on TEE, is primarily performed when the patient is under general anesthesia. Patients are almost always hemodynamically quite stable during the procedure. Therefore additional arterial or central venous lines for monitoring or infusions are often not needed. A urinary catheter is placed and removed 24 hours later. Because MR, and particularly functional MR, is dynamically affected by volume and systemic vascular resistance, those patient variables may be augmented to assess the degree of MR after placement of a MitraClip. Because the fasting state and general anesthesia can artificially lower systemic blood pressure, the patient may be challenged with a bolus dose of phenylephrine to raise the systemic blood pressure to at least the normotensive range before the interventionist decides about the end result of the MitraClip procedure.

During the case, prophylactic antibiotics are given, and after transseptal puncture unfractionated heparin is given to raise the activated clotting time above 250 seconds. Additional bolus doses of heparin are given to maintain this range. At the conclusion of the procedure, protamine is given to reverse the heparin. The venotomy site can be closed with a subcutaneous figure-eight stitch to achieve hemostasis **(Figure 11–8)**. The stitch is removed the next morning. Other closure methods include the use of manual compression or predeployment of 1 or 2 6F ProGlide sutures.

The transseptal puncture is a key part of the MitraClip procedure and is different than that performed for diagnostic, electrophysiologic, or mitral stenosis purposes. Since the MitraClip system is a mechanical one, the location of the transseptal puncture must be precise relative to the point of pathology of the mitral valve and its relationship to the atrial septum. The direction of the transseptal system arising from the inferior vena cava is usually through the center of the fossa ovalis in an anterior vector **(Figure 11–9, _dotted arrow_; Video 11–1).** However, for the MitraClip system to work efficiently, the MitraClip needs to be positioned over the line of coaptation of the mitral valve, which is a posterior structure. Therefore a transseptal position that is posterior is often desired **(Figure 11–9, _solid arrow_).** If an anterior transseptal puncture is performed, the MitraClip system can still work, but the complicated curves that are required on the catheter and Clip Delivery System make for a prolonged procedure **(Video 11–2).** Nevertheless, there occasionally is the unusual lie of the heart such that the mitral valve is anterior, and therefore a direct puncture

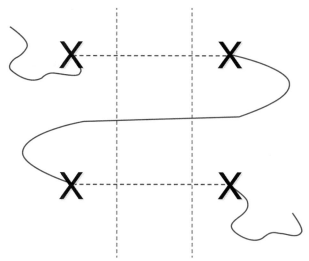

Figure 11–8 Figure-eight stich technique. This technique can be used to achieve hemostasis in the right femoral vein after removal of the 24F MitraClip guiding catheter. The vein is represented by the orange dotted lines. The suture is shown as a _blue line_. The suture is subcutaneous, as represented by the _blue dotted line,_ and external as shown by the _solid blue lines._ The X's represent the skin entry sites of the suture. The free ends of the suture are pulled tight, and after durable hemostasis is obtained, the suture is cut and removed (generally the next morning).

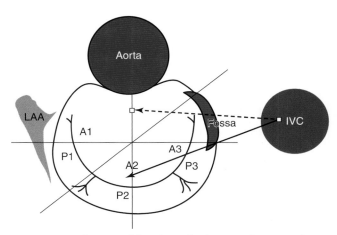

Figure 11–9 Schematic of the relationship between the points of transseptal puncture and the mitral valve. Note that the standard transseptal location through the fossa ovalis would create an anterior direction into the left atrium _(dotted line)._ In order to position the MitraClip system over the mitral valve, a more posterior direction to the transseptal is often desired _(solid line)._ (IVC, Inferior vena cava; LAA, left atrial appendage.)

through the center of the fossa ovalis will bring the catheter and MitraClip directly down onto the valve **(Video 11–3).** To determine this, the author preplans the transseptal puncture by using three-dimensional TEE. During the actual transseptal puncture, however, 2-dimensional TEE (and not on fluoroscopy) is used. A bicaval view first demonstrates fossa and septal anatomy, as well as tenting of the transseptal dilator against the septum. Then switch to a short axis view (≈45 degrees on the TEE multiplane) in which the tenting on the septum demonstrates its anterior/posterior relationship **(Video 11–4).** It is important to visualize the line of coaptation of the mitral valve and realize that this is posterior in most.

Again, because the MitraClip system is a mechanical system, it must be positioned a precise distance above the pathology on the mitral valve. The 4-chamber TEE view **(Video 11–5)** may be used to determine whether the point of tenting on the atrial septum is 4 cm above that location. It is also important to be aware that in restrictive leaflet pathology this point may be in the ventricle, as opposed to prolapse or flail in which it is in the atrium.

After placement of the MitraClip and Clip Delivery System into the left atrium, steering involves medial deflection using the "M" knob on the Clip Delivery System with anterior and posterior course corrections (counterclockwise and clockwise torque on the steerable guide). This is guided by short-axis, two-chamber, and left ventricular outflow tract (LVOT) views from the two-dimensional TEE **(Videos 11–6, 11–7, and 11–8)**. Alternatively, efficient guiding of the system through the left atrium can be accomplished using three-dimensional TEE imagery from the back of the left atrium. To standardize the three-dimensional view, the aortic valve is placed at the 12 o'clock position with the atrial septum at the 3 o'clock position **(Video 11–9)**. The settings are maximized to visualize both the mitral valve and as much of the far atrial walls as possible **(Video 11–10)**. In addition to guiding left atrial navigation of the MitraClip and Clip Delivery System, three-dimensional TEE is useful for orienting the MitraClip arms so that they are perpendicular to the line of mitral valve coaptation, which is necessary to facilitate a grab on the leaflets **(Video 11–11)**. **Video 11–12** shows the entire procedure in animation format.

POTENTIAL COMPLICATIONS AND MANAGEMENT

In the EVEREST randomized clinical trial, complications directly related to the MitraClip procedure were quite rare, and its safety profile was remarkable. Although complications may ensue from anesthesia or the TEE, careful attention to detail by all members of the heart valve team can help mitigate these. Relevant to the MitraClip delivery system, the venous access is 24F at the skin. Despite this large bore, venous vascular complications have not been reported. However, complications have ensued relative to the transseptal puncture, including pericardial effusions and tamponade related to puncturing the back wall of the atrium or anteriorly into the aortic root. Careful echocardiographic guidance (and reliance on echocardiography rather than fluoroscopy) can help prevent this as well as help the interventionist be alert for the appearance of a pericardial effusion. As in all left atrial procedures, air embolism is a risk. This may be mitigated by careful aspiration and flushing of the steerable guide, as well as having the Clip Delivery System attached to continuous flushes. It also is helpful to visualize the distal tip of the steerable guide to make sure that it is not up against tissue, in which case aspiration of air into the system upon withdrawal of the catheter can occur.

The MitraClip, being a mechanical system, can malfunction. Awareness of its parts and mechanical function is helpful for problem solving such mechanical malfunctions. With overtightening of the medial deflection cables on the Clip Delivery System (M knob actuation) past 90 degrees there is a risk of creating a permanent bend or set in the catheter, which can make the delivery of the MitraClip difficult. This can be noted by use of fluoroscopy with advancement of the clip into the ventricle. If degree of catheter set is pronounced, it is recommended to change out the system for a new one.

With all complications, the keys are awareness for their occurrence and having a backup plan available.

11.7 Summary

Just as the previous decade comprised a marked explosion in the utility and maturity of transcatheter interventions for coronary artery disease, the next decade will bear a similar focus on transcatheter approaches to heart valve disease. The MitraClip system represents a first generation step in this direction and is remarkable for its success as such. There is complexity both to the mechanical MitraClip system, as well as to the understanding of the mitral pathology. However, both can be mastered with time. As is true with many things, the pendulum of excitement for these novel technologies will initially swing a bit farther than where the real utility of these approaches will truly lie, and careful patient selection will be imperative.

REFERENCES

1. Jones EC, Devereux RB, Roman MJ, et al: Prevalence and correlates of mitral regurgitation in a population-based sample (the Strong Heart Study), Am J Cardiol 87(3):298–304, 2001.
2. Gammie JS, Sheng S, Griffith BP, et al: Trends in mitral valve surgery in the United States: results from the Society of Thoracic Surgeons Adult Cardiac Surgery Database, Ann Thorac Surg 87(5):1431–1437, 2009, discussion 1437–1439.
3. Fann JI, St Goar FG, Komtebedde J, et al: Beating heart catheter-based edge-to-edge mitral valve procedure in a porcine model: efficacy and healing response, Circulation 110(8):988–993, 2004.
4. St Goar FG, Fann JI, Komtebedde J, et al: Endovascular edge-to-edge mitral valve repair: short-term results in a porcine model, Circulation 108(16):1990–1993, 2003.
5. Herrmann HC, Kar S, Siegel R, et al: Effect of percutaneous mitral repair with the MitraClip device on mitral valve area and gradient, EuroIntervention 4(4):437–442, 2009.
6. Feldman T, Wasserman HS, Herrmann HC, et al: Percutaneous mitral valve repair using the edge-to-edge technique: six-month results of the EVEREST Phase I clinical trial, J Am Coll Cardiol 46(11):2134–2140, 2005.
7. Feldman T, Foster E, Glower DD, et al: Percutaneous repair or surgery for mitral regurgitation, N Engl J Med 364(15):1395–1406, 2011.
8. Feldman T, Kar S, Rinaldi M, et al: Percutaneous mitral repair with the MitraClip system: safety and midterm durability in the initial EVEREST (Endovascular Valve Edge-to-Edge REpair Study) cohort, J Am Coll Cardiol 54(8):686–694, 2009.
9. STS National Database. Mitral valve repair and replacement patients. Incidence of complications summary. Society of Thoracic Surgeons, Ann Thorac Surg 2009.
10. Gammie JS, O'Brien SM, Griffith BP, et al: Influence of hospital procedural volume on care process and mortality for patients undergoing elective surgery for mitral regurgitation, Circulation 115(7):881–887, 2007.
11. Whitlow PL, et al: MitraClip therapy in the EVEREST High Risk Registry: one year results, EuroIntervention 4:437–442, 2008.
12. Rogers JH, Yeo KK, Carroll JD, et al: Late surgical mitral valve repair after percutaneous repair with the MitraClip system, J Card Surg 24(6):677–681, 2009.

Chapter 12

Percutaneous Repair of Paravalvular Leaks

AMAR KRISHNASWAMY • E. MURAT TUZCU • SAMIR R. KAPADIA

Paravalvular leak (PVL) complicating mechanical or bioprosthetic surgical valve replacement is an uncommon but occasional occurrence. Various series have demonstrated an incidence of 2% to 12% after mitral valve replacement (MVR) and 1% to 5% after aortic valve replacement (AVR). Furthermore, transcatheter aortic valve replacement (TAVR) is a burgeoning technology, with moderate to severe aortic regurgitation (AR) in up to 17% of patients, the majority of whom have paravalvular AR (PAR).[1] Given the magnitude of individuals in the United States and worldwide who undergo each of these operations, there are a large number of patients each year who suffer from PVL.

Most patients with PVL need treatment within the first year after valve replacement.[2] These patients usually suffer from symptoms of congestive heart failure (CHF) (85%), though hemolysis is also common (13% to 47% of patients).[3] The risk for PVL is greater for mechanical prostheses, and it is higher among patients with calcified annuli, those undergoing valve replacement for infective endocarditis, and patients with a history of previous valve surgery in the same position. Each of these factors provides a predisposition to improper suturing of the valve ring into the annulus.

Whereas medical therapy of CHF and erythropoietic agents with periodic blood transfusion for anemia may be adequate therapy for some patients, a number of others remain significantly debilitated by PVL. Unfortunately, reoperation for PVL is fraught with a high recurrence rate and carries with it the inherent morbidity and mortality risks of redo open heart surgery (OHS). Furthermore, sick patients with CHF facing redo OHS face a much higher mortality from the operation than healthy patients undergoing a first valve surgery, and subsequent redo operations carry risk that is even higher still.

As a result, structural interventionalists have become increasingly interested in developing percutaneous methods for PVL closure. Since the first reports of the procedure in 1992, a number of series have been published with encouraging rates of procedural success and good clinical outcomes.[4–7] This chapter will provide an overview of the imaging, techniques, devices, and outcomes of percutaneous mitral and aortic PVL closure. Although not specifically addressed, closure of tricuspid valve ring or prosthetic leaks is feasible using similar methods and devices.

12.1 Imaging

As with all structural cardiac interventions, multimodality imaging is imperative to a safe and successful procedure. The mainstays of diagnosis are transthoracic echocardiography (TTE) and transesophageal echocardiography (TEE). During the percutaneous PVL closure procedure, two-dimensional (2D) and three-dimensional (3D) TEE, intracardiac echocardiography (ICE), fluoroscopy/angiography, and more recently computed tomography (CT)–fluoroscopy fusion may all be used.

PREPROCEDURAL ECHOCARDIOGRAPHY

For most patients, the diagnosis of valvular regurgitation and PVL is made by TTE. It should be noted, however, that because of shielding from prosthetic valves, regurgitation may not be well visualized on the TTE. Furthermore the eccentric nature of most PVLs makes diagnosis of regurgitation severity more difficult, because routine parameters such as size of the color-flow jet or the proximal isovolumic surface area may be significantly underestimated. Therefore further imaging either with TEE or angiography is recommended in cases when the clinical presentation and TTE are incongruent.

Performance of a percutaneous PVL closure requires precise definition of the leak origin in order to properly direct wires and devices to the area. Preprocedural echocardiography is therefore important not only to define the degree of PVL, but also to identify the exact origin of the regurgitant jet and allow for procedural planning before the patient's arrival in the catheterization lab or hybrid operating room.

Localization of Mitral Paravalvular Leak

For the sake of consistency in nomenclature, the mitral valve (MV) is viewed as a clock face, and leak origin defined by the position on the clock **(Figure 12–1).** Using TTE, the parasternal short-axis image is useful, displaying the MV as a clock face that allows an easy definition of the PVL origin **(Figure 12–2).** In a large surgical series, the most common location for mitral PVL was anteromedial (between hours 10 and 11) and posterolateral (between hours 5 and 6).[3] Similar analysis of a percutaneous series revealed the most common mitral PVLs between 10 and 2 o'clock (45%) and between 6 and 10 o'clock (37%).[6]

When using TEE, localizing the PVL requires a reconstruction of the clock face in the mind of the operator. **Figure 12–3** demonstrates the clock-face orientation of the MV with TEE angles listed around the periphery of the valve showing which parts of the MV are interrogated at each angle. Movement of the TEE probe cranial and caudal with anteflexion or retroflexion of the imaging crystal cuts the valve at planes parallel to those listed.

An example of PVL localization by TEE is given in **Figure 12–4:** In A, the leak origin is shown in the 120-degree view, with the leak in the anterior portion of the MVR; in B, the leak origin is shown in the 30-degree aortic short-axis view, just medial to the aortic valve (AV) (i.e., next to the left coronary cusp). The ultrasound beam at each of these TEE angles is applied to the MV clock-face view in C, with localization of the PVL at the intersection. D confirms the location where an Amplatzer ventricular septal occluder device (St. Jude Medical, St. Paul, Minn.) was subsequently placed.

Localization of Aortic Paravalvular Leak

Position along the perimeter of the aortic valve can also be referenced to a clock face, as shown in **Figure 12–1.** In a large series examining PVL closure, aortic leaks most commonly presented at the 7 to 11 o'clock position (46%), followed by the 11 to 3 o'clock position (36%).[6] Alternatively, operators may choose to identify the origin of the PVL with respect to the native cusp location (i.e., right, left, and noncoronary cusps). This is useful for procedural guidance and for assessing risk of coronary impingement with a device. Whereas the long-axis TTE and TEE views are helpful in defining the anteroposterior relationship of the leak, the short-axis view is most helpful in defining

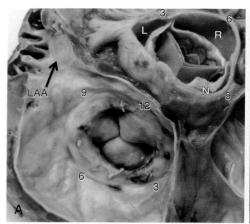
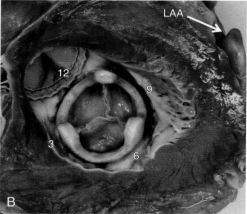

Figure 12–1 Clock-face designation of the mitral and aortic valves from the left atrial side **(A)** and left ventricular side **(B).** *L,* Left coronary cusp; *LAA,* left atrial appendage; *N,* noncoronary cusp; *R,* right coronary cusp.

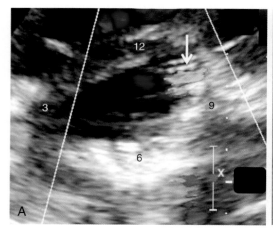
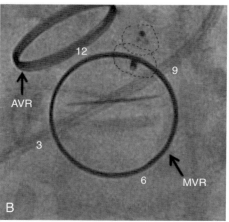

Figure 12–2 A, Transthoracic echocardiogram in a patient with mitral paravalvular leak (PVL). Parasternal short-axis view demonstrates the mitral clock face with the leak at 10 o'clock. **B,** The patient went on to have PVL closure using a 6-mm Amplatzer septal occluder device (left anterior oblique projection). *AVR,* aortic valve replacement; *MVR,* mitral valve replacement.

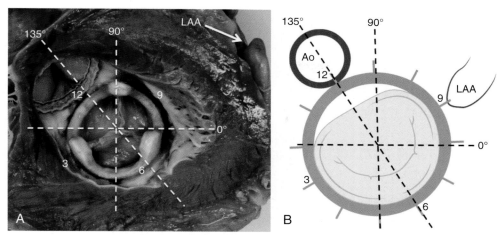

Figure 12–3 Mitral valve (MV) as viewed from the left ventricle. The angles shown refer to the cuts made by a transesophageal echocardiography imaging crystal. The numbers correspond to the clock face perspective of the MV (numbering is as viewed from the left atrium). *Ao,* Aorta; *LAA,* left atrial appendage.

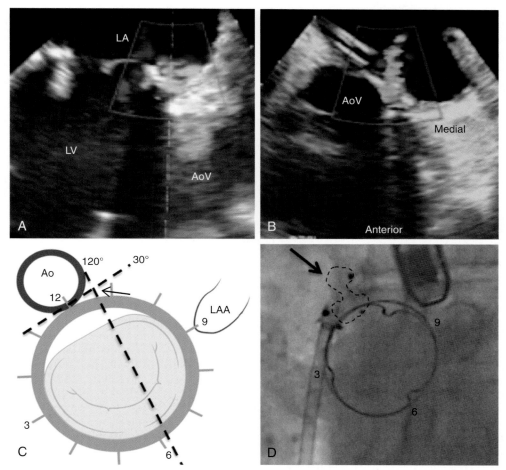

Figure 12–4 **Transesophageal echocardiography (TEE) analysis to determine location of mitral paravalvular leak (PVL). A,** TEE 120-degree view, and **B,** TEE 30-degree short-axis view. **C,** The TEE planes are shown on the mitral valve clock face (LV view) with the intersection *(arrow)* defining the PVL origin. **D,** Deployment of the Amplatzer muscular ventricular septal defect (VSD) occluder *(arrow)* confirms the initial leak localization by TEE (left anterior oblique projection). *AoV,* aortic valve; *LA,* left atrium; *LAA,* left atrial appendage; *LV,* left ventricle.

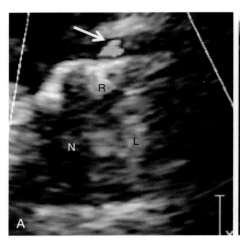

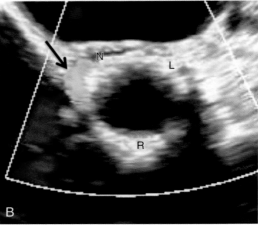

Figure 12–5 **Aortic paravalvular leak localization. A,** Transthoracic echocardiogram parasternal short-axis view, leak at native right coronary cusp. **B,** Transesophageal echocardiogram short-axis view (45°), leak at junction of right and noncoronary cusps. *L,* native left coronary cusp; *N,* native noncoronary cusp; *R,* native right coronary cusp.

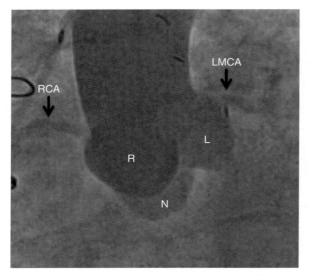

Figure 12–6 Aortic root angiogram in the left anterior oblique projection. *L,* left coronary cusp; *LMCA,* left main coronary artery; *N,* noncoronary cusp; *R,* right coronary cusp; *RCA,* right coronary artery.

the leak with respect to the cusps **(Figure 12–5)**. This relationship allows a simple translation to the fluoroscopic projection of the aortic root **(Figure 12–6)**.

PROCEDURAL ECHOCARDIOGRAPHY

Guidance of the percutaneous PVL closure procedure can be performed using TEE and/or ICE. The authors perform all PVL procedures using only conscious sedation and local anesthetic, and therefore try to minimize the duration of TEE use, instead favoring ICE to direct the procedure until TEE is absolutely necessary **(Figure 12–7)**. Generally, the TEE probe is placed after crossing the leak with a wire and before crossing it with a delivery sheath. In certain situations, ICE is ineffective at properly visualizing the mitral PVL and TEE guidance is necessary for crossing the leak. This is especially true in cases of lateral PVL, where the ICE catheter is furthest away from the leak. ICE is routinely used for transseptal (TS) puncture of the interatrial septum (IAS), and therefore it is already in

place for guidance during mitral PVL procedures that are performed via TS puncture. In patients requiring tricuspid or aortic PVL, an extra femoral venous sheath is placed to introduce the ICE catheter for procedural guidance.

TEE is also integral to the PVL procedure for wire/catheter guidance, evaluation of procedural success and need for additional device(s), and assessment of complications (such as valve impingement by the device). Since ICE and TEE are 2D imaging modalities, the entirety of wires and catheters may not be seen in the left atrium (LA) if the devices are off-axis to the imaging plane. Echocardiographic guidance of the equipment may therefore require constant adjustment of the ICE and/or TEE. On the other hand, real-time 3D TEE provides excellent image resolution and guidance of wires and devices to the site of PVL with minimal manipulation of the imaging probe **(Figure 12–8)**. Because not all probes and TEE machines are capable of real-time 3D imaging, it is important to assure that the proper equipment is on hand before commencing the procedure.

PROCEDURAL FLUOROSCOPY AND ANGIOGRAPHY

Fluoroscopic imaging is routine in catheterization lab procedures. Interventional cardiologists have become accustomed to manipulating wires, catheters, and other devices while observing their movements on the fluoroscopic screen. In the case of mechanical or bioprosthetic valve replacements, an additional degree of guidance is provided by the prosthetic valve/ring. In order to cross the PVL, orthogonal fluoroscopic views are necessary to assure appropriate wire placement in all planes. This is most easily done using a biplane system; in labs without biplane fluoroscopy, repetitively moving the C-arm to each view can be cumbersome but should be done. This is especially important after device deployment in the paravalvular space to assure that prosthetic leaflet motion is not hindered. For mitral PVL, the 30-degree right anterior oblique and left anterior oblique (LAO) caudal (spider) projections are most useful for device placement. For aortic PVL, a shallow LAO projection often provides adequate imaging.

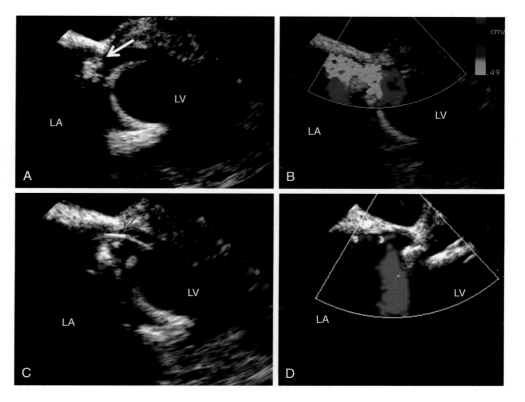

Figure 12–7 Use of intracardiac echocardiography to guide mitral paravalvular leak (PVL) closure. **A,** Two-dimensional view of the PVL *(arrow).* **B,** Color-flow Doppler demonstration of the leak. **C,** Wire across the leak *(arrow).* **D,** Minimal mitral regurgitation after deployment of closure device. *LA,* Left atrium; *LV,* left ventricle.

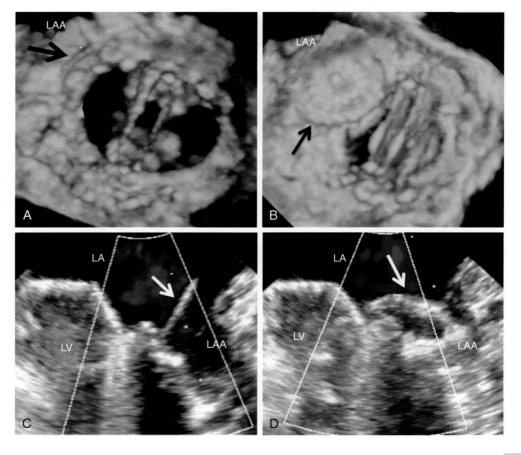

Figure 12–8 Transesophageal echocardiography (**TEE**) guidance of mitral paravalvular leak (**PVL**) closure. Three-dimensional TEE (LA view) shows the wire crossing the PVL (**A**) and the Amplatzer septal occluder device in position (partially in the left atrial appendage *[LAA]*) (**B**). **C** and **D,** Confirmation in two-dimensional TEE view. *LA,* Left atrium; *LV,* left ventricle.

In addition to echocardiography, angiography may be helpful in defining the location of a PVL for procedural guidance **(Figure 12–9)**. However, as the patients who need PVL closure are often sick with numerous comorbidities including chronic kidney disease, angiography is not often used.

PROCEDURAL COMPUTED TOMOGRAPHY–FLUOROSCOPY FUSION IMAGING

Fluoroscopy provides a 2D image of 3D structures. The operator must integrate the 2D and 3D images obtained echocardiographically into his or her mental picture of the intracardiac space to properly guide wires, catheters, and devices to the PVL for percutaneous closure under fluoroscopic guidance. In order to bridge this 2D-to-3D gap,

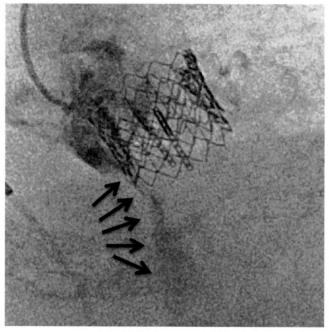

Figure 12–9 Aortic root angiography in a patient with aortic paravalvular leak (PVL) after transcatheter aortic valve replacement (left anterior oblique projection). Transesophageal echocardiography had demonstrated the leak at the junction of the right and noncoronary cusps. Angiography was helpful in delineating the PVL *(arrows)* for subsequent wiring. Closure is demonstrated in **Figure 12-16.**

technologies have been developed to overlay information taken from CT onto the real-time fluoroscopic image.[8]

A thorough description of the fusion process has been previously published (see reference 8), and an overview is given in **Figure 12–10.** In brief, after the initial identification of PVL origin using TTE and/or TEE, a mark is made on the preprocedural CT scan of the PVL. Markings of the proposed TS puncture location are also made to aid guidance of the Brockenbrough needle. CT markings are made of the prosthetic valve, the trachea, and/or other structures to provide assurance of proper image overlay. Upon the patient's arrival to the cardiac catheterization lab, a rotational CT-like image (Syngo DynaCT, Siemens Healthcare, Forchheim, Germany) is obtained to establish the patient orientation on the table. The preprocedural CT is then registered to the procedural DynaCT (3D-3D fusion), and the CT markings can be overlaid onto the real-time fluoroscopic images. This process is quite helpful in directing wires through the PVL, anecdotally reducing procedural time, radiation dose, and TEE duration.

12.2 Techniques for Paravalvular Leak Closure

The ultimate goal of percutaneous PVL closure is to cross the leak with a wire and deliver an occluding device. Many different approaches are employed depending on the location of the PVL, and many different devices are available, though none are designed specifically for this purpose and are repurposed from other settings (i.e., septal defect closure).

ACCESS SITE/APPROACH FOR PARAVALVULAR LEAK CLOSURE

In the case of mitral PVL, the operator must decide on the approach that will allow access to the leak and that provides enough support to deliver the bulky delivery sheath and device to the area. Potential routes for mitral PVL closure include:

1. TS Approach: TS puncture and antegrade access to the mitral PVL is from the LA via a femoral venous sheath. If there is inadequate support to place a delivery sheath with a wire passed into the left

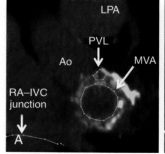
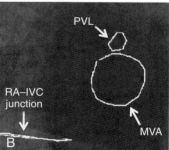
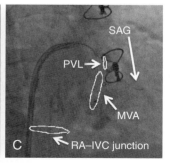

Figure 12–10 Fusion of preprocedural computed tomography (CT) markings to real-time fluoroscopy. **A,** Areas of interest are marked on the preprocedural CT (left anterior oblique [LAO] projection). **B,** The CT markings are overlaid onto the real-time fluoroscopic image in the catheterization lab (LAO). **C,** The PVL marking facilitates crossing the leak with a SAG (right anterior oblique projection). *Ao,* Aorta; *IVC,* inferior vena cava; *LPA,* left pulmonary artery; *MVA,* mitral valve anulus; *PVL,* paravalvular leak; *RA,* right atrium; *SAG,* stiff-angled Glidewire.

ventricle, the wire can be advanced to the descending aorta **(Figure 12–11, A)** (and also snared via the femoral artery if necessary) or snared via a transapical (TA) sheath **(Figure 12–11, B)**. TA snaring may be useful if snaring from the descending aorta results in impingement upon the prosthetic leaflets and hemodynamic compromise or in the presence of a mechanical aortic valve.

2. Femoral Artery Approach: A guiding catheter is advanced across the AV to the left ventricle and the PVL is wired retrograde. This may be accomplished with a Glidewire (Terumo Medical, Somerset, NJ) or even a 0.014-inch coronary wire that can often be "blown through" the mitral PVL. The retrograde wire is then snared via TS puncture and brought to a femoral venous sheath; devices are delivered in an antegrade fashion across the PVL via the femoral vein **(Figure 12–11, C)**. This approach is not feasible if the patient has a mechanical AVR.

3. TA Approach: Direct retrograde wiring is from the left ventricle via TA sheath placement. Devices may be delivered retrograde via a delivery sheath placed in the left ventricular (LV) apex **(Figure 12–11, D)** or in an antegrade fashion after snaring the wire via TS puncture (in order to minimize the LA apical sheath size) **(Figure 12–11, E)**.

The choice of the above approaches must be made on a patient-specific basis. The TS approach is usually favored over the TA approach in order to avoid direct LA apical trauma and the potential complications of sheath insertion therein. Generally, a PVL that is near the anterior and lateral aspects of the MV can be wired via the TS approach.

Leaks that are posterior and medial may be more difficult to engage from the LA because of the acute angles that are presented after TS puncture; therefore the apical or retrograde aortic approaches may be preferred. This is not to say that posterior/medial leaks cannot be fixed via TS puncture, but operators should be aware that failure to cross the PVL antegrade does not imply complete failure of the percutaneous approach in a given patient.

In some rare circumstances, a patient's IAS may be so calcified that TS puncture or advancement of a sheath across the IAS is not possible. Consideration may be given to the application of electrocautery energy to the Brockenbrough TS needle to facilitate puncture. If the TS approach is impossible, TA access or a retrograde femoral artery approach should be considered.

For patients with aortic PVL, the retrograde femoral artery approach is most commonly used. When this is not successful, consideration may be given to the TS or TA approaches. Patients with concomitant mechanical MVR are not candidates for the TS approach. Care must also be taken with the TS approach to avoid creating a taut loop of wire from the IAS to the aorta that can cause MV leaflet impingement (and hence MR) or tear the MV apparatus.

Sheath size is dictated by the choice of approach and expected devices to be delivered (discussed in the following paragraphs). Another consideration is whether multiple devices need to be delivered simultaneously. In this case, a large femoral sheath (i.e., 16F) may be placed to allow placement of two large delivery sheaths across the IAS at the same time.

Transseptal Approach to Mitral Paravalvular Leak Closure

The TS puncture is described in Chapter 4. With respect to PVL closure, however, the specific location of TS puncture should be carefully planned to allow easiest access to the leak. For leaks that are lateral, the usual puncture high on the IAS is reasonable. However, for patients with a more medial leak, a lower and more posterior TS puncture allows

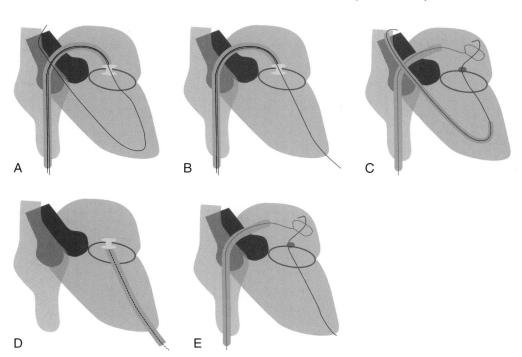

Figure 12–11 Approaches to mitral paravalvular leak closure. A, Antegrade wiring via transseptal (TS) puncture followed by advancement of the wire to the descending aorta. **B,** TS wire is snared via transapical (TA) puncture. **C,** Retrograde wiring from the left ventricle followed by TS puncture and delivery of devices via the antegrade TS approach. **D,** Retrograde wiring and device delivery via TA sheath. **E,** Retrograde wiring via TA approach followed by TS puncture to snare the wire and advance devices in an antegrade fashion. *(Adapted from Kapadia, SR., Tuzcu, EM. Plugging holes.* Circ Cardiovasc Interv *2011; 4: 308-10.)*

more direct/coaxial access to the PVL (**Figure 12–12**). After dilation of the IAS, we prefer to advance an Agilis NxT steerable guide catheter (St. Jude Medical, St. Paul, Minn.) to the LA. The Agilis is an 8.5F (internal diameter) catheter with a deflectable tip and is available with three distal curl options: (1) small (16.8 mm), (2) medium (22.4 mm), and (3) large (50.0 mm). The authors generally use the medium curve for most applications, though the presence of a severely dilated LA may necessitate the large curl, or a significantly acute angle from the IAS to the leak (in the case

of medial PVLs) may require a small curl. Some operators prefer to use a curved-tip guiding catheter such as the JR4, Berenstein, or Hockey Stick instead of the Agilis.

A 120-cm 4F angled glide catheter is then advanced via the Agilis into the LA. The telescopic combination of the angled glide catheter tip and articulation of the Agilis provides a wide range of directions to direct a wire across the leak.[9] A 0.035-inch stiff-angled Glidewire (SAG) is the first choice, but a hydrophilic 0.014-inch coronary wire may be used if the SAG is unsuccessful. Once the wire is across the leak, it is advanced further into the descending aorta. At this point the wire may be snared via femoral artery access if necessary, though simply advancing it to the distal aorta usually provides enough purchase and support for the procedure. If the operator chooses not to advance the wire to the aorta (i.e., in a patient with mechanical AVR), the angled Glide catheter can be advanced to the left ventricle and used to exchange the SAG wire for a stiffer support wire such as an Amplatz Extra Stiff (Cook Medical, Bloomington, Ind.) wire or Lunderquist wire (Cook Medical) if necessary. Care should be taken to make a broad curve on these wires to avoid trauma/perforation of the left ventricle.

The combination of the Agilis and Glide catheter is then removed. A delivery sheath is then advanced over the SAG that is in place across the PVL. Delivery sheath size is based on the size of the device needed. The authors usually use the 8F Amplatzer TorqVue 45-Degree Delivery System (St. Jude Medical). Alternatively, a 6F multipurpose guide catheter can be used, depending on the device that will be delivered to the leak. Once the TorqVue is advanced to the left ventricle, the SAG is removed and the occluder device is loaded into the sheath. The LV disc is then deployed and apposed to the LV side of the leak. The LA side of the device is then exposed. Careful evaluation should be made fluoroscopically and by echo for leak persistence and/or impingement of the device(s) on the prosthetic valve (discussed later). The TS approach is illustrated in **Figure 12–13**.

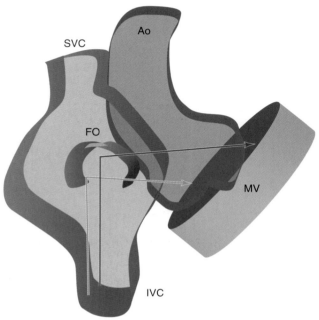

Figure 12–12 Location of transseptal puncture. Typical puncture at the fossa ovalis *(FO; green line)* allows access to the lateral mitral annulus. A low and posterior puncture *(yellow line)* is necessary for access to the medial mitral annulus. *Ao,* Aorta; *IVC,* inferior vena cava; *MV,* mitral valve; *SVC,* superior vena cava. *(Adapted from Yuksel, UC,. et al. Percutaneous closure of a postero-medial mitral paravalvular leak. Catheter Cardiovasc Interv 2011;77:281-5.)*

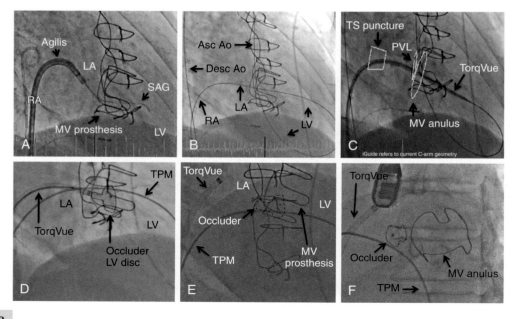

Figure 12–13 Mitral PVL closure via TS approach. A, Agilis steerable catheter in the LA (via right femoral vein), through which an angled glide catheter and SAG was used to cross the leak. **B,** The wire was advanced to the descending aorta for support. **C,** A 9F TorqVue delivery sheath was advanced across the leak to the left ventricle (markings made using DynaCT fusion are also shown). **D,** The LV side of the Amplatzer patent ductus artiosus (PDA) occluder was deployed. Final position of the occluder device in right anterior oblique (RAO) **(E)** and left anterior oblique (LAO) **(F)** projections. *Asc Ao,* Ascending aorta; *Desc Ao,* descending aorta; *LA,* left atrium; *LV,* left ventricle; *MV,* mitral valve; *RA,* right atrium; *PVL,* paravalvular leak; *SAG,* stiff-angled Glidewire; *TPM,* temporary pacemaker; *TS,* transseptal.

In situations where one device does not adequately close the PVL, two (or more) devices can be deployed. This is illustrated in **Figure 12–14.** Briefly, after crossing the leak with an SAG wire, the Agilis or other catheter (such as a 7F multipurpose guide) is advanced over the wire to the left ventricle and a second SAG wire is advanced to the aorta. Each wire can then accommodate a delivery sheath if necessary. If the operators prefer to deploy both devices simultaneously to assess the degree of PVL closure, a large enough femoral venous sheath (14F to 20F) is required to accommodate both delivery systems. For instance, two 6F coronary guides can be advanced across the defect to allow simultaneous deployment of two Amplatzer vascular plugs. Alternatively, operators may choose to advance an 0.014-inch wire via the TorqVue delivery sheath before advancing the occluder device, keeping wire access to the leak in case there is need for a second device **(Figure 12–15).**

Transseptal Approach to Aortic Paravalvular Leak Closure

The general principles of the aortic PVL closure via the TS approach are the same as those for the mitral procedure. As stated, patients with mechanical MVRs are not candidates for this approach, and care must be taken when creating the wire loop in the left ventricle to not cause trauma to the MV apparatus.

After standard TS puncture, a balloon-tipped catheter is floated through the MV to the left ventricle. This is then exchanged for a diagnostic catheter with a sharply curved tip (such as an internal mammary artery [IMA] catheter) that looks toward the AV. The leak is then crossed using a SAG wire (or hydrophilic 0.014-inch coronary wire) that is advanced to the descending aorta and snared for externalization at the femoral artery sheath. The delivery sheath and devices may be delivered either antegrade or retrograde, although the retrograde approach may be safer with respect to MV trauma. Care must also be taken when deploying the aortic disc to not impinge on the right or left coronary ostia.

Femoral Artery Approach to Mitral Paravalvular Leak Closure

To gain access to the MV via the femoral approach, the aortic valve must be crossed. Therefore this approach is not feasible in patients with a mechanical AVR. Furthermore, because of the difficulties associated with crossing the leak from this position, the femoral approach is not often used. If this approach is chosen, an acutely angled catheter (such as an IMA) or reversed-curve catheter (such as an AL-1) may be placed in the left ventricle to facilitate crossing the leak. The wire is then snared via TS puncture, and devices are advanced antegrade via the femoral venous sheath (as in the TS approach).

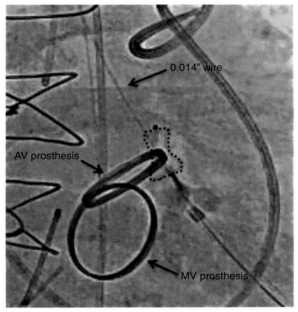

Figure 12–15 Securing the leak before device deployment. A 0.014-inch wire was advanced across the aortic paravalvular leak via the delivery sheath before deployment of the Amplatzer Vascular Plug I (AVP I) in case additional devices were needed for complete closure. The procedure was performed via the transapical approach. *AV,* aortic valve; *MV,* mitral valve.

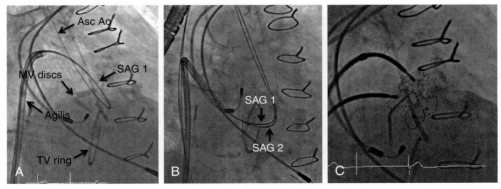

Figure 12–14 Double wiring of a large mitral paravalvular leak (PVL) to place two devices simultaneously. A, The PVL was crossed with a SAG wire via an Agilis catheter and advanced to the descending aorta. **B,** The Agilis was then advanced to the left ventricle and a second SAG was advanced to the descending aorta. **C,** The Agilis was removed, delivery sheaths were advanced over each wire, and two Amplatzer ventricular septal defect occluder devices were deployed in sequence. *Asc Ao,* Ascending; *MV,* mitral valve; *SAG,* stiff-angled Glidewire; *TV,* tricuspid valve.

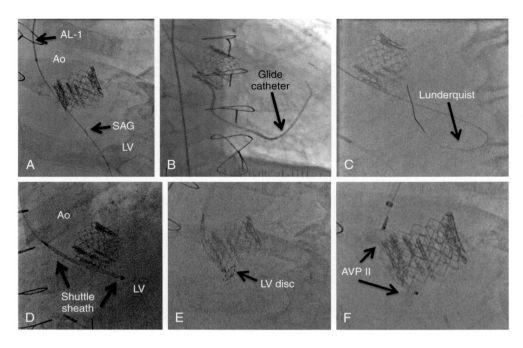

Figure 12–16 Aortic paravalvular leak after transcatheter aortic valve replacement closed via the retrograde approach. A, Cannulation of the leak using a SAG via a 5F AL-1 catheter. B, 4F Glide catheter advanced to the LV. C, Lunderquist wire advanced to the LV. D, 6F shuttle sheath advanced to the LV. E, LV portion of the 12-mm Amplatzer Vascular Plug II (AVP II) deployed. F, Aorta side of the device is deployed. Ao, Aorta; LV, left ventricle; SAG, stiff-angled Glidewire.

Femoral Artery Approach to Aortic Paravalvular Leak Closure

This is the most common approach to aortic PVLs and is illustrated in **Figure 12–16.** An easily directable catheter is used (e.g., Amplatz Left 1 [AL-1] or multipurpose [MP]) to wire the leak with a SAG wire (or hydrophilic 0.014-inch coronary wire if necessary). A multipurpose guide can easily engage the right and noncoronary cusps, whereas an AL-1 or AL-2 guide may be required to engage a PVL in the left coronary cusp. The wire is then exchanged in the left ventricle for a stiffer support 0.035-inch wire, such as an Amplatz Extra Stiff or Lunderquist. Again, care must be taken to make a broad loop on the wire to avoid LV trauma. In the rare circumstance that this does not provide enough support for device delivery sheath insertion, consideration may be given to snaring the wire via TS or TA approach to create a rail. Devices are chosen as appropriate for the leak, taking care not to impinge upon the coronary ostia. It may be prudent to perform coronary angiography before device release to confirm patency.

Transapical Approach to Mitral Paravalvular Leak Closure

When crossing the mitral leak from the antegrade TS approach is not possible (either because of technical difficulties in wiring or an inability to cross the IAS), the TA approach can be quite helpful. Before puncture of the LV apex, a left coronary angiogram should be taken to evaluate the position of the left anterior descending coronary artery (LAD) in order to avoid accidental coronary puncture with apical cannulation. Some investigators have advocated the use of preprocedural CT to plan the puncture, including evaluation of the course of the LAD and distance from the skin.[10]

Under fluoroscopic guidance the LV apex is cannulated using a micropuncture needle, and a 5F sheath is advanced to the left ventricle. Crossing the PVL is

accomplished using a SAG wire or hydrophilic 0.014-inch coronary wire. The rest of the procedure is dictated by the degree of support that is required to deliver an occluding device to the PVL. In many cases simply advancing the SAG wire distally into a pulmonary vein provides enough purchase and support to advance the delivery sheath across the PVL. If more support is necessary, the SAG can be exchanged for a stiffer 0.035-inch wire that is parked in the vein. Alternatively, the SAG can be snared after TS puncture and brought to the femoral vein, after which point devices can be advanced across the PVL in an antegrade fashion. This is the recommended approach if large devices/delivery sheaths are required in order to minimize the necessary sheath size at the LV apex.

Because all of these patients have undergone at least one OHS in the past, pericardial scarring is usually present. Therefore as long as sheath size is minimized (6F or less), simply withdrawing the sheath from the LV apex usually allows passive closure of the site. Before the patient leaves the procedure area, the pericardial space should be observed echocardiographically after sheath removal to evaluate to accumulating effusion. When larger sheaths are used, consideration may be given to off-label closure of the apical site using a suture device such as the Perclose (Abbott Vascular, Redwood City, Calif.), deployment of an Amplatzer duct occluder, or primary surgical closure (although this requires an incision).

Transapical Approach to Aortic Paravalvular Leak Closure

In patients for whom an aortic PVL cannot be crossed using the retrograde approach, the TA approach is usually considered next. The procedure is similar to that described for the mitral PVL, except that after crossing the leak the wire is either advanced to the descending aorta or snared in the aorta and externalized to the femoral artery. If large occluder devices are necessary, it is

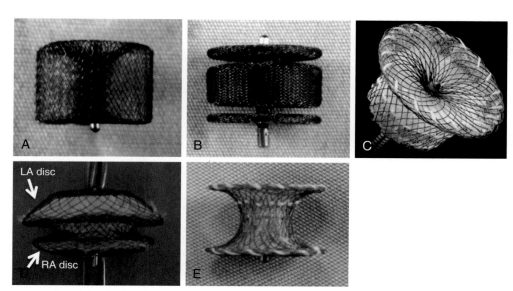

Figure 12–17 **Devices used for paravalvular leak closure. A,** Amplatzer vascular plug I (AVP I). **B,** Amplatzer vascular plug II (AVP II). **C,** Amplatzer patent ductus arteriosus occluder. **D,** Amplatzer septal occluder. **E,** Amplatzer muscular ventricular septal defect occluder. *LA,* left atrium; *RA,* right atrium.

recommended to advance these devices retrograde via a larger femoral artery sheath.

12.3 Available Devices for Paravalvular Leak Closure

There are no devices that are created specifically for PVL closure. As a result, a number of other devices have been used in an off-label fashion for this purpose **(Figure 12–17).** Because PVLs do not come in standard sizes, and because many of them are crescentic in shape, a great deal of thought in the planning phase should go into the decision about which and how many devices are necessary. Of course, it is not uncommon to have to readdress the intended plan midprocedure to either change the type or number of devices. An extra wire may be placed across the PVL before deployment of a device in case a second device is necessary for a successful closure. Furthermore, when choosing a device care should be taken to consider the proximity of the leak to surrounding structures including the coronary ostia and mechanical leaflets.

With respect to specific device choice, a number of factors must be considered, and there are no specific criteria to dictate device choice. Nevertheless, the following may be considered:

- The AVP I is a simple cylinder design, has large holes in the nitinol mesh, and does not have a fabric inner layer; this is therefore not used often.
- The AVP II is superior to the AVP I, given that the discs on either side of the cylindrical portion help create a better seal, and the nitinol mesh is more tightly woven. Other benefits include the fact that it can be delivered via smaller sheath sizes than the septal occluder devices and also has the largest experience. Lack of an inner fabric makes sealing less effective.
- The rectangular-shaped AVP III may have advantages over the other two AVPs, but it is not currently available in the United States. It is only available in smaller sizes and also has no inner fabric.

- The muscular ventricular septal defect (VSD) occluder has an inner fabric that is optimal for leak closure, but it is a stiff device and may cause more hemolysis than the others. It is beneficial for circular holes.
- The atrial septal defect (ASD) occluder is sometimes used and has the benefit of an inner fabric similar to the VSD device. The major issue with this device is the large discs on either side that may impinge on the valve, especially in patients with a tilting-disc mechanical prosthesis and a leak located at the hingepoint of the leaflets.
- The patent ductus arteriosus (PDA) occluder is an easily delivered device with an inner fabric and can be quite useful, but unfortunately it is available only in limited sizes.
- The available device sizes and necessary delivery sheath requirements are listed in **Tables 12–1 through 12–4**.

12.4 Complications of Paravalvular Leak Closure

In addition to the usual complications of any percutaneous intervention (such as vascular complications, stroke, and cardiac perforation), there are some that deserve special mention with respect to performance of percutaneous PVL closure procedures.

COMPLETE HEART BLOCK

The atrioventricular node occupies a position at the junction of the IAS and interventricular septum. As such, it sits close to the medial aspect of the AV and MV (between 1 and 3 o'clock on the MV clock face). Therefore complete heart block may occur with deployment of devices in this location. The patient in **Figure 12–13** faced this very complication, which is why a temporary pacing wire is seen after introduction of the PDA occluder into the medial mitral PVL (D-F). Whereas some patients undergoing PVL closure may already have a pacemaker in place, those without require special attention, and

TABLE 12–1

Amplatzer Septal Occluder Device and Recommended Sheath Size

Waist Diameter	LA Disc Diameter	RA Disc Diameter	Minimum Sheath Size
4 mm	16 mm	12 mm	6F-7F
5 mm	17 mm	13 mm	6F-7F
6 mm	18 mm	14 mm	6F-7F
7 mm	19 mm	15 mm	6F-7F
8 mm	20 mm	16 mm	6F-7F
9 mm	21 mm	17 mm	6F-7F
10 mm	22 mm	18 mm	6F-7F
11 mm	25 mm	21 mm	7F
12 mm	26 mm	22 mm	7F
13 mm	27 mm	23 mm	7F
14 mm	28 mm	24 mm	7F
15 mm	29 mm	25 mm	7F
16 mm	30 mm	26 mm	7F
17 mm	31 mm	27 mm	7F
18 mm	32 mm	28 mm	8F-9F
19 mm	33 mm	29 mm	8F-9F
20 mm	34 mm	30 mm	8F-9F
22 mm	36 mm	32 mm	9F
24 mm	38 mm	34 mm	9F
26 mm	40 mm	36 mm	10F
28 mm	42 mm	38 mm	10F
30 mm	44 mm	40 mm	10F
32 mm	46 mm	42 mm	10F
34 mm	50 mm	44 mm	12F
36 mm	52 mm	46 mm	12F
38 mm	54 mm	48 mm	12F

LA, left atrium; RA, right atrium.

TABLE 12–2

Amplatzer Muscular VSD Occluder Device Size and Recommended Sheath Size

Device Diameter	Device Length	Minimum Amplatzer TorqVue Delivery Sheath Size
4 mm	7 mm	5F 180° curve or 6F 45° curve
6 mm	7 mm	6F 45° or 180° curve
8 mm	7 mm	6F 45° or 180° curve
10 mm	7 mm	6F 45° or 180° curve
12 mm	7 mm	7F 45° or 180° curve
14 mm	7 mm	8F 45° or 180° curve
16 mm	7 mm	8F 45° or 180° curve
18 mm	7 mm	9F 45° or 180° curve

TABLE 12–3

Amplatzer Vascular Plug I Device and Recommended Sheath Size

Device Diameter	Device Length	Minimum Sheath Size	Minimum Guide Size
4 mm	7 mm	4F	5F
6 mm	7 mm	4F	5F
8 mm	7 mm	4F	5F
10 mm	7 mm	5F	6F
12 mm	8 mm	5F	6F
14 mm	8 mm	6F	8F
16 mm	8 mm	6F	8F

TABLE 12–4

Amplatzer Vascular Plug II Device and Recommended Sheath Size

Device Diameter	Device Length	Minimum Sheath Size	Minimum Guide Size
3 mm	6 mm	4F	5F
4 mm	6 mm	4F	5F
6 mm	6 mm	4F	5F
8 mm	7 mm	4F	5F
10 mm	7 mm	5F	6F
12 mm	9 mm	5F	6F
14 mm	10 mm	6F	8F
16 mm	12 mm	6F	8F
18 mm	14 mm	7F	9F
20 mm	16 mm	7F	9F

a temporary pacemaker wire and pacing box should be close at hand before device deployment.

INTERFERENCE WITH THE VALVE

Given the fact that there are no specific devices meant for PVL closure, selection of the available devices must take into consideration not only the size of the defect but also the location of the defect in relation to the prosthetic leaflets. In certain positions (e.g., leaks close to the insertion points of mechanical leaflet tilting discs), devices with significant overhang (i.e., atrial or ventricular septal occluders) may impinge on movement of the leaflets. This may cause the leaflets to either remain in a partially open or partially closed position, resulting in either severe valvular regurgitation or stenosis, respectively. To avoid this, care should be taken to observe the valve prosthesis function (both echocardiographically and fluoroscopically) with the device in place but before detachment from the delivery system. If necessary, the device may then be retracted and another device used **(Figure 12–18).**

IMPINGEMENT ON CORONARY OSTIA

For patients with aortic PVL, consideration should be given to the proximity of left main and right coronary ostia to the leak. Position of the leak should therefore be noted on the short-axis echo images to assess the relationship of the PVL with respect to the native coronary cusps. Additionally, distance can be measured from the leak to the coronary ostium on CT scan to determine whether coronary occlusion might be a risk with the procedure. After positioning of the device in the aortic PVL, but before detachment, a close inspection of the hemodynamic tracings and LV wall motion on echocardiography should be made. If there is any suggestion of coronary impingement by the device, the device should be withdrawn. Additionally, contrast injection can be performed via the delivery sheath to assess opacification of the coronary artery, or

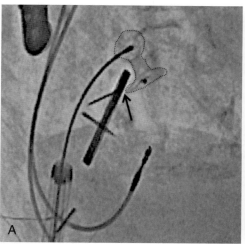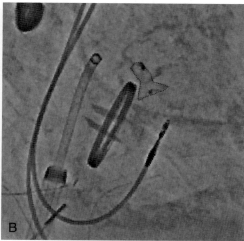

Figure 12–18 Mitral paraval-vular leak closure complicated by valve dysfunction. A, Interference of an Amplatzer muscular ventricular septal defect occluder with one disc of a mechanical mitral valve replacement *(arrow)* resulted in severe mitral stenosis. **B,** Proper valve function was restored with removal of the device and replacement with an Amplatzer ductal occluder.

a pigtail catheter can be positioned in the aortic root (via another arterial access) for root angiography.

DEVICE EMBOLIZATION

Embolization of the occluder devices is rare, occurring in fewer than 1% to 5% of large series.[6,11] Given the size of the devices, embolization to the great vessels of the aortic arch is rare. Instead, the devices either remain in the cardiac chambers (usually left ventricle), or embolize to the aortic bifurcation or proximal lower-extremity vessels. In most cases, the device is retrieved percutaneously with a snare. A bioptome may also be a successful method for peripheral arterial retrieval, although care must be taken if using a bioptome within a cardiac chamber to avoid perforation. Alternatively, if the device is permanently lodged within the left ventricle without significant risk for further mobilization, consideration can be given to leaving it in place with monitoring by CT or echocardiography during follow-up care.[6]

PERICARDIAL EFFUSION AND HEMOTHORAX

Puncture of the cardiac chambers either during TS puncture or LV apical puncture, or as a result of the manipulation of stiff wires in the left ventricle all may lead to pericardial effusion. As percutaneous PVL closure is performed using ICE and TEE guidance, the pericardial space should be carefully evaluated over the course of the procedure for evidence of accumulating effusion. After apical sheath removal, the LV apex should be examined for evidence of color flow into the pericardial space as well as accumulation of fluid. Similarly, hemothorax is a known complication of LV apical puncture, and postprocedural chest X-ray should be obtained in all patients undergoing PVL closure using the TA approach.

12.5 Clinical Outcomes of Percutaneous Paravalvular Leak Closure

The first series of percutaneous PVL closure was published by Hourihan and colleagues[4] in 1992. Since that

time, a number of case reports and series of varying size have provided encouraging outcomes and have stimulated interest in the procedure as an alternative to redo OHS.[5] Two groups with a large experience in PVL closure provided more comprehensive data on the procedure.

Sorajja and colleagues published their short-term outcomes of closing 141 defects (78% mitral, 22% aortic) in 115 patients.[11] Most patients suffered from CHF (93%), the majority of whom had New York Heart Association class III or greater (69%); a large number also had hemolysis (37%). Overall procedural success was achieved in 77% of cases (76% for mitral PVL and 80% for aortic PVL), with an 8.7% rate of major adverse events at 30 days (death, myocardial infarction, stroke, emergency surgery, and bleeding). There were no acute procedural deaths, and one patient required emergency surgery for valve interference where the device could not be retrieved percutaneously. Only 10% of patients had 3+ or higher levels of regurgitation. In cases that were not successful, the most commonly cited reason was residual regurgitation after device deployment (25 patients); five patients had valve interference by the device; a delivery sheath could not be advanced in two patients, and the defect could not be wired in one patient. The investigators also demonstrated a significant learning curve for PVL closure, with mean procedural time decreasing from a peak of over 160 minutes to less than 130 minutes.

The same authors also provided long-term data on 126 patients (including the group of patients discussed) who underwent closure of 154 PVLs.[7] The 3-year survival rate was 64%, with no difference based on degree of residual regurgitation, underlining the relatively comorbid state of patients who had clinically meaningful PVLs. Interestingly, among survivors, 64 of 89 patients who had CHF had no or minimal exertional dyspnea. On the other hand, 14 of 29 survivors had continued hemolysis that was unrelated to the degree of residual regurgitation; only one patient experienced worsening hemolysis after the procedure. The presence of hemolysis after PVL closure was found to have negative prognostic significance.

Ruiz and colleagues[6] performed 57 PVL procedures in 43 patients; 10 patients required two procedures, and two patients required three procedures. The leaks were predominantly mitral (38 out of 49), and procedural success was achieved in 86% of patients. The 30-day all-cause mortality rate of 5.4% compares quite favorably with that of a large surgical series of patients requiring reoperation (6%).[2] Even though 13 of 37 patients (35%) who had successful leak closure were discovered to have new or worsening hemolysis, the percentage of patients requiring erythropoietic agents or blood transfusion decreased from 56% to 5%.

Taken together, the above series and other case reports of percutaneous PVL closure demonstrate a reasonable and durable success rate with low to moderate levels of risk. Effectiveness of PVL closure for patients with symptoms of CHF is well established; the significance of this procedure on hemolysis (and the clinical relevance of postprocedural hemolysis) remains unclear. Given the fact that a large number of these patients are older, have a number of comorbidities, and have previously undergone OHS more than once, the percutaneous approach is an attractive alternative to redo valve surgery.

12.6 Paravalvular Leak in the Transcatheter Aortic Valve Replacement Era

The field of TAVR is growing at an exponential rate with increasing reports of its efficacy and safety in large registries and randomized trials. The current widely available valves include the self-expanding CoreValve ReValving system (Medtronic, Minneapolis, Minn.) and the balloon-expandable Edwards SAPIEN device (Edwards Lifesciences, Irvine, Calif.). With increasing experience, investigators have also become more aware of the clinical consequences of PAR that are often seen in patients after TAVR. As such, there have been a number of studies to help understand the factors that may predispose a patient to PAR and methods to improve PAR after valve implantation.

INCIDENCE AND OUTCOMES OF PARAVALVULAR AORTIC REGURGITATION AFTER TRANSCATHETER AORTIC VALVE REPLACEMENT

Valve undersizing, malpositioning of the aortic prosthesis (too aortic or too ventricular), or bulky calcification of the leaflets are all implicated as causes of PAR. In the group of patients randomized to TAVR (n = 348) versus surgical AVR (sAVR; n = 351) in the Placement of AoRTic TraNscathetER Valve (PARTNER) I trial, Kodali and colleagues noted that whereas the overall outcome was equivalent, the incidence of PAR was significantly greater in patients assigned to TAVR at 2 years (6.9% vs 0.9%, p < 0.001).[12] Similarly, Bleiziffer and colleagues demonstrated an 8% incidence of PAR among 227 patients treated with TAVR (using both the CoreValve ReValving system and the Edwards SAPIEN valve) at 2 years.[13] In a group of 667 patients undergoing TAVR with either valve prosthesis, Tamburino and colleagues reported an incidence of PAR of 21%.[14] Although the incidence of PAR is highly variable depending on the study and the criteria used, it is safe to say that it is a significant occurrence.

The significance of PAR has also been better understood with increasing experience with TAVR. In the PARTNER I group, the incidence of moderate or severe PAR was an independent predictor of mortality (hazard ratio [HR] 2.11).[12] Furthermore, any degree of PAR, even mild, was associated with worse mortality at 2 years' follow-up study. In the analysis by Tamburino and colleagues, moderate or severe PAR was also identified as a significant independent predictor of mortality (HR 3.8).[14] These analyses and others indicate that efforts should be concentrated to minimize the incidence of PAR during transcatheter valve replacement.

PREPROCEDURAL IMAGING FOR ANNULUS SIZING

Precise sizing of the aortic annulus is necessary to minimize both the aortic trauma that may result from valve oversizing and complications such as valve embolization or PAR that may result from valve undersizing. A number of studies have demonstrated that 2D echocardiography (TTE and TEE) provides an imprecise assessment of the elliptical aortic annulus when compared with surgical dilators or multidetector CT (MDCT). As such, MDCT has largely supplanted the role of echocardiography in assessing annulus size in a number of centers, since it provides a 3D perspective of the annulus.

In a study comparing 2D echocardiography to MDCT for annulus sizing, Jilaihawi and colleagues demonstrated the following differences in mean annulus measurements: 20.4 mm by TTE, 22.5 mm by TEE, 21.3 to 27.2 mm by MDCT (depending on method).[15] The discrepancy in annular size observed using echocardiography versus MDCT also has significant implications for procedural planning and resultant AR. In their analysis, the investigators also found that MDCT sizing was more predictive of post-TAVR PAR than echocardiographic measurements, and furthermore that prospective application of a CT-guided prosthesis-sizing approach resulted in a lower incidence of PAR.

PROCEDURAL APPROACHES TO REDUCE PARAVALVULAR AORTIC REGURGITATION

Although optimal prosthesis sizing in TAVR is the primary goal to reduce PAR, procedural variables including valve malpositioning and inadequate valve expansion are not uncommon occurrences. As such, a number of possible solutions to minimizing PAR exist.

Valve Deployment and Positioning

Great care should be taken when positioning and deploying the TAVR prosthesis. The SAPIEN valve is generally implanted in the middle of the annulus (50/50 aortic/ventricular). Most operators perform aortic root angiography to assure proper positioning before balloon dilation of the stented valve. A position either too aortic or too ventricular may result in improper sealing by the valve "skirt" and therefore PAR.

The CoreValve is usually positioned with the stented portion 3 to 5 mm into the LV outflow tract. In cases of deployment that is too ventricular, the valve can be snared and repositioned.

Postdilation of the Transcatheter Aortic Valve Replacement Prosthesis

If the prosthesis is well-positioned, one approach to treating post-TAVR PAR is to postdilate the valve. This may provide better apposition and "sealing" between the stented valve and the annulus, thereby reducing PAR. In the TAVR series mentioned previously, Tamburino and colleagues[14] performed postdilation of the valve in approximately 10% of cases. Caution must be taken not to be overaggressive in postdilation, however, because this could result in annular trauma or worsening of central AR as a result of malcoaptation of the prosthetic valve leaflets. The authors add 0.5 to 1.5 cc of saline to the SAPIEN balloon to perform postdilation. Postdilation is necessary in about 10% of patients, and this is currently reserved for moderate leak as determined by echo and hemodynamics. There is some suggestion that postdilation may be associated with higher periprocedural stroke, although this is still controversial. In patients undergoing treatment with the CoreValve ReValving system, postdilation using a routine valvuloplasty balloon is reasonable, and a balloon slightly larger than the annulus is reasonable.

Valve-in-Valve Implantation for Paravalvular Aortic Regurgitation after Transcatheter Aortic Valve Replacement

In cases of PAR that remains significant even after postdilation and is thought to be caused by malpositioning, or when central regurgitation increases with postdilation, deployment of a second valve-in-valve implant may be necessary. This is usually the case when the valve is deployed either too high or too low in the annulus, and it may be necessary not only to address PAR but also to stabilize the valve if prosthesis embolization is a concern. In the PARTNER I high-risk surgical cohort, 1.5% of patients required a valve-in-valve procedure as a result of significant PAR. The procedure for implanting a second SAPIEN prosthesis is similar to the first; the wire is left in place, and the second valve is deployed as necessary (either more aortic or more ventricular) with at least one set of overlapping stents. Care must be taken to not compromise the coronary ostia.

Paravalvular Leak Closure

As illustrated in **Figure 12–16,** there remain cases of PAR that are recalcitrant to postdilation or valve-in-valve implantation. In these situations it may be necessary to implant a device to close the PVL, as discussed in this chapter. Care must be taken to not damage the proximal or distal stent struts while crossing the leak with wires and delivery catheters or the device itself. There are unfortunately no large series demonstrating the results of this procedure, but given the clinical outcomes of significant PAR, closure should be considered in appropriate cases.

12.7 Summary

PVLs are a not uncommon complication after valve replacement. Reoperation is often quite risky and may not yield optimal results. Therefore closure of PVLs via the percutaneous approach has gained favor in recent years, and clinical outcomes are promising. With the proliferation of TAVR and concerns regarding postprocedural PVL, it is likely that percutaneous PVL closure will become even more common. Preprocedural imaging using echocardiography is imperative to properly define the PVL and determine a procedural strategy. Intraprocedural imaging consists predominantly of fluoroscopy, TEE, and ICE, although recent advances in fusion of CT and fluoroscopy hold great promise for guiding these procedures. Although there are a number of devices available for other applications that are used in an "off-label" fashion for PVL closure, devices specific to this setting are under development.

REFERENCES

1. Rodes-Cabau J: Transcatheter aortic valve implantation: current and future approaches, Nat Rev Cardiol 9:15–29, 2012.
2. Genoni M, Franzen D, Vogt P, et al: Paravalvular leakage after mitral valve replacement: improved long-term survival with aggressive surgery? Eur J Cardiothorac Surg 17:14–19, 2000.
3. De Cicco G, Russo C, Moreo A, et al: Mitral valve periprosthetic leakage: anatomical observations in 135 patients from a multicentre study, Eur J Cardiothorac Surg 30:887–891, 2006.
4. Hourihan M, Perry SB, Mandell VS, et al: Transcatheter umbrella closure of valvular and paravalvular leaks, J Am Coll Cardiol 20:1371–1377, 1992.
5. Kim MS, Casserly IP, Garcia JA, et al: Percutaneous transcatheter closure of prosthetic mitral paravalvular leaks: are we there yet? JACC Cardiovasc Interv 2:81–90, 2009.
6. Ruiz CE, Jelnin V, Kronzon I, et al: Clinical outcomes in patients undergoing percutaneous closure of periprosthetic paravalvular leaks, J Am Coll Cardiol 58:2210–2217, 2011.
7. Sorajja P, Cabalka AK, Hagler DJ, et al: Long-term follow-up of percutaneous repair of paravalvular prosthetic regurgitation, J Am Coll Cardiol 58:2218–2224, 2011.
8. Krishnaswamy A, Tuzcu EM, Kapadia SR: Three-dimensional computed tomography in the cardiac catheterization laboratory, Catheter Cardiovasc Interv 77:860–865, 2011.
9. Yuksel UC, Tuzcu EM, Kapadia SR: Percutaneous closure of a posteromedial mitral paravalvular leak: the triple telescopic system, Catheter Cardiovasc Interv 77:281–285, 2011.
10. Jelnin V, Dudiy Y, Einhorn BN, et al: Clinical experience with percutaneous left ventricular transapical access for interventions in structural heart defects a safe access and secure exit, JACC Cardiovasc Interv 4:868–874, 2011.
11. Sorajja P, Cabalka AK, Hagler DJ, et al: Percutaneous repair of paravalvular prosthetic regurgitation: acute and 30-day outcomes in 115 patients, Circ Cardiovasc Interv 4:314–321, 2011.
12. Kodali SK, Williams MR, Smith CR, et al: Two-year outcomes after transcatheter or surgical aortic-valve replacement, N Engl J Med 366;1686–1695, 2012.
13. Bleiziffer S, Mazzitelli D, Opitz A, et al: Beyond the short-term: clinical outcome and valve performance 2 years after transcatheter aortic valve implantation in 227 patients, J Thorac Cardiovasc Surg 143:310–317, 2012.
14. Tamburino C, Capodanno D, Ramondo A, et al: Incidence and predictors of early and late mortality after transcatheter aortic valve implantation in 663 patients with severe aortic stenosis, Circulation 123:299–308, 2011.
15. Jilaihawi H, Kashif M, Fontana G, et al: Cross-sectional computed tomographic assessment improves accuracy of aortic annular sizing for transcatheter aortic valve replacement and reduces the incidence of paravalvular aortic regurgitation, J Am Coll Cardiol 59:1275–1286, 2012.

Chapter 13

Valve-in-Valve Therapy

RONALD K. BINDER • JOHN G. WEBB

13.1 Key Points

- Transcatheter valve implantation is feasible in failing surgical aortic, mitral, pulmonic and tricuspid bioprostheses.
- Access may be transarterial (femoral, subclavian, axillary), transvenous (femoral, subclavian, jugular), transapical, transatrial, or direct transaortic.
- Paravalvular regurgitation (PR) must be distinguished from valvular regurgitation, because it will not respond to valve-in-valve (VIV) implants.
- The specific model and the labeled (external) diameter of the bioprosthesis must be confirmed.
- The internal diameter of the bioprosthesis must be determined from the manufacturer and noninvasive imaging.
- The transcatheter valve size must match or exceed the internal diameter of the surgical bioprosthesis.
- VIV implantation in very small surgical bioprostheses may lead to high transvalvular gradients.
- The radiographic and echocardiographic appearance of the surgical bioprosthesis posts and sewing ring should be understood.
- Transcatheter valves depend largely on anchoring within the sewing ring, not the stent posts.
- The durability of VIV implants is unknown at the present time.

Reoperative replacement of failing bioprosthetic heart valves carries a higher risk of morbidity and mortality than the initial valve replacement procedure. An alternative to reoperation is transcatheter VIV implantation. Transcatheter VIV implantation has been successfully performed for failing surgical bioprostheses in the aortic, mitral, pulmonic, and tricuspid positions. This chapter covers the practical challenges, selection criteria, techniques, and outcomes of VIV implantation.

13.2 Causes of Bioprosthetic Valve Failure

Bioprosthetic valves are derived from animal tissue (xenograft or heterograft) or from human tissue (homograft). The most commonly used biologic materials are porcine aortic valve and bovine pericardial tissue. In stented bioprostheses the leaflet tissue is suspended from a frame made of various alloys or plastics. The stent is seated on a basal ring, which may be circular or saddle shaped. Freedom from bioprosthetic valve failure is reportedly 70% to 90% at 10 years and 40% to 70% at 15 years.[1-5] Failure may occur because of stenosis, regurgitation, both of these, or a paravalvular leak.

A major contributor to bioprosthetic failure is calcification, which involves an interaction between phospholipids, glutaraldehyde collagen cross-linking, and circulating calcium.[6] Younger age at implantation, diabetes, renal failure, and abnormalities of calcium metabolism such as hyperparathyroidism are risk factors for accelerated valve calcification. Structural failure may also occur as a result of a leaflet tear, which may occur in the absence of calcification.[7] Typically this occurs in the area of the commissures, where the leaflet stress is highest. Whereas growth of host tissue onto the valve frame is part of a natural healing process, proliferative overgrowth with pannus restricts leaflet mobility. Additional mechanisms of structural valve failure include infective endocarditis and valve thrombosis, both contraindications for VIV procedures.

13.3 Patient Selection and Indications for Valve-in-Valve Therapy

Transcatheter VIV implantation may be considered in patients with failing surgical bioprostheses caused by severe regurgitation, stenosis, or both, regardless of surgical valve position. Significant PR has to be excluded, because it does not respond to VIV therapy. Endocarditis and valve thrombosis are generally considered contraindications. The lack of long-term durability data restricts VIV procedures to patients at high or prohibitive surgical risk. Furthermore, the internal diameter of the surgical bioprosthesis limits the size of the transcatheter heart valve (THV), which is of concern when dealing with a very small bioprosthesis. Patients need to undergo thorough

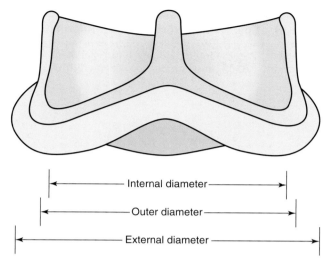

Figure 13–1   Schematic representation of a stented surgical biopros-thesis. The internal, outer, and external diameters all represent different dimensions of surgical bioprostheses. Whereas surgeons have to conform the size of the bioprosthesis to the diameter of the native valve annulus, operators performing valve-in-valve procedures have to fit the transcatheter heart valve to the internal diameter of the bioprosthesis. *(Reprinted with permission from Elsevier; Gurvitch, R, Cheung, A, Ye, J, et al: Transcatheter valve-in-valve implantation for failed surgical bioprosthetic valves. J Am Coll Cardiol 58:2196-2209, 2011.)*

screening to determine the most appropriate access site that allows safe and effective THV delivery. Comorbidities that may influence life expectancy should be taken into account before pursuing with VIV treatment.

DIMENSIONS OF SURGICAL BIOPROSTHETIC HEART VALVES

Surgical bioprostheses are usually referred to according to their labeled size, a number that roughly corresponds to the diameter in mm of the aortic annulus as determined by a surgeon intraoperatively. This labeled size does not refer to the internal diameter of the valve, which is the most important diameter to consider in VIV treatment **(Figure 13–1)**. In most cases the labeled size corresponds to the outer diameter of the stent; however, in the case of stentless valves it typically corresponds to the external diameter of the valve. Unfortunately valve size labeling varies by manufacturer and is not standardized; moreover, different models of valves with the same reported label size (external diameter) may have different internal diameters.

A surgical operative report or patient valve implant card should be obtained to verify the specific manufacturer, model, and labeled size of the valve actually implanted. The internal diameter should then be ascertained from the manufacturer. The dimensions of a range of commonly implanted surgical bioprostheses are found in **Tables 13–1 to 13–3.** The nominal external diameter of the THV for VIV implantation should match or exceed the internal diameter of the surgical bioprosthesis. Undersizing the THV may lead to intervalvular regurgitation or embolization. Excessive oversizing of the THV may result in underexpansion of the THV frame within the surgical

bioprosthesis and lead to compromised hemodynamics and leaflet durability. In the authors' experience, underexpansion up to 20% of the nominal THV diameter is generally acceptable.[8] However, sizing considerations should not only take into account the internal prosthesis diameter, but also the nature of surgical bioprosthetic valve failure. Highly calcified, stenotic valves or those with prominent pannus may have smaller internal diameters. Imaging findings from computed tomography or transesophageal echocardiography should be taken into account when assessing THV sizing. However, their accuracy and reproducibility have not been tested for this indication.

13.4 Transcatheter Heart Valves and Device Selection

The majority of experience with transcatheter VIV implantations has been obtained with the Edwards SAPIEN/SAPIEN XT (Edwards Lifesciences, Irvine, Calif.), CoreValve (Medtronic, Minn.), and Melody (Medtronic, Minn.) valves. Experience with some of the newer THVs is limited.

1. The Edwards SAPIEN and SAPIEN XT: The Edwards SAPIEN THV **(Figure 13–2)** is a balloon-expandable valve composed of a stainless steel frame with bovine pericardial leaflets. The inflow of the frame is covered with a fabric cuff to provide an annular seal. It comes in two sizes with external diameters of 23 mm and 26 mm. The successor is the SAPIEN XT valve **(Figure 13–2),** which has a cobalt chromium frame, bovine pericardial leaflets and is manufactured in four sizes with external diameters of 20 mm, 23 mm, 26 mm, and 29 mm. These valves have been successfully used for VIV procedures in the aortic, mitral, pulmonic, and tricuspid positions. Unlike self-expanding valves, balloon-expandable valves are suitable for both retrograde (e.g., transapical for mitral bioprostheses) as well as the antegrade (e.g., transjugular for tricuspid bioprostheses) procedures. For transarterial or transvenous approaches the valve is compressed onto the low profile NovaFlex delivery catheter and introduced through an 18F to 20F sheath (or 16F expandable sheath).
2. The Medtronic CoreValve: The CoreValve system is composed of a self-expandable nitinol frame with porcine pericardial leaflets **(Figure 13–3)**. The system is manufactured in four sizes with external annular diameters of 23 mm, 26 mm, 29 mm, and 31 mm. The self-expanding valve frame is deployed by retraction of a restraining sheath. The system may only be used in a retrograde transarterial orientation (transfemoral, subclavian, axillary, or transaortic), and the long frame prevents its use in mitral, tricuspid, and pulmonary prostheses. A potential advantage of this valve is that the leaflets are mounted relatively high (supraannular) within the stent frame, with the potential for larger valve orifice when implanted in small diameter surgical bioprostheses. (See also Chapter 7.)

TABLE 13–1

Valve Dimensions for Selected 18- to 23-mm Surgical Bioprostheses, as per Manufacturer Product Information

Valve Label Size	Valve Type/Model	External Sewing Ring Diameter (ED), mm	Stent Outer Diameter (OD), mm	Internal Stent Diameter (ID), mm
18	Soprano (Sorin)	26	21	17.8
19	Magna (Edwards Lifesciences)	24	19	18
	Perimount (Edwards Lifesciences)	26	19	18
	Mosaic (Medtronic)	25	19	17.5
	Hancock Ultra (Medtronic)	24	19	17.5
	Hancock II (Medtronic)	N/A	N/A	N/A
	Mitroflow (Sorin)	21	18.6	15.4
	Trifecta (St. Jude Medical)	24	19	N/a
	Epic/Bicor (St. Jude Medical)	N/A	N/A	N/A
	Epic Supra/Bicor Supra (St. Jude Medical)	N/A	N/A	N/A
20	Soprano (Sorin)	28	23	19.8
21	Magna (Edwards Lifesciences)	26	21	20
	Perimount (Edwards Lifesciences)	29	21	20
	Mosaic/Hancock II (Medtronic)	27	21	18.5
	Hancock/Hancock Ultra (Medtronic)	26	21	18.5
	Mitroflow (Sorin)	23	20.7	17.3
	Trifecta (St. Jude Medical)	26	21	N/A
	Epic/Bicor (St. Jude Medical)	N/A	21	19
	Epic Supra/Bicor Supra (St. Jude Medical)	N/A	21	21
22	Soprano (Sorin)	30	25	21.7
23	Magna (Edwards Lifesciences)	28	23	22
	Perimount (Edwards Lifesciences)	31	23	22
	Mosaic/Hancock II (Medtronic)	30	23	20.5
	Hancock/Hancock Ultra (Medtronic)	28	23	22
	Mitroflow (Sorin)	26	22.7	19
	Trifecta (St. Jude Medical)	28	23	N/A
	Epic/Biocor (St. Jude Medical)	N/A	23	21
	Epic Supra/Biocor Supra (St. Jude Medical)	N/A	23	23

(Reprinted with permission from Elsevier; Gurvitch, R, Cheung, A, Ye, J, et al: Transcatheter valve-in-valve implantation for failed surgical bioprosthetic valves. *J Am Coll Cardiol* 58:2196-2209, 2011.)

3. The Melody valve: The Melody transcatheter valve **(Figure 13–4)** is composed of a bovine jugular venous valve sutured within a platinum iridium stent. The system is manufactured in four sizes, including 23 mm, 26 mm, 29 mm, and 31 mm. The valve is designed for use in pulmonary circulation, mostly to treat dysfunctional right ventricular outflow tract conduits or other pulmonary bioprostheses in patients with congenital heart disease. It has also been used for the tricuspid,[9] aortic,[10] and mitral[10] positions. The functioning of this valve in a low-pressure environment is well established, but long-term durability in a high-pressure environment may be questionable. (See also Chapter 8.)

4. The Inovare valve: The Inovare valve (Braile Biomédica, Brazil) consists of a balloon expandable cobalt–chromium stent with bovine pericardial leaflets **(Figure 13–5)**. It was approved for transapical native aortic valve implantation in November, 2011, in Brazil. It is only available with a transapical delivery system, although a transfemoral system is under development. There is only very limited experience with VIV procedures[11] (personal communication Valter Lima MD, Porto Alegre, Brazil). Very similar in appearance to the SAPIEN valve, it may offer a lower cost alternative to the other valves.

ACCESS ROUTE

The access options for transcatheter valve implantation depend on the bioprosthetic position and the delivery systems available. Aortic bioprostheses can be approached the least invasively and with conscious sedation using transarterial (femoral, axillary) access. Transaortic or transapical access to the aortic valve may avoid the risk of arterial injury and facilitate positioning. Mitral bioprostheses can be easily approached retrogradely through the left ventricle using apical access. However, the transvenous–transseptal approach has also been used successfully. Although positioning may be more difficult, the need for thoracotomy,

TABLE 13–2

Valve Dimensions for Selected 24- to 29-mm Surgical Bioprostheses, as per Manufacturer Product Information

Valve Label Size	Valve Type/Model	Sewing Ring External Diameter (ED), mm	Stent Outer Diameter (OD), mm	Stent Internal Diameter (ID), mm
24	Soprano (Sorin)	32	27	23.7
25	Magna (Edwards Lifesciences)	28	23	22
	Perimount (Edwards Lifesciences)	31	23	22
	Mosaic/Hancock II (Medtronic)	30	23	20.5
	Mosaic Ultra/Hancock I Ultra (Medtronic)	30	25	22.5
	Mitroflow (Sorin)	29	25.1	21
	Trifecta (St. Jude Medical)	31	25	N/A
	Epic/Biocor (St. Jude Medical)	N/A	25	23
	Epic Supra (St. Jude Medical)	N/A	25	25
26	Soprano (Sorin)	35	29	25.6
27	Magna (Edwards Lifesciences)	32	27	26
	Perimount (Edwards Lifesciences)	35	27	26
	Mosaic/Hancock II (Medtronic)	36	27	24
	Mosaic Ultra/Hancock II Ultra (Medtronic)	32	27	24
	Mitroflow (Sorin)	31	27.3	22.9
	Trifecta (St. Jude Medical)	33	27	N/A
	Epic/Biocor (St. Jude Medical)	N/A	27	27
	Epic Supra (St. Jude Medical)	N/A	27	27
28	Soprano (Sorin)	38	31	27.6
29	Magna (Edwards Lifesciences)	34	29	28
	Perimount (Edwards Lifesciences)	37	29	28
	Mosaic/Hancock II (Medtronic)	39	29	26
	Mosaic Ultra/Hancock II Ultra (Medtronic)	34	29	26
	Mitroflow (Sorin)	33	29.5	24.7
	Trifecta (St. Jude Medical)	35	29	N/A
	Epic/Biocor (St. Jude Medical)	N/A	29	27
	Epic Supra (St. Jude Medical)	N/A	N/A	N/A

(Reprinted with permission from Elsevier; Gurvitch, R, Cheung, A, Ye, J, et al: Transcatheter valve-in-valve implantation for failed surgical bioprosthetic valves. *J Am Coll Cardiol* 58:2196-2209, 2011.)

TABLE 13–3

Valve Dimensions for Selected Stentless Valves, as per Manufacturer Product Information

Valve Label Size	Bioprosthesis	Company	Outer Diameter (OD), mm	Internal Diameter (ID), mm
19	Freestyle	Medtronic	19	16
	Prima Plus	Edwards	19	16
	3F Therapeutics	ATS Medical	19	17
	Toronto SPV	St. Jude Medial	N/A	
	Pericarbon Freedom	Sorin Biomedical	19	17
21	Freestyle	Medtronic	21	18
	Prima Plus	Edwards	21	18
	3F Therapeutics	ATS Medical	21	19
	Toronto SPV	St. Jude Medial	21	18
	Pericarbon Freedom	Sorin Biomedical	21	19
23	Freestyle	Medtronic	23	20
	Prima Plus	Edwards	23	20
	3F Therapeutics	ATS Medical	23	21
	Toronto SPV	St. Jude Medial	23	20
	Pericarbon Freedom	Sorin Biomedical	23	21
25	Freestyle	Medtronic	25	21
	Prima Plus	Edwards	25	21
	3F Therapeutics	ATS Medical	25	23
	Toronto SPV	St. Jude Medial	25	21
	Pericarbon Freedom	Sorin Biomedical	25	23

(Reprinted with permission from Elsevier; Gurvitch, R, Cheung, A, Ye, J, et al: Transcatheter valve-in-valve implantation for failed surgical bioprosthetic valves. *J Am Coll Cardiol* 58:2196-2209, 2011.)

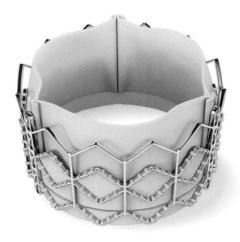
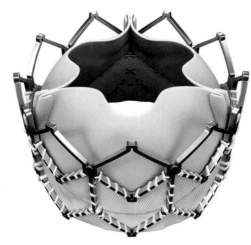

Figure 13–2   Edwards SAPIEN Transcatheter Heart Valve *(left)* **and Edwards SAPIEN XT Transcatheter Heart Valve** *(right)* **balloon expandable valves.** These balloon-expandable bovine pericardial tissue valves may be implanted antegrade or retrograde for valve-in-valve procedures in the aortic, mitral, pulmonic, and tricuspid positions. Accurate deployment mostly requires rapid ventricular pacing. *(Images published with permission of Edwards Lifesciences LLC, Irvine, Calif. Edwards SAPIEN and Edwards SAPIEN XT are trademarks of Edwards Lifesciences Corporation.)*

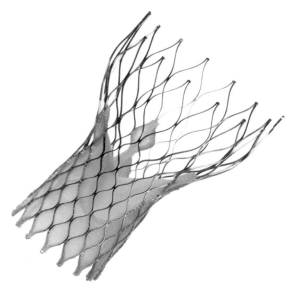

Figure 13–3   The CoreValve™ System. The CoreValve is a self-expandable nitinol porcine pericardial tissue valve. It was the first self-expandable valve used for a valve-in-valve procedure.[18] It is suitable only for the aortic position and only via a retrograde approach (e.g., transfemoral, transsubclavian, or direct transaortic). *(Courtesy of Medtronic, Minn.)*

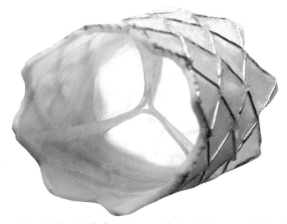

Figure 13–4   The Melody™ Transcatheter Pulmonary Valve. The Melody valve was the first transcatheter valve ever implanted in a human. It is most commonly used for stenotic or regurgitant right ventricle–pulmonary artery conduits in patients with congenital heart disease. The valve consists of a platinum iridium stent with a bovine jugular vein valve sewn inside. *(Courtesy of Medtronic, Minn.)*

POSITIONING PRINCIPLES AND DEPLOYMENT

Securely anchoring the THV is important to avoid device malposition, embolization, and paravalvular leaks. The THV has to be positioned so that its stent frame overlaps the prosthetic sewing ring **(Figure 13–6)**. Prostheses may be stented or stentless, have radiopaque markers or rings, or be radiolucent. The radiopaque markers may be placed at the top of the stent posts or close to the anatomic sewing ring at the basal portion of the bioprosthesis. Regardless, the exact type of bioprosthetic valve, its radiographic appearance, and the relationship of radiopaque markers to the sewing ring must be appreciated **(Figure 13–7)**.

To accurately place the THV, a coaxial view of the bioprosthesis is required. The fluoroscopically visible components and markers of the bioprosthesis should be used to determine the appropriate C-arm angulation for a perpendicular view. Rotating the C-arm until the basal ring appears as a straight line suggests perpendicularity to the valve plane and an appropriate implant view.

ventriculotomy, and possibly general anesthetic may be avoided. Pulmonary bioprostheses are best approached using transvenous access from the femoral, jugular, or subclavian vein. Tricuspid bioprostheses were initially approached using an open transatrial approach with direct puncture of the right atrium.[12] More recently, transvenous access from the femoral, jugular, or subclavian vein has been favored.

Whereas in the early experience with transcatheter valve implantation, vascular access implied surgical cut-down, percutaneous closure devices are rapidly turning transarterial and transvenous transcatheter valve replacement into a fully percutaneous procedure. Suture-based vascular closure can be accomplished with either the Perclose ProGlide or ProStar devices (Abbott Vascular, Abbott Park, Ill.).

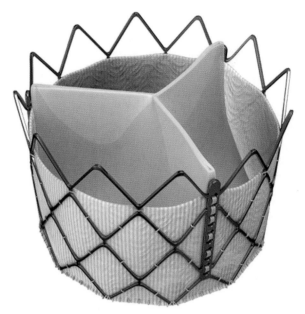

Figure 13–5 The Inovare Braile Biomédica Valve. The Inovare Braile Biomédica Valve is a balloon-expandable cobalt–chromium pericardial leaflet valve that had been used in about a dozen valve-in-valve procedures at the time of publication. *(Courtesy of Braile Biomédica, Brazil.)*

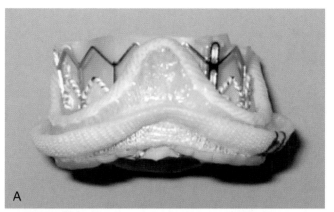

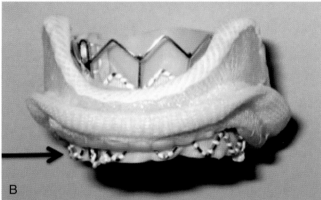

Figure 13–6 Positioning of the transcatheter heart valve inside a surgical bioprosthesis. Correct positioning of the transcatheter valve inside the surgical bioprosthesis is paramount for successful valve-in-valve procedures. In **A,** an Edwards SAPIEN valve inside a Carpentier-Edwards valve is implanted too high. This may result in intervalvular leak or valve embolization. The correct position is shown in **B,** where the transcatheter valve is anchored in the surgical sewing ring *(arrow).* *(Reprinted with permission from Elsevier; Gurvitch, R, Cheung, A, Ye, J, et al: Transcatheter valve-in-valve implantation for failed surgical bioprosthetic valves.* J Am Coll Cardiol 58:2196-2209, 2011.)

For valves without a radiopaque ring but markers at the top of the stent posts, aligning the three markers in one line leads to a perpendicular view. Aortic valves are typically slightly directed anterior and to the patient's right, so that either right anterior oblique–caudal or left anterior oblique–cranial views achieve perpendicularity. Mitral valves are typically directed to the left and anterior, so that a right anterior oblique C-arm angulation may achieve a perpendicular view. If the valve is radiolucent, other imaging modalities such as transesophageal echocardiography are critical for intraprocedural positioning.

PRESTENTING

Additional radial strength and reduction in the risk of stent fracture is achieved for the Melody valve by "prestenting" with a bare metal stent and is usually performed when pulmonic conduits are treated. Prestenting can also lengthen the landing zone and facilitate positioning, especially for THVs that are relatively short. In the tricuspid and pulmonary positions implantation of a longer bare metal stent may provide a landing zone for implantation of a relatively short SAPIEN/XT stent. Prestenting with a covered stent may be desirable when rupture of a small diameter pulmonary conduit is a possibility.

RAPID PACING

Rapid ventricular pacing at a rate between 160 to 200 bpm using a temporary transvenous right ventricular wire can effectively reduce transvalvular flow and cardiac motion. This may facilitate deployment of the THV, but it may impair hemodynamic stability. Rapid ventricular

pacing is usually applied for relatively short balloon-expandable valves (e.g., Edwards SAPIEN, SAPIEN XT, Inovare) and is more useful when the pulse pressure is high, as in the aortic or mitral position. Longer self-expandable THVs with retention mechanisms (e.g., CoreValve [Medtronic] or the Portico valve [St. Jude Medical]) are usually deployed without rapid pacing, although rapid pacing may still be helpful in occasional cases. The importance of high pulse pressure and transvalvular flow is less in the lower pressure right heart. However, even in the tricuspid or pulmonic position, rapid pacing may be helpful to reduce cardiac motion during valve deployment.

PREDILATION

Balloon predilation has been commonly used before transcatheter valve implantation in the setting of native valve stenosis. Similarly, predilation may facilitate crossing and positioning of stenotic bioprosthetic valves. However, predilation of bulky and friable degenerated bioprostheses may result in debris embolization, a concern

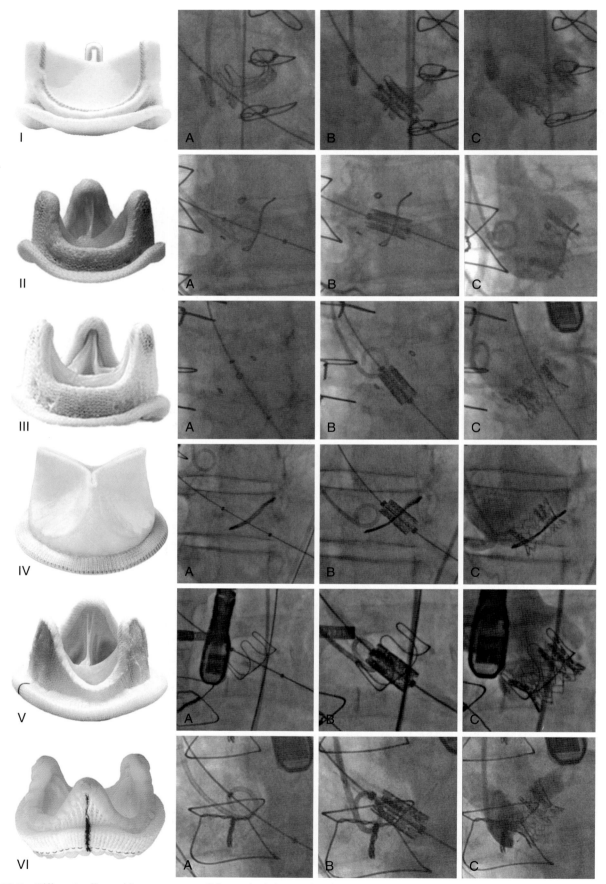

Figure 13–7 **Different radiographic appearances of bioprosthetic heart valves in the aortic position.** Commonly used surgical bioprosthetic valves are shown *(I-VI)* with their perpendicular radiographic appearance in the aortic position **(A),** the crimped transcatheter heart valve across the bioprosthesis with the correct implant height **(B),** and the postdeployment aortic root angiogram **(C).** *I,* Perimount 21 mm, SAPIEN 23 mm; *II,* Hancock 25 mm, SAPIEN 26 mm; *III,* Mosaic 21 mm, SAPIEN 23 mm; *IV,* Mitroflow 23 mm, SAPIEN 23 mm; *V,* Carpentier-Edwards 25 mm, SAPIEN 26 mm; *VI,* St. Jude Medical Epic 21 mm, SAPIEN 23 mm. *(Adapted and Reprinted with permission from Elsevier; Kempfert, J, Van Linden, A, Linke, A, et al: Transapical off-pump valve-in-valve implantation in patients with degenerated aortic xenografts.* Ann Thorac Surg *89:1934-1941, 2010; Gurvitch, R, Cheung, A, Ye, J, et al: Transcatheter valve-in-valve implantation for failed surgical bioprosthetic valves.* J Am Coll Cardiol *58:2196-2209, 2011.)*

especially for left-sided prostheses. Predilation may also cause tears in degenerated, friable bioprosthetic leaflets, resulting in acute severe regurgitation. Consequently, predilation is increasingly avoided except when difficulty is anticipated with retrograde crossing of a severely stenosed or calcified bioprostheses.

CORONARY OBSTRUCTION

When considering VIV implantation in the aortic position the risk of coronary obstruction has to be appraised. The relation of the failing bioprosthesis to the coronary ostia, the bulkiness and calcification of the leaflets, the distance of the ostia from the annular plane, the dimensions of the sinuses, and the characteristics of the surgical bioprosthesis have to be taken into account. The leaflet tissue of most surgical bioprostheses is mounted internal to the stent frame. This ensures that the leaflet tissue will not be displaced external to the valve posts. However, coronary occlusion has been observed after VIV implantation within stented bioprosthesis that have externally mounted pericardial leaflets that can be displaced outwards and within nonstented bioprostheses.[13] Each case must be evaluated on an individual basis, as VIV implants have been successful in both settings where the anatomy is suitable.

HEMODYNAMICS AFTER VALVE-IN-VALVE IMPLANTATION

Although valvular and intervalvular regurgitation is uncommon after VIV interventions, a high residual transvalvular gradient may sometimes cause concern. THV expansion after VIV procedures is limited by the internal diameter of the failing bioprostheses and the relatively undilatable sewing ring. Underexpansion and patient prosthesis mismatch may significantly impair hemodynamics.[14] Therefore postprocedure gradients across VIV implants are significantly higher than those in bioprostheses implanted for native valve disease. Whereas postprocedural mean gradients across THVs implanted in native aortic stenosis mostly range around 7 to 10 mmHg, the transaortic mean gradient after VIV procedures are around 10 to 20 mmHg and higher in small bioprostheses. This may be acceptable in patients who cannot undergo surgery, but it may be prohibitive in operable patients with longer life expectancy. Although CoreValve VIV implantation is limited to the aortic valve using a retrograde approach, it has been suggested that transvalvular gradients may be positively influenced by its supraannular leaflets.

REGURGITATION AFTER VALVE-IN-VALVE IMPLANTATION

Transcatheter aortic valve replacement for native aortic stenosis is generally associated with some degree of PR, although it is usually mild. Because the circular sewing ring of surgical bioprostheses facilitates intervalvular sealing, PR is rarely an issue with VIV procedures.

There are three potential sources of regurgitation after VIV implantation.[8]

1. PR: Regurgitation is located between the native annulus and the surgical bioprosthesis. VIV implantation will not affect this leak, and paravalvular leak closure with a dedicated device (e.g., Amplatzer vascular plug; St. Jude Medical, St. Paul, Minn.) should be considered.[15]

2. Intervalvular regurgitation: Regurgitation arises from a leak between the surgical bioprosthesis and the transcatheter valve. Undersizing of the transcatheter valve and heavy irregular calcifications of the surgical bioprosthesis account for this form of regurgitation. Postdilation of the THV may alleviate this leak. Intervalvular regurgitation is rarely an issue because of good annular sealing between the THV and surgical bioprostheses.

3. Transvalvular regurgitation: Regurgitation is located inside the new THV. Immediately after deployment, the guidewire or delivery system across the valve may cause transvalvular regurgitation. Deformation and overexpansion of the THV may also contribute. Transvalvular regurgitation does not seem to be a major issue in the literature on VIV procedures.[2]

13.5 Considerations for Valve-in-Valve Implantation in Different Positions

VALVE-IN-VALVE IMPLANTATION IN AORTIC POSITION

Of all heart valves, the aortic valve has the highest incidence of surgical valve replacement. Therefore failing bioprostheses in the aortic position are increasingly encountered as a target for VIV procedures. Registry data on aortic VIV procedures are shown in **Table 13–4**. A common access is the retrograde transfemoral approach, which may be performed without general anesthesia and with fluoroscopic guidance. Antegrade transapical aortic VIV implantation allows more direct access to the valve, facilitating positioning, and together with the direct transaortic approach is a valuable alternative when vascular access is poor. However, both techniques imply thoracotomy and general anesthesia, which may be avoided by a transsubclavian or transaxillary approach. Both the SAPIEN/XT valves and the CoreValve device have been used with good early results, although later follow-up study is limited. Although the Melody valve has also been used in the aortic position,[10] its long-term durability in high-pressure environments is questionable, and parts of the valve have to be resected before implantation. As depicted in **Figure 13–4,** all stent cells of the Melody valve are covered by vein wall tissue. To allow blood flow into the sinuses and to the coronaries, a portion of the vein wall must be manually resected, creating open cells in THV frame. For these reasons, the Melody valve is least suitable for aortic VIV procedures.

TABLE 13–4

Aortic Valve-in-Valve Reports

Publication	Number of Valves Reported	THV Implanted	Surgical Implant	Access	Residual Transvalvular Gradient	30-Day Survival
Khawaja, et al[20]	4	CoreValve	CE, Mitroflow, Cryolife-O'Brien,	3 transfemoral 1 subclavian	PG 30-39 mmHg	100%
Maroto, et al[21]	2	Edwards SAPIEN	Hancock	Transapical	PG 13 and 17 mmHg	Not reported
Pasic, et al[22]	14	Edwards SAPIEN	CE, Hancock, Mosaic, Freestyle, Homograft	Transapical	MG 13.1 ± 6.4 mmHg	86%
Seiffert, et al[23]	4	Edwards SAPIEN	Hancock, St. Jude Biocor	Transapical	MG 19.0 ± 12.4 mm Hg	75%
Kempfert, et al[19]	11	Edwards SAPIEN	CE, Hancock, SJM Epic, Mitroflow, Mosaic, Perimount	Transapical	MG 11 ± 4 mmHg	100%
Gotzmann, et al[24]	5	CoreValve	Hancock, CE, Labcor Santiago	Transfemoral	MG 16.4 ± 3.6 mmHg	100%
Latib, et al[25]	17	Edwards SAPIEN SAPIEN XT	CE, SJM, Mosaic, Mitroflow, Bravo, Pericarbon, Hancock, Freestyle, Xenomedica	16 transfemoral 1 transapical 1 transaxillary	MG 13.4 ± 4.8 mmHg	100%
Webb, et al[26]	10	Edwards SAPIEN	CE, Ionescu Shiley, Shelhigh, Freestyle, Mosaic	8 transapical 2 transfemoral	MG 20.2 ± 6.7 mmHg	100%

CE, Carpentier-Edwards; MG, mean gradient; THV, transcatheter heart valve; PG, peak gradient; SJM, St. Jude Medical.

VALVE-IN-VALVE IMPLANTATION IN MITRAL POSITION

The most commonly used access for mitral VIV procedures is the retrograde transapical approach. This technique allows straightforward access for the bioprosthesis but requires a thoracotomy and general anesthesia. If these are to be avoided, an antegrade femoral transvenous approach may be pursued. However, this access is not straightforward, and valve positioning through a transseptal puncture may be challenging. The CoreValve is not suited for the mitral position. The Melody valve has been used in the setting of mitral prosthetic failure[10]; however, its durability is questionable in the setting of the high pressures encountered in the left heart. Most centers have used the Edwards SAPIEN or the SAPIEN XT for mitral VIV procedures with encouraging results. Results of mitral VIV implantations are shown in **Table 13–5.**

VALVE-IN-VALVE IMPLANTATION IN TRICUSPID POSITION

Surgical tricuspid valve replacement is a rarity compared with aortic, mitral, or pulmonic procedures. The tricuspid VIV literature consists of isolated case reports and small series **(Table 13–6, Figure 13–8).** Initially, direct right transatrial access has been used, although this has been supplanted by transvenous access. Antegrade percutaneous access from the internal jugular vein or the subclavian vein has been advocated to facilitate direct engagement of the superiorly tilted tricuspid valve. Transfemoral venous access is feasible, but the angle between the inferior vena cava and the tricuspid valve may or may not be favorable. Only the balloon-expandable SAPIEN, SAPIEN XT, and Melody valves have been successfully used in this position. Because a temporary pacing wire placed in the right ventricle would get trapped between the THV and the surgical bioprosthesis, the procedure is either done without rapid ventricular pacing, or with right atrial, pericardial, or left ventricular pacing.

VALVE-IN-VALVE IMPLANTATION IN PULMONIC POSITION

The first in-human transcatheter valve implantation ever was performed in a failing pulmonic valve conduit in 2000 using the Melody valve. Since then VIV procedures have become the preferred treatment strategy in failing right ventricle–pulmonary artery conduits in patients with congenital heart disease **(Table 13–7, Figure 13–9).** The valve most commonly used in this position is the Melody valve, which is usually implanted using a transvenous femoral approach. Late stent fracture of the Melody valve may occur in up to one quarter of patients, although prestenting conduits may reduce the risk of stent fracture and reintervention.[16,17] The SAPIEN valve with its stainless steel frame and thicker bovine pericardial leaflets has been utilized in the setting of pulmonary VIV implants without documented stent fracture; however, follow-up study remains limited.

TABLE 13–5
Mitral Valve-in-Valve Reports

Publication	Number of Valves Reported	Transcatheter Heart Valve Implanted	Surgical Implant	Access	Residual Transvalvular Mean Gradient	30-Day Survival
Cheung, et al[27]	11	Edwards SAPIEN	Various manufacturers	Transapical	7 mmHg	100%
Seiffert, et al[23]	1	Edwards SAPIEN	Carpentier-Edwards	Transapical	3 mmHg	0%
De Weger, et al[28]	1	Edwards SAPIEN	Mosaic	Transapical	4 mmHg	100%
Van Garsse, et al[29]	1	Edwards SAPIEN	Perimount	Transapical	3 mmHg	100%
Gaia, et al[11]	1	Inovare Braile Biomedical	Not reported	Transapical	5 mmHg	0%
Hammerstingl, et al[15]	1	SAPIEN XT Simultaneous paravalvular leak closure Amplatzer vascular plug III	Hancock, Medtronic	Transapical	Not reported	100%
Himbert, et al[30]	1	SAPIEN XT	mitral annuloplasty ring	Transfemoral, transseptal, antegrade	8 mmHg	100%
Dvir, et al[31]	2	Edwards SAPIEN	Not reported	Transapical	Not reported	100%
Seiffert, et al[32]	1	Edwards SAPIEN	Carpentier-Edwards	Transapical	4 mmHg	100%
Montorfano, et al[33]	1	SAPIEN XT	Carpentier-Edwards	Transfemoral, transseptal, antegrade	3 mmHg	100%
Cerillo, et al[34]	3	Edwards SAPIEN	Hancock, Perimount	Transapical	4-9mmHg	66%

TABLE 13–6
Tricuspid Valve-in-Valve Reports

Publication	Number of Valves	Transcatheter Heart Valve Implanted	Surgical Implant	Access	Residual Transvalvular Mean Gradient	30-Day Survival
Hon, et al[12]	1	Edwards SAPIEN	Mosaic	Transatrial	4 mmHg	100%
Weich, et al[35]	1	SAPIEN XT	Perimount	Transjugular	3 mmHg	100%
Jux, et al[9]	1	Melody	Not reported	Transfemoral	Not reported	100%
Roberts, et al[36]	15	Melody	CE, Hancock, Mosaic, Homograft, Sorin Bicarbon	11 transfemoral 4 transjugular	3.9 mmHg	93%
Webb, et al[26]	1	Edwards SAPIEN	Mosaic	Transatrial	4 mmHg	100%
Cerillo, et al[34]	1	Edwards SAPIEN	Hancock	Transjugular	9 mmHg	100%
Eicken, et al[37]	1	Melody	Homograft	Transfemoral	2-3 mmHg	100%
Gewillig, et al[38]	1	SAPIEN XT	CE	Transjugular	None	100%
Riede, et al[39]	1	Melody	Edwards Perimount	Transfemoral	Not reported	Not reported
Kenny, et al[40]	1	Edwards SAPIEN	Edwards Perimount	Transfemoral	Not reported	Not reported
Nielsen, et al[41]	1	Edwards SAPIEN	CE	Transatrial	Not reported	Not reported
Van Garsse, et al[42]	1	Edwards SAPIEN	CE	Transjugular	2 mmHg	Not reported

CE, Carpentier-Edwards.

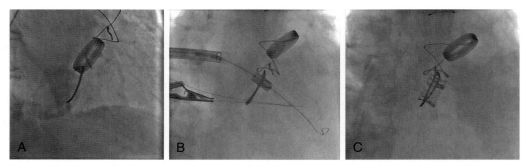

Figure 13–8   Tricuspid valve-in-valve. A, A stenosed and regurgitant Mitroflow 27-mm valve in tricuspid position. This stentless bioprosthesis has a radiopaque basal ring, which is shown coaxial and therefore represents a line. A bileaflet mechanical valve in the mitral position is seen above it. **B,** An Edwards SAPIEN 26-mm valve is being positioned via a direct transatrial approach (mini right thoracotomy). **C,** The final postdeployment fluoroscopic view. *(Reprinted with permission from Elsevier; Gurvitch, R, Cheung, A, Ye, J, et al: Transcatheter valve-in-valve implantation for failed surgical bioprosthetic valves. J Am Coll Cardiol 58:2196-2209, 2011.)*

TABLE 13–7
Pulmonic Valve-in-Valve Reports

Publication	Number of Valves Reported	Transcatheter Heart Valve Implanted	Surgical Implant	Access	Residual Transvalvular Mean Gradient	30-Day Survival
Zahn, et al[16]	34	Melody	Homografts, valved conduits, tube grafts	Transfemoral	17.3 ± 7.3 mmHg	100%
Khambadkone, et al[43]	59	Early version of the Melody valve	Homografts	Transfemoral	19.5 ± 15.3 mmHg	100%
Boone, et al[44]	7	Edwards SAPIEN	Homografts	Transfemoral	14.9 ± 6.9 mmHg	100%
Nordmeyer, et al[45]	20	Melody	Homografts	Transfemoral	Not reported	100%
Jux, et al[9]	1	Melody	Homograft	Transfemoral	Not reported	100%
McElhinney, et al[46]	124	Melody	Homografts, not specified bioprostheses	Transfemoral	Peak gradient 12 mmHg	99%

13.6 Summary

Transcatheter VIV procedures for failing surgical bioprostheses offer an alternative to reoperative surgical valve replacement. Short-term durability seems adequate for many high-risk patients, but long-term durability is unknown. Early but encouraging results in patients with aortic, mitral, pulmonic, and tricuspid bioprostheses suggest that this may well become standard therapy in this setting.

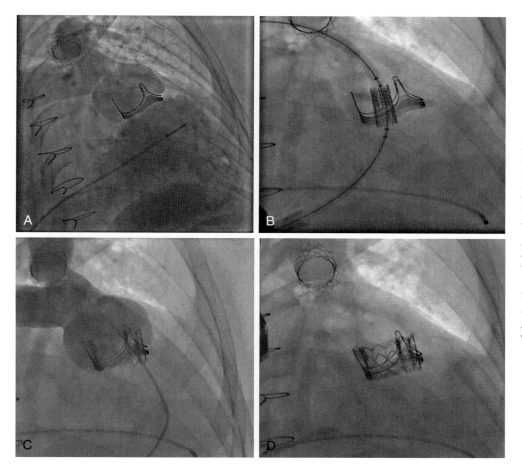

Figure 13-9 **Pulmonic valve-in-valve. A,** A severely regurgitant Carpentier-Edwards Perimount 27-mm valve in pulmonic position in a 21-year-old man with repaired tetralogy of Fallot (a left pulmonary artery stent is also seen). **B,** An Edwards SAPIEN 26-mm valve is being positioned. **C,** The post-deployment pulmonary angiogram demonstrates no residual regurgitation. **D,** The final fluoroscopic result. *(Reprinted with permission from Elsevier; Gurvitch, R, Cheung, A, Ye, J, et al: Transcatheter valve-in-valve implantation for failed surgical bioprosthetic valves. J Am Coll Cardiol 58:2196-2209, 2011.)*

REFERENCES

1. Schoen FJ, Levy RJ: Calcification of tissue heart valve substitutes: progress toward understanding and prevention, *Ann Thorac Surg* 79:1072–1080, 2005.
2. van Geldorp MW, Eric Jamieson WR, Kappetein AP, et al: Patient outcome after aortic valve replacement with a mechanical or biological prosthesis: weighing lifetime anticoagulant-related event risk against reoperation risk, *J Thorac Cardiovasc Surg* 137:881–886, 2009. 6e1-5.
3. Jamieson WR, Miyagishima RT, Burr LH, et al: Carpentier-Edwards porcine bioprostheses: clinical performance assessed by actual analysis, *J Heart Valve Dis* 9:530–535, 2000.
4. Ruel M, Kulik A, Rubens FD, et al: Late incidence and determinants of reoperation in patients with prosthetic heart valves, *Eur J Cardiothorac Surg* 25:364–370, 2004.
5. Jamieson WR, Rosado LJ, Munro AI, et al: Carpentier-Edwards standard porcine bioprosthesis: primary tissue failure (structural valve deterioration) by age groups, *Ann Thorac Surg* 46:155–162, 1988.
6. Schoen FJ, Fernandez J, Gonzalez-Lavin L, et al: Causes of failure and pathologic findings in surgically removed Ionescu-Shiley standard bovine pericardial heart valve bioprostheses: emphasis on progressive structural deterioration, *Circulation* 76:618–627, 1987.
7. Butany J, Leask R: The failure modes of biological prosthetic heart valves, *J Long Term Eff Med Implants* 11:115–135, 2001.
8. Gurvitch R, Cheung A, Ye J, et al: Transcatheter valve-in-valve implantation for failed surgical bioprosthetic valves, *J Am Coll Cardiol* 58:2196–2209, 2011.
9. Jux C, Akintuerk H, Schranz D: Two melodies in concert: transcatheter double-valve replacement, *Catheter Cardiovasc Interv*, 80:997–1001, 2011.
10. Hasan BS, McElhinney DB, Brown DW, et al: Short-term performance of the transcatheter Melody valve in high-pressure hemodynamic environments in the pulmonary and systemic circulations, *Circ Cardiovasc Interv* 4:615–620, 2011.
11. Gaia DF, Palma JH, de Souza JA, et al: Transapical mitral valve-in-valve implant: an alternative for high risk and multiple reoperative rheumatic patients, *Int J Cardiol* 154:e6–e7, 2012.
12. Hon JK, Cheung A, Ye J, et al: Transatrial transcatheter tricuspid valve-in-valve implantation of balloon expandable bioprosthesis, *Ann Thorac Surg* 90:1696–1697, 2010.
13. Gurvitch R, Cheung A, Bedogni F, et al: Coronary obstruction following transcatheter aortic valve-in-valve implantation for failed surgical bioprostheses, *Catheter Cardiovasc Interv* 77:439–444, 2011.
14. Seiffert M, Conradi L, Baldus S, et al: Impact of patient-prosthesis mismatch after transcatheter aortic valve-in-valve implantation in degenerated bioprostheses, *J Thorac Cardiovasc Surg* 143:617–624, 2012.
15. Hammerstingl C, Nickenig G, Endlich M, et al: Treatment of a severely degenerated mitral valve bioprosthesis with simultaneous transapical paravalvular leak closure and valve-in-valve implantation, *Eur Heart J* 33:1976, 2012.
16. Zahn EM, Hellenbrand WE, Lock JE, et al: Implantation of the Melody transcatheter pulmonary valve in patients with a dysfunctional right ventricular outflow tract conduit early results from the U.S. clinical trial, *J Am Coll Cardiol* 54:1722–1729, 2009.
17. McElhinney DB, Cheatham JP, Jones TK, et al: Stent fracture, valve dysfunction, and right ventricular outflow tract reintervention after transcatheter pulmonary valve implantation: patient-related and procedural risk factors in the US Melody Valve Trial, *Circ Cardiovasc Interv* 4:602–614, 2011.
18. Wenaweser P, Buellesfeld L, Gerckens U, et al: Percutaneous aortic valve replacement for severe aortic regurgitation in degenerated bioprosthesis: the first valve-in-valve procedure using the CoreValve Revalving system, *Catheter Cardiovasc Interv* 70:760–764, 2007.
19. Kempfert J, Van Linden A, Linke A, et al: Transapical off-pump valve-in-valve implantation in patients with degenerated aortic xenografts, *Ann Thorac Surg* 89:1934–1941, 2010.

20. Khawaja MZ, Haworth P, Ghuran A, et al: Transcatheter aortic valve implantation for stenosed and regurgitant aortic valve bioprostheses CoreValve for failed bioprosthetic aortic valve replacements, J Am Coll Cardiol 55:97–101, 2010.

21. Maroto LC, Rodriguez JE, Cobiella J, et al: Transapical off-pump aortic valve-in-a-valve implantation in two elderly patients with a degenerated porcine bioprosthesis, Eur J Cardiothorac Surg 37: 738–740, 2010.

22. Pasic M, Unbehaun A, Dreysse S, et al: Transapical aortic valve implantation after previous aortic valve replacement: clinical proof of the "valve-in-valve" concept, J Thorac Cardiovasc Surg 142:270–277, 2011.

23. Seiffert M, Franzen O, Conradi L: Series of transcatheter valve-in-valve implantations in high-risk patients with degenerated bioprostheses in aortic and mitral position, Catheter Cardiovasc Interv 76:608–615, 2010.

24. Gotzmann M, Mugge A, Bojara W: Transcatheter aortic valve implantation for treatment of patients with degenerated aortic bioprostheses: valve-in-valve technique, Catheter Cardiovasc Interv 76:1000–1006, 2010.

25. Latib A, Ielasi A, Montorfano M, et al: Transcatheter valve-in-valve implantation with the Edwards SAPIEN in patients with bioprosthetic heart valve failure: the Milan experience, EuroIntervention 7:1275–1284, 2012.

26. Webb JG, Wood DA, Ye J, et al: Transcatheter valve-in-valve implantation for failed bioprosthetic heart valves, Circulation 121: 1848–1857, 2010.

27. Cheung AW, Gurvitch R, Ye J, et al: Transcatheter transapical mitral valve-in-valve implantations for a failed bioprosthesis: a case series, J Thorac Cardiovasc Surg 141:711–715, 2011.

28. de Weger A, Tavilla G, Ng AC, et al: Successful transapical transcatheter valve implantation within a dysfunctional mitral bioprosthesis, JACC Cardiovasc Imaging 3:222–223, 2010.

29. van Garsse LA, Gelsomino S, van Ommen V, et al: Emergency transthoracic transapical mitral valve-in-valve implantation, J Interv Cardiol 24:474–476, 2011.

30. Himbert D, Brochet E, Radu C, et al: Transseptal implantation of a transcatheter heart valve in a mitral annuloplasty ring to treat mitral repair failure, Circ Cardiovasc Interv 4:396–398, 2011.

31. Dvir D, Assali A, Vaknin-Assa H, et al: Transcatheter aortic and mitral valve implantations for failed bioprosthetic heart valves, J Invasive Cardiol 23:377–381, 2011.

32. Seiffert M, Baldus S, Conradi L, et al: Simultaneous transcatheter aortic and mitral valve-in-valve implantation in a patient with degenerated bioprostheses and high surgical risk, Thorac Cardiovasc Surg 59:490–492, 2011.

33. Montorfano M, Latib A, Chieffo A, et al: Successful percutaneous anterograde transcatheter valve-in-valve implantation in the mitral position, JACC Cardiovasc Interv 4:1246–1247, 2011.

34. Cerillo AG, Chiaramonti F, Murzi M, et al: Transcatheter valve-in-valve implantation for failed mitral and tricuspid bioprosthesis, Catheter Cardiovasc Interv 78:987–995, 2011.

35. Weich H, Janson J, van Wyk J, et al: Transjugular tricuspid valve-in-valve replacement, Circulation 124:e157–e160, 2011.

36. Roberts PA, Boudjemline Y, Cheatham JP, et al: Percutaneous tricuspid valve replacement in congenital and acquired heart disease, J Am Coll Cardiol 58:117–122, 2011.

37. Eicken A, Fratz S, Hager A, et al: Transcutaneous Melody valve implantation in "tricuspid position" after a Fontan Bjork (RA-RV homograft) operation results in biventricular circulation, Int J Cardiol 142:e45–e47, 2010.

38. Gewillig M, Dubois C: Percutaneous re-revalvulation of the tricuspid valve, Catheter Cardiovasc Interv 77:692–695, 2011.

39. Riede FT, Dahnert I: Implantation of a Melody valve in triscuspid position, Catheter Cardiovasc Interv, 80:474–476, 2012.

40. Kenny D, Hijazi ZM, Walsh KP: Transcatheter tricuspid valve replacement with the Edwards SAPIEN valve, Catheter Cardiovasc Interv 78:267–270, 2011.

41. Nielsen HH, Egeblad H, Klaaborg KE, et al: Transatrial stent-valve implantation in a stenotic tricuspid valve bioprosthesis, Ann Thorac Surg 91:e74–e76, 2011.

42. Van Garsse LA, Ter Bekke RM, van Ommen VG: Percutaneous transcatheter valve-in-valve implantation in stenosed tricuspid valve bioprosthesis, Circulation 123:e219–e221, 2011.

43. Khambadkone S, Coats L, Taylor A, et al: Percutaneous pulmonary valve implantation in humans: results in 59 consecutive patients, Circulation 112:1189–1197, 2005.

44. Boone RH, Webb JG, Horlick E, et al: Transcatheter pulmonary valve implantation using the Edwards SAPIEN transcatheter heart valve, Catheter Cardiovasc Interv 75:286–294, 2010.

45. Nordmeyer J, Coats L, Lurz P, et al: Percutaneous pulmonary valve-in-valve implantation: a successful treatment concept for early device failure, Eur Heart J 29:810–815, 2008.

46. McElhinney DB, Hellenbrand WE, Zahn EM, et al: Short- and medium-term outcomes after transcatheter pulmonary valve placement in the expanded multicenter U.S. Melody Valve Trial, Circulation 122:507–516, 2010.

Alcohol Septal Ablation for Obstructive Hypertrophic Cardiomyopathy

RICHARD G. BACH • GAGAN D. SINGH • JEFFREY A. SOUTHARD

14.1 Key Points

- In appropriate patients with hypertrophic cardiomyopathy (HCM), alcohol septal ablation using contrast echocardiographic guidance causes targeted necrosis, thinning of the basal interventricular septum, and widening of the left ventricular outflow tract (LVOT) and relieves outflow tract obstruction.
- Alcohol septal ablation is indicated as an alternative option for septal reduction therapy for patients with HCM who have significant symptoms refractory to medical therapy and attributable to severe LVOT obstruction that results from asymmetric septal hypertrophy (ASH) and systolic anterior motion (SAM) of the mitral valve.
- Patients at higher risk for surgical myectomy, including older patients and those with comorbidities, and symptomatic patients who have not obtained a satisfactory result after septal myectomy, may be excellent candidates for alcohol septal ablation.
- Alcohol septal ablation may be complicated by high-degree atrioventricular (AV) block, requiring permanent pacemaker (PPM) implantation in approximately 10% of patients and ventricular tachyarrhythmias in up to 3% of patients and should be performed in experienced centers.

HCM is the most common cardiovascular genetic disorder, characterized by unexplained cardiac hypertrophy involving a nondilated left ventricle in the absence of other identifiable cardiac or systemic causes. The location and extent of myocardial hypertrophy can vary among patients with HCM, but the most common phenotype involves ASH of the basal interventricular septum that may be accompanied by dynamic obstruction of the LVOT. Although there is wide anatomic and physiologic heterogeneity among patients with HCM and variability in the clinical manifestations, the presence of dynamic LVOT obstruction has been related to symptomatic status and a higher risk of death.[1,2] In patients with appropriate anatomic features and significant dynamic LVOT obstruction associated with severe and limiting symptoms refractory to medical therapy, treatment with septal reduction therapy may be considered to improve quality of life. Septal reduction for patients with HCM can be accomplished by one of two procedures: (1) surgical septal myectomy or (2) percutaneous transcatheter alcohol septal ablation. Whereas septal myectomy has been recommended as a preferred method of septal reduction for many patients (especially younger patients), for patients at higher surgical risk or who prefer to avoid surgery, alcohol septal ablation represents an effective treatment option that can provide similarly successful symptom relief and improved quality of life.[3]

14.2 Background

ALCOHOL SEPTAL ABLATION: HISTORICAL CONSIDERATIONS

Alcohol septal ablation was first reported by Ulrich Sigwart in 1995.[4] Sigwart had made the seminal observation that the degree of LVOT obstruction in patients with HCM responded favorably to ischemia caused by temporary balloon occlusion of a major septal artery, but that it returned to baseline after balloon deflation.

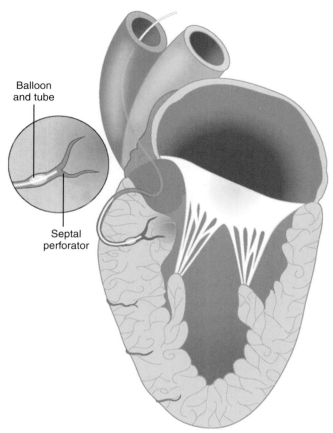

Figure 14–1 Transcatheter alcohol septal ablation. The illustration shows an inflated angioplasty balloon occluding the first septal perforator branch of the left anterior descending artery (LAD) with a targeted area of necrosis in the perfused basal septum caused by injection of alcohol via the balloon catheter.

Balloon and tube

Septal perforator

In this first report, in three cases he was able to successfully and durably reduce the LVOT obstruction by inducing targeted necrosis of the basal interventricular septum via selective injection of alcohol into a septal artery and achieve sustained relief of symptoms that had previously been refractory to medical management. The conceptual approach is illustrated in **Figure 14–1.** In subsequent reports of early experience with alcohol septal ablation in relatively small case series, successful LVOT gradient reduction and improvement in symptoms was demonstrated, although it was associated with a relatively high incidence (30% to 40%) of high-degree AV block, requiring PPM insertion.[5-8] After the initial series of patients, a technical advance was recognized, whereby intraprocedural contrast echocardiographic mapping of the perfusion territory of the candidate septal artery was incorporated into the procedure,[9] allowing more selective and precise localization of the target territory appropriate for ablation. This was associated with reduction in the rate of complications, including AV block. Since its introduction, alcohol septal ablation has been used successfully worldwide to treat a large number of severely symptomatic patients with HCM and LVOT obstruction,

including patients who have undergone a previously unsuccessful surgical myectomy.[10]

OUTCOMES

With respect to procedural success and outcomes, several studies have confirmed that significant reduction of the LVOT gradient and improvement of symptoms are accomplished by alcohol septal ablation in 90% or more of patients.[11,12] Recent meta-analysis and reports with longer-term follow-up periods have supported immediate, short-term and sustained long-term gradient reduction and symptomatic improvement after alcohol septal ablation.[13-17] Despite the absence of randomized trial data, comparisons of contemporary case series suggest that the symptomatic improvements after alcohol septal ablation appear similar to those reported after myectomy, although alcohol septal ablation is associated with a somewhat higher posttreatment LVOT gradient and higher risk of PPM implantation. A systematic review[18] of 42 published studies analyzing results from 2959 patients undergoing alcohol septal ablation from 1996 to 2005, with an average follow-up time of about 1 year, reported a sustained reduction of the resting LVOT gradient from 65 mmHg to 16 mmHg and of the provoked LVOT gradient from 125 mmHg to 32 mmHg, associated with a significant improvement in exercise capacity and New York Heart Association (NYHA) functional class (from a mean of 2.9 to 1.2).

Long-term follow-up data from a substantial number of patients undergoing alcohol septal ablation have been reported from several centers since 2008. Welge et al[19] reported that for 347 patients who underwent alcohol septal ablation at one center in Germany, at a follow-up period of over nearly 5 years 89% were symptomatically improved with NYHA class I or II symptoms, 74% were free of LVOT obstruction at rest, and 60% did not exhibit any provocable LVOT obstruction. Fernandes and colleagues[14] reported long-term outcomes of alcohol septal ablation performed in 629 patients at two centers in the United States from 1996 to 2007. The mean follow-up period was 4.6 ± 2.5 years and ranged from 3 months to 10.2 years. In that series, there appeared to be a progressive decline in the LVOT gradient over the long-term follow-up period, with the mean resting gradient at baseline of 77 ± 31 mmHg decreasing to 26 ± 27 mmHg at 3 months, 20 ± 24 mmHg at 1 year, and less than 10 mmHg in those tested after 5 years (p < 0.001). During follow-up study, NYHA functional class decreased from the baseline of 2.8 ± 0.6 to 1.2 ± 0.5 (p < 0.001); Canadian Cardiovascular Society (CCS) angina class decreased from 2.1 ± 0.9 to 1.0 ± 0 (p < 0.001); and exercise time increased from 4.8 ± 3.3 to 8.2 ± 1.0 minutes (p < 0.001) **(Figure 14–2).** The survival estimates were favorable at 1, 5, and 8 years at 97%, 92%, and 89%, respectively. The rate of new pacemakers required for high-degree heart block was 9.7%. Within this cohort, 14% underwent repeat alcohol septal ablation and 4% underwent myectomy for unsatisfactory initial results. Sorajja et al[20] reported outcomes from 138 patients who underwent alcohol septal ablation at the Mayo Clinic from 1999 to 2006. In that

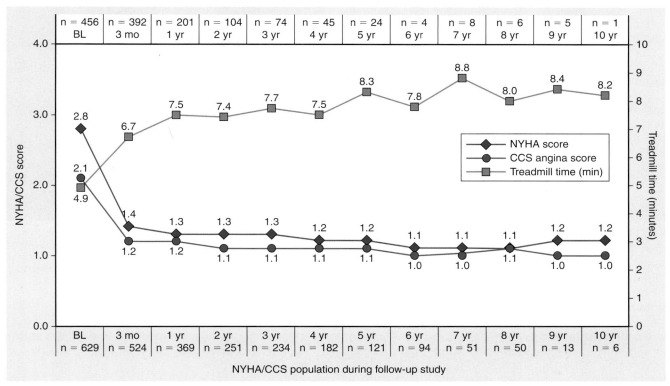

Figure 14–2 Long-term follow-up study after alcohol septal ablation among 629 patients with hypertrophic cardiomyopathy including functional score (NYHA heart failure class and CCS angina class) and treadmill exercise time showing marked early improvement of heart failure symptoms, angina, and treadmill exercise time at 3 months that persisted during the follow-up period. (*BL*, Baseline; *CCS*, Canadian Cardiovascular Society; *NYHA*, New York Heart Association.) (*Reproduced with permission from Fernandes, VL, Nielsen, C, Nagueh, SF, et al: Follow-up of alcohol septal ablation for symptomatic hypertrophic obstructive cardiomyopathy the Baylor and Medical University of South Carolina experience, 1996 to 2007. JACC Cardiovasc Interv 1:561-70, 2008.*)

series, the 4-year survival rate free of death and severe NYHA class III/IV symptoms after alcohol septal ablation was 76.4%, and 71 patients (51%) became asymptomatic. They noted, however, from a nonrandomized comparison, that the rate of procedural complications appeared higher than in age- and gender-matched patients who had undergone septal myectomy at the Mayo Clinic, especially among younger patients. Jensen and colleagues[21] recently reported long-term outcomes of alcohol septal ablation among 279 patients with HCM, many of whom had significant comorbidities, performed from 1999 to 2010 in four Scandinavian centers. In their experience, the median LVOT gradient at rest was reduced by alcohol septal ablation from 58 to 12 mmHg at 1-year (p < 0.001), and the gradient provoked by Valsalva maneuver was reduced from 93 to 21 mmHg (p < 0.001). The proportion of patients with NYHA class III/IV symptoms was reduced from 94% to 21% (p < 0.001), and the proportion of patients with syncope was reduced from 18% to 2% (p < 0.001). In-hospital mortality was low at 0.3%. The 1-, 5- and 10-year survival rates were 97%, 87%, and 67%, respectively (p < 0.06 vs. an age- and sex-matched background population).

A report of a large-scale North American registry[13] has provided additional important information from a multicenter experience involving 874 patients undergoing alcohol septal ablation at nine centers from 2000 to 2010. Before the procedure nearly 80% of patients had NYHA class III or IV heart failure symptoms; 43% of patients had CCS class III or IV angina; and 29% reported syncope. After the procedure, there was significant symptomatic improvement, with fewer than 5% of patients having NYHA class III or IV heart failure, less than 1% of patients having CCS class III angina (none had class IV), and only 2.9% of patients with syncope. Among the patients in the registry, survival estimates at 1, 5, and 9 years were 97%, 86%, and 74%, respectively. The authors noted that the overall survival rate at 1 year after alcohol septal ablation (97% vs. 98%) was similar to that seen in a disease-free general population, and survival at 1, 5, and 9 to 10 years appeared better after alcohol septal ablation compared with patients reported in other series, who had HCM and did not undergo septal reduction therapy.[22]

Despite the high success rate of alcohol septal ablation, a small proportion (<10%) of patients may not achieve adequate hemodynamic or clinical response. Among several potential causes, insufficient necrosis and thinning of the basal septal hypertrophy may be the most common etiology. Patients who undergo alcohol septal ablation and are found at follow-up study to have significant residual LVOT gradients, and unrelieved or recurrent symptoms may benefit from a second septal reduction procedure. Among patients in the reported series, approximately 6% to 14% underwent repeat alcohol septal ablation, with reportedly favorable hemodynamic and symptomatic outcomes,[13,18,19,21,23,24] and 2% to 3% underwent surgical myectomy, also with favorable outcomes but a possibly higher risk of postoperative pacemaker requirement caused by AV block, compared with patients undergoing myectomy without a prior history of septal ablation.[25] It should be noted, however, that in the North American registry, multivariate analysis suggested that repeat alcohol septal ablation procedures may be associated with higher long-term mortality risk.[13]

14.3 Typical Patient Presentation

Patients with HCM and LVOT obstruction often have one or more of three cardinal symptom complexes: (1) dyspnea on exertion, (2) anginal chest pain, and/or (3) syncope and near syncope. These symptoms are not specific for HCM or LVOT obstruction and are shared by other, more common cardiovascular disorders, suggesting that the clinician must have an adequate index of suspicion to establish an accurate diagnosis, and the evaluation should include imaging studies to differentiate the varied possible etiologies. Furthermore, the relationships among cardiac anatomy, physiology, and symptoms are not always straightforward for patients with HCM, posing challenges to diagnosis and selection of treatment. Patients may note an exacerbation of symptoms after meals, and this characteristic may be a clue to alert the clinician to the possibility of HCM with LVOT obstruction. Syncope and episodes of near syncope are also not uncommon in patients with HCM and may have one of a number of etiologies, but they also should raise the index of suspicion for significant LVOT obstruction.

14.4 Patient Evaluation

The diagnosis of HCM generally relies on high-quality echocardiographic detection of the characteristic asymmetric left ventricular (LV) hypertrophy. HCM is diagnosed when maximal LV wall thickness is 15 mm or greater in the absence of other identifiable causes, whereas wall thickness of 13 to 14 mm may be considered borderline.[3] The most common phenotype of HCM relevant for consideration of septal reduction includes disproportionate hypertrophy of the basal interventricular septum (ASH), such that the ratio of the septal to posterior wall thickness is greater than 1:3 **(Figure 14–3).** This basal septal hypertrophy typically narrows the LVOT and may be accompanied by SAM of the anterior mitral valve leaflet. During ventricular systole, as flow accelerates across the basal hypertrophied septum, drag forces and a Venturi effect are created where the anterior leaflet of the mitral valve is directed towards that segment of the septum, resulting in mitral–septal contact. In a substantial proportion of patients, ASH and SAM contribute to significant dynamic LVOT obstruction, although the

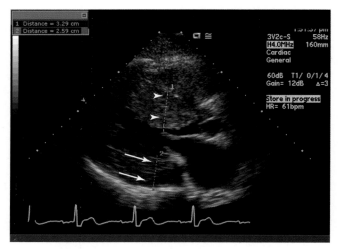

Figure 14–3 Parasternal long-axis view indicates an asymmetrically thickened left ventricular myocardium. The septal myocardium (arrowheads) is thickened at approximately 3.3 cm, whereas the posterior wall (arrows) is thickened at 2.6 cm. The ratio of the septal to posterior wall is approximately 1:3.

degree of obstruction to LV outflow varies across a wide spectrum. It has been estimated that one quarter to one third of patients show LVOT obstruction at rest, although when adequate provocative testing is performed, the majority of patients with HCM (≥70%) are found to have significant resting or provocable obstruction.[26]

The evaluation of patients with HCM for consideration of eligibility for septal reduction therapy includes two-dimensional echocardiography, employing a protocol that fully investigates these relevant anatomic and physiologic features. This includes a focused assessment of LV morphology, septal thickness, and dynamic LVOT obstruction at rest and with stress. The examination may be best accomplished with a specialized stress echocardiogram protocol, providing an objective assessment of exercise tolerance and an assessment of LVOT velocity at peak physiologic stress. Dynamic LVOT obstruction is most commonly quantified using Doppler echocardiographic interrogation of the LVOT, with care to avoid contaminating the spectral display with accelerated velocity from mitral regurgitation, which can confound accurate estimation of the LVOT gradient **(Figure 14–4).** With LVOT obstruction in HCM the spectral Doppler display shows a characteristic accelerated velocity with a late-peaking dagger-shaped appearance **(Figure 14–5).** Because intraventricular obstruction can be present from other causes such as fixed subaortic stenosis or midventricular obstruction in the setting of cavity obliteration, care is warranted in identifying the site and etiology of obstruction. The systolic pressure gradient resulting from LVOT obstruction is proportional to the peak instantaneous LVOT velocity and can be reliably estimated using the modified Bernoulli formula. Because LVOT obstruction is dynamic and may not be present at rest in many patients, provocative maneuvers are necessary for a comprehensive evaluation of LVOT obstruction in patients with symptoms suspected because of HCM. Doppler imaging during Valsalva maneuver and

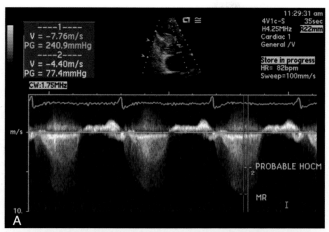

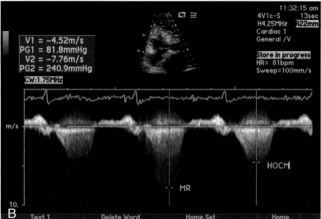

Figure 14–4 **A,** Continuous wave pulse Doppler through the left ventricular outflow tract (LVOT) can often be difficult, because the mitral regurgitant velocities can interfere with measurement. **B,** Moving the site of Doppler analysis at the time of recording can help differentiate mitral regurgitant velocities from LVOT velocity. Resting LVOT gradient is approximately 80 mmHg.

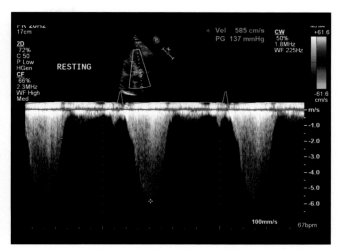

Figure 14–5 Continuous wave Doppler through the LVOT. The accelerated velocity has a characteristic late-peaking dagger-shaped appearance. The Doppler signal demonstrates a resting gradient of 137 mmHg.

amyl nitrite inhalation can elicit a provoked gradient, although upright exercise with immediate assessment of the peak LVOT velocity likely represents the most physiologically sound method to estimate the relevant peak provocable LVOT gradient. Combining a formal exercise stress protocol with immediate postexercise Doppler echocardiography is the authors' preferred method for determining the presence and quantifying the degree of physiologically relevant provocable LVOT obstruction, and it is especially useful in evaluating patients with symptoms who do not have resting outflow obstruction or whose degree of resting LVOT obstruction is only mild to moderate (i.e., <50 mmHg).[26] For patients who cannot exercise, graded dobutamine infusion has been used as a method to estimate peak provocable gradients by a readily reproducible protocol, but because of concerns regarding its potential lack of specificity and physiologic relevance, its use in selection of patients for septal reduction has been controversial.

Transesophageal echocardiography (TEE) also has an important role in the evaluation of patients with HCM to assess coincident mitral regurgitation and mitral valve morphology and to exclude any form of fixed LVOT obstruction that may be unexpectedly present in a small number of patients carrying a diagnosis of HCM referred for septal reduction.[27] TEE can help define mitral valve, chordal and papillary muscle anatomy, and the degree and etiology of mitral regurgitation. For patients in whom severe mitral regurgitation is observed, some features of the visualized regurgitant jet (e.g., eccentricity and posterior direction, responsiveness to pharmacologic maneuvers) and mitral valve morphology can be helpful in determining whether the mitral regurgitation is likely secondary to LVOT obstruction and SAM (when it is likely to improve with relief of LVOT obstruction) or whether it is the result of independent mitral valve pathology, when indications favoring surgical valvular intervention may also be present.[28] With respect to any suspicion of fixed LVOT obstruction, also termed *discrete subaortic stenosis*, the subaortic ridge or membrane may not be visible on two-dimensional echocardiographic images, whereas coincident septal hypertrophy may resemble traditional HCM, leading to mistaken diagnosis and treatment.[27] Clues to the presence of a subaortic membrane or some form of fixed LVOT obstruction on two-dimensional imaging include absence of SAM or an accelerated LVOT velocity that is early peaking despite absence of morphologic features of aortic stenosis, often associated with mild to moderate aortic insufficiency. When suspected, additional imaging by TEE or cardiac magnetic resonance imaging is strongly recommended to exclude fixed LVOT obstruction before consideration of alcohol septal ablation.

Cardiac catheterization is also routinely performed in the evaluation of candidacy for septal reduction therapy, providing an angiographic assessment of coincident coronary artery disease and septal artery anatomy and allowing a thorough catheter-based assessment of the dynamic intraventricular obstruction, any of which may affect management strategy. In patients with anginal chest pain, coronary angiography is essential to assess the presence of coincidental coronary artery disease. The catheter-based evaluation of ventricular hemodynamics may also be especially important when the results of rest or provoked gradient assessment by Doppler echocardiography are equivocal or unobtainable. Hemodynamic assessment can be readily performed using small-caliber catheters and two transducers to measure simultaneous intraventricular and aortic or femoral artery pressure. For intraventricular measurements, a pigtail catheter should be avoided because of side holes extending several centimeters along the distal end, potentially crossing the site of obstruction and artifactually lowering the LVOT gradient, and end-hole catheters raise a theoretical concern of catheter entrapment and artifactually increased intraventricular pressure. Catheters with end and side holes limited to the distal 1 to 2 cm (e.g., multipurpose A-2 or Halo pigtail catheter) may be best suited for this evaluation. Simultaneous LV and aortic or femoral artery pressures are measured at rest, after ventricular extrasystoles, during Valsalva maneuver, and after amyl nitrite inhalation to fully profile the resting and provocable LVOT gradients. The Brockenbrough-Braunwald-Morrow sign, a simultaneous increase in the LVOT systolic gradient associated with a diminished aortic pulse pressure after a ventricular extrasystole that is likely the result of postextrasystolic potentiation of LV contractility, is the classic manifestation of the dynamic LV–aortic gradient, and remarkably high gradients can be seen **(Figures 14–6 and 14–7)**. A careful pullback can demonstrate the intraventricular location of the systolic gradient and confirm the absence or measure the amount of any aortic valve–related systolic gradient in the presence of coincident aortic valve stenosis **(Figure 14–8)**.

INDICATIONS AND PATIENT SELECTION FOR ALCOHOL SEPTAL ABLATION

Transcatheter alcohol septal ablation is indicated as an option for septal reduction to improve symptoms that are attributable to LVOT obstruction in patients with severe functional class III to IV symptoms despite appropriate medical therapy. The most common symptoms indicating septal reduction are NYHA class III or IV dyspnea on exertion and/or CCS class III to IV angina pectoris. Some patients may also have disabling syncopal episodes or frequent presyncope associated with severe LVOT obstruction. The 2011 ACCF/ACC Guideline for the Diagnosis and Treatment of Hypertrophic Cardiomyopathy[3] specifically recommends (class IIb, Level of Evidence B) that alcohol septal ablation, when performed in experienced centers, may be considered as an alternative to surgical myectomy for eligible adult patients with HCM with severe drug-refractory symptoms and LVOT obstruction when after a balanced and thorough discussion, the patient expresses a preference for septal ablation. Appropriate candidates for alcohol septal ablation **(Box 14–1)** should have: (1) ASH with adequate septal thickness (≥15 to 18 mm); (2) a documented resting or provocable outflow tract gradient of 50 mmHg or greater that is caused by ASH and SAM of the mitral valve (and

not from systolic cavity obliteration); and (3) suitable septal artery anatomy.[3]

When weighing options for septal reduction for an individual patient, certain considerations favor surgical intervention. The effectiveness of alcohol septal ablation is uncertain in patients with HCM with marked septal hypertrophy (i.e., >30 mm),[23] and guideline recommendations specifically state that the procedure should be discouraged in such patients (class IIb, level of evidence: C).[3] Other conditions that favor surgical intervention include younger age, unusual valve or papillary muscle abnormalities that can structurally contribute to LVOT obstruction,[29-31] and coincident cardiac disease that would independently prompt surgical repair (e.g., intrinsic mitral valve pathology or complex coronary artery disease). In experienced hands, surgical myectomy can provide excellent hemodynamic results. Since atrial fibrillation is poorly tolerated in patients with HCM, patients with HCM who experience severe symptoms and paroxysmal or sustained atrial fibrillation may be considered candidates for a surgical approach that includes septal myectomy combined with a Maze procedure to reduce the likelihood of recurrent atrial fibrillation, although reported experience is limited[32] and the long-term outcomes of this approach are not yet well defined. In contrast, patients at high risk of surgical morbidity or mortality, including older patients and those with other comorbidities that pose higher surgical risk or will likely limit long-term survival, are excellent candidates for alcohol septal ablation. In addition, patients with symptoms who have not obtained a satisfactory result after surgical myectomy may also be considered candidates for septal ablation.[33,34]

All patients undergoing evaluation for septal reduction therapy should also be screened for risk factors for sudden cardiac death (SCD).[35] If there are risk factors identified, such patients may be candidates for prophylactic implantable cardioverter-defibrillator (ICD) implantation. Of note, for patients who elect to undergo alcohol septal ablation, prior implantation of a dual-chamber pacemaker ICD can facilitate the procedure by obviating the need for temporary pacing and the potential associated risks and prolonged bedrest.

14.5 Alcohol Septal Ablation: Procedural Technique

Left coronary angiography first performed in the right anterior oblique cranial view is useful to identify candidate proximal septal perforator arteries for potential ablation and to assess their angles of origin to anticipate technical difficulty and guide equipment selection. Septal arteries may originate from the left anterior descending, diagonal, median ramus, and left main arteries, although most target vessels arise from the proximal to midleft anterior descending artery **(see Figure 14–6 and Figure 14–9, A)**. The most proximal significant septal artery is most likely to provide perfusion to the target territory, although septal artery anatomy and perfusion distribution is quite variable,

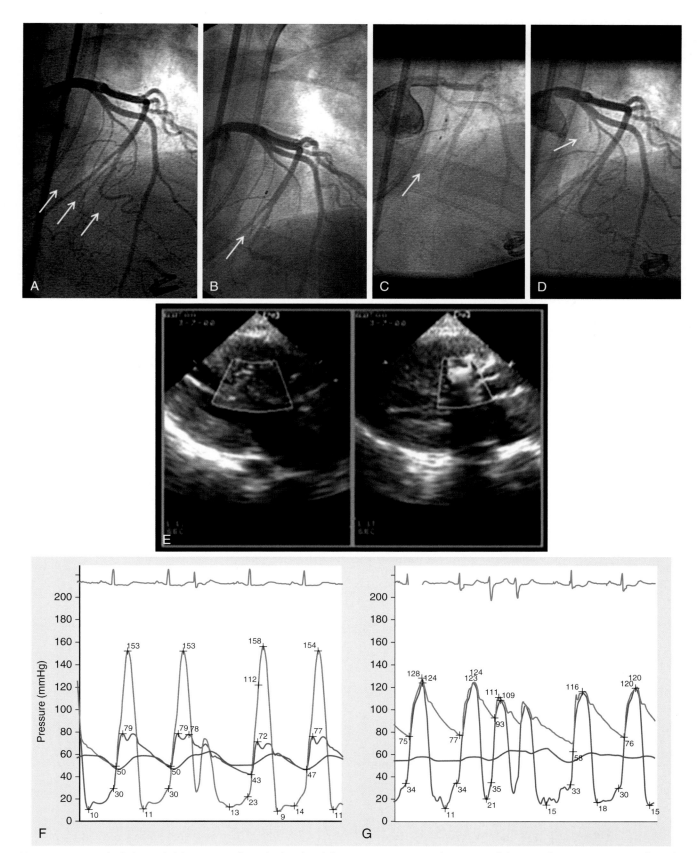

Figure 14–6 **A,** Alcohol septal ablation procedure: the baseline left coronary angiogram shows 3 candidate septal arteries originating from the proximal LAD *(arrows)*. **B,** The second septal artery is cannulated with a balloon *(arrow),* but contrast echo imaging via the inflated balloon shows enhancement of the midseptum remote from the ASH and SAM (*E, left*). **C,** The balloon is then repositioned into the first septal artery and inflated *(arrow),* and repeat contrast echo (with power harmonic) imaging shows enhancement of the basal septum at the site of septal–SAM contact (*E, right*). **D,** Then 2.5 cc of alcohol is injected over 10 minutes; after later balloon removal, repeat angiography shows typical proximal occlusion of the ablated first septal *(arrow).* The lower graphs show the patient's LVOT hemodynamics with and without ventricular extrasystoles before **(F)** and immediately after **(G)** alcohol septal ablation, showing immediate near elimination of the resting and provoked LVOT gradient by alcohol septal ablation.

and at times the second or even third septal branch or a septal branch originating from the first diagonal or ramus arteries perfuses the appropriate target location. It is not recommended to ablate more than two septal arteries during a single setting; instead midterm results may be evaluated over the subsequent 3 to 12 months. Often the gradient decreases over time as myocardial fibrosis occurs with regression in wall thickness. Occasionally, extreme angulation of the origin of a candidate septal artery may suggest an inability to wire the vessel using conventional wiring techniques, in which case use of alternative techniques, such as tip-deflecting catheters or magnetic navigation for vessel wiring[36] may be anticipated.

Once suitability for alcohol septal ablation has been determined, a temporary transvenous pacing catheter is positioned in the right ventricular (RV) apex for demand pacing during and after the procedure because of the risk of procedural heart block. Because the pacing catheter may be required for several days after the procedure, the operator should consider placing the transvenous pacing catheter from the internal jugular vein, allowing greater comfort for the patient by avoiding prolonged femoral venous access. For baseline hemodynamics including resting and peak provocable intraventricular systolic gradient measurement, an appropriate catheter is placed into the left ventricle that is maintained for continuous hemodynamic and LVOT gradient assessment

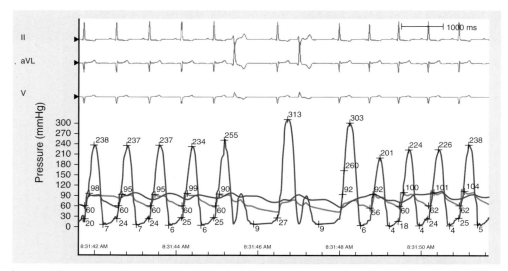

Figure 14–7 Simultaneous left ventricular (LV)–aortic measurement indicates a peak–peak gradient of approximately 150 mmHg at rest. Post-premature ventricular contraction, peak systolic aortic pressure and aortic pulse pressure decrease, whereas peak LV pressure increases. This generates an inducible gradient of approximately 235 mmHg. This phenomenon is referred to as the Brockenbrough-Braunwald-Morrow sign, and is likely the result of postextrasystolic potentiation. The *blue line* is the LV pressure; the *gold line* is the aortic pressure; and the *green line* is the respirometer.

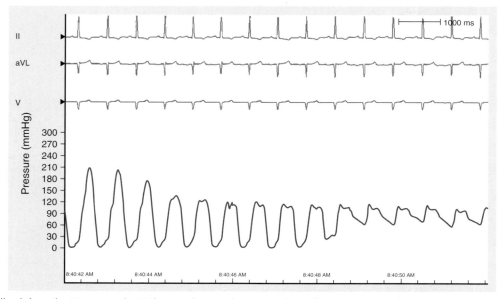

Figure 14–8 Pullback from the LV apex to the LV base and across the aortic valve indicates that most of the gradient exists between the LV apex and the base, consistent with LVOT disease. Note the absence of a gradient between the LV base and the aorta.

throughout the procedure. A catheter that can be positioned stably within the LV cavity, measures pressure from inwardly directed side holes within a 1-cm helical tip, and has been shown to have a reduced likelihood of ectopy[37] is the Halo pigtail catheter (AngioDynamics, Queensbury, N.Y.). This catheter is positioned via a sheath in the contralateral femoral artery. Alternately, a Langston dual lumen multipurpose catheter (Vascular Solutions, Minneapolis, Minn.) can be used for simultaneous LV–aortic pressure measurements. For the actual ablation, a transfemoral approach using guiding catheters with reasonably firm degrees of backup support

ASH, Asymmetric septal hypertrophy; *CCS,* Canadian Cardiovascular Society; *LVOT,* left ventricular outflow tract; *NYHA,* New York Heart Association; *SAM,* systolic anterior motion.

(such as XB LAD, XB, Q, or EBU curves) to allow wire and balloon advancement around the severe angulation of the origin of the septal arteries is typical, although a transradial approach has been successfully used.[38] The patient's blood is then anticoagulated, typically with unfractionated heparin.

Depending on the septal artery anatomy, wiring the selected candidate septally is often the most challenging step of the procedure, and guidewire characteristics appear to make a significant difference in the ease or difficulty of wiring. Often, a standard workhorse 0.014-inch guidewire can be used successfully. In more challenging cases, the 0.014-inch Whisper moderate support wire (Abbott Vascular, Abbott Park, Ill.) tracks well into the desired branch once it has been cannulated, despite the angle of entry, and supports balloon catheter advancement, although other hydrophilically coated 0.014-inch wires may be used as well. To cannulate the septal origin typically requires an extreme bend at the wire tip, on the order of a double 45-degree bend with the length of the secondary bend proportional to the diameter of the left anterior descending artery (LAD). The wire is preloaded into a short over-the-wire balloon (the shortest length available, 6 or 8 mm, is advantageous) that is slightly oversized compared with the diameter (typically 1.5 to 2.25 × 6 mm balloons) of the selected candidate's septal artery **(see Figures 14–6 and 14–9, *B*)**. For septal arteries that bifurcate proximally, it can be helpful to view the angiographic course in left anterior oblique cranial view to select the septal subbranch with a leftward course in an attempt to selectively target the left endocardial septum.

After wiring the septal artery, the balloon is then tracked into the proximal septal artery and inflated to an adequately occlusive pressure. Additional angiography is performed via the guiding catheter to confirm complete occlusion of the septal artery by the inflated balloon **(see Figures 14–6 and 14–9, *C*)**. If any antegrade flow around the balloon is noted, the balloon should be exchanged for a larger balloon until complete occlusion is documented. The guidewire is then withdrawn and contrast is injected via the inflated balloon catheter to

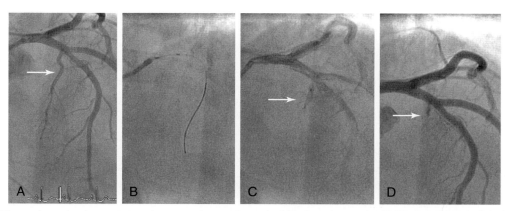

Figure 14–9 **A,** Cineangiography demonstrates a large septal artery *(arrow)* arising from the proximal LAD. **B,** A 0.014-inch hydrophilic wire with an over-the-wire balloon is then successfully advanced into the septal artery. **C,** The balloon is then expanded in the proximal septal artery, and lack of contrast flow confirms absence of anterograde flow down the septal artery. **D,** After septal ablation and removal of wire and balloon, contrast angiography demonstrates an occluded septal artery.

confirm the distal angiographic distribution of the septal artery, exclude presence of collaterals to remote vessels, and reconfirm absence of backflow leakage. A serious complication is reflux of alcohol into the LAD that can result in a significant anterior myocardial infarction (MI). This is an uncommon complication, but all operators should be aware of this possibility. With the balloon inflated, echocardiographic contrast (Optison [GE Healthcare, Piscataway, NJ] or Definity [Lantheus Medical Imaging, N. Billerica, Mass.] diluted in saline, in our experience at a ~ of 1:3-1:5 ratio) is then injected via the balloon catheter with simultaneous two-dimensional contrast echo imaging to define the perfusion territory of the target septal artery **(see Figure 14–6 and Figure 14–10)** and exclude angiographically invisible connections to remote vessels or territories. Diluted agitated contrast can also be injected into the septal artery and visualized by echocardiography. Multiple views, including parasternal long-axis, short-axis, and apical 3- and 4-chamber views **(see Figure 14–10, A and B),** allow the operator to fully image the area perfused, its coverage of the asymmetric septal bulge, and relationship to the site of septal–SAM contact. As additional safety steps, imaging in an apical 4-chamber view is performed during contrast injection to exclude enhancement of RV myocardial structures, and mid to apical ventricular imaging is performed in short-axis view to visualize the papillary muscles during echo contrast injection to exclude any perfusion of a papillary muscle by the target septal artery. The perfusion area defined by echo contrast enhancement may be suboptimal for several reasons. Contrast may enhance a segment of the septum that does not encompass the basal septal bulge adjacent to the site of septal–SAM contact, in which case ablation is unlikely to be effective in gradient reduction. In that circumstance, the balloon should be repositioned into another candidate septal artery and imaging repeated. Contrast may also enhance the appropriate target region but also a remote region(s) because of preexistent collaterals or connections from the septal artery to other vessels, posing a serious risk of remote infarction during alcohol injection. The area of contrast enhancement may also extend beyond the target area intended for ablation, for example, into a segment of RV myocardium. In these circumstances, the wire may be reinserted to reposition the balloon selectively into a subbranch to repeat imaging and potentially isolate an acceptable territory.

Once the appropriate septal artery has been selected and an appropriate target perfusion territory confirmed by echo contrast imaging, ablation is then performed. The syringe containing alcohol should be clearly labeled and kept separate from other syringes in the work area to prevent inadvertent use. The balloon catheter is first flushed clear of echo contrast agent with saline, followed by slow injection of 1.5 to 3 cc (depending on septal artery size/distribution) of pharmaceutical grade absolute dehydrated ethanol; the first milliliter is injected slowly over the first 60 to 180 seconds, and the remainder is injected over the next several minutes for a total injection period of up to 10 minutes. A good general rule is no more than 0.5 cc per minute. It is essential that the alcohol be injected slowly and deliberately to give it time to disperse into the septal tissue. Administering it too quickly can increase the chance of AV block or ventricular arrhythmias or that the alcohol will be forced through collaterals and result in infarct in a related non-target vessel. If AV block or ventricular ectopy is encountered, the rate of injection is slowed. The sonographer continues imaging during alcohol injection; the alcohol causes bright echo reflectivity of the infused tissue to give immediate feedback that the alcohol depot is infusing the intended area. If persistent ventricular ectopy develops, an immediate intravenous (IV) lidocaine bolus is administered and a continuous IV infusion started. The patient will often complain of chest pain, and ST elevation may be seen. Adequate sedation and use of morphine sulfate is often required. After completion of the alcohol injection the inflated balloon is left in place for an additional 10 minutes without flushing. Before removal, the balloon can be flushed with a small amount of normal saline while inflated to remove the remaining alcohol from the lumen. After that the balloon is deflated and carefully but quickly withdrawn, and repeat left coronary angiography performed to document proximal occlusion of the target septal artery **(see Figures 14–6 and 14–9, D)** and patency of all other coronary vessels. LVOT hemodynamics are then reassessed at rest and after provocation. The temporary pacemaker is sutured

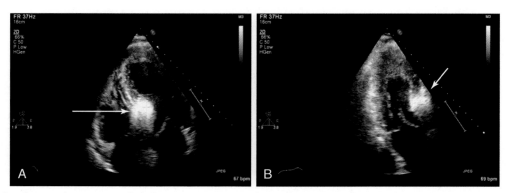

Figure 14–10   After the septal artery is occluded using an appropriately sized over-the-wire angioplasty balloon, echocardiographic contrast is administered via end-hole injection. Simultaneous transthoracic echocardiography demonstrates the basal septum being "highlighted" in the apical 4-chamber **(A)** and apical 3-chamber **(B)** views.

in position. The procedure concludes with echo imaging to exclude any pericardial effusion and briefly assess the immediate echocardiographic results. The patient is then transferred to the cardiac intensive care unit (CICU) for at least 24 hours of monitoring. During this period AV nodal blocking agents are withheld, although in the absence of any signs of AV block they are usually restarted at lower doses within 48 hours. If signs of trifascicular block (usually right bundle branch block (RBBB) with left anterior or posterior fascicular block and first degree AV block) become evident on serial electrocardiographs (ECGs) or if transient or persistent high-degree AV block develops, the temporary pacemaker is maintained and the patient is monitored in the CICU longer. If prolonged bed rest is necessary, attention to anticoagulation for deep venous thrombosis prophylaxis is recommended. Serial cardiac biomarkers are measured every 6 to 8 hours, similar to an acute MI protocol. After completing CICU observation the patient is transferred to a telemetry unit and monitored for an additional 3 to 4 days, because complete heart block or ventricular arrhythmias can develop abruptly but with diminishing likelihood during the first 4 days after the procedure. Most patients who were severely symptomatic report symptom benefit even in this early recovery period. For any patient developing bradycardia as a result of high-degree AV block, a dual chamber pacemaker (with or without ICD capabilities, determined based on presence of risk factors for SCD) is implanted as soon as feasible. Of note, echocardiographic assessment during the in-hospital recovery period does not appear useful in assessing procedural results or predicting the degree of later septal thinning or hemodynamic results.

During follow-up study, patients are monitored clinically, and a standardized HCM protocol treadmill stress echocardiogram (identical to the baseline stress echo evaluation) is repeated at 3 months and then yearly after alcohol septal ablation. At the 3-month point, septal thinning is evident **(Figure 14–11)** and can be quantified along with residual LVOT gradients at rest and with exercise, Valsalva, and amyl nitrite, although maximum benefit may not have been achieved at this point. It should be recognized that additional LV remodeling and improvement in the LVOT gradient has been observed between 3 months and 1 to 2 years after the procedure.[24]

COMPLICATIONS

Several complications related to alcohol septal ablation have been reported and require careful attention for any operator planning to perform the procedure. The single-center and multicenter registry reports provide a combined experience of alcohol septal ablation in over 4000 patients. Across centers, in-hospital mortality rates ranging from 0% to 4% have been reported with alcohol septal ablation, whereas in the larger scale North American and Scandinavian multicenter registries the procedure-related mortality was 0.3% to 0.6%.[13,21] The pooled results of the reported studies suggest a 1.5% to 3% incidence of in-hospital ventricular fibrillation or ventricular tachycardia, a 0.7% to 1.8% incidence of dissection or thrombosis of the LAD (that appeared more common in early experience), and a 0.5% to 1.4% incidence of pericardial effusion or hemopericardium, a proportion of which caused cardiac tamponade and required urgent pericardial drainage. Unwanted myocardial infarction distant from the planned septal infarction, resulting either from alcohol back leakage from lack of adequate occlusiveness of the septal balloon catheter or from collateral vessels connecting the target septal artery to a remote territory is a serious but rare and potentially avoidable complication. Conduction abnormalities including high-degree AV block represent the most common complication of alcohol septal ablation. New RBBB occurs in about 35% to 60% of patients undergoing alcohol septal ablation.[39,40] Results reported since the common use of myocardial contrast echocardiographic guidance suggest the rate of high-degree or complete heart block requiring PPM insertion is in the range of 9% to 17%,[13,14,19-21,39] although in the most experienced centers of the North American registry it decreased to 6.5%.[13] In a multivariable logistic regression analysis of 224 patients in the Baylor database,[41] independent

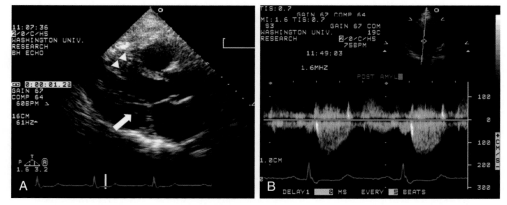

Figure 14–11 Echocardiographic follow-up image (of the patient shown in Figure 14–6) 3 months after alcohol septal ablation. A, The parasternal long-axis view shows marked thinning of the basal septal hypertrophy *(arrowheads)* and no SAM of the mitral valve *(arrow)*. B, Continuous wave Doppler shows a near normal velocity signal even after amyl nitrite inhalation, consistent with no significant resting or provoked LVOT systolic gradient. The patient reported significantly improved exercise tolerance, with near resolution of exertional dyspnea and chest tightness.

predictors of complete heart block and the need for a PPM after alcohol septal ablation included female gender, bolus injection of alcohol, injection of more than one septal artery, preexistent left bundle branch block (LBBB) and first-degree AV block on the baseline ECG. Of note, in their analysis the patients who required permanent pacemaker placement after alcohol septal ablation had similar improvement in NYHA functional class and exercise capacity when compared with patients who did not require pacing.

The mechanism of septal thinning by alcohol septal ablation involves creation of scar tissue in the basal interventricular septum at the site of ablation. This has raised concern of a potentially increased risk of serious late ventricular arrhythmias after alcohol septal ablation. Although some single-center case series have suggested potentially increased rates of adverse arrhythmic events after alcohol septal ablation, others have not confirmed these rates or supported these concerns. In a study that included over 5 years of follow-up care at one center, among 91 patients who underwent alcohol septal ablation, 7% of patients reportedly died of SCD, and 12% survived one or more episodes of ventricular tachyarrhythmia.[42] This cohort had a high prevalence of conventional risk factors for SCD at baseline. Noseworthy et al[43] examined the rates of SCD among 89 patients treated with alcohol septal ablation at their institution, and the rate of ventricular tachycardia or ventricular fibrillation, appropriate ICD therapy, or cardiac arrest among those with implanted ICDs or PPMs (n = 42). Patients were classified as either high risk or low risk on the basis of established clinical indications for ICD implantation. Importantly, there was no mortality attributable to SCD in their cohort at a mean follow-up period of 5 years. When events that occurred only after hospital discharge were examined, the annual event rate for ventricular tachycardia or appropriate ICD therapy was 2.1% per year in low-risk patients, and 10.7% per year in high-risk patients. From the observed rates and historical comparisons, the authors concluded that the rate of ventricular arrhythmias observed in their high-risk patients after alcohol septal ablation was not significantly different from what would be expected in a similar cohort with high-risk features and likely reflected the natural history of the disease. Their analysis also suggested that a less successful hemodynamic outcome with higher postablation residual LVOT gradient may be associated with a higher arrhythmic risk. Cuoco et al[44] prospectively studied 123 consecutive patients with HCM who underwent alcohol septal ablation and had an ICD implanted for primary prevention of SCD. They found that the annual rate of ICD intervention over a 3-year period was 2.8%, a rate lower than previously reported for primary prevention of SCD in HCM, consistent with a lack of proarrhythmia resulting from alcohol septal ablation. In the North American registry, among 94 patients who had ICD implantation after alcohol septal ablation for clinical indications, appropriate ICD discharge for ventricular arrhythmias occurred in 11 patients over the follow-up period, resulting in an average annual ICD discharge

rate of 1.2%.[13] Finally, in a meta-analysis by Leonardi et al[17] focused on mortality and SCD after alcohol septal ablation compared with surgical septal myectomy among over 4000 patients, the rates of all-cause mortality and SCD after both alcohol septal ablation and surgical myectomy were similarly low. In that analysis, after adjustment for baseline characteristics, the odds ratios for treatment effect on all-cause mortality and SCD appeared lower in alcohol septal ablation cohorts compared with surgical myectomy cohorts.

14.6 Sample Case 1

A patient with symptomatic obstructive HCM is referred for alcohol septal ablation (see Figure 14–6). The patient reports significant and lifestyle-limiting decreased exercise tolerance owing to exertional dyspnea and chest tightness despite maximum medical therapy. Invasive hemodynamic assessment demonstrates a resting gradient of 70 mmHg with a provoked gradient of 80 mmHg. Selective coronary angiography demonstrates at least three candidate septal arteries. The second septal artery is successfully cannulated and balloon-occluded. Echo contrast is delivered via end-hole injection with simultaneous two-dimensional echocardiography demonstrating enhancement of the midseptum, an area remote from the area of septal–mitral contact. The wire and balloon are removed, and the first septal artery is cannulated and balloon-occluded. End-hole contrast injection now demonstrates basal septum enhancement at the site of septal–mitral contact. Alcohol administration is initiated as described in this chapter. Final angiographic images demonstrate typical proximal occlusion of the first septal branch. Invasive hemodynamic measurements indicate complete elimination of resting and provoked LVOT gradient.

At 3-month follow-up study the patient reports near resolution of exertional dyspnea and chest tightness. Two-dimensional echocardiography demonstrates a markedly thinned basal septum and an absence of SAM of the mitral valve. Doppler echocardiography confirms a resolved outflow tract gradient even in the presence of amyl nitrate (see Figure 14–11).

14.7 Sample Case 2

A 77-year-old male was referred for consideration of alcohol-based septal reduction therapy. Asymmetric and obstructive HCM was first diagnosed 12 years before referral, which was based on a murmur auscultated during a routine physical examination. A transthoracic echocardiogram demonstrated an asymmetrically thickened left ventricle with an inducible outflow tract gradient. Three years before referral, the patient had a resting gradient of 56 mmHg that increased to 104 mmHg with exercise. A year before referral, the exercise gradient increased to 171 mmHg. During each evaluation, the patient's medical therapy was successfully titrated to maximum tolerable doses. Six months before referral, the patient described onset of exertional dyspnea after walking his dogs for more than 100 yards. Two weeks before referral, the patient could not take his garbage to the street (≈10 yards) without significant dyspnea.

A current echocardiogram confirmed an asymmetrically thickened LV myocardium **(see Figure 14–3).** Additional views with Doppler echocardiography **(Video 14–1)** confirmed moderate mitral regurgitation secondary to SAM of the anterior mitral valve leaflet. Continuous wave Doppler demonstrated a resting LVOT gradient of 137 mmHg **(see Figure 14–5).** Given findings on echocardiogram and the degree of symptoms on maximum tolerable doses of medical therapy, septal reduction therapy was indicated; given his age, the patient had a strong preference in proceeding with alcohol-based septal reduction therapy. The patient was referred to the cardiac catheterization lab.

Invasive hemodynamic assessment indicated a resting gradient of 150 mmHg and postextrasystolic potentiation increased the gradient to 235 mmHg **(see Figure 14–7).** Coronary angiography did not demonstrate any obstructive coronary disease. A moderately sized single septal perforator was identified and selected as a target for alcohol septal ablation **(see Figure 14–9, A).** After placement of a temporary pacemaker within the RV apex, alcohol septal ablation as described in this chapter is completed **(Videos 14–2 and 14–3).**

The first septal perforator was wired with a 300-cm ASAHI Prowater wire (Abbott Laboratories, Abbott Park, Ill) using a 2 × 8 mm over-the-wire balloon as support **(see Figure 14–9, B and Video 14–2, B).** The balloon was then advanced into proximal portion of the septal artery and inflated. With the wire removed, coronary angiography was then performed to ensure lack of anterograde flow down the septal artery **(see Figure 14–9, C and Video 14–2, C).** Next, echocardiographic contrast was administered via end-hole injection, and simultaneous transthoracic echocardiography was performed **(see Figure 14–10).** Contrast echocardiography demonstrates that only the basal septum was supplied by this particular septal artery. There was lack of echo contrast within adjacent RV myocardium, and there was no echo contrast in the remainder of the LV wall segments **(see Video 14–3).** Once it was determined that this is an appropriate target, a total of 3 cc of absolute ethanol over 20 minutes was administered via end-hole injection. At the 8.5-minute mark, the patient's ECG demonstrated widening QRS with ST deviations; the pattern is consistent with development of a left bundle branch block. The patient remained hemodynamically stable, and the infusion of alcohol was continued. At the end of the procedure, the left bundle branch block had persisted. Once the alcohol had been administered, repeat continuous Doppler wave echocardiography and invasive hemodynamics were measured; postablation resting and provoked gradients are shown in **Figure 14–12. Table 14–1** summarizes

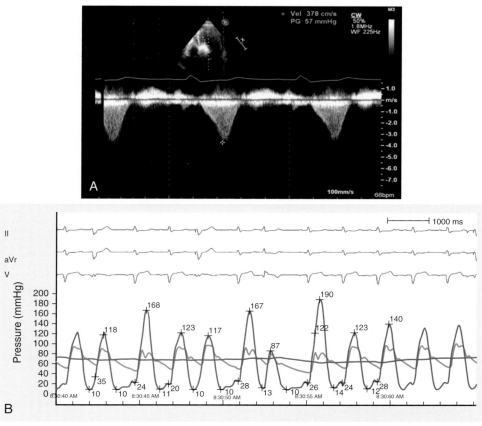

Figure 14–12 **A,** Continuous wave Doppler echocardiography shows a postablation resting gradient of 57 mmHg. **B,** Invasive hemodynamic measurements show a resting gradient of approximately 40 mmHg with postextrasystolic potentiation of 110 mmHg.

TABLE 14–1

Sample Case 2: Pre- and post-ablation left ventricular outflow tract ingredients

	Before Ablation	After Ablation
Resting	150 mmHg	40 mmHg
Post-PVC	235 mmHg	110 mmHg

PVC, Premature ventricular contraction.

the pre- and postablation gradients. Final angiographic images demonstrate complete occlusion of the large first septal perforator with excellent coronary flow down the LAD **(see Figure 14–9, *D* and Video 14–2).**

Shortly after arriving to the CICU, the patient was noted to be in complete heart block and was pacer dependent; this condition persisted into hospital day 3. Patient underwent ICD implantation before discharge home. At a 2-month visit, the patient's transthoracic echo showed dramatic thinning of his basal septum, and his mitral regurgitation had decreased in character and severity when compared with his preprocedure images **(Video 14–4).** The patient reported that he had returned to walking his dogs for 100 yards at a time, and could go for brisk walks with a 2% to 3% incline without any exertional chest pain or dyspnea.

14.8 Summary

Alcohol septal ablation represents an effective alternative nonsurgical treatment option when performed by experienced operators for carefully selected patients with HCM and severe symptoms attributable to severe LVOT obstruction refractory to medical therapy. Compared with septal myectomy, alcohol septal ablation can provide similarly successful short- and long-term symptom relief and improved quality of life.

REFERENCES

1. Wigle ED, Rakowski H, Kimball BP, et al: Hypertrophic cardiomyopathy. Clinical spectrum and treatment, *Circulation* 92:1680–1692, 1995.
2. Maron MS, Olivotto I, Betocchi S, et al: Effect of left ventricular outflow tract obstruction on clinical outcome in hypertrophic cardiomyopathy, *N Engl J Med* 348:295–303, 2003.
3. Gersh BJ, Maron BJ, Bonow RO, et al: 2011 ACCF/AHA Guideline for the diagnosis and treatment of hypertrophic cardiomyopathy: a report of the American College of Cardiology Foundation/American Heart Association Task Force on Practice Guidelines. Developed in collaboration with the American Association for Thoracic Surgery, American Society of Echocardiography, American Society of Nuclear Cardiology, Heart Failure Society of America, Heart Rhythm Society, Society for Cardiovascular Angiography and Interventions, and Society of Thoracic Surgeons, *J Am Coll Cardiol* 58:e212–e260, 2011.
4. Sigwart U: Nonsurgical myocardial reduction for hypertrophic obstructive cardiomyopathy, *Lancet* 346:211–214, 1995.
5. Seggewiss H, Gleichmann U, Faber L, et al: Percutaneous transluminal septal myocardial ablation in hypertrophic obstructive cardiomyopathy: acute results and 3-month follow-up in 25 patients, *J Am Coll Cardiol* 31:252–258, 1998.
6. Knight C, Kurbaan AS, Seggewiss H, et al: Nonsurgical septal reduction for hypertrophic obstructive cardiomyopathy: outcome in the first series of patients, *Circulation* 95:2075–2081, 1997.
7. Lakkis NM, Nagueh SF, Dunn JK, et al: Nonsurgical septal reduction therapy for hypertrophic obstructive cardiomyopathy: one-year follow-up, *J Am Coll Cardiol* 36:852–855, 2000.
8. Lakkis N, Kleiman N, Killip D, et al: Hypertrophic obstructive cardiomyopathy: alternative therapeutic options, *Clin Cardiol* 20:417–418, 1997.
9. Faber L, Seggewiss H, Gleichmann U: Percutaneous transluminal septal myocardial ablation in hypertrophic obstructive cardiomyopathy: results with respect to intraprocedural myocardial contrast echocardiography, *Circulation* 98:2415–2421, 1998.
10. Faber L, Welge D, Hering D, et al: Percutaneous septal ablation after unsuccessful surgical myectomy for patients with hypertrophic obstructive cardiomyopathy, *Clin Res Cardiol* 97:899–904, 2008.
11. Nagueh SF, Ommen SR, Lakkis NM, et al: Comparison of ethanol septal reduction therapy with surgical myectomy for the treatment of hypertrophic obstructive cardiomyopathy, *J Am Coll Cardiol* 38:1701–1706, 2001.
12. Qin JX, Shiota T, Lever HM, et al: Outcome of patients with hypertrophic obstructive cardiomyopathy after percutaneous transluminal septal myocardial ablation and septal myectomy surgery, *J Am Coll Cardiol* 38:1994–2000, 2001.
13. Nagueh SF, Groves BM, Schwartz L, et al: Alcohol septal ablation for the treatment of hypertrophic obstructive cardiomyopathy: a multicenter North American registry, *J Am Coll Cardiol* 58:2322–2328, 2011.
14. Fernandes VL, Nielsen C, Nagueh SF, et al: Follow-up of alcohol septal ablation for symptomatic hypertrophic obstructive cardiomyopathy the Baylor and Medical University of South Carolina experience 1996 to 2007, *JACC Cardiovasc Interv* 1:561–570, 2008.
15. Agarwal S, Tuzcu EM, Desai MY, et al: Updated meta-analysis of septal alcohol ablation versus myectomy for hypertrophic cardiomyopathy, *J Am Coll Cardiol* 55:823–834, 2010.
16. Alam M, Dokainish H, Lakkis NM: Hypertrophic obstructive cardiomyopathy-alcohol septal ablation vs. myectomy: a meta-analysis, *Eur Heart J* 30:1080–1087, 2009.
17. Leonardi RA, Kransdorf EP, Simel DL, et al: Meta-analyses of septal reduction therapies for obstructive hypertrophic cardiomyopathy: comparative rates of overall mortality and sudden cardiac death after treatment, *Circ Cardiovasc Interv* 3:97–104, 2010.
18. Alam M, Dokainish H, Lakkis N: Alcohol septal ablation for hypertrophic obstructive cardiomyopathy: a systematic review of published studies, *J Interv Cardiol* 19:319–327, 2006.
19. Welge D, Seggewiss H, Fassbender D, et al: Long-term follow-up after percutaneous septal ablation in hypertrophic obstructive cardiomyopathy [German], *Dtsch Med Wochenschr* 133:1949–1954, 2008.
20. Sorajja P, Valeti U, Nishimura RA, et al: Outcome of alcohol septal ablation for obstructive hypertrophic cardiomyopathy, *Circulation* 118:131–139, 2008.
21. Jensen MK, Almaas VM, Jacobsson L, et al: Long-term outcome of percutaneous transluminal septal myocardial ablation in hypertrophic obstructive cardiomyopathy: a Scandinavian multicenter study, *Circ Cardiovasc Interv* 4:256–265, 2011.
22. Ommen SR, Maron BJ, Olivotto I, et al: Long-term effects of surgical septal myectomy on survival in patients with obstructive hypertrophic cardiomyopathy, *J Am Coll Cardiol* 46:470–476, 2005.
23. Faber L, Welge D, Fassbender D, et al: One-year follow-up of percutaneous septal ablation for symptomatic hypertrophic obstructive cardiomyopathy in 312 patients: predictors of hemodynamic and clinical response, *Clin Res Cardiol* 96:864–873, 2007.
24. Seggewiss H, Rigopoulos A, Welge D, et al: Long-term follow-up after percutaneous septal ablation in hypertrophic obstructive cardiomyopathy, *Clin Res Cardiol* 96:856–863, 2007.
25. Nagueh SF, Buergler JM, Quinones MA, et al: Outcome of surgical myectomy after unsuccessful alcohol septal ablation for the treatment of patients with hypertrophic obstructive cardiomyopathy, *J Am Coll Cardiol* 50:795–798, 2007.
26. Maron MS, Olivotto I, Zenovich AG, et al: Hypertrophic cardiomyopathy is predominantly a disease of left ventricular outflow tract obstruction, *Circulation* 114:2232–2239, 2006.
27. Bruce CJ, Nishimura RA, Tajik AJ, et al: Fixed left ventricular outflow tract obstruction in presumed hypertrophic obstructive cardiomyopathy: implications for therapy, *Ann Thorac Surg* 68:100–104, 1999.

28. Yu EH, Omran AS, Wigle ED, et al: Mitral regurgitation in hypertrophic obstructive cardiomyopathy: relationship to obstruction and relief with myectomy, J Am Coll Cardiol 36:2219–2225, 2000.
29. Prifti E, Frati G, Bonacchi M, et al: Accessory mitral valve tissue causing left ventricular outflow tract obstruction: case reports and literature review, J Heart Valve Dis 10:774–778, 2001.
30. Maron BJ, Nishimura RA, Danielson GK: Pitfalls in clinical recognition and a novel operative approach for hypertrophic cardiomyopathy with severe outflow obstruction due to anomalous papillary muscle, Circulation 98:2505–2508, 1998.
31. Reis RL, Bolton MR, King JF, et al: Anterior-superior displacement of papillary muscles producing obstruction and mitral regurgitation in idiopathic hypertrophic subaortic stenosis. Operative relief by posterior-superior realignment of papillary muscles following ventricular septal myectomy, Circulation 50:II181–II188, 1974.
32. Chen MS, McCarthy PM, Lever HM, et al: Effectiveness of atrial fibrillation surgery in patients with hypertrophic cardiomyopathy, Am J Cardiol 93:373–375, 2004.
33. Joyal D, Arab D, Chen-Johnston C, et al: Alcohol septal ablation after failed surgical myectomy, Catheter Cardiovasc Interv 69:999–1002, 2007.
34. Juliano N, Wong SC, Naidu SS: Alcohol septal ablation for failed surgical myectomy, J Invasive Cardiol 17:569–571, 2005.
35. Spirito P, Seidman CE, McKenna WJ, et al: The management of hypertrophic cardiomyopathy, N Engl J Med 336:775–785, 1997.
36. Bach RG, Leach C, Milov SA, et al: Use of magnetic navigation to facilitate transcatheter alcohol septal ablation for hypertrophic obstructive cardiomyopathy, J Invasive Cardiol 18:76–178, 2006.
37. Caracciolo EA, Kern MJ, Collis WC, et al: Improved left ventriculography with the new 5F helical-tip Halo catheter, Am Heart J 128:724–732, 1994.
38. Cuisset T, Franceschi F, Prevot S, et al: Transradial approach and subclavian wired temporary pacemaker to increase safety of alcohol septal ablation for treatment of obstructive hypertrophic cardiomyopathy: the TRASA trial, Arch Cardiovasc Dis 104:444–449, 2011.
39. Talreja DR, Nishimura RA, Edwards WD, et al: Alcohol septal ablation versus surgical septal myectomy: comparison of effects on atrioventricular conduction tissue, J Am Coll Cardiol 44:2329–2332, 2004.
40. Valeti US, Nishimura RA, Holmes DR, et al: Comparison of surgical septal myectomy and alcohol septal ablation with cardiac magnetic resonance imaging in patients with hypertrophic obstructive cardiomyopathy, J Am Coll Cardiol 49:350–357, 2007.
41. Chang SM, Nagueh SF, Spencer WH 3rd, et al: Complete heart block: determinants and clinical impact in patients with hypertrophic obstructive cardiomyopathy undergoing nonsurgical septal reduction therapy, J Am Coll Cardiol 42:296–300, 2003.
42. ten Cate FJ, Soliman OI, Michels M, et al: Long-term outcome of alcohol septal ablation in patients with obstructive hypertrophic cardiomyopathy: a word of caution, Circ Heart Fail 3:362–369, 2010.
43. Noseworthy PA, Rosenberg MA, Fifer MA, et al: Ventricular arrhythmia following alcohol septal ablation for obstructive hypertrophic cardiomyopathy, Am J Cardiol 104:128–132, 2009.
44. Cuoco FA, Spencer WH 3rd, Fernandes VL, et al: Implantable cardioverter-defibrillator therapy for primary prevention of sudden death after alcohol septal ablation of hypertrophic cardiomyopathy, J Am Coll Cardiol 52:1718–1723, 2008.

Chapter 15

Percutaneous Approach to Pericardial Window

MITUL PATEL • EHTISHAM MAHMUD

15.1 Background

The management of chronic pericardial effusions by cardiologists and cardiothoracic surgeons poses significant challenges and is burdened with limitations because of the generally moribund state of patients stricken with this condition. Malignancy and infection most commonly cause pericardial effusions in developed countries representing 23% and 27% of cases, respectively.[1]

In the case of malignant pericardial effusions, recurrence rates after pericardiocentesis range from 13% to 50%.[2-4] Likewise, recurrence risk after subxiphoid pericardial windowing is nearly 5%. Neither treatment has been shown to reduce mortality rates, and, in the setting of advanced malignancy with associated malnourished and immunocompromised states, surgical windows pose significant perioperative risks including infection and prolonged hospitalization.[5]

Percutaneous balloon pericardiotomy (PBP) was initially described by Palacios and colleagues in 1991.[6] They presented their experience and technique in eight patients, all of whom were hospitalized with recurrent, malignant pericardial effusions after initial pericardiocentesis had been performed to relieve cardiac tamponade. In a subsequent multicenter registry of 50 patients, a 92% success rate with PBP in treating malignant pericardial effusions was reported.[7] The technique has since evolved to include a double-balloon technique and the use of an Inoue balloon.[8,9] Although the predominant experience with PBP has involved recurrent, malignant pericardial effusions, the procedure has also been successfully performed in cases of cardiac tamponade that occurred as a result of purulent effusions, pulmonary hypertension, uremic pericarditis, and congenital heart disease.[10-13]

Success rates and short- or long-term outcomes of PBP have not been directly compared with surgical pericardial window, sclerosing agents, or radiation therapy. This is mostly attributable to the patient population in whom the procedure is applicable, because it is a moribund group with limited life expectancy, poor functional status, and overall poor quality of life.

15.2 Indications

The procedure can be considered in most cases of recurrent pericardial effusion after initial diagnostic and therapeutic pericardiocentesis. However, the majority of practice has been limited to cases of recurrent, malignant pericardial effusions. Although PBP has been performed on effusions of alternative etiologies,[10-13] caution should be exercised in infectious etiologies, because PBP may lead to the development of an empyema. Both the patient and family also need to understand the grave nature of the patient's condition, because the procedure is usually palliative.

15.3 Preoperative Evaluation and Checklist

1. Informed consent: Explain possible complications, including a pain and management plan, as well as potential damage to coronary arteries, atrial or ventricular perforation, pneumothorax, infection, bleeding, need for emergency surgery, potential arrhythmias, and death.
2. Preprocedural laboratories: Tests for complete blood count, electrolytes and renal function (given potential contrast administration and possible uremia-induced platelet dysfunction), and coagulation parameters should all be assessed.
3. Prophylactic antibiotics: Antibiotic prophylaxis with either cephazolin or vancomycin is reasonable, because most patients are immunocompromised and antibiotics have been shown to reduce the incidence of postprocedural fevers.[7]

4. Sedation/pain management: Barring significant hemodynamic compromise, judicious use of analgesics and sedatives is required. Intravenous fentanyl and midazolam work well for moderate conscious sedation. Subcutaneous lidocaine (Xylocaine) should be administered in close proximity to the pericardium as well. In addition, if renal function is not compromised, intravenous ketorolac works well to reduce both pain and the associated inflammatory response to the procedure.

5. Imaging: Adjunctive transthoracic echocardiography to determine optimal viewing windows and to aid in confirming intrapericardial position of the initial access before PBP is strongly recommended.

15.4 Procedural Technique

The procedure is best performed in the cardiac catheterization laboratory with use of both echocardiographic and fluoroscopic guidance. Initially, transthoracic echocardiography should be used to assure the presence of a large, circumferential effusion that can be accessed from the subxiphoid approach **(Figure 15–1).** Loculated effusions are best managed surgically. The ideal window is one where fluid accumulation is greatest, the pericardium is closest to the chest wall, and proximity to structures between the chest wall and the pericardium (i.e., liver, spleen) is limited or completely avoided.

The patient should be appropriately sedated with the combination of a benzodiazepine and opiates. In addition, extensive local administration of lidocaine (Xylocaine), ideally with infiltration of the parietal pericardium, is required. Intravenous ketorolac may also provide adjunctive pain relief, especially in the setting of pericardial inflammation.

Access to the pericardium is then obtained using a micropuncture needle. Once the dilator in the micropuncture

kit is placed, agitated saline can be infused via the dilator and visualized on echocardiography to assure positioning in the pericardial space **(Figure 15–2).** Alternatively, a small amount of contrast can be injected and visualized under fluoroscopy. Sequential dilations are then performed, and ultimately, a 7F sidearm sheath is placed in the pericardium. After the sheath is in place, two separate 0.035-inch wires are introduced through the sheath. The course of the wires should be confirmed on fluoroscopy to ensure ample intrapericardial wire position for support when advancing the balloons for dilation **(Figure 15–3).** Soft-tipped, stiff-shaft 0.035-inch wires like the Amplatz (Cook Medical, Bloomington, Ind.)

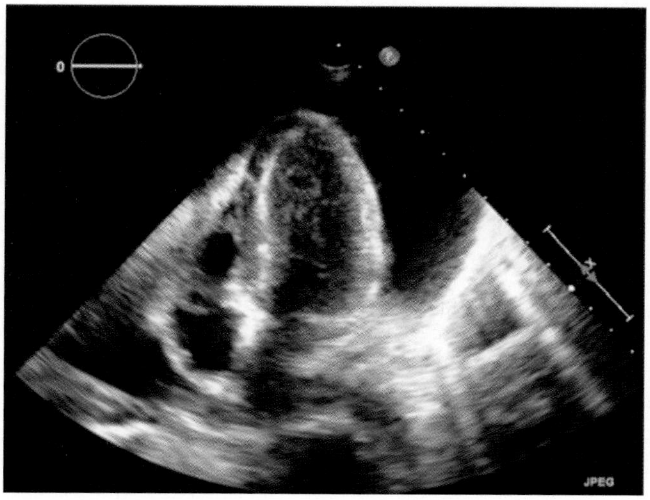

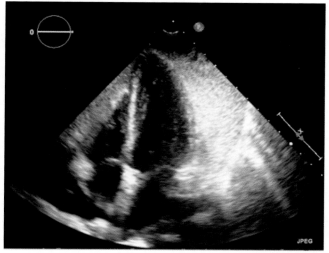

Figure 15–2 Echocardiogram from the apical view during injection of agitated saline into the pericardial space, demonstrating appropriate access.

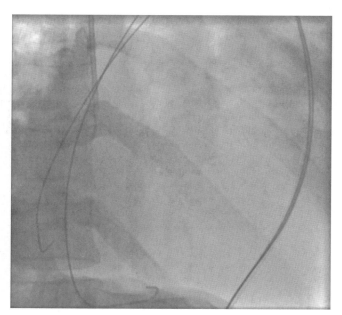

Figure 15–3 Fluoroscopy demonstrating appropriate wire position with two 0.035-inch wires in the pericardial space.

Figure 15–1 Echocardiogram from the apical view revealing a large, circumferential pericardial effusion.

or Supracore wires (Abbott Vascular, Santa Clara, Calif.) provide optimal support.

With both wires in place, the 7F sheath is removed and replaced with two separate 6F or larger sheaths (depending on patient size and thus the planned balloon size) over each individual wire. Next, an 8- to 12-mm × 2-cm balloon (Charger, Boston Scientific, Natick, Mass.) is advanced over one of the wires while a second 8- to 12-mm × 4-cm balloon is advanced over the second wire. Under fluoroscopy, it is easy to visualize the location where the two wires start to separate from each other. This location represents the parietal pericardium. The balloons are then advanced sequentially to the point that they both straddle the pericardium evenly. Care should be taken to ensure that the proximal edges of both balloons have passed through the subcutaneous space so as not to traumatize the subcutaneous tissue with the inflation.

After carefully positioning the balloons fluoroscopically, each balloon is sequentially inflated. These initial inflations should only be partial inflations in order to ensure the balloons are free of the subcutaneous space and are evenly straddling the pericardium. If these two conditions are not met, the balloons should be advanced or retracted accordingly. Once optimal positions are reached, both balloons should be inflated simultaneously until their waists disappear **(Figure 15–4)**. Next, the longer balloon should be anchored in place while the shorter balloon is advanced and retracted across the pericardium several times to assure an adequately sized window **(Figures 15–5 and 15–6)**.

Then, both balloons are removed and a standard 6F pigtail catheter is advanced over either wire into the pericardial space. Subsequently, either diluted contrast or agitated saline should be infused through the pigtail catheter and imaged with fluoroscopy or echocardiography. This step is to ensure that the pericardiotomy will allow for adequate and active drainage into the pleural space. Once this is confirmed, the pigtail catheter should be used to actively drain the remaining

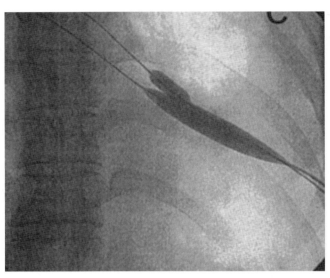

Figure 15–5 Fluoroscopy demonstrating advancement of the shorter balloon into the pericardial space. *(Reprinted with permission from Hsu KL, Tsai CH, Chiang FT, et al: Percutaneous balloon pericardiotomy for patients with recurrent pericardial effusion: using a novel double-balloon technique with one long and one short balloon. Am J Cardiol 80:1635-1637, 1997.)*

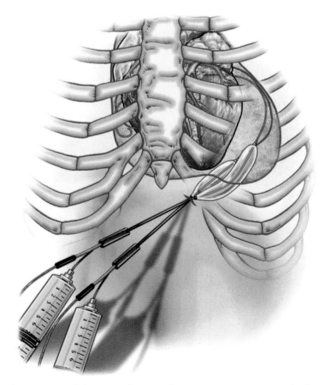

Figure 15–4 Schematic diagram demonstrating appropriate balloon position and inflation for double balloon pericardiotomy.

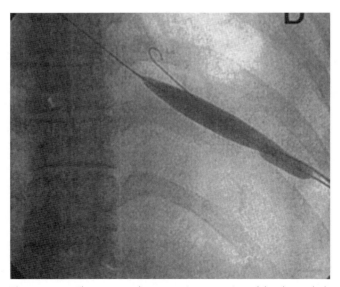

Figure 15–6 Fluoroscopy demonstrating retraction of the shorter balloon outside the pericardial space. *(Reprinted with permission from Hsu KL, Tsai CH, Chiang FT, et al: Percutaneous balloon pericardiotomy for patients with recurrent pericardial effusion: using a novel double-balloon technique with one long and one short balloon. Am J Cardiol 80:1635-1637, 1997.)*

effusion, and subsequently the other 0.035-inch wire can be removed. After confirming complete drainage with a final echocardiographic image, the pigtail catheter should be sutured or adhered in place and remain attached to suction. Once the drainage from the pigtail is less than 50 cc over 24 hours it can be removed. A postprocedure chest x-ray to assure the absence of a pneumothorax is required.

VARIABLES AND KEY POINTS

1. Sheath size: Sheath sizing should be determined based on the patient's body habitus and planned balloon size. Check the inventory in the catheterization lab and sheath-size requirements for available balloon inventory.
2. Deploy balloon before draining to ensure cushion between balloons and visceral pericardium: It is important to have an adequately sized effusion before PBP in order to avoid potential damage to subcutaneous tissues, the epicardial coronary vessels, and the myocardium. Thus PBP is most safely performed before draining the effusion.
3. Double balloon versus single balloon versus Inoue: The double-balloon technique creates an adequately sized window that most single balloons cannot provide. In addition, the double-balloon PBP is better tolerated from a pain standpoint compared with PBP using the single Inoue balloon. Also, larger balloons may rupture more easily than two smaller balloons. If a balloon ruptures subcutaneously, retracting the balloon can become difficult and there is a chance of retained balloon fragments.
4. Complete the procedure with agitated saline or contrast injection to assure outflow to the pleural cavity: This is an important step to assure procedural success. Although contrast injection is more easily visualized, if echocardiographic windows are optimal, agitated saline might be safer and lower contrast use.

5. Echocardiographic surveillance: Perform follow-up echocardiography before consideration of drain removal and 24 hours after drain removal to assure there has been no reaccumulation.

REFERENCES

1. Corey GR, Campbell PT, Van Trigt P, et al: Etiology of large pericardial effusions, Am J Med 95:209–213, 1993.
2. Kopecky SL, Callahan JA, Tajik AJ, et al: Percutaneous pericardial catheter drainage: report of 42 consecutive cases, Am J Cardiol 58:633–635, 1986.
3. Markiewicz W, Borovik R, Ecker S: Cardiac tamponade in medical patients: treatment and prognosis in the echocardiographic era, Am Heart J 111:1138–1142, 1986.
4. Patel AK, Kosolcharoen PK, Nallasivan M, et al: Catheter drainage of the pericardium: practical method to maintain long-term patency, Chest 92:1018–1021, 1987.
5. Mills SA, Julian S, Holliday RH, et al: Subxiphoid pericardial window for pericardial effusive disease, J Cardiovasc Surg (Torino) 30:768–773, 1989.
6. Palacios IF, Tuzcu EM, Ziskind AA, et al: Percutaneous balloon pericardial window for patients with malignant pericardial effusion and tamponade, Cathet Cardiovasc Diagn 22:244–249, 1991.
7. Ziskind AA, Pearce AC, Lemmon CC, et al: Percutaneous balloon pericardiotomy for the treatment of cardiac tamponade and large pericardial effusions: description of technique and report of the first 50 cases, J Am Coll Cardiol 21:1–5, 1993.
8. Chow WH, Chow TC, Yip AS, et al: Inoue balloon pericardiotomy for patients with recurrent pericardial effusion, Angiology 47:57–60, 1996.
9. Wang HJ, Hsu KL, Chiang FT, et al: Technical and prognostic outcomes of double-balloon pericardiotomy for large malignancy-related pericardial effusions, Chest 122:893–899, 2002.
10. Aqel R, Mehta D, Zoghbi GJ: Percutaneous balloon pericardiotomy for the treatment of infected pericardial effusion with tamponade, J Invasive Cardiol 18:E194–197, 2006.
11. Aqel RA, Aljaroudi W, Hage FG, et al: Left ventricular collapse secondary to pericardial effusion treated with pericardiocentesis and percutaneous pericardiotomy in severe pulmonary hypertension, Echocardiography 25:658–661, 2008.
12. Chouhan NS, Mukharjee S, Chandra P: Percutaneous balloon pericardiotomy in a patient with end stage renal disease with recurrent pericardial effusion and pericardial tamponade, Indian Heart J 62:87–89, 2010.
13. Forbes TJ, Horenstein SM, Vincent JA: Balloon pericardiotomy for recurrent pericardial effusions following fontan revision, Pediatr Cardiol 22:527–529, 2001.

Chapter 16

Transcatheter Left Atrial Appendage Occlusion

MARK REISMAN • CINDY J. FULLER

Atrial fibrillation (AF) is the most common cardiac arrhythmia, and a major cause of stroke in the elderly.[1] An estimated 12 to 16 million Americans will have a diagnosis of AF by 2050.[2] The risk of stroke attributable to AF increases with age from 1.5% in the 50- to 59-year-old age group to 23.5% in the 80- to 89-year-old age group.[1] The annual incidence of stroke in persons with untreated AF is 4.5%.[3] Adjusted odds ratios for mortality in AF are 1.9 in women and 1.5 in men,[4] and 1.71 overall.[5] Women have strokes later in life, and they are more likely than men to have long-term disability and poor functional status poststroke.[6]

Oral anticoagulation is recommended for prevention of stroke in AF (class I, level of evidence A)[7]; however, warfarin treatment requires frequent monitoring to maintain International Normalized Ratio (INR) between 2 and 3.[7] In addition, a significant number of drugs commonly used by this population can potentiate warfarin action, including amiodarone, simvastatin, and omeprazole.[8] Patients taking warfarin must also adhere to a consistent intake of vitamin K and avoid a number of dietary supplements that can affect coagulation. For example, fish oil potentiates coagulation, whereas ginseng can inhibit warfarin action.[8] The direct thrombin inhibitor dabigatran does not require regular monitoring as does warfarin, but it has a similar risk of hemorrhage as warfarin at the higher dose of 150 mg two times daily.[9] In addition, dabigatran and the direct Factor Xa inhibitor rivaroxaban are primarily excreted by the kidney; therefore dosages need to be adjusted in persons with chronic kidney disease.[10] Alternative therapies are warranted, particularly in patients who are not candidates for anticoagulant therapy or who are at high risk of bleeding.

The left atrial appendage (LAA) is a prominent source of thrombi in AF, accounting for 90% of thrombi observed in patients undergoing cardioversion.[11] In a small number of patients (3%), the LAA may be a source of focal atria tachycardia.[12] As a result, surgical and transcatheter techniques have been explored to reduce the risk of stroke in persons with AF by occluding the LAA. The percentage of complete closure or occlusion is dependent on the modality employed[13,14] and the selection of appropriate anatomy. The high variability of LAA anatomy[15] does not allow for a "one device fits all" paradigm. Thus several devices are under clinical evaluation or preclinical assessment.

This chapter will review the risk of stroke in AF; discuss the role of the LAA in the etiology of AF-related stroke; and examine surgical, combined epicardial/endovascular, and endovascular LAA occlusion procedures in comparison with oral anticoagulant therapy. LAA occlusion in concert with electrophysiological AF ablation will also be briefly discussed. Real-world procedural considerations will be presented because there is a steep learning curve to negotiate to avoid adverse outcomes.

16.1 Risk of Ischemic Stroke in Atrial Fibrillation

History of stroke and/or transient ischemic attack (TIA) was the major predictor of stroke in patients with AF in one analysis (relative risk 2.5; 95% confidence interval [CI] 1.8 to 3.5),[16] in addition to diabetes, hypertension, and increasing age. Several scoring systems have been proposed to assess risk of stroke in AF. The most widely used system in clinical practice is the **C**ongestive heart failure, **H**ypertension, **A**ge >75 years, **D**iabetes, and **S**troke score ($CHADS_2$),[17] which combines several risk predictors into a 7-point scale **(Box 16–1).** Patients with a $CHADS_2$ score of 1 or higher were more likely to have left atrium or LAA thrombus or sludge than those with a $CHADS_2$ score of 0 (3.9% vs. 0%, p < 0.01), and the prevalence of left atrial spontaneous echocardiographic contrast (SEC) increased with increasing $CHADS_2$ score (24% with score of 0; 83% with score of 4 to 6, p < 0.01).[18] Obesity is also a risk factor for left atrial and LAA thrombus in AF. Patients with a body mass index (BMI) of

Questionnaires for the Assessment of Stroke Risk in Atrial Fibrillation

CHADS$_2$

- **C**ongestive heart failure: 1 point
- **H**ypertension: 1 point
- **A**ge >75 years: 1 point
- **D**iabetes: 1 point
- History of **S**troke or TIA: **2** points

CHA$_2$DS$_2$-VASc

- **C**ongestive heart failure or left ventricular ejection fraction ≤40%: 1 point
- **H**ypertension: 1 point
- **A**ge ≥75 years: **2** points
- **D**iabetes: 1 point
- **S**troke/TIA/thromboembolism: **2** points
- **V**ascular disease (myocardial infarction, peripheral arterial disease, or aortic plaque): 1 point
- **A**ge 65 to 74 years: 1 point
- **S**ex **c**ategory female: 1 point

TIA, Transient ischemic attack.

27.0 kg/m^2 or higher have a greater prevalence of nonparoxysmal AF (37% vs. 21%, $p < .001$) and CHADS$_2$ score of 1 or higher (68% vs. 49%, $p < .001$).[19] A higher CHADS$_2$ score was also associated with increased risk of hemorrhagic stroke and death in the RE-LY trial,[20] which compared dabigatran and warfarin in AF patients. The American College of Chest Physicians recommends no medical intervention for AF patients with a CHADS$_2$ score of 0.[21]

The CHADS$_2$ score has been modified to accommodate other risk factors for stroke in AF. Data from the Euro Heart Survey on Atrial Fibrillation were used to develop the 10-point (0 to 9) CHA$_2$DS$_2$-VASc score.[22] Determinants of this score are listed in **Box 16–1.** Low risk is categorized as a CHA$_2$DS$_2$-VASc score of 0, intermediate risk as a score of 1, and high risk as a score 2 or greater. Increased CHA$_2$DS$_2$-VASc score was associated with increased risk of thromboembolic events at 1 year, with 0 events per patient year in the low-risk group, 0.46 events per patient year in the intermediate-risk group, and 1.71 events per patient year in the high-risk group ($p < .0001$).[23] The European Society for Cardiology has recommended that the CHA$_2$DS$_2$-VASc scoring system be used if the CHADS$_2$ score is 0 to 1 or when a more detailed assessment of stroke risk is indicated.[24] Patients with a CHA$_2$DS$_2$-VASc score of 0 had no differences in stroke risk in a population-based study, regardless of medication use.[25] These scoring systems for stroke risk in AF are highly important because they guide selection of medical treatment or interventions.

In addition to comorbid conditions, endothelial dysfunction and platelet activation may play a role in stroke risk in AF. These characteristics are interrelated and may be associated with the obesity, hypertension, and diabetes seen in patients with metabolic syndrome.[26] Plasma levels of von Willebrand factor (vWF) were increased in persons with AF relative to those in sinus rhythm,

whereas the levels of the vWF protease, a disintegrin and metalloproteinase with a thrombospondin-type 1 motif member 13 (ADAMTS13), were decreased in AF.[27] In this study, the vWF/ADAMTS13 ratio was negatively correlated with LAA flow velocity (r = −0.345, $p = .002$).[27] Plasma soluble CD40 ligand, a marker of platelet activation, was correlated with extent of SEC (r = 0.377, $p = .02$); however, levels of soluble CD40 ligand were not associated with warfarin use.[28] Soluble P-selectin and fibrin D-dimer levels, indicative of prolonged platelet activation and coagulability respectively, were increased in 17 patients with AF relative to 34 patients in a sinus rhythm control group.[29] Endothelial dysfunction and platelet activation are thus further risk factors for stroke in AF, especially because of their potential for interaction with a prosthetic device in the LAA.

16.2 The Left Atrial Appendage

ANATOMIC CONSIDERATIONS

The LAA is derived from the embryonic left atrium.[30] It is a blind pouch lying on the anterior surface of the heart. Normal anatomic variation in LAA morphology is shown in **Figure 16–1.** An autopsy study[31] showed that 54% of LAAs examined (n = 500) have two lobes, with 23%, 20%, and 3% having three, one, and four lobes, respectively. In addition to multiple lobes, the pectinate muscles create a trabecular structure that may promote thrombus formation.[30] In another autopsy study,[15] 220 casts of the LAA from patients with known medical histories were examined for the course of the principal axis and the number of lobes and finer structures. Ninety-two (42%) casts had an "extremely bent and extremely spiral" course, whereas only 16 casts (7%) had a straight course. The number of lobes and finer structures were significantly correlated with LAA volume and ostium diameter. Hearts from patients who had AF had larger LAA volumes and ostial diameters (both $p < .01$) and a lower number of lobes ($p < .05$) than hearts from patients who were in sinus rhythm before death.[15]

The ostium of the LAA is elliptical in shape,[15,31] which may have consequences for the design of occlusion devices.[32] The diameter and area of the LAA ostium increase progressively with the severity of AF.[33] The pectinate muscles within the LAA may be misread as thrombi on two-dimensional (2D) transesophageal echocardiography (TEE),[34] and they may hinder the success of LAA ligation or occlusion. Use of real-time three-dimensional (3D) TEE can help distinguish between pectinate muscles and thrombi[35]; however, a poor 2D image often predicts an inconclusive real-time 3D TEE result. In addition, 2D TEE underestimates the size of the LAA ostium relative to real-time 3D TEE,[33] which can impact the choice of device size.

DIAGNOSTIC CONSIDERATIONS

TEE and computed tomography angiography (CTA) are effective modalities to assess left atrial and LAA anatomic

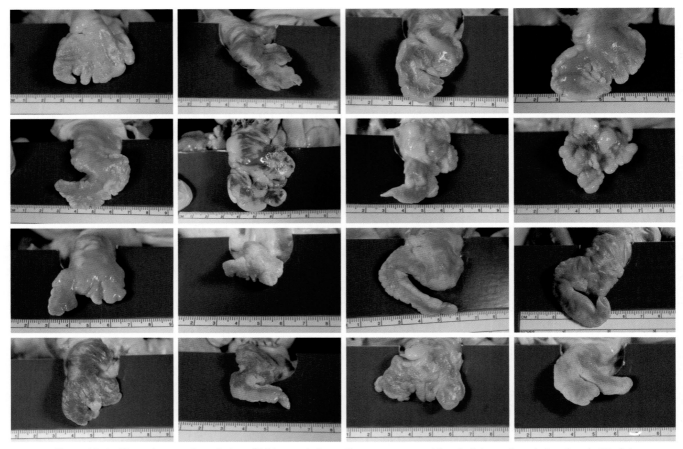

Figure 16–1 Normal anatomic variation of LAA morphology. *(Images courtesy of Seattle Science Foundation, Seattle, Wash.)*

and functional features that may increase thrombogenesis in AF.[11] SEC on TEE, which may reflect microemboli, is increased in AF.[36] The highest amount of SEC is negatively correlated with LAA velocity.[36,37] Patients with AF and thrombus have lower LAA velocity than patients without thrombus (no thrombus, 32 ± 21 cm/sec; with thrombus, 9 ± 6 cm/sec; $p < .001$.[36] AF patients with a history of stroke also have larger LAA depth and neck dimensions.[38] Increased left atrial volume index (odds ratio [OR] 1.02; $p = .018$) and lower left ventricular ejection fraction (OR 1.02; $p = .05$) on TEE measurement can predict LAA thrombus formation. Transthoracic echocardiography (TTE) with measurement of LAA wall velocity (LAWV) was used to assess risk of recurrent stroke in AF patients.[39] In this study, patients with TTE-LAWV less than 8.7 cm/sec were more likely to experience recurrent cerebrovascular events (hazard ratio 5.05; 95% CI 2.25 to 11.36).[39] The combination of low LAA flow velocity, endothelial dysfunction, platelet activation, and procoagulant state may thus set up an ideal environment for thrombus formation in the LAA.

CTA has become an important tool to assess LAA morphology. The image quality may be compromised at times by poor timing of contrast appearance in the LAA. CTA gives an excellent 3D understanding of the orientation of the appendage relative to the pulmonary artery, the number of lobes, and the shape of the appendage as well as

the orientation of the appendage—posterior, lateral, or anterior.[40] CTA has become essential in the deployment of the SentreHEART LARIAT device (SentreHEART, Palo Alto, Calif.). Wang et al[41] have categorized LAA morphology into four categories based on CTA analysis: (1) wind sock (one long, dominant lobe; 46.7% of patients studied); (2) cauliflower (short length with complex internal structure; 29.1%); (3) chicken wing (one prominent bend in LAA; 18.3%); and (4) cactus (dominant central lobe with secondary lobes; 5.9%). The ostium shape and LAA location relative to the left superior pulmonary vein can also be categorized by CTA.[41] Patients who have AF with the chicken wing LAA morphology are less likely to have a history of stroke or TIA than the other LAA morphologies (OR 0.21, 95% CI 0.05 to 0.91; $p = 0.04$).[42]

INDICATIONS FOR LEFT ATRIAL APPENDAGE OCCLUSION AND PATIENT SELECTION

The primary drug used for medical management of stroke risk in AF has been warfarin. As discussed, for many patients warfarin is either not tolerated or interferes with other medications or lifestyle. Major gastrointestinal bleeding and hemorrhagic stroke are principal adverse events with warfarin or the newer oral anticoagulants. Two bleeding risk scales have been validated for patients on oral anticoagulant therapy, with the acronyms

Questionnaires for the Assessment of Bleeding Risk in Patients with Atrial Fibrillation on Oral Anticoagulant Therapy

HEMORR₂HAGES[43]

Unless otherwise indicated, each item in the mnemonic receives 1 point.

- **H**epatic or renal disease
- **E**thanol abuse
- **M**alignancy
- **O**lder (age >75 years)
- **R**educed platelet count or function
- **R**ebleeding risk: **2** points
- **H**ypertension (uncontrolled)
- **A**nemia
- **G**enetic factors associated with increased bleeding propensity
- **E**xcessive fall risk
- **S**troke

HAS-BLED [44]

Unless otherwise indicated, each item in the mnemonic receives 1 point.

- **H**ypertension (uncontrolled, >160 mmHg systolic)
- **A**bnormal renal or liver function: 1 point each, maximum 2 points
- **S**troke
- **B**leeding history or predisposition (anemia)
- **L**abile INR (<60% of time in therapeutic range)
- **E**lderly (age >65 years)
- Concomitant **D**rug use (antiplatelet agents, NSAIDs) or ethanol abuse: 1 point each, maximum 2 points

INR, International normalized ratio; *NSAIDs,* nonsteroidal antiinflammatory drugs.

HEMORR₂HAGES[43] and HAS-BLED.[44] The constituents of these scales are listed in **Box 16–2.** The HAS-BLED scale outperformed the HEMORR₂HAGES scale in the SPORTIF trial of the direct thrombin inhibitor ximelagatran and warfarin in showing a stepwise increase in rates of major bleeding with higher scores.[45] Patients with a high risk of bleeding are natural choices for LAA occlusion, with the caveat that these devices are noninferior to warfarin regarding stroke prevention.[46]

As mentioned above, the CHADS₂ and CHADS₂-VASc scores provide essential information on stroke risk in patients with AF and should be used when considering an intervention such as epicardial or endovascular LAA occlusion. The complex integration of risk of stroke, risk of procedure, risk of bleeding, and quality of life is essential to developing a strong clinical trial, where the results can be interpreted and applied to real-world patients.

16.3 Left Atrial Appendage Exclusion Modalities

Although anticoagulant therapy is recommended to reduce stroke risk in AF,[7] alternative strategies are needed for patients who have contraindications to use of anticoagulants. Hence, exclusion of the LAA has emerged as a treatment option. Three approaches have been developed to exclude the LAA. Open surgery for LAA exclusion or removal has been relegated at this time to combined coronary artery bypass graft (CABG) or valve surgery. Epicardial LAA occlusion via ligation has been used, as well as a hybrid epicardial/endovascular approach. Finally, several endovascular LAA occlusion devices are currently under evaluation **(Figure 16–2).** The rates of complete occlusion are highly variable[47,48]; additionally, periprocedural adverse event rates may be dependent on operator experience.[49]

OPEN SURGICAL APPROACHES

Surgical ligation or excision of the LAA can be performed in patients with AF who are deemed at high risk for stroke and are undergoing concurrent CABG or mitral valve surgery. The literature consists mostly of retrospective case series or case reports.

The Left Atrial Appendage Occlusion Study (LAAOS)[13] was the first randomized, single-center study of surgical LAA occlusion in patients undergoing concurrent CABG with staples or sutures versus a control group. Seventy-seven patients were randomized either to undergo occlusion (n = 52) or the control group (no occlusion; n = 25); only 11 (14%) had a history of AF. TEE was used to test degree of occlusion at 8 postoperative weeks in 44 of 52 (85%) patients. Occlusion was successful in 29 (66%) patients, more so when stapling was employed (72%) rather than sutures (45%, *p* = .14). Two patients, both in the occlusion group, had thromboembolic events during hospitalization. One patient with AF, patent foramen ovale, and bilateral carotid stenosis had an intraoperative stroke; the other patient had a TIA on the third postoperative day. Importantly, after a follow-up period of 13 ± 7 months, no additional stroke events were reported in either occlusion or control groups.[13]

In one retrospective series,[50] six females with AF underwent LAA occlusion concurrently with mitral or aortic valve surgery. The LAA was occluded with running sutures, and no TEE was performed intraoperatively. At follow-up TEE (23 to 159 postoperative days), only one of the patients had complete closure of the LAA ostium. All of the other five patients had postoperative SEC within the LAA, which was more serious than it was before the occlusion in two patients. One patient with incomplete occlusion of the LAA had a stroke 4 weeks postoperatively despite having an INR of 5.9.[50] The authors concluded that intraoperative TEE was necessary to assure complete closure of the LAA and reduce risk of postoperative stroke. The primary issue limiting the use of surgical LAA occlusion is the variability of complete closure, ranging from 17% to 93%.[51] It should be noted that there is a difference between the anatomical ostium and the TEE-defined ostium of the LAA[31] that may adversely affect occlusion regardless of the approach. Inadequate TEE visualization of the ostium during surgery may result in incomplete closure of the LAA, which allows continued formation of thrombus within the structure.

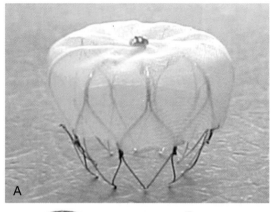

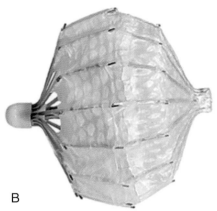

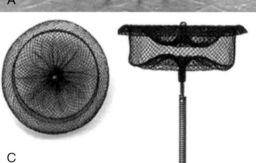

Figure 16–2   **LAA occlusion devices discussed in this review. A,** WATCHMAN device. **B,** PLAATO device. **C,** Amplatzer cardiac plug. *(Adapted from Sievert H, Lesh MD, Trepels T, et al: Percutaneous left atrial appendage transcatheter occlusion to prevent stroke in high-risk patients with atrial fibrillation: early clinical experience,* Circulation *105(16):1887-1889, 2002.)*

A major concern is whether incomplete occlusion is worse than no occlusion, given that reduced blood flow velocity in the LAA may enable more thrombus formation than in the fully patent situation. Kanderian et al[52] performed a retrospective analysis of 137 patients who underwent surgical LAA occlusion and had TEE evaluation 8 ± 12 months after surgery. Excision resulted in a 73% successful closure rate, compared with 23% for suture exclusion and 0% for stapler exclusion ($p < .001$). Thrombus was visualized within the LAA in 28 of 68 (41%) patients who had unsuccessful closure after suture or stapler exclusion; however, 11% of patients who had successful closure versus 15% of patients who had unsuccessful closure suffered a stroke or TIA after surgery ($p = .61$). Based on these findings, the authors identified four outcomes of surgical LAA closure: (1) successful closure; (2) patent LAA, defined as persistent communication of the LAA with left atrium as a result of dehiscence; (3) excluded LAA with persistent flow, defined as color-flow jet between LAA and left atrium despite appearance of closure; and (4) remnant LAA with pouch greater than 1 cm in length. The authors concluded that anticoagulation therapy should not be discontinued until successful closure is confirmed by TEE evaluation.[52]

EPICARDIAL LEFT ATRIAL APPENDAGE OCCLUSION

Epicardial methods for LAA occlusion are in development, and some devices are being used clinically. Procedures can be performed concurrent with open surgery or via endovascular techniques. The AtriCure AtriClip system (Cincinnati, OH) **(Figure 16–3)** was used in 34 patients with AF who were undergoing concurrent CABG or valve replacement.

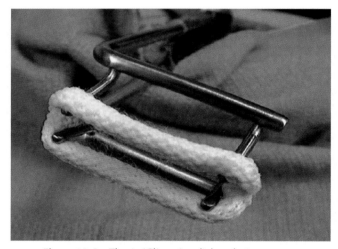

Figure 16–3   The AtriClip epicardial occlusion system.

The LAA was successfully occluded in all patients after 3 months, as assessed by TEE.[53] Epicardial exclusion of the LAA may have other beneficial effects in AF. In a small case series (N=10) utilizing the AtriClip system[54] in concert with pulmonary vein isolation and off-pump coronary artery bypass, 100% of patients achieved acute electrical isolation of the LAA. The Aegis system (Aegis Medical Innovations, Inc., Vancouver, Canada), a percutaneous device, consists of a "grabber" with integrated electrodes to identify the LAA under fluoroscopic guidance, and a ligator (hollow suture) to cinch the LAA at the base. Ligation of the LAA was successful in five out of six dogs in a preclinical study.[55] Necropsy after 2 to 3 months revealed an atretic remnant LAA in the animals. A silicone band delivered via a percutaneous system (Cardioblate; Medtronic, Minneapolis, Minn.) resulted in complete occlusion of the LAA in 15 out of 15 dogs studied.[56]

A combination epicardial/endovascular procedure, consisting of the LARIAT suture delivery device and magnetic-tipped guidewires with a balloon-tipped endovascular catheter, was initially tested in 10 dogs.[57] Balloon inflation to confirm the position of the LAA resulted in complete closure in five out of five dogs, whereas a residual proximal LAA was seen in three of four dogs without balloon inflation ($p = .05$). A larger study involving 26 dogs demonstrated complete LAA closure in 100% of the dogs.[58] A subset of 10 dogs was studied for 7 days (n = 3), 1 month (n = 3), and 3 months (n = 4). Histological examination demonstrated an atretic LAA with complete endothelialization at the closure site by day 7.[58] A small (n = 13) nonrandomized study[59] has been completed on LAA ligation using the SentreHEART system. The majority (11/13, 85%) of these patients underwent concurrent catheter ablation, and the remaining two patients (15%) underwent concurrent mitral valve replacement. Ten of the 11 patients undergoing catheter ablation and both of those with mitral valve replacement achieved successful ligation of the LAA. Follow-up TEE performed 60 days after ligation in six patients revealed complete closure in four (67%); the remaining two patients had color-flow jet less than 2 mm on color flow Doppler.[59]

A larger, single-center observational study consisting of 119 patients assessing the efficacy of LAA closure and procedural safety with the SentreHEART system has been reported.[60] Sixteen patients were excluded by computed tomography because of LAA orientation behind the pulmonary artery or LAA diameter larger than 40 mm. Fourteen patients were excluded as a result of thrombus identified during TEE or adhesions. Of the 85 patients undergoing LAA ligation with the LARIAT suture delivery device, 96% of the LAA ligations resulted in complete closure, with the remaining patient having a leak less than 2 mm as seen by Doppler echocardiography at the 1-year follow up examination. There were no device-related complications. Three access-related complications occurred in three patients. The adverse events included chest pain (24%), pericarditis (2.4%), late pericardial effusion (1.2%), and late thrombus formation (1.2%).[60] LAA ligation with the LARIAT suture device appears to be effective at excluding the LAA with acceptably low access rate of complications. However, none of the epicardial procedures discussed have been assessed for long-term reduction of stroke risk in humans with AF.

ENDOVASCULAR APPROACHES

Percutaneous catheter-based techniques offer the advantages of familiar techniques for the interventionalist and visibility of the LAA on TEE, because of a volume-filled heart, for direct assessment of degree of occlusion in the catheterization lab. The devices are delivered via percutaneous 12F to 14F catheters from the femoral vein and then through transseptal puncture. The delivery catheters are designed to engage the LAA. Great care is taken when manipulating catheters into the LAA because of the

risk of perforation. The devices are shown in **Figure 16–2.** Two devices for transcatheter occlusion have been tested in large prospective clinical trials: Percutaneous Left Atrial Appendage Transcatheter Occlusion (PLAATO; ev3, Plymouth, Minn.; **Figure 16–2, B),** which was tested in a nonrandomized trial[61]; and WATCHMAN (Atritech division of Boston Scientific, Plymouth, Minn.; **Figure 16–2, A),** which has been tested in a randomized trial against warfarin therapy.[46] The Amplatzer device (AGA Medical, Golden Valley, Minn.; **Figure 16–2, C)** has been used for LAA occlusion and is presently being evaluated in a phase I Investigational Device Exemption (IDE) randomized trial. A very small (N = 5) case series of the Amplatzer device has been published.[62] No periprocedural adverse events were reported, and TEE at 30 days after the index procedure showed no flow into the LAA and no thrombus formation on the atrial surface of the device.

16.4 Clinical Data

The PLAATO system, the first endovascular device designed specifically for LAA occlusion, was deployed in patients with contraindications to warfarin treatment.[63] The occluder consists of a self-expanding nitinol cage covered with polytetrafluoroethylene **(see Figure 16–2, B).** Three rows of anchors along the maximum circumference secure the cage within the LAA ostium. Results of the original PLAATO trial and subsequent long-term follow-up evaluations are detailed in **Table 16–1.** Deployment of the device was successful in the first 15 patients, with no evidence of thrombi or residual atrial shunt after septal puncture.[63] Results of the European and North American prospective feasibility studies were published in 2005.[61] Occlusion was successful in 108 of 111 (97%) patients, and the average duration of follow-up study was 9.8 months (90.7 implant years). There were seven major adverse events (MAEs) in five patients, including two strokes and four cardiac/neurological deaths. Three TIAs occurred. After up to 5 years of follow-up study, the annualized stroke/TIA rate was 3.8%, compared with an anticipated rate of 6.6% using the CHADS$_2$ score.[64] In a single-center study of 73 patients,[65] no patients suffered a stroke in 2 years of follow-up evaluation. The European PLAATO Study[14] included 180 patients. One hundred forty patients had follow-up TEE 2 months after deployment, and 126 (90%) had total occlusion. The stroke rate at 129 patient years of follow-up study was 2.3%. There were 16 MAEs in 12 patients (12.4%), eight of which were procedure-related. The authors pointed out in the discussion that the PLAATO device needs to be oversized by 20% to 50% relative to the LAA ostial diameter to guarantee stable placement and occlusion.[14] The manufacturer has not pursued subsequent trials of the device. Despite the noncommercialization of the PLAATO device, it showed the potential of mechanically closing the LAA for patients needing an alternative to antithrombotic treatment, both safely and what appeared to be effectively when compared with historical controls. Additionally, it gave many operators experience navigating the left atrium and the LAA.

TABLE 16–1 ■

Percutaneous Left Atrial Appendage Transcatheter Occlusion (PLAATO) Trial Reports*

	First Author (year)			
	Ostermayer (2005)[61]	Park (2009)[65]	Block (2009)[64]	Bayard (2010)[14]
Number of patients/number of study sites	111/14	73/1	64/10	180/18
Age, years	71 ± 9	73 ± 10	73 (range 43-90)	70 ± 10
Male	66 (59%)	37 (51%)	39 (61%)	118 (62%)
CHADS$_2$ score	2.5 ± 1.3	2.5 ± 1.4	2.6 ± 1.3	3.1 ± 0.8
Percutaneous LAA occlusion success	108 (97%)	71 (97%)	61 (94%)	162 (90%)
Duration of follow-up study	9.8 months (mean)	2 years	5 years	9.6 ± 6.9 months
Number of strokes/annual stroke rate	2/2.2%	0/0%	8/3.8%	3/2.3%
Adverse events:		1 (1.4%)	0 (0%)	2 (1.1%)
Device embolization	0 (0%)	1 (1.4%)	0 (0%)	5 (2.8%)
Pericardial effusion	2 (1.8%)	0 (0%)	1 (1.6%)	6 (3.7%)
Cardiac tamponade	2 (1.8%)			

LAA, left atrial appendage.
*Data are presented as mean ± standard deviation or frequency (percent).

TABLE 16–2 ■

Results of the PROTECT AF Trial*[46]

	Device Group	Control Group	Risk Ratio (Device/Control)
Intention-to-treat analysis (device n = 463, control n = 244)			
Composite primary efficacy endpoint	3.0 (1.9-4.5)	4.9 (2.8-7.1)	0.62 (0.35-1.25)
Composite primary safety endpoint	7.4 (5.5-9.7)	4.4 (2.5-6.7)	1.69 (1.01-3.19)
Per-protocol analysis (device n = 389, control n = 241)			
Composite primary efficacy endpoint	1.9 (1.0-3.2)	4.6 (2.6-6.8)	0.40 (0.19-0.91)
Composite primary safety endpoint	1.5 (0.7-2.8)	4.4 (2.5-6.7)	0.35 (0.15-0.80)

*Data are presented as rate per 100 patient years, with 95% credible interval in parentheses. Refer to text for definitions of endpoints.

The WATCHMAN device **(see Figure 16–2, A)** has incremental benefits in terms of delivery and recapture compared with the PLAATO device. WATCHMAN is a self-expanding, open-ended, nitinol cage with tines to anchor the device in place. The body of the device, specifically the aspect exposed to the left atrium, is covered in a permeable polytetrafluoroethylene membrane.[66]

PROTECT AF was a prospective, randomized controlled trial to assess noninferiority of the WATCHMAN device to warfarin therapy.[46] Patients with nonvalvular AF were eligible for inclusion if they had CHADS$_2$ scores of 1 or higher and had no contraindications to warfarin treatment. The randomization ratio was 2 intervention (device)/1 control (warfarin to achieve INR of 2 to 3). A total of 408 patients received a device, and 241 patients received warfarin. The composite primary efficacy endpoint consisted of ischemic or hemorrhagic stroke, cardiovascular or unexplained death, or systemic embolism; the composite primary safety endpoint consisted of excessive bleeding or procedure-related complications.

Table 16–2 shows the results of the PROTECT AF trial. The intention-to-treat (ITT) analysis included all randomized patients (n = 463 device, n = 244 control), whereas the successful treatment (per protocol) group included device patients who were able to discontinue warfarin after device implantation (n = 389) and control patients at the start of warfarin treatment (n = 241). At 45 days

postimplantation, 349 of 408 (86%) patients in the device group were able to discontinue warfarin per protocol, and this increased to 355 of 385 (92%) patients at 6 months. The composite primary efficacy endpoint was not significantly different between groups in the ITT analysis (rate ratio [RR] = 0.62, 95% credible interval [CrI] 0.35 to 1.25); however, the composite primary safety RR was not favorable toward device implantation (1.69, 95% CrI 1.01 to 3.19). This was because of 22 pericardial effusions (4.8%), four air emboli (0.9%), and three device embolizations (0.6%) in the device group. Most of these events occurred periprocedurally or shortly after implantation. For the per-protocol analysis, the composite primary efficacy and safety endpoints favored device implantation (efficacy RR = 0.4, 95% CrI 0.19 to 0.91; safety RR = 0.35, 95% CrI 0.15 to 0.80). The control group had a higher prevalence of major bleeding and hemorrhagic stroke relative to the device group (per-protocol analysis: major bleeding, control 4.1% vs. device 3.5%; hemorrhagic stroke, control 2.5% vs. device 0.2%). The control group had INR within therapeutic range (2 to 3) only 66% of the time,[46] which has been seen in other studies of warfarin.[67]

The results of the PROTECT AF trial need to be taken within the context of the population enrolled.[46] First, a high proportion of patients in both groups had CHADS$_2$ scores of 1 (device n = 157 [34%]; control n = 66 [27%]), indicative of a low-risk population that could be managed with anticoagulant or antiplatelet therapy. Many of the adverse events in the device group occurred early in the trial, indicative of an operator learning curve. A registry (Continued Access to PROTECT AF [CAP]) tracked nonrandomized patients who received the WATCHMAN device. Safety analysis of both PROTECT AF and CAP showed significant reductions in procedure time (62 ± 34 vs. 50 ± 21 min, respectively; $p < .001$) and in the rate of procedure- or device-related safety events within 7 days of the procedure, compared with PROTECT AF, to 3.7% of patients versus 7.7% of patients experiencing events ($p = .007$). The CAP registry also had lower rates of serious pericardial effusions relative to PROTECT AF (2.2% vs. 5.0%, respectively; $p = .019$).[49]

A second randomized trial, Prospective Randomized EVAluation of the WATCHMAN LAA Closure Device In Patients with Atrial Fibrillation versus Long-Term Warfarin Therapy (PREVAIL; clinicaltrials.gov NCT01182441), is being analyzed at the time of this writing. The PREVAIL trial design is similar to PROTECT AF; however, inclusion/exclusion criteria have been changed. Patients will be excluded from PREVAIL if their CHADS$_2$ scores are 1 unless they have one of the following characteristics: (1) female aged 75 years or older; (2) left ventricular ejection fraction between 30% and 34.9%; (3) aged 65 to 74 years with diabetes or coronary artery disease; or (4) aged 65 years and older with documented congestive heart failure.

Amplatzer devices have been used for LAA occlusion in nonrandomized trials. The first study[68] involved off-label use of the occluder used for patent foramen ovale or atrial septal defect closure in 16 patients with AF. With the exception of one device embolization, complete occlusion of the LAA was observed in all subjects in 5 patient years of follow-up study. Two patients with AF received the Amplatzer Cardiac Plug implant **(see Figure 16–2, C)**, as described in another report.[69] No adverse events were seen at 1 month postprocedure in either patient. Eighty-six patients with moderate to high risk of stroke (CHADS$_2$ score 2.6 ± 1.2) were implanted with the Amplatzer Cardiac Plug.[47] Total procedural complications were low (5.7%), and follow-up evaluation of 69 patients (25.9 patient years) revealed no stroke or peripheral vascular thromboembolism. LAA closure was complete in 67 of 69 patients.[47] A phase I clinical trial (NCT01118299) was initiated, and results are pending at this writing.

As is the case with inadequate surgical ligation,[52] inadequate endovascular LAA occlusion may be a risk for thromboembolic events. The PROTECT AF protocol[46] performed TEE at 45 days and at 6 and 12 months postimplantation to assess peridevice leak. If the leak was less than 5 mm at 45 days, patients discontinued warfarin. Patients remained on clopidogrel for 6 months postimplantation and on aspirin permanently. In long-term follow-up study of patients in the PROTECT AF trial who were implanted with the WATCHMAN device,[48] the prevalence of peridevice flow as measured by TEE and color Doppler decreased (40.9% at 45 days to 32.1% at 12 months; $p < .001$). There was no association between peridevice flow and adverse clinical events (i.e., stroke,

peripheral embolism, or death) in the cohort regardless of continued anticoagulant therapy ($p = .857$)[48]; therefore patients with peridevice leaks were not at increased risk.

16.5 Procedural Considerations

SENTREHEART

Preprocedure

The results of the 3D CTA are reviewed to assess the anatomy and determine pericardial access. CTA is helpful to define the shape and size of the appendage. If the width of the appendage is greater than 40 mm, then the device will not be able to get over the body of the appendage to ligate the neck or ostium of the appendage. The CTA also provides information as to the orientation of the appendage and thus how lateral or anterior the guide sheath needs to be to have the straightest vector to achieve launching over the distal end of the appendage and to the ostium. Finally, CTA helps the interventionalist determine where to place the endovascular LAA wire so that the optimal orientation for capture is achieved.

An overview of the procedure is shown in **Video 16–1.** A baseline TEE is performed to check for visual thrombus, pericardial thickening, or pericardial effusion **(Video 16–2).** Presence of LAA thrombus is a contraindication for the procedure. The TEE views can confirm how many lobes are present. In contrast to endovascular prostheses like the WATCHMAN, many intracardiac characteristics are not as important for the LARIAT, with the exception of defining clot, which is much better appreciated on TEE than CTA. Use of TEE in this procedure can also help delineate the extent of the pectinate muscles and the orientation of the os of the appendage. Pectinate muscles that appear to be proximal to the true appendage may serve as a persistent nidus of thrombus and thus a risk for stroke. Postprocedure, TEE is used to assess ligation success.

Procedure

In the majority of institutions, general anesthesia is used because of the placement of the TEE probe for an extended time. The patient should be off anticoagulation therapy if clinically acceptable; antibiotic prophylaxis should be used. Once the patient is prepped and draped, the first step is to get access to the pericardial space. The "dry tap" is done with the Pajunk needle (Pajunk Medical Systems, Norcross, Ga.) **(Video 16–3),** and accessed using contrast confirmation and then advancement of a 0.035-inch guidewire into the pericardium. Once this is achieved, either over this wire or a stiffer wire the SofTIP guide catheter (SentreHEART) is advanced and positioned in the pericardial space **(Video 16–4).** TEE should be used to confirm that the catheter is not causing compression of the right ventricle and that there is no pericardial effusion. If an effusion does occur, drainage can be done via a pigtail catheter through the sheath, or a second pericardial access can be performed for drainage.

The next step is to gain access to the left atrium using a conventional transseptal approach. The fossa should be crossed in the central position or slightly superior and posterior. The entry to the os of the LAA is anterior to the fossa and best achieved when the catheter has a straight vector towards the LAA (Video 16–5). Using a pigtail catheter for careful access to the LAA or directly with a guidewire and then a pigtail catheter, a left atriogram can be obtained. This can also be done through the transseptal catheter (Videos 16–6 and 16–7).

Once left atrial access is obtained, a 0.025-inch FindrWIRE (SentreHEART) with a small curve approximately 2 to 3 cm from the tip is backloaded into the catheter; both are navigated to the apex of the LAA under fluoroscopic guidance. The proximal marker of the balloon should be placed just distal to the coronary sinus or circumflex artery based on TEE. The FindrWIRE should be in the distal apex (preferably of an anterior lobe) of the LAA. The 0.035-inch wire is introduced through the pericardial guide cannula, directed to the endovascularly placed FindrWIRE, and connected end-to-end by opposite-pole magnetic tips under fluoroscopic guidance (Videos 16–8 and 16–9).

Once the wires have been connected, the LARIAT is placed over the wire. The LARIAT is advanced toward the LAA; the snare is reopened and advanced over the LAA. The distal snare loop of the LARIAT should align with the proximal marker of the EndoCATH balloon (SentreHEART). The balloon is inflated with a 50:50 mixture of contrast and saline (Video 16–10). The origin of the LAA and the epicardial surface is determined using TEE (Video 16–11). The LARIAT snare is then closed completely (Video 16–12). TEE and atriogram are used to identify correct placement of the snare. If not adequate, the snare is reopened and repositioned and then the balloon is deflated.

The 0.025-inch FindrWIRE is retracted to the tip of the balloon. This should be done while holding tension on the epicardial wire, so that the epicardial wire does not lurch forward. The EndoCATH and FindrWIRE are removed as a single unit from the LAA. Once the placement is deemed satisfactory, the LARIAT suture is released and tightened until resistance is met (Videos 16–13 and 16–14). Two final tightenings are then performed with a suture-tension force gauge, the TenSURE device (SentreHEART).

Color duplex TEE is used to confirm adequacy of closure; confirm with atriograms (30° right anterior oblique [RAO] ±10° cranial and 30° left anterior oblique) (Videos 16–15 and 16–16). Once the LAA is completely excluded, the red suture-release tab is cut and withdrawn from over the LAA with snare completely open. Both LARIAT and FindrWIRE are then withdrawn completely from guide cannula, and the remnant suture tail is cut with a remote suture cutter, SureCUT (SentreHEART) (Video 16–17).

Postprocedure Care

Postprocedure care is focused on managing issues surrounding pericardial access. Often the patient will not have any drainage from the delivery catheter, and there is no effusion noted on TEE. In cases where there is a "clean" entry into the pericardial space, the delivery sheath can be removed in the catheterization lab or, for additional precautions, in the recovery area. If there is evidence of effusion or an inadvertent entry into the right ventricle, a pigtail catheter should be left in the pericardial space to drain overnight. The catheter should be removed once there is certainty that there is no reaccumulation.

Pain is common after the procedure, probably because of irritation of the pericardial tissue. Management is typically with analgesics, often nonsteroidal antiinflammatory drugs. The pain can be quite debilitating and should be managed aggressively. Some operators have used direct injection of lidocaine into the pericardial space. The benefits of this treatment have not been studied rigorously, however.

Weekly follow-up evaluation by phone is important. The patient should be asked about chest pain, dyspnea, or any changes in respiratory status. Late cases of hemothorax have been seen that may not have been recognized earlier. These may be related to the initial pericardial access.

Although there is no rigorous protocol for TEE follow-up examination, imaging by 90 days postprocedure is highly recommended.

WATCHMAN

Preprocedure

The WATCHMAN is an investigational device at the time of this writing. The workup to determine whether or not the patient is a candidate is based on the eligibility criteria of the PREVAIL trial. The $CHADS_2$ score should be 2 or higher unless the patient is a female aged 75 years or older, has a baseline left ventricular ejection fraction between 30% and 35%, or is aged 65 years or older and has diabetes, coronary artery disease, or congestive heart failure. In contrast to the LARIAT device, the WATCHMAN workup only requires a TEE to assess the LAA. Anatomical exclusion criteria include high-risk patent foramen ovale, implanted valve prosthesis, mitral valve stenosis, or mobile atheroma in the aortic arch or descending aorta.

Procedure

An overview of the procedure is illustrated in Video 16–18. A traditional transseptal puncture is achieved to provide an orientation that optimizes access to not only the os of the LAA, but orients towards the lobe in which the operator ultimately wants to place the delivery catheter (DC) for the WATCHMAN device. Once the transseptal puncture is performed (either directly with the Amplatz Super Stiff guidewire or using a multipurpose catheter), the Super Stiff guidewire should be placed in the left upper pulmonary vein to be used as a rail. Once positioned there, the double- or single-curve WATCHMAN DC (Figure 16–4) is inserted and the Amplatz Super Stiff guidewire can be removed as the DC is positioned in the left atrial cavity. Through the catheter, a 6F pigtail is advanced up the DC and placed in the LAA. Access into the LAA in the majority

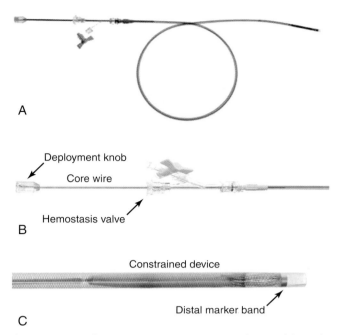

Figure 16–4 **A,** The WATCHMAN DC. **B,** Proximal view of the catheter. **C,** Distal view of catheter showing constrained device and marker band.

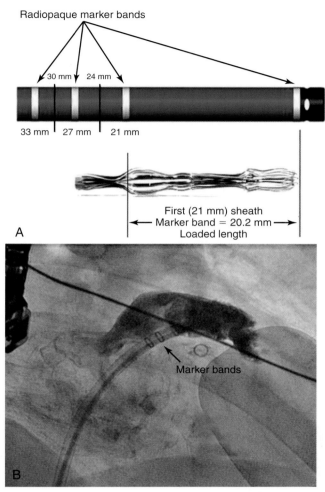

Figure 16–5 **A,** Association of radiopaque marker bands on WATCHMAN DC with size of device. **B,** Fluoroscope shot of delivery catheter with markings at ostium of the left atrial appendage.

of cases is via a counterclockwise or anterior rotation of the pigtail catheter and/or the DC. Once the pigtail catheter is in the LAA, LAA images are obtained. The best working view is RAO 30° oblique and 30° caudal, which correlates with the TEE image at 135°. A simple RAO view correlates with the TEE image at 45° or 90°, whereas the cranial RAO correlates with the TEE image at 0°.

Once the pigtail catheter is in the optimal position and provides the best access, which is often the lobe that allows optimal orientation of the WATCHMAN with relation to the os and that the length of the device is accommodated, the DC is placed distally into the LAA over the pigtail catheter. Additional angiography is done at this point to assure positioning and to be certain that the DC is not against the LAA wall. TEE is used continuously during the procedure to assist in positioning the catheters and to reassess LAA dimensions. It is important to be certain that the patient is euvolemic during the procedure so that true LAA measurements can be obtained. The marker bands on the DC define where the various devices will land proximally; therefore it is critical to determine which device will be placed and to make sure that the marker band corresponding to that device is located at or near the os of the LAA **(Figure 16–5).**

The device size is chosen to be 2 to 4 mm greater than the maximum LAA ostium diameter **(Table 16–3).** WATCHMAN devices come in 21-, 24-, 27-, 30-, and 33-mm sizes. For example, if the maximum LAA ostium diameter is 26 mm, a 30-mm device is selected. Once the correct size WATCHMAN device is selected and prepared, the 6F pigtail catheter is removed while keeping the DC in position with the correct sizing marker band at the os. The delivery system is inserted carefully until the distal marker band of the delivery system is lined up with the distal marker band of the DC under fluoroscopy.

TABLE 16–3

WATCHMAN Device Size-Selection Table

Maximum LAA Ostium (mm)	Device Size (mm) (Uncompressed Diameter)
17-19	21
20-22	24
23-25	27
26-28	30
29-31	33

LAA, Left atrial appendage.

Once the marker bands are lined up, the delivery system is held in place and the access sheath **(Figure 16–6)** is retracted and snapped onto the delivery catheter (AS/DC assembly; **Figure 16–7).** The position of the DC tip needs to be confirmed before deployment **(Figure 16–8).**

The implant is slowly unsheathed within the LAA. The device is deployed by holding the deployment knob stationary while retracting the AS/DC assembly slowly to deploy the device completely. Leaving the core wire attached, the AS/DC assembly is withdrawn to a few centimeters from the device, allowing the device to align with the LAA **(Figure 16–9)**. The WATCHMAN device should meet all four of the device release criteria, abbreviated as PASS:

1. **P**osition: The plane of maximum diameter of the device should be at or just distal to the LAA ostium and span it completely. This is confirmed via TEE and fluoroscopy.

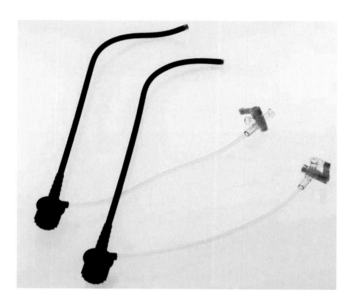

Figure 16–6 The WATCHMAN single-(lower right) and double-curve (upper left) access sheaths, with detail of the distal end showing the marker band.

2. **A**nchor or Stability: The AS/DC assembly is withdrawn a few centimeters from the device.
Gently pull back and then release deployment knob. The device and the LAA should move in unison. This is also confirmed via TEE and fluoroscopy.
3. **S**ize: The plane of maximum diameter of device is measured and should be 80% to 92% of original size, as measured under TEE.
4. **S**eal: All lobes must be distal to device and sealed under TEE.

If any of the release criteria are not met, the device can always be recaptured. A partial recapture and redeployment can be done if the device was initially distal and did not cover all of the LAA lobes. If the initial position is too proximal, a full recapture is performed. In this situation, the DC would be repositioned and deployment of a new device would be attempted. Once the operator is satisfied with placement and the device release criteria are met, the deployment knob is rotated counterclockwise three to five full turns to release the device.

Postprocedure Care

Standard-of-care procedures should be used to control postprocedure bleeding at the access site. Patients should remain on warfarin (INR 2 to 3) and 81 mg aspirin for a minimum of 45 days after implantation. At 45 days, device placement should be confirmed with TEE. Cessation of warfarin at this point is at physician discretion. Patients who discontinue warfarin should begin 75mg clopidogrel and aspirin daily through 6 months postimplant and remain on daily aspirin indefinitely. Appropriate endocarditis prophylaxis should be followed for

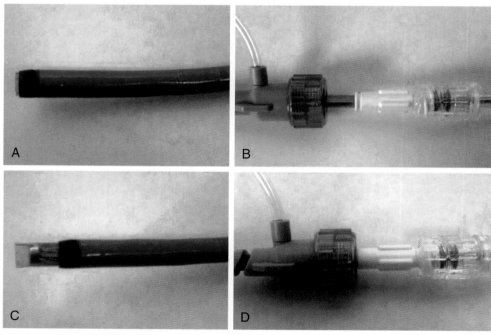

Figure 16–7 The WATCHMAN assembly sheath/delivery catheter (AS/DC) assembly. Panels **A** and **B** represent the respective positions of the distal and proximal AS/DC after advancement into the left atrial appendage (LAA). It is important for the interventionist to retract the sheath rather than advance the catheter to avoid perforation of the LAA. The resulting proper positions are shown in panels **C** and **D**.

6 months after device implant. Continuing endocarditis prophylaxis beyond 6 months is at physician discretion.

16.6 Potential Complications and Their Prevention

The three major complications of the PROTECT AF trial were: (1) pericardial effusion (6.5%), (2) intraprocedural stroke (1.1%, mostly because of air embolism),

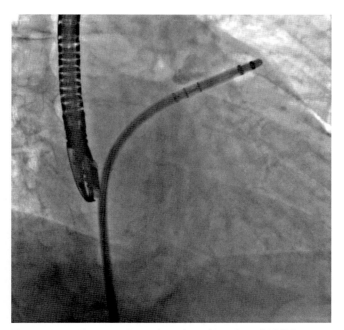

Figure 16–8 Fluoroscopic confirmation of location of AS/DC assembly at the ostium of the left atrial appendage.

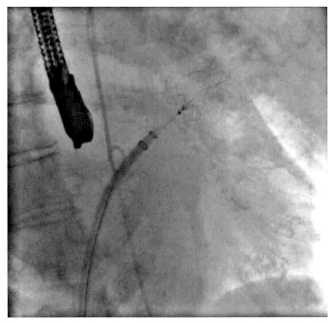

Figure 16–9 Deployment of the WATCHMAN device in the left atrial appendage before release.

and (3) device embolization (0.6%).[46] These complications were much less prevalent in CAP,[49] indicative of the learning curve for this procedure. Continuous TEE monitoring is essential to assure proper device placement and to avoid puncture of the distal LAA. Catheters need to be completely flushed with saline to avoid air emboli. Finally, scrupulous attention to the device release criteria is needed before releasing the device.

While SentreHEART has not been tested for LAA occlusion in a randomized trial, hemopericardium of less than 50 mL was observed in one (9%) patient who underwent the procedure.[59] An additional patient who had pectus excavatum required thoracoscopic removal of the snare because of compression by the concave sternum.[59] A complication of this type can be avoided by thorough evaluation of the mediastinal space by 3D CTA before the procedure.

16.7 Summary

Occlusion of the LAA via surgical, epicardial, or endovascular approaches may reduce risk of stroke in patients with AF. In the PROTECT AF study, endovascular LAA occlusion was not inferior to warfarin therapy in stroke prevention. However, adequate operator training is essential to avoid periprocedural adverse events such as pericardial effusion. Additional trials involving device and procedural refinements are in progress or under consideration to ascertain whether LAA occlusion can replace anticoagulation in patients with nonvalvular AF to reduce risk of stroke.

REFERENCES

1. Wolf PA, Abbott RD, Kannel WB: Atrial fibrillation as an independent risk factor for stroke: the Framingham Study, *Stroke* 22(8): 983–988, 1991.
2. Miyasaka Y, Barnes ME, Gersh BJ, et al: Secular trends in incidence of atrial fibrillation in Olmsted County, Minnesota, 1980 to 2000, and implications on the projections for future prevalence, *Circulation* 114(2):119–125, 2006.
3. Risk factors for stroke and efficacy of antithrombotic therapy in atrial fibrillation: analysis of pooled data from five randomized controlled trials, *Arch Intern Med* 154(13):1449–1457, 1994.
4. Benjamin EJ, Wolf PA, D'Agostino RB, et al: Impact of atrial fibrillation on the risk of death: the Framingham Heart Study, *Circulation* 98(10):946–952, 1998.
5. Smith EE, Shobha N, Dai D, et al: Risk score for in-hospital ischemic stroke mortality derived and validated within the Get With the Guidelines-Stroke Program, *Circulation* 122(15):1496–1504, 2010.
6. Petrea RE, Beiser AS, Seshadri S, et al: Gender differences in stroke incidence and poststroke disability in the Framingham heart study, *Stroke* 40(4):1032–1037, 2009.
7. Fuster V, Ryden LE, Cannom DS, et al: ACC/AHA/ESC 2006 guidelines for the management of patients with atrial fibrillation—executive summary: a report of the American College of Cardiology/American Heart Association Task Force on Practice Guidelines and the European Society of Cardiology Committee for Practice Guidelines (Writing Committee to Revise the 2001 Guidelines for the Management of Patients With Atrial Fibrillation), *J Am Coll Cardiol* 48(4):854–906, 2006.
8. Holbrook AM, Pereira JA, Labiris R, et al: Systematic overview of warfarin and its drug and food interactions, *Arch Intern Med* 165(10):1095–1106, 2005.
9. Eikelboom JW, Wallentin L, Connolly SJ, et al: Risk of bleeding with 2 doses of dabigatran compared with warfarin in older and younger patients with atrial fibrillation: an analysis of the randomized evaluation of long-term anticoagulant therapy (RE-LY) trial, *Circulation* 123(21):2363–2372, 2011.

10. Walenga JM, Adiguzel C: Drug and dietary interactions of the new and emerging oral anticoagulants, *Int J Clin Pract* 64(7):956–967, 2010.

11. Thambidorai SK, Murray RD, Parakh K, et al: Utility of transesophageal echocardiography in identification of thrombogenic milieu in patients with atrial fibrillation (an ACUTE ancillary study), *Am J Cardiol* 96(7):935–941, 2005.

12. Wang YL, Li XB, Quan X, et al: Focal atrial tachycardia originating from the left atrial appendage: electrocardiographic and electrophysiologic characterization and long-term outcomes of radiofrequency ablation, *J Cardiovasc Electrophysiol* 18(5):459–464, 2007.

13. Healey JS, Crystal E, Lamy A, et al: Left atrial appendage occlusion study (LAAOS): results of a randomized controlled pilot study of left atrial appendage occlusion during coronary bypass surgery in patients at risk for stroke, *Am Heart J* 150(2):288–293, 2005.

14. Bayard YL, Omran H, Neuzil P, et al: PLAATO (percutaneous left atrial appendage transcatheter occlusion) for prevention of cardioembolic stroke in nonanticoagulation eligible atrial fibrillation patients: results from the European PLAATO study, *EuroIntervention* 6(2):220–226, 2010.

15. Ernst G, Stollberger C, Abzieher F, et al: Morphology of the left atrial appendage, *Anat Rec* 242(4):553–561, 1995.

16. Hart RG, Pearce LA, Albers GW, et al: Independent predictors of stroke in patients with atrial fibrillation: a systematic review, *Neurology* 69(6):546–554, Aug 7 2007.

17. Gage BF, Waterman AD, Shannon W, et al: Validation of clinical classification schemes for predicting stroke: results from the National Registry of Atrial Fibrillation, *JAMA* 285(22):2864–2870, 2001.

18. Puwanant S, Varr BC, Shrestha K, et al: Role of the CHADS$_2$ score in the evaluation of thromboembolic risk in patients with atrial fibrillation undergoing transesophageal echocardiography before pulmonary vein isolation, *J Am Coll Cardiol* 54(22):2032–2039, 54 2009.

19. Tang RB, Liu XH, Kalifa J, et al: Body mass index and risk of left atrial thrombus in patients with atrial fibrillation, *Am J Cardiol* 104(12):1699–1703, 2009.

20. Oldgren J, Alings M, Darius H, et al: Risks for stroke, bleeding, and death in patients with atrial fibrillation receiving dabigatran or warfarin in relation to the CHADS$_2$ score: a subgroup analysis of the RE-LY trial, *Ann Intern Med* 155(10):660–667, Nov 15 2011. W204.

21. You JJ, Singer DE, Howard PA, et al: Antithrombotic therapy for atrial fibrillation: Antithrombotic Therapy and Prevention of Thrombosis, 9th ed: American College of Chest Physicians evidence-based clinical practice guidelines, *Chest* 141(2 Suppl):e531S–575S, 2012.

22. Lip GY, Nieuwlaat R, Pisters R, et al: Refining clinical risk stratification for predicting stroke and thromboembolism in atrial fibrillation using a novel risk factor-based approach: the euro heart survey on atrial fibrillation, *Chest* 137(2):263–272, 2010.

23. Lip GY, Frison L, Halperin JL, et al: Identifying patients at high risk for stroke despite anticoagulation: a comparison of contemporary stroke risk stratification schemes in an anticoagulated atrial fibrillation cohort, *Stroke* 41(12):2731–2738, 2010.

24. Camm AJ, Kirchhof P, Lip GY, et al: Guidelines for the management of atrial fibrillation: the Task Force for the Management of Atrial Fibrillation of the European Society of Cardiology (ESC), *Eur Heart J* 31(19):2369–2429, 2010.

25. Taillandier S, Olesen JB, Clementy N, et al: Prognosis in patients with atrial fibrillation and CHA$_2$DS$_2$-VASc Score = 0 in a community-based cohort study, *J Cardiovasc Electrophysiol* 23(7):708-713, 2012.

26. Vaidya D, Szklo M, Cushman M, et al: Association of endothelial and oxidative stress with metabolic syndrome and subclinical atherosclerosis: multiethnic study of atherosclerosis, *Eur J Clin Nutr* 65(7):818–825, 2011.

27. Uemura T, Kaikita K, Yamabe H, et al: Changes in plasma von Willebrand factor and ADAMTS13 levels associated with left atrial remodeling in atrial fibrillation, *Thromb Res* 124(1):28–32, 2009.

28. Duygu H, Barisik V, Kurt H, et al: Prognostic value of plasma soluble CD40 ligand in patients with chronic nonvalvular atrial fibrillation, *Europace* 10:210–214, 2008.

29. Alberti S, Angeloni G, Tamburrelli C, et al: Platelet-leukocyte mixed conjugates in patients with atrial fibrillation, *Platelets* 20(4):235–241, Jun 2009.

30. Al-Saady NM, Obel OA, Camm AJ: Left atrial appendage: structure, function, and role in thromboembolism, *Heart* 82(5):547–554, 1999.

31. Veinot JP, Harrity PJ, Gentile F, et al: Anatomy of the normal left atrial appendage: a quantitative study of age-related changes in 500 autopsy hearts: implications for echocardiographic examination, *Circulation* 96(9):3112–3115, 1997.

32. Su P, McCarthy KP, Ho SY: Occluding the left atrial appendage: anatomical considerations, *Heart* 94(9):1166–1170, 2008.

33. Nucifora G, Faletra FF, Regoli F, et al: Evaluation of the left atrial appendage with real-time 3-dimensional transesophageal echocardiography: implications for catheter-based left atrial appendage closure, *Circ Cardiovasc Imaging* 4(5):514–523, 2011.

34. Willens HJ, Qin JX, Keith K, et al: Diagnosis of a bilobed left atrial appendage and pectinate muscles mimicking thrombi on real-time 3-dimensional transesophageal echocardiography, *J Ultrasound Med* 29(6):975–980, Jun 2010.

35. Marek D, Vindis D, Kocianova E: Real time 3-dimensional transesophageal echocardiography is more specific than 2-dimensional TEE in the assessment of left atrial appendage thrombosis, *Biomed Pap Med Fac Univ Palacky Olomouc Czech Repub* 157:22–26, 2013.

36. Fatkin D, Kelly RP, Feneley MP: Relations between left atrial appendage blood flow velocity, spontaneous echocardiographic contrast and thromboembolic risk in vivo, *J Am Coll Cardiol* 23(4):961–969, 23 1994.

37. Handke M, Harloff A, Hetzel A, et al: Left atrial appendage flow velocity as a quantitative surrogate parameter for thromboembolic risk: determinants and relationship to spontaneous echocontrast and thrombus formation: a transesophageal echocardiographic study in 500 patients with cerebral ischemia, *J Am Soc Echocardiogr* 18(12):1366–1372, 2005.

38. Beinart R, Heist EK, Newell JB, et al: Left atrial appendage dimensions predict the risk of stroke/TIA in patients with atrial fibrillation, *J Cardiovasc Electrophysiol* 22(1):10–15, 2011.

39. Tamura H, Watanabe T, Nishiyama S, et al: Prognostic value of low left atrial appendage wall velocity in patients with ischemic stroke and atrial fibrillation, *J Am Soc Echocardiogr* 25(5):576–583, 2012.

40. Abbara S, Mundo-Sagardia JA, Hoffmann U, et al: Cardiac CT assessment of left atrial accessory appendages and diverticula, *AJR Am J Roentgenol* 193(3):807–812, 2009.

41. Wang Y, Di Biase L, Horton RP, et al: Left atrial appendage studied by computed tomography to help planning for appendage closure device placement, *J Cardiovasc Electrophysiol* 21(9):973–982, 2010.

42. Di Biase L, Santangeli P, Anselmino M, et al: Does the left atrial appendage morphology correlate with the risk of stroke in patients with atrial fibrillation? Results from a multicenter study, *J Am Coll Cardiol* 60(6):531–538, 2012.

43. Gage BF, Yan Y, Milligan PE, et al: Clinical classification schemes for predicting hemorrhage: results from the National Registry of Atrial Fibrillation (NRAF), *Am Heart J* 151(3):713–719, 2006.

44. Pisters R, Lane DA, Nieuwlaat R, et al: A novel user-friendly score (HAS-BLED) to assess 1-year risk of major bleeding in patients with atrial fibrillation: the Euro Heart Survey, *Chest* 138(5):1093–1100, 2010.

45. Lip GY, Frison L, Halperin JL, et al: Comparative validation of a novel risk score for predicting bleeding risk in anticoagulated patients with atrial fibrillation: the HAS-BLED (hypertension, abnormal renal/liver function, stroke, bleeding history or predisposition, labile INR, elderly, drugs/alcohol concomitantly) score, *J Am Coll Cardiol* 57(2):173–180, 2011.

46. Holmes DR, Reddy VY, Turi ZG, et al: Percutaneous closure of the left atrial appendage versus warfarin therapy for prevention of stroke in patients with atrial fibrillation: a randomised noninferiority trial, *Lancet* 374(9689):534–542, 2009.

47. Guerios EE, Schmid M, Gloekler S, et al: Left atrial appendage closure with the Amplatzer cardiac plug in patients with atrial fibrillation, *Arq Bras Cardiol* 98(6):528–536, 2012.

48. Viles-Gonzalez JF, Kar S, Douglas P, et al: The clinical impact of incomplete left atrial appendage closure with the WATCHMAN device in patients with atrial fibrillation: a PROTECT AF (percutaneous closure of the left atrial appendage versus warfarin therapy for prevention of stroke in patients with atrial fibrillation) substudy, *J Am Coll Cardiol* 59(10):923–929, 2012.

49. Reddy VY, Holmes D, Doshi SK, et al: Safety of percutaneous left atrial appendage closure: results from the WATCHMAN Left Atrial Appendage System for Embolic Protection in Patients with AF (PROTECT AF) clinical trial and the Continued Access Registry, *Circulation* 123(4):417–424, 2011.

50. Schneider B, Stollberger C, Sievers HH: Surgical closure of the left atrial appendage: a beneficial procedure? *Cardiology* 104(3):127–132, 2005.

51. Dawson AG, Asopa S, Dunning J: Should patients undergoing cardiac surgery with atrial fibrillation have left atrial appendage exclusion? *Interact Cardiovasc Thorac Surg* 10(2):306–311, 2010.

52. Kanderian AS, Gillinov AM, Pettersson GB, et al: Success of surgical left atrial appendage closure: assessment by transesophageal echocardiography, *J Am Coll Cardiol* 52(11):924–929, 2008.

53. Salzberg SP, Plass A, Emmert MY, et al: Left atrial appendage clip occlusion: early clinical results, *J Thorac Cardiovasc Surg* 139(5):1269–1274, 2010.

54. Starck CT, Steffel J, Emmert MY, et al: Epicardial left atrial appendage clip occlusion also provides the electrical isolation of the left atrial appendage, *Interact Cardiovasc Thorac Surg* 15(3):416–418, 2012.

55. Bruce CJ, Stanton CM, Asirvatham SJ, et al: Percutaneous epicardial left atrial appendage closure: intermediate-term results, *J Cardiovasc Electrophysiol* 22(1):64–70, 2011.

56. McCarthy PM, Lee R, Foley JL, et al: Occlusion of canine atrial appendage using an expandable silicone band, *J Thorac Cardiovasc Surg* 140(4):885–889, 2010.

57. Singh SM, Dukkipati SR, d'Avila A, et al: Percutaneous left atrial appendage closure with an epicardial suture ligation approach: a prospective randomized preclinical feasibility study, *Heart Rhythm* 7(3):370–376, 2010.

58. Lee RJ, Bartus K, Yakubov SJ: Catheter-based left atrial appendage (LAA) ligation for the prevention of embolic events arising from the LAA: initial experience in a canine model, *Circ Cardiovasc Interv* 3(3):224–229, 2010.

59. Bartus K, Bednarek J, Myc J, et al: Feasibility of closed-chest ligation of the left atrial appendage in humans, *Heart Rhythm* 8(2):188–193, 2011.

60. Bartus K, Han FT, Bednarek J, et al: Percutaneous left atrial appendage suture ligation using the LARIAT device in patients with atrial fibrillation: initial clinical experience, *J Am Coll Cardiol* 62(2):108–118, 2013.

61. Ostermayer SH, Reisman M, Kramer PH, et al: Percutaneous left atrial appendage transcatheter occlusion (PLAATO system) to prevent stroke in high-risk patients with nonrheumatic atrial fibrillation: results from the international multicenter feasibility trials, *J Am Coll Cardiol* 46(1):9–14, 2005.

62. Montenegro MJ, Quintella EF, Damonte A, et al: Percutaneous occlusion of left atrial appendage with the Amplatzer cardiac plug in atrial fibrillation, *Arq Bras Cardiol* 98(2):143–150, 2012.

63. Sievert H, Lesh MD, Trepels T, et al: Percutaneous left atrial appendage transcatheter occlusion to prevent stroke in high-risk patients with atrial fibrillation: early clinical experience, *Circulation* 105(16):1887–1889, 2002.

64. Block PC, Burstein S, Casale PN, et al: Percutaneous left atrial appendage occlusion for patients in atrial fibrillation suboptimal for warfarin therapy: 5-year results of the PLAATO (percutaneous left atrial appendage transcatheter occlusion) study, *JACC Cardiovasc Interv* 2(7):594–600, 2009.

65. Park JW, Leithauser B, Gerk U, et al: Percutaneous left atrial appendage transcatheter occlusion (PLAATO) for stroke prevention in atrial fibrillation: 2-year outcomes, *J Invasive Cardiol* 21(9):446–450, 2009.

66. Sick PB, Schuler G, Hauptmann KE, et al: Initial worldwide experience with the WATCHMAN left atrial appendage system for stroke prevention in atrial fibrillation, *J Am Coll Cardiol* 49(13):1490–1495, 2007.

67. Hankey GJ: Replacing aspirin and warfarin for secondary stroke prevention: is it worth the costs? *Curr Opin Neurol* 23(1):65–72, Feb 2010.

68. Meier B, Palacios I, Windecker S, et al: Transcatheter left atrial appendage occlusion with Amplatzer devices to obviate anticoagulation in patients with atrial fibrillation, *Catheter Cardiovasc Interv* 60(3):417–422, 2003.

69. Rodes-Cabau J, Champagne J, Bernier M: Transcatheter closure of the left atrial appendage: initial experience with the Amplatzer cardiac plug device, *Catheter Cardiovasc Interv* 76(2):186–192, 2010.

Chapter 17

Percutaneous Closure of Congenital, Acquired, and Postinfarction Ventricular Septal Defects

NOA HOLOSHITZ • QI-LING CAO • ZIYAD M. HIJAZI

Ventricular septal defects (VSDs) are the most common congenital heart disease, accounting for 25% of all congenital heart defects and occurring in 3 to 3.5 infants per 1000 live births.[1] Congenital VSDs often close spontaneously in childhood or are otherwise treated. However, they may be left undiagnosed until adulthood. Previously undiagnosed VSDs can present in adulthood with a murmur, bacterial endocarditis, or cyanosis and exercise intolerance secondary to pulmonary hypertension. Alternatively, a VSD can be acquired during adulthood either after a myocardial infarction (MI), as a complication of cardiac surgery, or rarely after trauma to the chest. Classification and nomenclature of VSDs can be confusing to the nonpediatric practitioner. For simplicity, this chapter will refer to them by their most commonly used names. **Figure 17–1** depicts the types of VSDs based on their location.

Perimembranous VSDs account for approximately 75% of all congenital VSDs. They are located in the midportion of the upper region of the ventricular septum and are related to the aortic and pulmonic valve. The second most common type of VSDs are the muscular VSDs, which are located entirely within the muscular portion of the septum; they account for approximately 10% of congenital VSDs. Although they may be found anywhere within the muscular septum, the majority are found in the midmuscular region. Anterior muscular defects are often multiple and may be referred to as "Swiss cheese" defects.[2] Small VSDs, which are sometimes referred to as Henri-Louis Roger's defects, are typically considered to be those defects that are less than one third the size of the aortic root. Because of their small size, little shunting occurs, and even if the defect does not close spontaneously, closure (surgical or percutaneous) may not be necessary. Other, less common VSDs such as supracristal

(subarterial [aortic] or subpulmonic) and inlet defects are not discussed here, because they are not amenable to percutaneous closure.

Acquired VSDs are much less common than congenital VSDs. However, in the adult population, most congenital VSDs will have already been addressed in childhood. Therefore acquired VSDs do make up a substantial proportion of VSDs diagnosed during adulthood. In the largest study published on VSD closure in the adult population, 61% of the 28 patients had unrepaired congenital defects, 18% had postoperative residual patch margin defects, and 21% had acquired VSDs (either iatrogenic postoperative defects or defects that were secondary to trauma).[3] Post-MI VSDs were not included in that study; however, another study from the same group published a few years earlier reported an additional 18 patients with post-MI VSDs who underwent transcatheter closure attempts.[4]

VSDs secondary to MI septal rupture are much less common in the postreperfusion therapy era, occurring in only 0.2% to 0.34% of patients receiving thrombolysis for acute MI in the Global Utilization of Streptokinase and Tissue Plasminogen Activator for Occluded Coronary Arteries (GUSTO-I) trial.[5] These patients are usually acutely ill and may be in cardiogenic shock. If left untreated, almost 50% of patients die within the first week[6]; ultimately the mortality for patients treated medically approaches 100%.[7] Early identification of the postinfarct VSD before the onset of irreversible organ failure caused by a low output state is crucial and requires a high index of suspicion. Transcatheter closure of these defects is feasible but offers a variety of challenges that will be discussed later in this chapter.

Iatrogenic VSDs are a rare entity that can be seen after surgical aortic or mitral valve replacement.[8] These

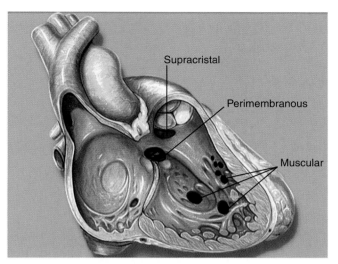

Figure 17-1 Locations of the common types of VSDs.

defects are usually located in the membranous septum and are usually hemodynamically insignificant. However, if closure of the defect is indicated, it is usually preferable to do so percutaneously, because repeat surgery can be complicated and associated with increased morbidity and mortality. An unusual type of iatrogenic VSD is a communication between the left ventricle and right atrium that is also known as the Gerbode defect.[9] This type of communication can rarely be seen congenitally and has been described after mitral and aortic valve surgery, as well as secondary to infective endocarditis and trauma to the chest.[10] These defects have historically been closed surgically; however, in cases of postsurgical Gerbode defects, repeat surgery can be challenging and it is possible to close the communication safely percutaneously. VSDs occurring after surgical myectomy in patients with hypertrophic obstructive cardiomyopathy have also been described, and closure of these defects percutaneously has been successful.[11,12] Along the same lines, it is possible to have residual VSDs after surgical patch repair. The incidence of residual shunting after surgical repair can be anywhere between 5% and 25%, depending on the type of VSD repaired.[13] These residual defects can be perimembranous, muscular, or apical, and if they are associated with a hemodynamically significant shunt, they need to be closed. Percutaneous closure offers a safe way to avoid the added morbidity and mortality associated with repeat sternotomy.[13]

17.1 History of Ventricular Septal Defect Closure

Surgical closure has long been the gold standard for treatment of VSDs. However, despite advances in surgical technique, it continues to be associated with significant morbidity and mortality,[14,15] especially when multiple defects are present or when repeat surgery is needed.

In 1987 the first percutaneous closure of a VSD was performed[16] using the Rashkind double-umbrella device.

The Rashkind device is a double disc composed of polyurethane foam on a hexagonal stainless steel frame.[17] The device was initially designed for closure of patent ductus arteriosus or atrial–septal defects (ASDs). The authors were the first to attempt closure of post-MI VSDs and congenital VSDs with this device. They crossed the VSD from the left ventricle and advanced a guidewire to the right heart and then delivered the device via a delivery sheath from the venous route. Of the three patients with congenital VSDs, one patient died, one still had significant left-to-right shunt, and only one 44-year-old patient with a 5-mm VSD had a complete closure. After this first report, several other studies have shown that although this device could reduce the left-to-right shunting, the overall success rate and closure results were not satisfactory.[18]

Other devices that have been used in the past included button devices, which have been shown to have a lower rate of complete closure and longer fluoroscopy time.[19] The Bard Clamshell umbrella, which was originally designed for ASD closure, was also used for VSD closure. The device was redesigned by the manufacturer (Nitinol Medical Technologies, Boston, Mass.) and renamed the CardioSEAL device. The U.S. registry for this device showed good outcomes with a 92% success rate for 55 patients and only 8% adverse events.[20] The U.S. Food and Drug Administration (FDA) has approved this device for use to close muscular VSDs in patients at high risk for surgical repair; however, the manufacturer of the device has gone out of business.

The Amplatzer muscular VSD occluder (St. Jude Medical, Plymouth, Minn.) is the most commonly used percutaneous VSD occlusion device **(Figure 17–2).** It was first used experimentally in dog models in 1999,[21] and use in humans quickly followed.[22] It is a self-expandable, double-disc device made from a nitinol wire mesh. The wire thickness ranges from 0.003 to 0.005 inch. The two discs are linked together by a short (7-mm) cylindrical waist with a diameter that corresponds to the size of the VSD. The Amplatzer muscular VSD occluder is currently available in sizes ranging from 4 to 18 mm in 2-mm increments. The left and right ventricle discs are 8 mm larger than the waist (except for the 4-mm device, in which the discs are 9 mm in diameter). The discs and waist are filled with polyester fabric that is securely sewn to the device by a polyester thread. Outcomes with this device have been very promising. The U.S. registry reported a success rate approaching 90% for implantation and 92% for complete closure at one year.[23,24] The device received FDA approval for closure of muscular VSDs in patients at high surgical risk.

The Amplatzer postinfarct VSD occluder is available in waist diameters 16 to 24 mm in 2-mm increments. It has a slightly different design from the muscular device. In the postinfarct device, the connecting waist is 10 mm long (to correspond to the thickness of the septum in adult patients) and the left- and right-sided discs are equal in size and 10 mm larger than the waist. The device has larger discs than the standard device in order to cover more of the friable ventricular septum and avoid device dislodgement and embolization. It is only available through the humanitarian device exemption (HDE) via the FDA for emergency or compassionate use in the United States.

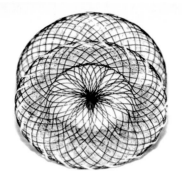
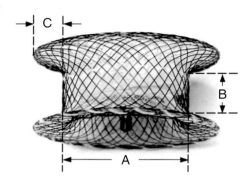

Figure 17–2 **Amplatzer muscular VSD occluder 2.** *A* corresponds to device diameter; *B* corresponds to length of the waist (7 mm for the muscular device, 10 mm for the postinfarct device); *C* corresponds to the ventricular side diameter (4 mm for the muscular device, 5 mm for the postinfarct device).

The older Amplatzer membranous device has an asymmetric design with the two discs offset from each other. It was available in diameters of 4 to 18 mm in 1-mm increments to allow for more precise sizing. However, because of problems with complete heart block when using this original device, the continued use of this device in clinical trials has ceased. The European registry reported a complete heart block rate of 5%[25]; however, some centers have cited a rate as high as 22%.[26] The Amplatzer membranous occluder 2 **(Figure 17–3)** is a new membranous occluder device that is undergoing clinical trials outside the United States with the hope that its new design will have a lower rate of impact on the conduction system and subsequent heart block. In the new model, the left disc has an elliptical and concave shape that adapts to the left ventricular outflow tract (LVOT) and provides stability. In addition, the nitinol wire is considerably thinner, which decreases the rigidity of the device. The waist length was increased from 1.5 to 3 mm, and polyester patches were sewn into the discs to ensure rapid occlusion. The device is available in 9 waist diameters (from 4 to 10 mm in 1-mm increments, plus 12 and 14 mm).[27]

17.2 Indications

The guidelines for VSD closure are listed in **Box 17–1.** The 2008 American College of Cardiology (ACC)/American Heart Association (AHA) guidelines for adults with congenital heart disease[1] give percutaneous closure of VSDs a IIb recommendation:

> *Device closure of a muscular VSD may be considered, especially if the VSD is remote from the tricuspid valve and the aorta, if the VSD is associated with severe left-sided heart chamber enlargement, or if there is pulmonary arterial hypertension.* (*Level of evidence:* C).

Indications that favor transcatheter closure include residual defects after prior attempts at surgical closure, trauma, or iatrogenic defects after surgical replacement of an aortic valve. Because most hemodynamically significant shunts are diagnosed and treated in childhood, significant shunting is a less likely indication for closure in the adult population than it is in young children.

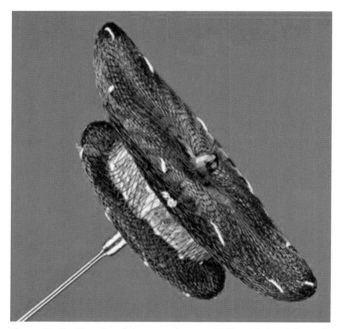

Figure 17–3 **New Amplatzer membranous VSD occluder.** It is available in two configurations: (1) eccentric, with a 1-mm superior rim and a 2-mm inferior rim, and (2) concentric (as shown), with 3-mm superior and inferior rims. The device is available in 9 waist diameters (ranging from 4 to 10 inches in 1-mm increments, plus 12 and 14 mm).

However, with age, progressive left ventricular dilation and symptoms of heart failure may develop even in the presence of a small shunt. In fact, the most common indications for closure of VSDs in the adult population by either transcatheter or surgical technique are symptoms of left ventricular dysfunction.[3,28]

17.3 Technique

ASSESSMENT OF VENTRICULAR SEPTAL DEFECT

Before the procedure it is very important to get an accurate evaluation of the defect and degree of shunting. Echocardiographic assessment of the size, number, and location of the VSDs is crucial for planning the interventional procedure. The parasternal long-axis view is the best view to

BOX 17–1

Guidelines for Ventricular Septal Defect Closure[1]

Class I

1. Surgeons with training and expertise in CHD should perform VSD closure operations. (Level of evidence: C)
2. Closure of a VSD is indicated when there is a pulmonary–to–systemic blood flow ratio (Qp/Qs) of 2 or more and clinical evidence of LV volume overload. (Level of evidence: B)
3. Closure of a VSD is indicated when the patient has a history of infective endocarditis. (Level of evidence: C)

Class IIa

1. Closure of a VSD is reasonable when net left-to-right shunting is present at a Qp/Qs greater than 1.5 with PA pressure less than two thirds of systemic pressure and PVR less than two thirds of systemic vascular resistance. (Level of evidence: B)
2. Closure of a VSD is reasonable when net left-to-right shunting is present at a Qp/Qs greater than 1.5 in the presence of LV systolic or diastolic failure. (Level of evidence: B)

Class IIb

1. Device closure of a muscular VSD may be considered, especially if the VSD is remote from the tricuspid valve and the aorta, if the VSD is associated with severe left-sided heart chamber enlargement, or if there is PAH. (Level of evidence: C)

Class III

1. VSD closure is not recommended in patients with severe irreversible PAH. (Level of evidence: B)

CHD, Congenital heart disease; *LV,* left ventricular; *PA,* pulmonary artery; *PVR,* pulmonary vascular resistance; *PAH,* pulmonary arterial hypertension; *VSD,* ventricular septal defect.

demonstrate membranous VSDs. In the short-axis view just below the aortic valve level, the defect is seen in a 10-o'clock position inferior to the right coronary cusp of the aortic valve and adjacent to the septal leaflet of the tricuspid valve. Muscular VSDs are best viewed in the short-axis view of the left ventricle or in the apical four-chamber view **(Figures 17–4 and 17–5).** It is critical to assess the VSD fully before starting the procedure to ensure that it is technically feasible to close it percutaneously.

SETUP AND ACCESS

Percutaneous VSD closure is performed when the patient is under general anesthesia in a catheterization lab with biplane angiography capabilities if possible. However, the procedure can be performed with the patient under conscious sedation and also using a single-plane fluoroscopic system. Intraprocedural echocardiography is usually needed, and this can be done by transesophageal, intracardiac, or transthoracic imaging. The main concept behind the procedure is the creation of an arteriovenous loop with a wire entering through the arterial side, into the left ventricle across the VSD, and externalized out the venous circulation. The authors usually use a Judkins right coronary catheter (Manufactured by multiple companies, such as Cordis Corporation, Bridgewater, N.J., or a Glidecath Cobra Catheter; Terumo Medical Corporation, Somerset, N.J.) to cross the VSD and then a Terumo Glidewire (Terumo Medical Corporation) to advance the catheter to either the pulmonary artery (PA) or superior vena cava. Alternatively, a venovenous loop can be used, with the wire crossing from the right atrium to the left atrium (via an existing defect or transseptal puncture), to the left ventricle, to the right ventricle, to the right atrium. Then the wire is snared from the femoral vein or the jugular vein depending on the location

APICAL-FOUR CHAMBER VIEW

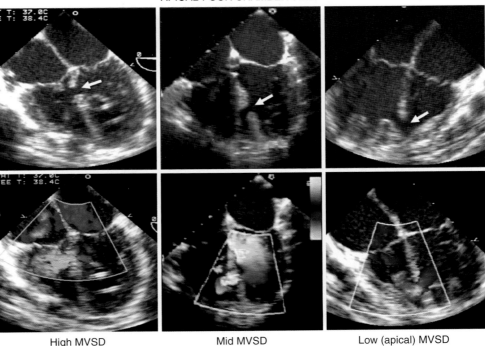

Figure 17–4 Apical four-chamber views of muscular VSDs *(arrows)* by TEE. *(MVSD,* Muscular VSD.)

High MVSD   Mid MVSD   Low (apical) MVSD

SHORT-AXIS VIEW

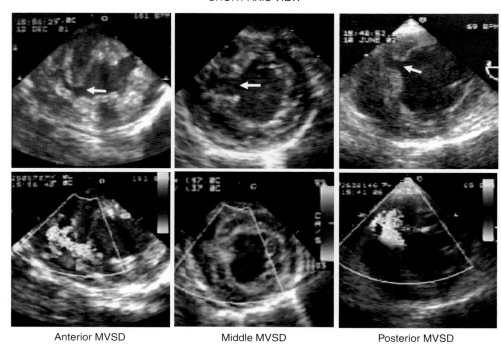

Anterior MVSD   Middle MVSD   Posterior MVSD

Figure 17–5 Short-axis views of muscular VSDs *(arrows)* by TEE. (*MVSD,* Muscular VSD.)

of the VSD. Alternatively, some defects can be closed without the need for an arteriovenous loop by simply crossing the defect in a retrograde fashion from the left ventricle, placing the delivery sheath over this wire, and delivering the appropriately sized device. If the device is delivered from the venous side, it can be delivered from the internal jugular or femoral vein based on the location of the defect. In general, defects that are higher and anteriorly located in the ventricular septum can be approached from the femoral vein, and defects in the apical, midmuscular, and basal locations are more easily closed from the internal jugular vein.[29,30]

RIGHT AND LEFT HEART CATHETERIZATION

Right and left heart catheterization should be performed in all patients to assess hemodynamics and pulmonary vascular resistance and to calculate a shunt fraction. A left-ventricular angiogram should be performed to rule out any additional defects and to create a road map to aid in accessing the defect from the left-ventricular side. This should be done in a single plane at a 35° left anterior oblique (LAO)/35° cranial view to profile the muscular septum. For perimembranous VSDs, 60° LAO/15 to 20° cranial angulation best profiles such VSDs. A complete transesophageal echocardiography (TEE, or intracardiac echo) is performed. It is important to pay attention to the cardiac structures near the VSD, such as papillary muscles, chordae tendineae, and moderator band. Echocardiographic monitoring of the steps of closure is crucial even for single VSDs. On rare occasions entanglement of the anterior mitral valve leaflet can occur, and the only way to detect this is by echocardiography **(Figure 17–6).**

DEVICE SIZING

Correct sizing of the closure device is important to prevent device embolization. The standard practice is to choose a device that is 1 to 2 mm larger than the VSD size as assessed by TEE or angiography measured at end diastole. Balloon sizing of the defect should not be done. For post-MI VSDs (because of the continued increase [maturation] in the size of defect), it is advisable to size the device 50% larger than the diameter of the measured VSD to prevent embolization or residual shunting. On rare occasions, a large Amplatzer septal occluder may be used to close a large post-MI VSD. However, because of the short waist, the interventionist should be careful in positioning this device across the defect.

DEVICE INSERTION AND DEPLOYMENT

The key step in successful VSD closure is the creation of a stable arteriovenous loop to provide a supportive frame for delivery sheath insertion. This is usually done by advancing a curved 4F to 5F end-hole catheter (Judkins right or Cobra) from the left ventricle across the VSD into the right ventricle. An exchange-length 0.035-inch J-tipped guidewire is advanced through the VSD into the right ventricle and into either the branch PA or the superior vena cava. There is not really much control as to where the wire will advance. Obviously it is easier to snare a wire from the superior vena cava than from the branch PA. This wire is then snared using a 15- to 25-mm gooseneck snare and externalized through either the femoral or internal jugular vein. A 6F to 8F long Mullins sheath (Cook Medical, Bloomington, Ind.) (or a TorqVue [St. Jude Medical, St. Paul, Minn.] sheath) is then advanced from the venous side to the right ventricle, through the defect,

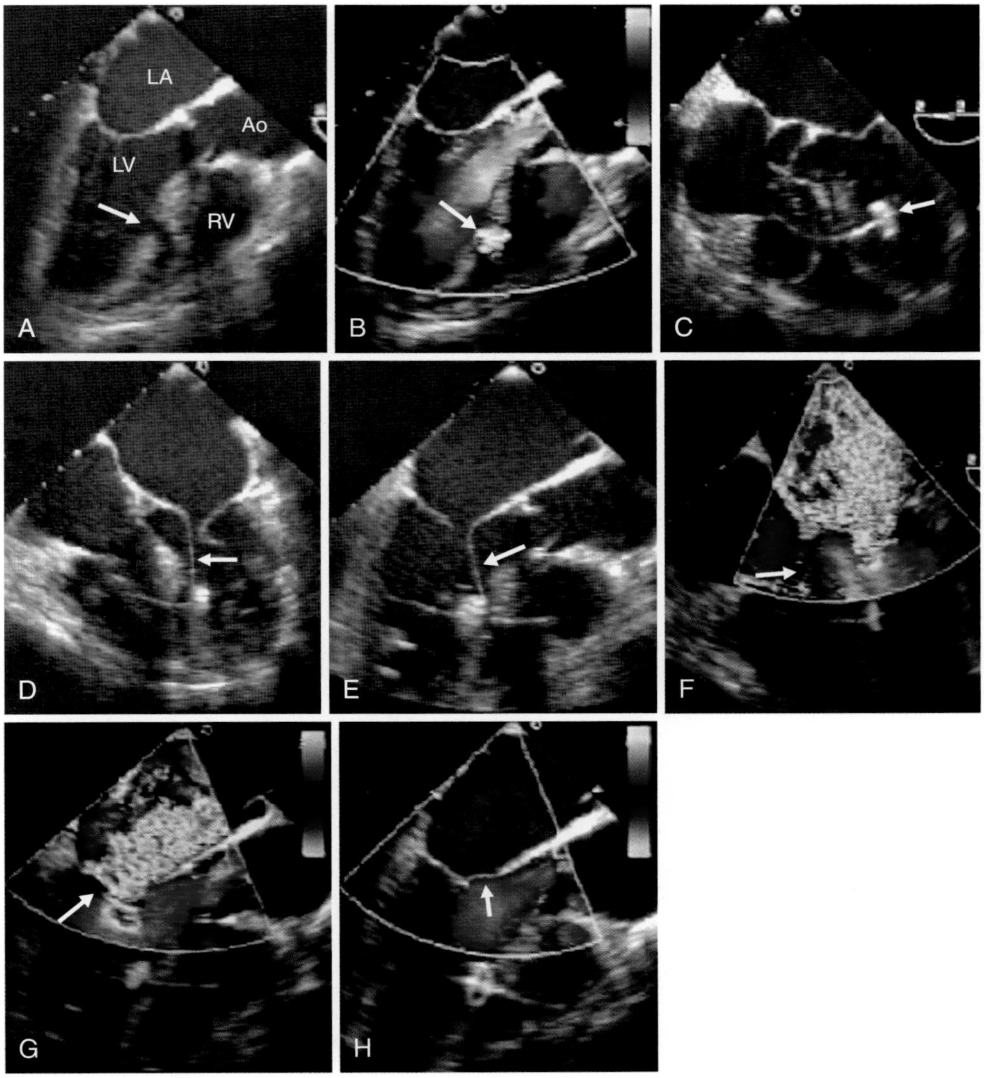

Figure 17–6 Complications of VSD closure: acute mitral regurgitation. A and **B,** TEE demonstrating a midmuscular VSD *(arrows).* **C,** The left ventricular disc was deployed *(arrow)* and pulled back to the septum. **D** and **E,** The chordae of the anterior leaflet of the mitral valve became entangled in the device *(arrows).* **F** and **G,** This led to severe acute mitral regurgitation and hemodynamic instability *(arrows).* **H,** Once this was recognized, the disc was repositioned, and the mitral regurgitation was eliminated *(arrow).* (*Ao,* Aorta, *LA,* left atrium; *LV,* left ventricle; *RV,* right ventricle.)

and positioned in the left ventricle. The dilator and the wire are removed, and the sheath is allowed to bleed back. If bleeding through the sheath is free, the sheath can be flushed with saline. The appropriately sized closure device is then screwed onto the delivery cable and brought inside a loader; the loader is then flushed with saline. The device is then introduced through the delivery sheath with the help of the loader and slowly advanced by pushing the cable. Once the device reaches the tip of the sheath in the left ventricle, the left-sided disc is extruded slowly under direct fluoroscopic and echocardiographic guidance **(Figures 17–7 and 17–8, Videos 17–1 and 17–2).** Once the left-sided disc is fully deployed, the device and sheath are pulled back to approximate the left-sided disc to the ventricular septum. When the left-sided disc is in good position, retracting the delivery sheath over the delivery cable deploys the remainder of the waist and the right-sided disc in their respective locations. On rare occasions, especially with anteriorly located VSDs, a wire is left alongside the device so that if device position is not accurate, recrossing the VSD will be easier.

DEVICE RELEASE AND IMAGING

After the device has been completely deployed, LV angiography is performed. If the position of the device is adequate by angiography and echocardiography, the device can be released from the delivery cable by counterclockwise rotation of the cable using the pin vise. The cable is then withdrawn into the sheath, and the sheath is pulled back into the right atrium. The orientation of the device may change after it is fully released from the delivery cable and all tension is released.

POSTPROCEDURE MANAGEMENT AND FOLLOW-UP CARE

Patients generally receive a dose of an appropriate antibiotic during the procedure and two additional doses 8 hours apart. After an overnight inpatient stay, they are usually discharged home the next day and must take aspirin for 6 months. Patients are instructed to avoid contact sports for 1 month, and endocarditis prophylaxis is recommended for 6 months.[31] Follow-up

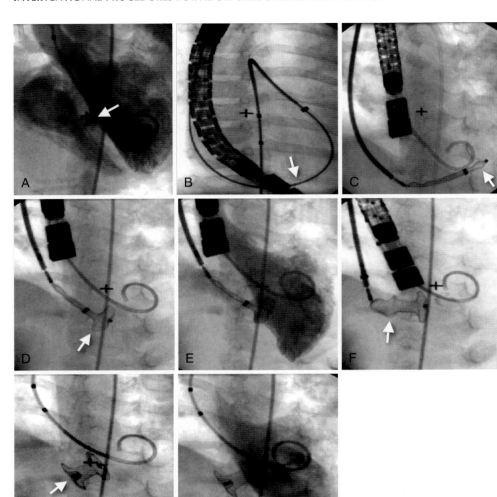

Figure 17–7 Fluoroscopic step-by-step approach to closure of a midmuscular VSD. A, The location of the defect is characterized by left ventricular angiography *(arrow)*. **B,** An arteriovenous loop is formed through the VSD *(arrow)*. **C,** The device is inserted through the VSD over the wire *(arrow)*, and **D,** the left ventricular disc is deployed *(arrow)*. **E,** Once left-ventricular angiography demonstrates good position of the left-sided disc, the right-sided disc can be deployed **(F,** *arrow***)** and the device can be released **(G,** *arrow***). H** shows the final angiography after device deployment with only a trivial residual shunt.

echocardiogram, chest x-ray, and electrocardiograph are performed at 6 months postclosure and then on a yearly basis.

ALTERNATE PROCEDURAL PROTOCOLS

It is possible to use a venovenous loop to insert the device (as opposed to an arteriovenous loop). In this technique, a catheter is inserted through the femoral vein, into the right atrium and through an atrial communication such as an ASD or a transseptal puncture into the left atrium. The catheter is then advanced through the VSD, and a wire is inserted through the catheter and into the right ventricle. A Mullins-type delivery sheath or a TorqVue sheath can be advanced over this wire, and delivery of the device can be done this way, or the wire can be snared from the jugular vein or the contralateral femoral vein, and a sheath can be advanced over this loop with delivery of the device.

Another rarely used technique is the retrograde delivery of the device via the femoral artery. In this technique, the defect is crossed from the left ventricular side, and

the delivery sheath is advanced over the wire from the femoral artery.

PERVENTRICULAR TECHNIQUE

Perventricular closure of VSDs is a technique reported in small infants. This technique allows hybrid device closure in very small infants and even neonates whose vessels are too small for a percutaneous approach but does not have the morbidity and mortality associated with cardiopulmonary bypass.[32,33] This technique is rarely performed in the adult population and is not discussed here in detail.

17.4 Complications

Percutaneous closure of VSD can be a safe procedure in the hands of an experienced operator. A wide spectrum of complications have been reported including vascular complications, complete heart block, tachyarrhythmias, air embolus, hypotension, injury to the aortic valve,

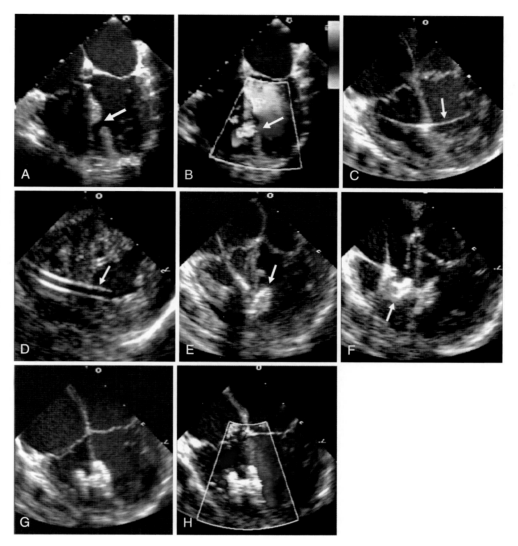

Figure 17–8 Echocardiographic step-by-step approach to closure of a midmuscular VSD. The defect can be visualized by two-dimensional (**A,** *arrow*) and color Doppler (**B,** *arrow*) echocardiography. **C,** Once the wire crosses the defect *(arrow),* an arteriovenous loop is formed and the device is inserted from the right ventricular side (**D,** *arrow*). **E,** The left-sided disc is deployed first *(arrow)* and is followed by the right-sided disc (**F,** *arrow*). **G,** Once good position is confirmed, the device can be released. **H** demonstrates color Doppler with no evidence of a residual shunt.

cardiac perforation, device embolization, hemolysis, hemodynamic instability, and death.[4,23-25,34-37]

The listed complications are serious; however, most can be avoided and/or treated. Vascular complications can be decreased by careful vascular access technique and proper hemostasis. It is not advisable to use a large-bore arterial sheath, and it is important to keep the activated clotting time (ACT) around 250 seconds during the procedure.

The risk of device embolization has been reported to be as low as 1.2% and is thought to be related to the level of operator expertise.[25] The device can migrate to the left ventricle and ascending aorta or alternatively to the right ventricle and PA. Embolization can be substantially reduced by correct utilization of TEE. The defect must be measured accurately, and careful attention must be paid to ensure optimal device placement. Before release of the device, thorough assessment of its position is critical. If device embolization does occur, it may be possible to percutaneously snare it; however, if the device becomes entangled in the chordae of either atrioventricular valve, surgical removal may be preferable. It is recommended that labs performing percutaneous VSD closures should

be stocked with all the appropriate types and sizes of snaring equipment. Operators performing VSD closures should be skilled at the use of snaring equipment, and it is recommended to have a congenital cardiac surgeon available in-house for back-up. Because of the recessed microscrew of the device, it is somewhat difficult to snare the VSD device; however, attempts should be made to snare it from the microscrew. If not possible, the middle of the device can be snared and attempt made to pull it inside a larger sheath. It is not recommended to pull the device through important structures (valves or small vessels).

Complete heart block has been one of the more common complications, particularly with the Amplatzer membranous device. The reported rate is between 5% and 22%.[25,27] A possible risk factor has been proposed to be a higher occluder-to-VSD size ratio.[26] Sizing of defects is a particular problem, because the morphology of a defect can be heterogeneous, and variation in measurements between color Doppler and two-dimensional imaging during TEE may lead to choice of the largest recorded measurement and therefore oversizing. Recovery of heart block has been reported with early treatment with high-dosage aspirin and high-dosage steroid use[38] or early surgical removal of the membranous occluder.[39] However, for most patients and physicians the risks of long term ventricular pacing are unacceptable, particularly when rates of complete heart block after surgical closure have been reported to be less than 1%.[40] Unlike patients who have had surgery, the timing of presentation of heart block with transcatheter closure is difficult to predict, and therefore uncontrolled presentation leading to syncope and potential death are a concern. As an alternative, the Amplatzer muscular occluder has been used for perimembranous VSDs with the distance of defect to aortic valve greater than 4 mm or in those with associated aneurysmal tissue surrounding the defect.[41] This approach in theory may either reduce the mechanical motion of the asymmetric nitinol occluder from exerting pressure on the conducting system or avoid it completely when positioned within the aneurysm away from both the conduction tissue and the aortic valve. Since the original Amplatzer membranous device has been withdrawn from the market, a new device has been designed by St. Jude and is undergoing clinical studies.

17.5 Postinfarction Ventricular Septal Defect: Special Considerations

Percutaneous closure of VSDs secondary to septal rupture after MI offers a unique set of patient-related and technical difficulties. Septal rupture usually occurs within the first week after MI and often within the first 24 hours.[7] There is little room for conservative management, because these patients tend to be very ill and are often in cardiogenic shock. Sudden hemodynamic deterioration as well as an increase in the VSD size is common, even in patients who initially may appear to be clinically stable.[42] The first large series of post-MI percutaneous VSD closure was reported by Landzberg and Lock in 1998.[43] They performed percutaneous closure of post-MI VSDs in 18 patients using the Clamshell double umbrella and later the CardioSEAL device. Eleven of the 18 patients had prior attempted surgical VSD closure. Of the seven patients treated with primary percutaneous closure, the 1-week mortality was 57%. The survivors had chronic VSDs that were treated late after the initial MI after fibrosis had occurred. In 2004, Holzer et al reported a series of 18 patients with post-MI VSDs who underwent percutaneous closure attempts with the Amplatzer postinfarct VSD device.[4] The procedure was successful in 16 of the 18 patients, and the 30-day mortality was 28%.

Closing these defects percutaneously presents technical difficulties as well. Crossing the VSDs with a glide wire may be problematic, because the wire may perforate the necrotic myocardium rather than the true defect; therefore, attempts at crossing with a balloon-tipped catheter may be preferable. The surrounding tissue undergoes lysis and necrosis and therefore may enlarge. It is advisable to use a device that is 50% larger than the defect to allow for enlargement. It has been suggested that the closure device itself may increase the size of the defect by compressing the surrounding tissue.[5]

REFERENCES

1. Warnes CA, Williams RB, Bashore TM, et al: ACC/AHA 2008 Guidelines for the management of adults with congenital heart disease: a report of the American College of Cardiology/American Heart Association task force on practice guidelines, Circulation 118:714, 2008.
2. Gersony WM, Rosenbaum MS: Congenital heart disease in the adult. New York, 2002, McGraw Hill. pp 27–45.
3. Al-Kashkari A, Balan P, Kavinsky CJ, et al: Percutaneous device closure of congenital and iatrogenic ventricular septal defects in adult patients, Catheter Cardiovasc Interv 77:260, 2011.
4. Holzer R, Balzer D, Amin Z, et al: Transcatheter closure of postinfarction ventricular septal defects using the new Amplatzer muscular VSD occluder: results of a U.S. registry, Catheter Cardiovasc Interv 61:196, 2004.
5. Birnbaum Y, Fishbein MC, Blanche C, et al: Ventricular septal rupture after acute myocardial infarction, New Engl J Med 347:1426, 2002.
6. Fox AC, Glassman E, Isom OW: Surgically remediable complications of myocardial infarction, Prog Cardiovasc Dis 21:461, 1979.
7. Crenshaw BS, Granger CB, Birnbaum Y, et al: Risk factors, angiographic patterns and outcomes in patients with ventricular septal defect complicating acute myocardial infarction, Circulation 101:27, 2000.
8. Holzer R, Latson L, Hijazi ZM: Device closure of iatrogenic membranous ventricular septal defects after prosthetic aortic valve replacement using the Amplatzer membranous ventricular septal defect occluder, Catheter Cardiovasc Interv 62:276, 2004.
9. Wasserman SM, Fann JI, Atwood JE, et al: Acquired left-ventricular-right atrial communication Gerbode-type defect, Echocardiography 19:67, 2002.
10. Sinisalo JP, Sreeram N, Jokinen E, et al: Acquired left ventricular-right atrium shunts, Eur J Cardiothorac Surg 39:500, 2011.
11. Spies C, Ujivari F, Schraeder R: Transcatheter closure of a ventricular septal defect following myectomy for hypertrophic obstructive cardiomyopathy, Cardiology 112:31, 2009.
12. Kilicgedik A, Karabay CY, Aung SM, et al: A successful percutaneous closure of ventricular septal defect following septal myectomy in patients with hypertrophic obstructive cardiomyopathy, Perfusion 27:253, 2012.
13. Dua JS, Carminati M, Lucente M, et al: Transcatheter closure of postsurgical residual ventricular septal defects: early and mid-term results, Catheter Cardiovasc Interv 75:246, 2010.
14. Serral A, Lacour-Gayet F, Bruniaux J, et al: Surgical management of isolated multiple ventricular septal defects, J Thorac Cardiovasc Surg 103:437, 1992.
15. Kitagawa T, Durham LA, Mosea RS, et al: Techniques and results in the management of multiple ventricular septal defects, J Thorac Cardiovasc Surg 115:848, 1998.
16. Lock JE, Block PC, McKay RG, et al: Transcatheter closure of ventricular septal defects, Circulation 78:361, 1988.
17. Du AD, Hijazi ZM: Transcatheter closure of ventricular septal defect. Federacion Argentina de Cardiologia FAC Available online at, http://www.fac.org.ar/scvc/llave/pediat/hijazi/hijazii.htm#tabla1.
18. Bridges ND, Perry SB, Keane JE, et al: Preoperative transcatheter closure of congenital muscular ventricular septal defects, N Engl J Med 324:1312, 1991.
19. Sideris EB, Walsh KP, Haddad JL, et al: Occlusion of congenital ventricular septal defects by the buttoned device: "buttoned device" clinical trials international register, Heart 77(3):276, 1997.
20. Lim DS, Forbes TJ, Rothman A, et al: Transcatheter closure of high-risk muscular ventricular septal defects with the CardioSEAL occluder: initial report from the CardioSEAL VSD registry, Catheter Cardiovasc Interv 70:740, 2007.
21. Amin Z, Gu X, Berry JM, et al: Periventricular closure of ventricular septal defects without cardiopulmonary bypass, Ann Thorac Surg 68:149, 1999.
22. Tofeig M, Patel RG, Walsh KP: Transcatheter closure of a mid-muscular ventricular septal defect with an Amplatzer VSD occlusion device, Heart 81:438, 1999.
23. Hijazi AM, Hakim F, Al-Fadley F, et al: Transcatheter closure of single muscular ventricular septal defects using the Amplatzer muscular VSD Occluder: initial results and technical considerations, Catheter Cardiovasc Interv 49:167, 2000.

24. Holzer R, Balzer D, Cao QL, et al: Device closure of muscular ventricular septal defects using the Amplatzer muscular ventricular septal defect occluder, *J Am Coll Cardiol* 43:1257, 2004.

25. Carminati M, Butera G, Chessa M, et al: Investigators of the European VSD registry: transcatheter closure of congenital ventricular septal defects: results of the European registry, *Eur Heart J* 28:2361, 2007.

26. Predescu D, Chaturvedi RR, Benson LN, et al: Occluder closure of hemodynamically significant perimembranous ventricular septal defects, *Catheter Cardiovasc Interv* 70:S6, 2007.

27. Velasco-Sanchez D, TzikasA, Ibrahim R, et al: Transcatheter closure of perimembranous ventricular septal defects: initial human experience with the Amplatzer membranous VSD occluder 2. *Catheter Cardiovasc Interv* 2012. [Epub ahead of print].

28. Mongeon FP, Burkhart HM, Ammash NM, et al: Indications and outcomes of surgical closure of ventricular septal defect in adults, *JACC Cardiovasc Interv* 3:290, 2010.

29. Hijazi ZM: Device closure of ventricular septal defects, *Catheter Cardiovasc Interv* 60:107, 2003.

30. Amin Z, Cao QL, Hijazi ZM, et al: Closure of muscular ventricular septal defects: transcatheter and hybrid techniques, *Catheter Cardiovasc Interv* 72:102, 2008.

31. Wilson W, Taubert KA, Gewitz M, et al: Prevention of infective endocarditis: guidelines from the American Heart Association, *Circulation* 116:1736, 2007.

32. Bacha EA, Cao QL, Starr JP, et al: Periventricular device closure of muscular ventricular septal defects on the beating heart: technique and results, *J Thorac Cardiovasc Surg* 126:1718, 2003.

33. Michel-Behnke I, Ewert P, Koch A, et al: Device closure of ventricular septal defects by hybrid procedures: a multicenter retrospective study, *Catheter Cardiovasc Interv* 77:242, 2011.

34. Waight DJ, Bacha EA, Kahana M, et al: Catheter therapy of Swiss cheese ventricular septal defects using the Amplatzer muscular VSD occluder, *Catheter Cardiovasc Interv* 55:355, 2002.

35. Hijazi ZM, Hakim F, Haweleh AA, et al: Catheter closure of perimembranous ventricular septal defects using the new Amplatzer membranous VSD occluder: initial clinical experience, *Catheter Cardiovasc Interv* 56:508, 2002.

36. Holzer R, DeGiovanni J, Walsh KP, et al: Transcatheter closure of perimembranous ventricular septal defects using the Amplatzer membranous VSD occluder: immediate and midterm results of an international registry, *Catheter Cardiovasc Interv* 68:620, 2006.

37. Fu YC, Bass J, Amin Z, et al: Transcatheter closure of perimembranous ventricular septal defects using the new Amplatzer membranous VSD occluder: results of the US phase I trial, *J Am Coll Cardiol* 47:319, 2006.

38. Walsh MA, Bialkowski J, Szkutnik M, et al: Atrioventricular block after transcatheter closure of perimembranous ventricular septal defects, *Heart* 92:1295, 2006.

39. Ovaert C, Dragulescu A, Sluysmans T, et al: Early surgical removal of membranous ventricular septal occluder might allow recovery of atrioventricular block, *Pediatr Cardiol* 29:971, 2008.

40. Tucker EM, Pyles LA, Bass JL, et al: Permanent pacemaker for atrioventricular conduction block after operative repair of perimembranous ventricular septal defect, *J Am Coll Cardiol* 50:1196, 2007.

41. Szkutnik M, Qureshi SA, Kusa J, et al: Use of the Amplatzer muscular ventricular septal defect occluder for closure of perimembranous ventricular septal defects, *Heart* 93:355, 2007.

42. Topaz O, Taylor AL: Interventricular septal rupture complicating acute myocardial infarction: from pathophysiologic features to the role of invasive and noninvasive diagnostic modalities in current management, *Am J Med* 93:683, 1992.

43. Landzberg MJ, Lock JE: Transcatheter management of ventricular septal rupture after myocardial infarction, *Semin Thorac Cardiovasc Surg* 10:128, 1998.

Chapter 18

Percutaneous Closure of Aortic, Coronary, and Ventricular Pseudoaneurysms and Coronary Fistulae

STEFAN C. BERTOG • JENNIFER FRANKE • LAURA VASKELYTE •
ILONA HOFMANN • HORST SIEVERT

Although many transcatheter closure techniques are closely related, aortic, ventricular, and coronary pseudoaneurysms each involve unique approaches. Likewise, coronary fistulas are discussed separately. Most closure techniques are improvisations of methods applied in more commonly encountered congenital defects (e.g., atrial septal defects [ASD] and ventricular septal defects [VSD]). There is no standard approach to either of these conditions because the location and relation to surrounding structures varies considerably.

18.1 Left Ventricular Pseudoaneurysms

There are three types of ventricular aneurysms: (1) true aneurysms that are outpouchings of ventricular segments (dyskinesis) involving the entire wall without disruption; (2) pseudoaneurysms that are disruptions of the entire ventricular free wall with blood extravasation into an extracardiac space with containment usually caused by overlying adhesive pericardium; and (3) pseudopseudoaneurysms (rare) that are partial disruptions of the ventricular wall, causing blood to enter and exit the ventricular wall.[1-3]

Pseudoaneurysms may be iatrogenic (previous thoracic surgery, most commonly mitral valve replacement), traumatic (e.g., stab wounds to the chest), secondary to infection (endocarditis), or in most cases, the consequence of myocardial infarction.[4] Postinfarction rupture of the free wall usually results in pericardial hemorrhage and abrupt hemodynamic compromise and death,[5] can

be seen in 2% to 4% of myocardial infarctions, and is found in 23% of patients with fatal myocardial infarction at autopsy.[6] Its occurrence seems to have a bimodal distribution with peaks early after the infarction (within 24 hours) and after 3 to 5 days. The incidence has decreased significantly in recent decades, likely the result of timely pharmacologic or mechanical reperfusion. In some cases, however, free wall rupture leads to a contained (by the fibrous adhesive parietal pericardium) extravasation of blood that may not be immediately apparent clinically and can be diagnosed years after the infarction. Although the main clinical concern is that pseudoaneurysms may rupture, there are no studies clarifying the natural history of pseudoaneurysms, particularly in patients in whom it is discovered years after the infarct. Additional concerns are heart failure related to ineffective delivery of blood into a noncontractile cavity, resulting in a compromise of forward cardiac output, and embolic events from thrombi located in the pseudoaneurysm cavity.[7,8]

The first challenge when faced with an outpouching of the left ventricular wall is the distinction between a pseudoaneurysm and true aneurysm. This can be difficult because on clinical grounds there are no features unique to either of the two entities that would allow confident distinction. Likewise, echocardiography will show dyskinetic myocardial motion in both cases and not uncommonly it is unclear whether the integrity of the myocardium is disrupted, particularly if thrombus is present within the cavity. It has been suggested that the ratio of the ostium of the cavity to the maximal cavity size may help in distinction between aneurysms and pseudoaneurysms with a ratio of less than 1:2 in favor of the latter and a ratio greater than 1:2 of the former. However, this criterion is less than perfect, and measurement of the ostium can be challenging echocardiographically. For example, in the largest analysis of pseudoaneurysms to date, the median ostium-to-pseudoaneurysm diameter ratio was 0.23, with a wide range (0.02 to 1.04), and less than 0.5 in only 75% of patients.[4] Conventional coronary angiography together with left ventriculography may be helpful. Overlying coronary arteries are often seen in true aneurysms, whereas typically they are absent on the surface of a pseudoaneurysm.[9] More recently, cardiac magnetic resonance imaging (MRI) has been reported useful,[10-12] particularly in the distinction of thrombus from myocardium,[12] and this should be part of the imaging work-up unless contraindicated or if other imaging modalities are diagnostic. It is also helpful in the assessment of the exact location, size, and characteristics of the ostium.[10] Pseudoaneurysms are more commonly located posterior than anterior or apical.[4]

The natural history of pseudoaneurysms is unknown. Observational studies with limited numbers of patients suggest high mortality rates for untreated pseudoaneurysms.[5,13,14] However, a selection bias does not allow definitive conclusions. For example, it is conceivable that patients with favorable clinical characteristics were selected for surgery, and those with prohibitive comorbidities associated with poor outcomes regardless of treatment were managed conservatively. The clinical presentation is variable, and some patients are incidentally found to have a pseudoaneurysm many years after the underlying myocardial infarction. In these patients the natural history may be much more favorable than in symptomatic patients with a pseudoaneurysm discovered shortly after the infarction. Traditionally, surgery has been considered the mainstay of therapy.[15-17] In the largest series published to date, in 107 patients who underwent surgical pseudoaneurysm repair, follow-up study demonstrated that 23% of patients died at a median of 3 days after surgery.[4] In 23 patients treated conservatively, the mortality was 48%. Deaths occurred early (median of 1 week after the infarct), and some patients were alive at 10 years' follow-up study. At the writing of this chapter, there are no studies that compare outcomes after surgical and percutaneous repair, and data on percutaneous repair are limited to case reports.[18-20]

Suitability for percutaneous repair depends mainly on anatomical features. Most importantly, it must be determined whether the muscular rim surrounding the aneurysm neck is large enough to securely anchor a closure device. All closure devices are nitinol discs connected by a waist (ASD or VSD occluders such as Amplatzer septal occluders or ventricular septal occluders; St Jude Medical, St. Paul, Minn.); these are described more in detail in the respective chapters on ASD and VSD closure. Note that vascular plugs are typically not used because they do not offer the same stability for pseudoaneurysm closure as septal occluders or perimembranous VSD occluders—most vascular plugs do not have a sufficient waist. They are delivered via a guide catheter or sheath positioned into the pseudoaneurysm cavity. The minimum-access caliber depends on the anticipated device type and size

and can be obtained by review of the manufacturer's instructions for use. The waist diameter of the occluder should match or be slightly larger (1 to 2 mm) than the estimated diameter of the aneurysm neck, and the disc diameter should be at least 5 to 10 mm larger than the aneurysm neck. Attention to proper sizing allows secure anchoring without oversizing, which results in tension on surrounding structures including the pseudoaneurysm cavity or valvular apparatus. Femoral venous access is obtained, and after transseptal puncture, a soft-tipped, 0.035-inch, curved J-wire with a stiff or superstiff body is positioned into the pseudoaneurysm cavity. Alternatively, after femoral arterial access, a catheter is placed into the left ventricle and the wire positioned into the pseudoaneurysm cavity. Anticoagulation with intravenous heparin maintaining an anticoagulation time above 250 seconds is recommended. Subsequently, the guide catheter or delivery sheath is advanced over the wire into the pseudoaneurysm cavity. It is important never to be tempted to advance the guide catheter or sheath without a J-tipped wire positioned in the cavity to avoid injury of the containing aneurysm wall. Contrast injection into the pseudoaneurysm cavity will confirm appropriate sheath or catheter position and allow characterization of the aneurysm dimensions. Concomitantly, preferably three-dimensional transesophageal or intracardiac echocardiography should be considered to complement fluoroscopic imaging and to help with real-time device positioning. With the catheter or guide tip far enough in the pseudoaneurysm cavity, the wire is removed and the occluder is advanced to the distal sheath or catheter tip via a delivery cable. The sheath or catheter is slowly withdrawn while maintaining occluder position via the delivery cable until the distal occluder disc is desheathed. A gentle tug is applied to assure secure anchoring, and if confirmed, the sheath or catheter is withdrawn further, maintaining position of the delivery cable to allow the proximal disc to unfold. At this point contrast injection into the left ventricle is performed to assess device positioning, and adequate position is further confirmed via echocardiography. If the position is suboptimal, the occluder can be retrieved into the sheath and redeployed or a different occluder used. If the position is good, the occluder can be released by counterclockwise rotation of the delivery cable. Final cineangiography will confirm a successful occluder position. When an occluder is implanted into the inferior, posterior, or lateral wall, attention should be directed at the mitral apparatus and degree of mitral regurgitation before release because impingement on the mitral support structure can cause mitral regurgitation. In this case retrieval and repositioning or use of a different occluder type or size may be an alternative. It is important not to expect complete closure immediately because this may take weeks or months to occur. Complications include those related to access (e.g., subcutaneous, retroperitoneal, or rectus sheath hematomas; arteriovenous fistulae; pseudoaneurysms); embolic events secondary to insufficiently deaired guide catheters, sheaths, or devices, or to equipment-attached thrombi and thrombi originating from the pseudoaneurysm cavity; and cardiac perforations (e.g., of the aorta or left atrium during transseptal puncture or of the pseudoaneurysm cavity). The only possible treatment of a ruptured pseudoaneurysm cavity is emergency surgery with pericardiocentesis while preparing for emergency surgery. The risk of this complication depends on the age of the pseudoaneurysm and is more likely to occur with fresher pseudoaneurysms, the walls of which are more friable than those that have been present for many years. **Figures 18–1 and 18–2** are examples of percutaneous repair of left ventricular pseudoaneurysms.

18.2 Aortic Pseudoaneurysms

Similar to pseudoaneurysm elsewhere, aortic pseudoaneurysms are ruptures with blood extravasation contained by overlying tissue, an unusual scenario. Traditionally this has been treated surgically. However, more recently percutaneous repair has become an option. The natural history of aortic pseudoaneurysms is unclear; however, compression of surrounding structures and rupture (which is almost invariably fatal) are concerns. Percutaneous approaches depend on the location of the aneurysm and involvement or proximity to important branches. Imaging is best performed with a combination of modalities (transesophageal echocardiography, computed tomography [CT] or MRI, and conventional angiography) to define the location, size, and neck diameter, as well as origin of surrounding branches. When the pseudoaneurysm is located with sufficient distance to important branches, thereby allowing a proximal and distal landing zone, aortic endoprostheses covering the pseudoaneurysm orifice similar to the exclusion of a true aortic aneurysm is an option. Alternatively, placement of an occluder (e.g., ASD or patent foramen ovale occluder) is an option. In this case, after femoral arterial access (access and sheath/catheter caliber depends on the anticipated closure device), a guide catheter or sheath is advanced retrogradely over a 0.035-inch J-tipped wire close to the entry point of the pseudoaneurysm. The wire is then carefully advanced into the pseudoaneurysm cavity, followed by the guide catheter or sheath, with care not to advance the sheath without a wire. Angiography is performed to define the aneurysm cavity and neck. Subsequently the occluder is advanced to the tip of the sheath or guide. The sheath or guide is withdrawn, maintaining occluder position with the delivery cable until the distal disc unfolds. Gentle tugging confirms secure positioning. The guide or sheath is then further withdrawn, allowing the proximal disc to deploy. Aortography is performed to confirm the desired device position and exclude compromise of flow to surrounding branches, and when the result is optimal, the device is released. **Figure 18–3** demonstrates percutaneous closure of an ascending thoracic aortic pseudoaneurysm.

18.3 Coronary Pseudoaneurysms

Coronary pseudoaneurysms are rare and almost exclusively the result of prior iatrogenic coronary manipulation (most commonly prior bypass surgery or percutaneous coronary interventions complicated by contained perforations) or trauma. If the pseudoaneurysm arises from a coronary or graft feeding no significant or minor myocardial tissue (so vessel occlusion is not expected to cause significant myocardial infarction), the best approach is embolization of the feeding graft **(Figure 18–4)**. This can be achieved with coils, or if the feeding vessel is large (as demonstrated in **Figure 18–4**), with a vascular plug. If the pseudoaneurysm arises from a coronary or graft that supplies important myocardial tissue, the pseudoaneurysm ostium can be closed with a covered stent placed in the feeding vessel. However, covered stents are fraught with a high risk of thrombosis or restenosis, and hence a surgical alternative should be considered first.

18.4 Coronary Artery Fistulae

Coronary fistulae are uncommon abnormal connections between coronary arteries and cardiac chambers, the coronary sinus, or the pulmonary artery, bypassing arterioles, capillaries, and venules. They may be congenital or the result of previous surgery (e.g., cardiac transplantation or right heart biopsies) or trauma. The most common feeding coronary artery is the right (52%), followed by the left anterior descending (30%) artery, and then the left circumflex coronary artery.[21] The receiving structure is most commonly the right ventricle, followed by the right atrium, coronary sinus, left ventricle, and pulmonary artery.[22] Occasionally, multiple fistulous tracts are encountered.[23] Although there is significant variability, when the fistula originates from the distal left anterior descending coronary artery and drains into the left ventricle, or when it connects the proximal right coronary artery to the coronary sinus, its course is often more tortuous than if it originates from the proximal coronaries and enters the right atrium.[24]

Fistulae are often asymptomatic and discovered during childhood related to a murmur on routine examinations. The murmur may have resemblance to that of a patent ductus arteriosus; however, it is typically located more caudally, and the peak intensity tends to be toward mid to late diastole. When symptoms occur they are most commonly related to high-output heart failure,[25,26] ischemia (the consequence of a steal phenomenon),[27] or thrombus formation with distal embolization.[28] In addition, ventricular or atrial arrhythmias[21] and infectious endocarditis[29] have been reported, as has rupture (rarely).[30] With the exception of small fistulae (e.g., those that are commonly encountered after right heart biopsies or heart transplantation), most can be visualized with cardiac echocardiography, CT angiography, and MRI; however, conventional angiography best outlines the fistula course. Adequate contrast opacification of the fistulous tract may be difficult because of the fistula size and high-flow characteristics. In this case, the use of a large guide catheter and power injector for delivery of larger contrast boluses or the use of a pigtail catheter positioned in the fistula origin (if this accommodates the pigtail tip) may be helpful.

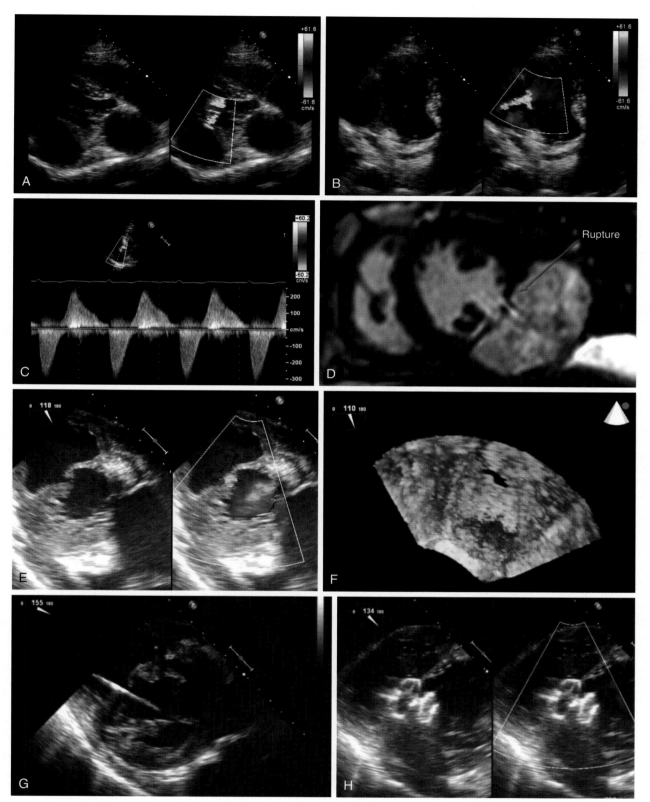

Figure 18–1 This is the case of a 65-year-old male with prior coronary artery bypass surgery and coronary stenting on multiple previous occasions, as well as an inferior wall myocardial infarction treated with thrombolysis. The patient experienced chest pain and heart failure symptoms and was found to have a large left ventricular pseudoaneurysm with the entry point located in the posterior wall. Bypass grafts were patent on coronary angiography (not shown here). **A** and **B** demonstrate a parasternal long axis and an apical two-chamber view of the pseudoaneurysm respectively. The typical pattern of flow into and out of the aneurysm during systole and diastole is seen on Doppler interrogation in **C**. The pseudoaneurysm cavity is further assessed by cardiac magnetic resonance imaging (**D**) and transesophageal echocardiography (**E**), both of which are helpful in the assessment of the rim surrounding the neck as well as the neck diameter. **F** is the complementary three-dimensional en-face image of the pseudoaneurysm neck. In **G**, a superstiff 0.035-inch wire has been positioned into the pseudoaneurysm cavity, and in **H**, appropriate occluder position is confirmed with the muscular rim surrounding the pseudoaneurysm neck sandwiched between the two occluder discs.

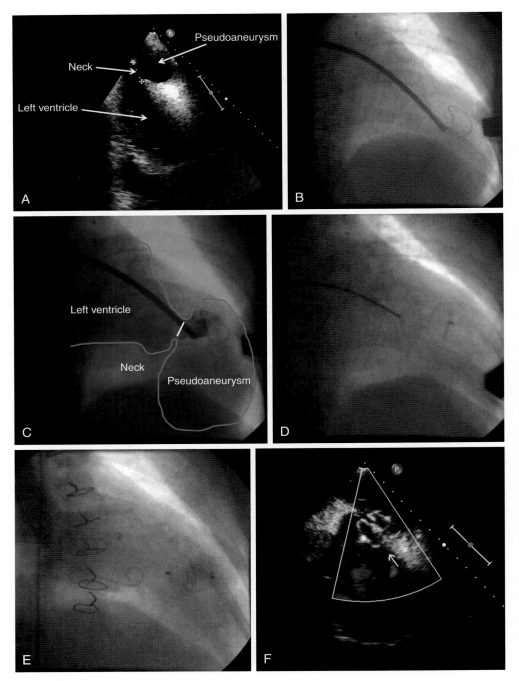

Figure 18–2 This is the case of a 42-year-old male who had undergone surgical left ventricular mass removal complicated by apical pseudoaneurysm formation that was subsequently closed with a Gore-Tex patch. Follow-up imaging demonstrated pseudoaneurysm enlargement and persistent extravasation of blood into the pseudoaneurysm cavity. **A** demonstrates a transesophageal echo view of the pseudoaneurysm, the left ventricle, and the neck. After venous access and transseptal puncture, a long sheath was placed into the left ventricular apex. **B,** A 0.035-inch J-tipped wire was positioned into the pseudoaneurysm cavity, and the sheath was advanced over the wire into the cavity. **C,** Contrast is injected into the pseudoaneurysm cavity. A 24-mm atrial septal defect occluder was released in a stepwise fashion with both discs sandwiching the rim of the aneurysm neck. **D,** A gentle tug is applied to the delivery cable to assure secure occluder position before release. **E,** The occluder is released and final left ventriculography performed with a pigtail catheter. **F,** Transesophageal echo demonstrates the occluder to be in a secure position.

Figure 18–3 This is a case of a 71-year old-female with a giant expanding ascending thoracic aortic pseudoaneurysm with comorbidities prohibitive for conventional surgery. **A** demonstrates the pseudoaneurysm on computed tomography (CT) before repair. **B,** After femoral arterial access, ascending aortic and arch angiography is performed with a pigtail catheter. This delineates the arch anatomy. Subsequently, the pigtail catheter is exchanged over a wire for a multipurpose catheter, the tip of which is positioned close to the pseudoaneurysm neck, and a 0.035-inch hydrophilic angled wire is advanced into the pseudoaneurysm catheter. **C,** The multipurpose catheter is advanced into the pseudoaneurysm cavity over the wire, and contrast is injected. **D,** A compliant sizing balloon is inflated at low pressure—just enough to allow a subtle waist—and the neck diameter is measured. **E,** Over the wire, a long sheath is advanced into the pseudoaneurysm cavity and contrast is injected; the wire is removed, and a 24-mm atrial septal defect occluder is advanced to the distal sheath tip. The distal sheath tip is withdrawn, unfolding the distal disc **(F),** and after secure positioning with a gentle tug is confirmed, the proximal disc is deployed **(G). H,** Angiography is performed via the sheath, confirming an optimal occluder position and patent arch vessels. **I,** Finally, the occluder is released by counterclockwise rotation of the delivery cable, and final angiography is performed to assess the position of the released occluder once again. **J,** Follow-up CT demonstrates complete thrombotic occlusion of the pseudoaneurysm.

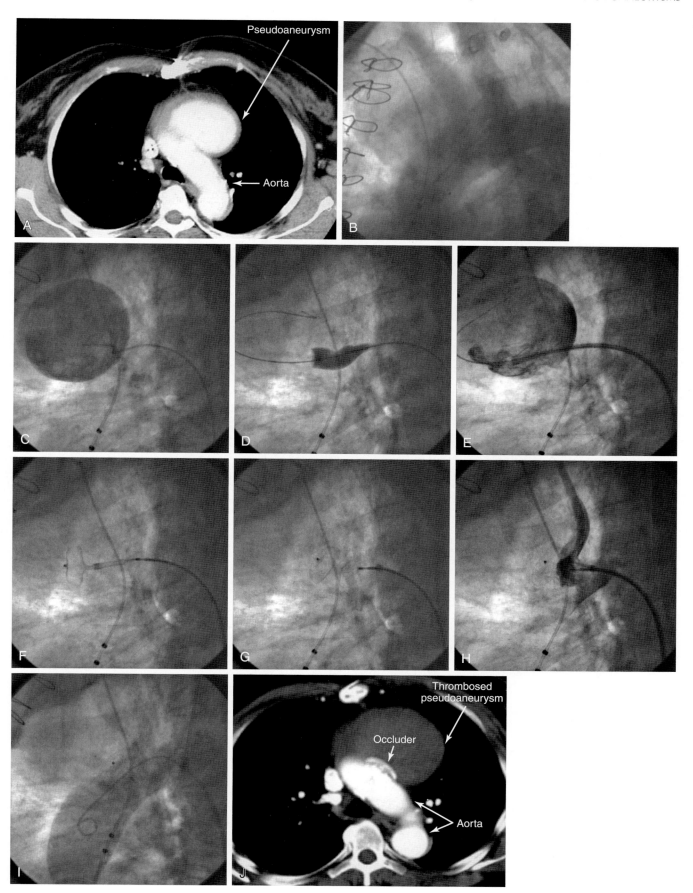

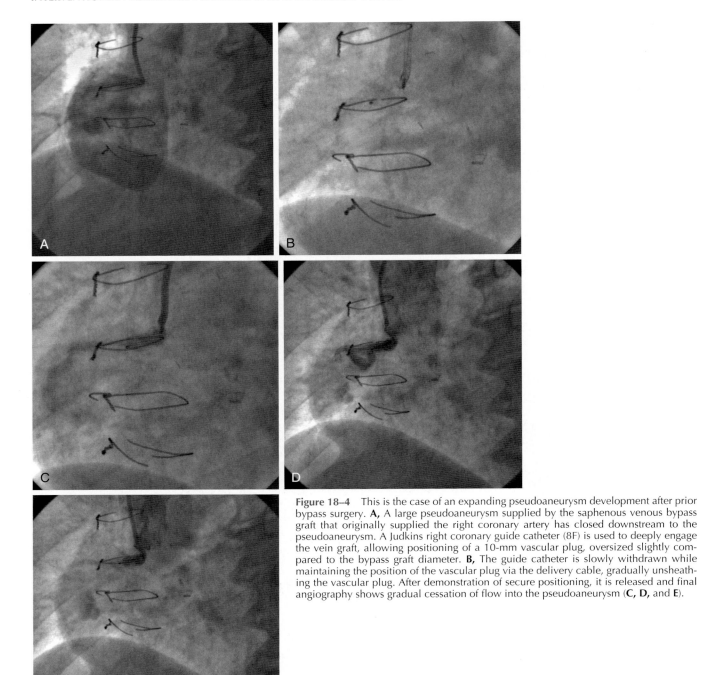

Figure 18–4 This is the case of an expanding pseudoaneurysm development after prior bypass surgery. **A,** A large pseudoaneurysm supplied by the saphenous venous bypass graft that originally supplied the right coronary artery has closed downstream to the pseudoaneurysm. A Judkins right coronary guide catheter (8F) is used to deeply engage the vein graft, allowing positioning of a 10-mm vascular plug, oversized slightly compared to the bypass graft diameter. **B,** The guide catheter is slowly withdrawn while maintaining the position of the vascular plug via the delivery cable, gradually unsheathing the vascular plug. After demonstration of secure positioning, it is released and final angiography shows gradual cessation of flow into the pseudoaneurysm (**C, D,** and **E**).

Though the identification and characterization of a coronary fistula is usually straightforward, the decision whether or not a fistula requires treatment can be difficult and controversial. No formal guidelines exist. However, small asymptomatic fistulae (e.g., small biopsy-related fistulae) that are not associated with signs of volume overload (e.g., chamber enlargement) are best left alone with clinical and echocardiographic follow-up examinations. Most would probably agree that symptomatic

fistulae and those that progressively increase in size or cause significant cardiac chamber enlargement should be considered for treatment. The first option, if this is technically feasible, is percutaneous closure. The approach depends on the anatomic characteristics.

Smaller fistulae (<5 mm) can be occluded with coils. These can be delivered by a guide catheter if this can be safely positioned into the fistula. If there is concern of injury to the coronary artery feeding the fistula, then

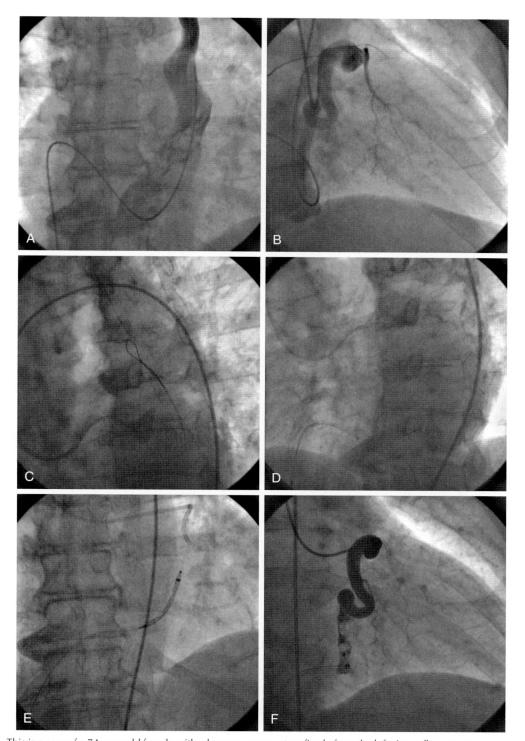

Figure 18–5   A, This is a case of a 74-year-old female with a large coronary artery fistula from the left circumflex coronary artery to the confluence of a persistent left superior vena cava and coronary sinus. **B** illustrates the fistula. Because of the rather large fistula size, a vascular plug was chosen for closure. Femoral arterial and venous access were obtained. The coronary artery was engaged with a 6F AL-2 guide catheter, and a venous sheath was advanced into the left persistent superior vena cava over a 0.035-inch J-tipped wire **(A).** Subsequently a 0.014-inch coronary guidewire was advanced via the fistula into the persistent right superior vena cava, snared with a 20-mm Gooseneck (ev3, Plymouth, Minn.) **(C)** and pulled into the venous sheath for support **(D).** The coronary wire loop then allowed advancement of the venous sheath in a retrograde fashion into the fistula tract. **E,** Finally, a 10-mm Amplatzer vascular plug was delivered via the venous sheath and deployed in the distal fistula tract, achieving near complete cessation of flow **(F).**

a delivery catheter (e.g., 4F to 5F coronary catheter or 2F to 3F microcatheter, depending on the size and tortuosity of the feeding vessel) can be positioned into the fistula over a guidewire or coronary wire and the coils placed via the delivery catheter. The sizes and characteristics of coils are usually described by three numbers: the first indicates the profile expressed in thousands of an inch; the second represents the unconstrained diameter (when it is allowed to assume its usual coil form) in millimeters; and the third is the length in its stretched state (when it is pulled apart into a straight line) in centimeters. Thus an 18-4-5 coil has a 0.018-inch profile, a 4-mm diameter in its unconstrained state, and a 5-cm length when pulled apart. Coils should be slightly oversized with respect to the target vessel diameter. For example, when the fistulous tract has a diameter of 4 mm, a coil with an unconstrained diameter of 5 to 6 mm should be chosen. The larger size will wedge the coil in position and minimize the risk of distal embolization. When placed via a delivery catheter, the coils are usually pushed into the vessel by a pusher wire. However, some coils (controlled release or detachable) can be delivered into the desired location, and if a size mismatch is recognized or the position is suboptimal, they can be removed before release. The choice of delivery method depends on the coil size and the anticipated coil location. A 7F or 8F guide catheter with a 4F or 5F delivery catheter is required for most large (0.035-inch) coils, whereas a 6F guide catheter can be used for delivery of smaller (0.018-inch) coils. When more distal delivery of the coils is desirable, it may be best to use a 7F or 8F guide catheter with a 5F catheter that can be advanced more distally and a 2F to 3F microcatheter for coil delivery. The mechanism by which the coils eventually cause occlusion of the fistulous tract is vessel (endothelial) injury and thrombogenicity of the coil itself rather than flow limitation because of the coils. Most coils are composed of nitinol or stainless steel. In addition, some have attached fibers to promote thrombosis. It is important to recognize that it may take some time for a vessel to close after coiling. Hence allowing some time before final angiography may prevent overzealous coiling. There is usually no need for reversal of anticoagulation. Of note, not all coils are compatible with MRI, and if an MRI is necessary, it is recommended to clarify compatibility with the manufacturer. Alternatively, placement of a covered stent across the origin of the fistula can be considered. However, currently available coronary covered stents are bulky, which can cause problems with delivery, particularly into more distal coronaries or through tortuous segments. More importantly, however, covered stents are associated with significant risks of in-stent restenosis and thrombosis and therefore should be considered only if all other alternatives are not feasible.

Medium sized and large fistulae (>5 mm) often require a different approach. Embolization with vascular plugs or large profile coils is often necessary **(Figure 18–5)**. The most commonly used plugs are Amplatzer vascular plugs, which are composed of self-expandable, multilayered, double-lobed nitinol mesh. The size is chosen approximately 30% larger than the vessel diameter to allow secure anchoring. The vascular plugs are attached to a delivery wire and are positioned into the fistula via a guide catheter or sheath. When the desired position is confirmed, they are released by counterclockwise rotation of the delivery wire via a microscrew. If the position is suboptimal or the size is inappropriate, as long as the plug is not released it can be pulled back into the guiding catheter or sheath and repositioned or removed entirely. The size of the guide catheter or sheath required depends on the profile of the vascular plug. Some newer generation plugs can be delivered via 4F or 5F guide catheters.[31] There are two basic delivery techniques. The plugs can be delivered antegradely through a guide catheter positioned via the feeding coronary into the fistula or retrogradely via a guide catheter positioned into the distal aspect of the fistula. The latter approach is chosen when significant risk of injury of the native feeding vessel is anticipated (e.g., when the fistula is very tortuous and guide positioning may create unwanted friction in the feeding coronary). Positioning vascular plugs or coils retrogradely into the distal fistula via a guide catheter can be challenging because there may be difficulties establishing and maintaining a secure guide or sheath position in the distal fistula. In this case, provided the draining chamber is the right atrium, ventricle, or coronary sinus, a guide catheter can be positioned in the coronary feeding the fistula, and a wire can be advanced through the fistula into the draining chamber where it is snared via a guide catheter or sheath positioned in the draining chamber. This loop then offers more support for a delivery catheter or sheath positioned in the distal fistula.

The most feared complications using coils or vascular plugs are inadvertent obstruction of the feeding native coronary artery and embolization into unwanted vascular territories. If the coil position is anticipated in the more proximal fistula segment close to the native coronary, balloon occlusion of the anticipated segment can be considered to assess whether ischemia will occur. In case of embolization, most coils and vascular plugs can usually be retrieved.[32]

Because of the rare occurrence of coronary fistulas that require percutaneous treatment and great variability in fistula anatomy, there are no official statements that guide postprocedural management. After closure of small fistulas, long-term antiplatelet therapy may be considered. In those patients with a persisting aneurysm stump or severe aneurysmatic dilation of the coronary vessel that originally fed the fistula, oral anticoagulation may be considered. Although infection of a coronary fistula has been reported, reported infection of the occluding device was not found by these authors. Nevertheless, after closure of fistulae larger than 3 to 4 mm in diameter double-bolus antibiotics (e.g., cephalosporin) are routinely administered on the day of the procedure. Thereafter antibiotic prophylaxis is not routinely administered. Although recurrent symptoms should guide reevaluation with noninvasive or invasive imaging, routine follow-up evaluation to assess for coronary ischemia may be considered, particularly in patients in whom ischemia was demonstrated before closure.

REFERENCES

1. Alessandrini F, De Bonis M, Lapenna E, et al: Posterior-septal pseudopseudoaneurysm with limited left-to-right shunt: an unexpected easy repair, J Cardiovasc Surg (Torino) 40:539–541, 1999.
2. Savage MP, Hopkins JT, Templeton JY 3rd, et al: Left ventricular pseudopseudoaneurysm: angiographic features and surgical treatment of impending cardiac rupture, Am Heart J 116:864–866, 1988.
3. Yvorra S, Desfossez L, Panagides D, et al: [False pseudoaneurysm of the left ventricle after myocardial infarction: recognition by transesophageal echocardiography], Arch Mal Coeur Vaiss 87:395–398, 1994.
4. Frances C, Romero A, Grady D: Left ventricular pseudoaneurysm, J Am Coll Cardiol 32:557–561, 1998.
5. Van Tassel RA, Edwards JE: Rupture of heart complicating myocardial infarction: analysis of 40 cases including nine examples of left ventricular false aneurysm, Chest 61:104–116, 1972.
6. Pollak H, Nobis H, Mlczoch J: Frequency of left ventricular free wall rupture complicating acute myocardial infarction since the advent of thrombolysis, Am J Cardiol 74:184–186, 1994.
7. Gueron M, Wanderman KL, Hirsch M, et al: Pseudoaneurysm of the left ventricle after myocardial infarction: a curable form of myocardial rupture, J Thorac Cardiovasc Surg 69:736–742, 1975.
8. Shabbo FP, Dymond DS, Rees GM, et al: Surgical treatment of false aneurysm of the left ventricle after myocardial infarction, Thorax 38:25–30, 1983.
9. Spindola-Franco H, Kronacher N: Pseudoaneurysm of the left ventricle: radiographic and angiocardiographic diagnosis, Radiology 127:29–34, 1978.
10. Harrity P, Patel A, Bianco J, et al: Improved diagnosis and characterization of postinfarction left ventricular pseudoaneurysm by cardiac magnetic resonance imaging, Clin Cardiol 14:603–606, 1991.
11. Hsu YH, Chiu IS, Chien CT: Left ventricular pseudoaneurysm diagnosed by magnetic resonance imaging in a nine-year-old boy, Pediatr Cardiol 14:187–190, 1993.
12. Duvernoy O, Wikstrom G, Mannting F, et al: Pre- and postoperative CT and MR in pseudoaneurysms of the heart, J Comput Assist Tomogr 16:401–409, 1992.
13. Vlodaver Z, Coe JI, Edwards JE: True and false left ventricular aneurysms: propensity for the altter to rupture, Circulation 51:567–572, 1975.
14. Davidson KH, Parisi AF, Harrington JJ, et al: Pseudoaneurysm of the left ventricle: an unusual echocardiographic presentation; review of the literature, Ann Intern Med 86:430–433, 1977.
15. Gueron M, Hirsch M, Venderman K, et al: Pseudoaneurysm of left ventricle. Report of a case diagnosed by angiography and successfully repaired, Br Heart J 35:663–665, 1973.
16. Smith RC, Goldberg H, Bailey CP: Pseudoaneurysm of the left ventricle: diagnosis by direct cardioangiography; report of two cases successfully repaired, Surgery 42:496–510, 1957.
17. Yakierevitch V, Vidne B, Melamed R, et al: False aneurysm of the left ventricle: surgical treatment, J Thorac Cardiovasc Surg 76:556–558, 1978.
18. Dudiy Y, Jelnin V, Einhorn BN, et al: Percutaneous closure of left ventricular pseudoaneurysm, Circ Cardiovasc Interv 4:322–326, 2011.
19. Vignati G, Bruschi G, Mauri L, et al: Percutaneous device closure of iatrogenic left ventricular wall pseudoaneurysm, Ann Thorac Surg 88:e31–e33, 2009.
20. Harrison W, Ruygrok PN, Greaves S, et al: Percutaneous closure of left ventricular free wall rupture with associated false aneurysm to prevent cardioembolic stroke, Heart Lung Circ 17:250–253, 2008.
21. McNamara JJ, Gross RE: Congenital coronary artery fistula, Surgery 65:59–69, 1969.
22. Levin DC, Fellows KE, Abrams HL: Hemodynamically significant primary anomalies of the coronary arteries: angiographic aspects, Circulation 58:25–34, 1978.
23. Reidy JF, Anjos RT, Qureshi SA, et al: Transcatheter embolization in the treatment of coronary artery fistulas, J Am Coll Cardiol 18:187–192, 1991.
24. Qureshi SA: Coronary arterial fistulas, Orphanet J Rare Dis 1:51, 2006.
25. Khan MD, Qureshi SA, Rosenthal E, et al: Neonatal transcatheter occlusion of a large coronary artery fistula with Amplatzer duct occluder, Catheter Cardiovasc Interv 60:282–286, 2003.
26. Wilde P, Watt I: Congenital coronary artery fistulae: six new cases with a collective review, Clin Radiol 31:301–311, 1980.
27. Oshiro K, Shimabukuro M, Nakada Y, et al: Multiple coronary LV fistulas: demonstration of coronary steal phenomenon by stress thallium scintigraphy and exercise hemodynamics, Am Heart J 120:217–219, 1990.
28. Ramo OJ, Totterman KJ, Harjula AL: Thrombosed coronary artery fistula as a cause of paroxysmal atrial fibrillation and ventricular arrhythmia, Cardiovasc Surg 2:720–722, 1994.
29. Alkhulaifi AM, Horner SM, Pugsley WB, et al: Coronary artery fistulas presenting with bacterial endocarditis, Ann Thorac Surg 60:202–204, 1995.
30. Bauer HH, Allmendinger PD, Flaherty J, et al: Congenital coronary arteriovenous fistula: spontaneous rupture and cardiac tamponade, Ann Thorac Surg 62:1521–1523, 1996.
31. Mordasini P, Szucs-Farkas Z, Do DD, et al: Use of a latest-generation vascular plug for peripheral vascular embolization with use of a diagnostic catheter: preliminary clinical experience, J Vasc Interv Radiol 21:1185–1190, 2010.
32. Tan CA, Levi DS, Moore JW: Embolization and transcatheter retrieval of coils and devices, Pediatr Cardiol 26:267–274, 2005.

RECOMMENDED READING

Berry RB, Brooks R, Gamaldo CE, et al: The AASM Manual for the Scoring of Sleep and Associated Events: Rules, Terminology and Technical Specifications, Version 2.0. www.aasmnet.org, Darien, Illinois: American Academy of Sleep Medicine, 2012.

Chapter 19

Percutaneous Treatment of Pulmonary Vein Stenosis

OLUSEUN ALLI • DAVID HOLMES, JR

Atrial fibrillation (AF) remains the most common arrhythmia encountered in clinical practice; it is estimated that by the year 2050 the number of patients in the United States may exceed 12 million.[1] Traditionally, AF has been treated medically with the aim of either restoring sinus rhythm or slowing down the arrhythmia to levels tolerated by the cardiovascular system. More recently, catheter mapping and utilization of surgically or catheter-based ablation strategies to the left atrial wall and pulmonary veins (PVs) have been developed and are quite successful in restoring sinus rhythm to a significant number of patients with this arrhythmia.[2-5] However, this does not eliminate the issue of thromboembolic events. Currently 40,000 to 50,000 ablation procedures are performed yearly in the United States, and this number is expected to increase.

PV stenosis (PVS) has emerged as a rare but serious complication of AF ablation. The emergence of this entity altered the way ablative procedures are now performed. Initial studies of PV ablation were performed with focal ablation within the PVs; this led to a high incidence of PVS. Subsequently, segmental ostial PV ablation was proposed and performed with the aim of isolating the PVs and avoiding ablation within the veins. This reduced but did not eliminate PVS, thereby leading to modification of the ablation technique. Currently, most ablative procedures are performed within the left atrium (LA), where the PVs are isolated by ablating around the PV using wide encircling lesions. Despite this technique of avoiding the PVs in their entirety, PVS remains a complication of AF ablation, but the incidence has been reduced considerably.[3]

19.1 Incidence and Prevalence of Pulmonary Vein Stenosis

The true incidence and prevalence of PVS remain undetermined; this is in part dependent on the diagnostic technique used for ascertainment. Rates have varied based on the technique of AF ablation, as mentioned previously. In the early series in which PV isolation was performed within the PVs, an incidence of 42.4% was documented.[6] With improvements in procedural techniques the incidence of PVS has fallen. A worldwide survey of 188 centers performing AF ablation revealed the incidence of PVS to be around 1.3%.[7]

19.2 Pulmonary Venous Anatomy

Good understanding of pulmonary venous anatomy is crucial for interventionalists wishing to undertake PV interventions. In a study using gadolinium-enhanced magnetic resonance imaging (MRI), Kato et al[8] examined PV anatomy in 28 patients with AF and 27 control patients. They found that there was significant variability in PV anatomy, with 38% of patients demonstrating variant anatomy. Typical PV anatomy involves four PVs with separate ostia: two left superior and inferior PVs, and two right superior and inferior PVs. In some patients the left superior and inferior PVs drain into a common antrum/ostia, which may have a short or long trunk. Another variant involves the right PV, in which there are one or two right middle veins. Occasionally, in addition to the right superior and inferior PVs, there is a right middle PV and a right "upper" PV that arises above the right superior PV (RSPV) **(Figure 19–1)**. This variability was also shown by Marom et al[9] In their study involving 201 patients who underwent computed tomography (CT) scanning, they found that 71% of patients had two right PVs: the RSPV and the right inferior PV (RIPV); 28% of patients had 3 to 5 PVs on the right side secondary to the middle PV, and 2% had a single PV on the right. The majority of patients (86%) had two ostia on the left: the left superior PV (LSPV) and the left inferior PV (LIPV), and the remainder (24%) had single ostia draining the two PVs on the left.[9]

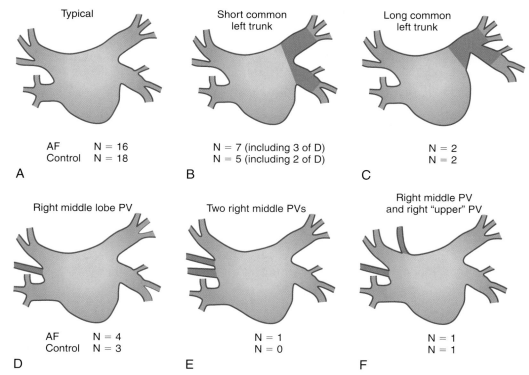

Figure 19–1 Branching pattern of the pulmonary veins (PVs) in patients with atrial fibrillation (AF) and in a control group. *Shaded portions* indicate parts different from typical anatomy. **A,** Typical branching pattern. **B,** Short common left trunk. **C,** Long common left trunk. **D,** Right middle PV. **E,** Two right middle PVs. **F,** Right middle and right "upper" PVs. *(From Kato R, et al: Pulmonary vein anatomy in patients undergoing catheter ablation of atrial fibrillation: lessons learned by the use of magnetic resonance imaging. Circulation 107;2004-2010, 2003. Reprinted with permission from Wolters Kluwer Health.)*

Other findings by Kato et al[8] include close proximity between the ostia of the right and left PV; separation of the mouth of the LSPV from the left atrial appendage by a thin rim of tissue; and no differentiation of size in the diameters of the PV with little variation in size of the PV in a given patient. They also found that the left PV has a longer neck, and that the PV ostia are usually oblong with the anteroposterior diameter less than the superoinferior diameter.[8]

19.3 Clinical Presentation

There is significant variability in clinical symptomatology of patients with PVS, ranging from an absence of symptoms to significant life-threatening disease. This variability is based on several factors, including the number of PVs involved, the severity of stenosis, the response of the pulmonary vasculature to the lesion, the time course of stenosis, the clinical setting, and the presence/extent of collaterals.[10-13] In a study by Packer et al,[13] symptomatic patients most commonly experienced dyspnea on exertion (83%), followed by dyspnea at rest (30%), recurrent cough (39%), chest pain (26%), flulike symptoms (13%), and hemoptysis (13%). Given the variability and lack of specificity of a particular symptom, detection of PVS requires a high index of suspicion on the part of the clinician. The diagnosis may be missed, or the symptoms may be attributed to another illness such as bronchopneumonia or interstitial lung disease. Routine screening and surveillance for symptoms that may herald the onset of PVS are very important.

19.4 Imaging Modalities

The best imaging modality for the assessment of PVS is yet to be determined. Thus a combination of imaging techniques is usually used to assess anatomic and physiologic impact of PVS. Modalities include chest X-ray, ventilation/perfusion (V/Q) scan, CT scan, transesophageal echocardiography (TEE), magnetic resonance angiography (MRA), and pulmonary venography.

COMPUTED TOMOGRAPHY AND MAGNETIC RESONANCE IMAGING

CT is one of the most commonly used imaging tools for making the diagnosis of PVS because it provides accurate definition of PV anatomy. There are some caveats to the use of CT imaging. A detailed knowledge of PV anatomy is required by the radiologist reading the images. Secondly, occasionally there may be the appearance of stenosis of the LIPV when there is "pseudostenosis." This was demonstrated in a study by Yamaji et al,[14] in which they performed CT imaging of the PV in 116 patients undergoing PV isolation for AF preablation and postablation. They found that in 11 patients there was more than 50% stenosis in the LIPV when the CT was performed in the supine position. This was not seen when the patients were imaged on the same day in the prone position. Occasionally when CT imaging is used for diagnosis, the PV may be interpreted as being completely occluded, but on subsequent PV angiography a small orifice may be seen. This was identified by Prieto et al[11] in their study of 44 patients with 80 stenosed PVs. Twenty-seven of the 80 stenosed PVs were identified on

CT as being 100% occluded; subsequent PV angiography demonstrated a small lumen in 13 of the 27 PVs. At the Mayo Clinic, CT is the modality of choice for imaging the PVs. A study performed at the Mayo Clinic[13] revealed that the mean PV orifice was 17.3 mm (with a range of 12 to 24 mm), the baseline diameter at the point of stenosis was 3 ± 2 mm, and the stenosis began 1 to 2 mm distal to the PV orifice and extended for variable lengths 7 to 35 mm **(Figure 19–2)**.

MRI is also an acceptable diagnostic modality **(Figure 19–3)**. An important caveat with MRI of the PVs is that there may be substantial changes in the size and location of the PV orifice during the cardiac cycle. Lickfett and colleagues examined this issue in a study.[15] They found that the largest orifice diameter was in late atrial diastole with a mean decrease of 32.5% during atrial systole. They also noted location changes of the PV orifice of up to 7 mm and that the orifice was larger in the coronal (lateral–medial) than the sagittal (anteroposterior) direction. MR perfusion imaging can also be reliably used to detect anatomic and functional impact of PVS. Kluge et al[16] examined this in a study of 110 patients after AF ablation. MR perfusion imaging was compared with single-photon emission CT perfusion imaging, and 51 patients with PVS were subsequently studied. They found that MRI detected 20 of 21 perfusion defects with

a sensitivity of 95.2% and a specificity of 100%. They also showed a cut-off of 6 mm diameter as being significant. A PV with a diameter of less than 6 mm had substantial decrease in perfusion compared with PVs greater than 6 mm in diameter. MRA has also been used to predict the occurrence of PVS after AF ablation. In a study of 104 patients undergoing AF ablation, MRA was performed preablation and postablation. It was shown that a relative reduction in PV diameter on the day after the procedure of 25% or more was predictive of the development of PVS using multivariate analysis, with a hazard ratio of 7.1 (p < 0.0001).[17]

TRANSESOPHAGEAL ECHOCARDIOGRAPHY

TEE is another method that may be used to aid the diagnosis of PVS, although it is not as accurate when compared with CT or MRI and is operator dependent. TEE can give accurate assessment of PV ostial anatomy and PV blood flow and is able to detect more severe stenosis of the PV as seen by changes in Doppler flow velocity. The usefulness of TTE for diagnosis of PVS was examined in a study by Jander et al.[18] They showed that TEE can be reliably used to diagnose or exclude PVS if the diagnosis is restricted to a combination of elevated peak velocity (>110 cm/sec) with turbulence and little

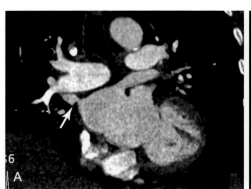
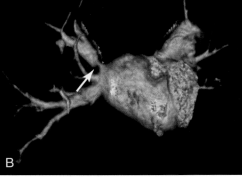

Figure 19–2 **A,** Computed tomography image showing tight stenosis involving the right superior pulmonary vein *(arrow)*. **B,** Three-dimensional volume rendering of the right superior pulmonary vein stenosis *(arrow)*.

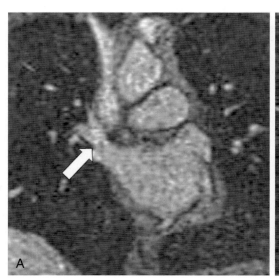
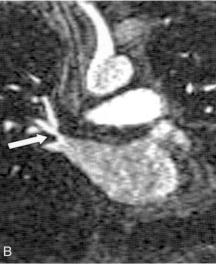

Figure 19–3 **Magnetic resonance image of the right upper pulmonary vein preablation and postablation for atrial fibrillation. A,** Normal-caliber right superior pulmonary vein (RSPV) *(arrow)* preablation, and **(B)** stenosed RSPV postablation *(arrow)*.

flow variation. TEE is limited by its inability to image deeply into all four PVs and is less useful in establishing the extent and location of PVS.

VENTILATION/PERFUSION SCAN

V/Q scan is a useful technique for assessing the hemodynamic significance of PVS. It is an ideal screening tool for patients suspected of having PVS because it is widely available and easy to interpret when compared with CT or MRI scans. VQ scans can be used to characterize the physiology of blood flow within the distribution of the PVS. Under normal conditions the apparent blood flow to one third of the lung ranges from 15% to 30%. A perfusion mismatch is seen with PVS in the range of 65% to 75%, and the level of perfusion to the affected lung is seen to have diminished to less than 25% of the expected perfusion; thus with severe stenosis the blood flow within the affected PV can be decreased to as low as 3% to 4%. In a study by Nanthakumar et al,[19] comparison between functional imaging using V/Q scan, anatomic imaging using CT or pulmonary venography, and hemodynamic assessment of PVS was performed. PVS resulted in decreased perfusion of the affected lobe when the resting PV–LA pressure gradient was at least 5 mmHg or when there was 80% luminal stenosis by venography or CT. When there was less than 50% stenosis, no perfusion defects were seen. **Figure 19–4** shows decreased perfusion of the entire left lung in a patient with stenosis involving the left upper and lower PVs.

PULMONARY VEIN ANGIOGRAPHY

PV angiography provides direct visualization of the degree of stenosis but is limited by its invasiveness, streaming, anatomic complexity, and high cost. A good baseline PV angiogram is required in multiple views before PV intervention. **Figure 19–5, A** shows a PV angiogram with stenosis involving the LSPV, and **Figure 19–5, B** shows the result of PV intervention.

19.5 Patient Selection

Patients with symptoms of PVS should be treated with PV dilation with or without stent placement. This is based on data showing feasibility and success of PV dilation and stenting in a majority of patients.[11-13,20] The time frame between the PV isolation procedure and development of symptoms is quite variable. In a report by Packer et al,[13] in which 23 patients with 34 PV stenoses were studied pre-AF and post–AF ablation, the mean time to the development of symptoms was 103 ± 100 days. In another study, the mean time to the development of symptoms after the diagnosis of PVS was 13.5 months.[21]

Treatment of asymptomatic patients with PVS is a little more controversial. It has been shown that patients with 100% occlusion of a single PV may be asymptomatic. In a study by Di Biase et al,[22] data from 18 patients with at least one complete occlusion of a PV were analyzed. Four (22%) patients were completely asymptomatic; reasons for lack of symptoms were attributed to

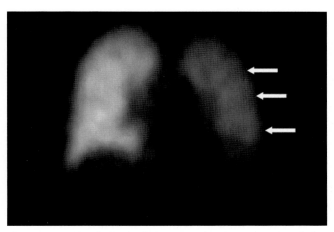

Figure 19–4 Ventilation/perfusion scan showing reduced perfusion of the left lung in a patient with stenosis involving the left upper and lower pulmonary veins *(arrows)*.

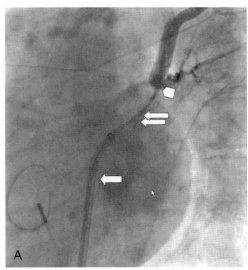
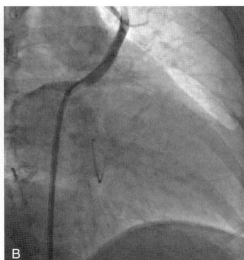

Figure 19–5 A, Stenosis involving the left superior pulmonary vein (LSPV) preintervention. The *single arrow* shows the SL-1 sheath, the *double arrows* show the multipurpose catheter, and the *arrowhead* is pointing to the stenosis at the LSPV ostium. **B,** Good flow through the previously stenosed orifice postintervention.

activation of compensatory mechanisms and absence of stenosis in the remaining ipsilateral PVs. In asymptomatic patients studied over time, PVS has been known to progress, leading to eventual thrombotic occlusion and decrease in pulmonary arterial flow to the affected lung segment. The decline in arteriovenous gradient after PVS and decline in arterial perfusion leads to ischemia and edema of the surrounding alveoli, eventually resulting in atelectasis, pulmonary infarction, or susceptibility to infections. Treatment options in asymptomatic patients with significant PVS include PV dilation (with or without stent placement) to prevent the consequences described or close follow-up care with immediate intervention upon development of symptoms (see **Figure 19–6** for a treatment algorithm for PVS).

19.6 Interventional Procedure

EQUIPMENT

Wires

1. 0.032-inch straight-tip (soft) wire
2. 0.035-inch J-tipped, stiff Amplatz exchange-length wire (Cook Medical, Bloomington, Ind.)
3. 0.035-inch Storq wire (Cordis Corporation, Miami Lakes, Fla.) for probing the PVs

Sheaths

1. 8.5F SL-1 sheath (St. Jude Medical, St. Paul, Minn.) through which the multipurpose catheter and eventually the percutaneous transluminal coronary angioplasty balloon will be advanced. For the right PVs, an SRO sheath (St. Jude Medical) or an Agilis sheath (St. Jude Medical) may be needed to cannulate the vein.
2. 9F 30-cm sheath for introduction of the intracardiac echocardiography (ICE) catheter (Siemens Medical, Mountain View, Calif.) via the left femoral vein
3. 4F or 5F sheath for placement of a pigtail catheter into the ascending aorta to guide transseptal puncture and also for arterial pressure monitoring
4. 7F sheath placed in the right femoral vein for transseptal puncture

Pressure Transducers

- For aortic pressure
- For LA pressure (through Mullins sheath)
- For PV pressure (through multipurpose catheter)

Catheters

- 4F or 5F pigtail catheter in the ascending aorta (to guide transseptal puncture and provide arterial pressure monitoring)
- Multipurpose catheter with end holes (to engage the PV)

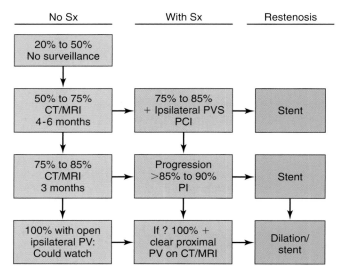

Figure 19–6 Treatment algorithm for PVS. (*CT,* Computed tomography; *MR,* magnetic resonance; *PI,* percutaneous intervention; *PV,* pulmonary vein; *PVS,* pulmonary vein stenosis; *Sx,* symptoms.) *(From Holmes D, et al: Pulmonary vein stenosis complicating ablation for atrial fibrillation: clinical spectrum and interventional considerations.* JACC Cardiovasc Interv 2;267-276, 2009. *Reprinted with permission from Elsevier.)*

- 4F Glide catheter to cannulate the PV in case the multipurpose catheter fails

Intracardiac Echocardiography

1. Intracardiac echo probe
2. Probe sterile cover
3. Intracardiac echo machine (draped)

PREMEDICATION

1. Aspirin 325 mg
2. Clopidogrel 75 mg dose
3. Heparin 100 units/kg after successful transseptal puncture

PROCEDURE

1. The procedure is performed with the patient under conscious sedation using fentanyl and midazolam.
2. The arterial and venous sheaths are placed after the patient is prepared and draped. A 9F 30-cm venous sheath is placed in the left femoral vein for the ICE catheter, a 4F or 5F arterial sheath is placed in the left femoral artery for arterial pressure monitoring, and a 7F venous sheath is placed in the right femoral vein.
3. Transseptal puncture is performed under biplane fluoroscopy using standard techniques with ICE guidance.
4. To ensure adequate access and reach the PVs that lie posterior in the LA, the SLO, SL-1, or SRO

(St. Jude Medical, St. Paul, Minn.) catheters are favored over the traditional Mullins sheath and dilator assembly. A Mullins sheath can complicate access into the RSPV and RIPV, and the other catheters are more maneuverable. Occasionally a steerable catheter (Agilis NxT catheter, St. Jude Medical, St. Paul, Minn.) is required for accessing the right-sided PVs. A standard Brockenbrough needle is still used for transseptal puncture.

5. Crossing at the level of the fossa ovalis is optimal; a puncture that is too high or too posterior makes access to the PVs more challenging. Access to the RIPV is aided by a septal puncture that is more anterior, whereas access to the LSPV or LIPV is aided by a more posterior septal puncture. Because these patients have previously had transseptal punctures, the atrial septum is occasionally thickened and fibrotic, resulting in the transseptal needle sliding superiorly towards the limbus and thereby creating a high puncture. In these cases the curve of the needle may have to be manually shaped to ensure access at the fossa ovalis. Other cases of difficult transseptal puncture are aided with the use of the SafeSept needle (Pressure Products, San Pedro, Calif.) or use of a radiofrequency needle (Bayliss Medical, Montreal, Canada).

6. Once access is obtained into the LA, the sheath is aspirated and flushed with heparinized saline. Unfractionated heparin at 100 units/Kg is administered and maintained to keep the activated clotting times (ACTs) between 250 and 300 seconds.

7. Typically a 6F multipurpose A-1 or A-2 catheter is used for entry into each PV **(see Figure 19–5).** Occasionally, in cases of severe PVS when the multipurpose catheter is unable to enter into the PV, a Storq wire with a soft tip is used to probe for the PV orifice. When there is difficulty accessing the PV, the LA can be evaluated with intracardiac ultrasound to identify aliasing color flow from the veins, with or without increased flow velocity (**Figure 19–7**). In addition, in some patients a subselective pulmonary arteriogram with delayed filming may allow visualization of the venoatrial junction.

8. Once the multipurpose catheter is in the PV distal to the stenosis, a transstenotic gradient is measured. This varies depending on lesion length and severity of stenosis, but it is usually in the range of 10 to 12 mmHg.

9. Selective pulmonary venography is then performed using hand contrast injection through either the multipurpose catheter or the transseptal sheath. This documents stenosis severity, lesion length, and the presence of affected branches.

10. Simultaneously, intracardiac ultrasound is used to interrogate the PV of interest and assessment of translesional velocity is performed. Usually the translesional velocity is 1 to 1.6 m/sec, although occasionally in the presence of severe stenosis it may be less than 1.0 m/sec **(see Figure 19–7).**

Preintervention

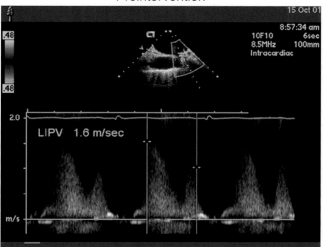

Postintervention

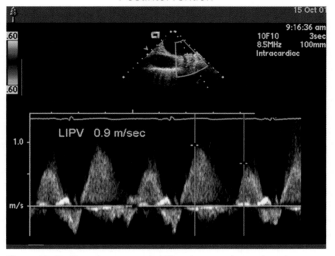

Figure 19–7 Doppler patterns in PV preintervention and postintervention images. *(From Holmes D, et al: Pulmonary vein stenosis complicating ablation for atrial fibrillation: clinical spectrum and interventional considerations.* JACC Cardiovasc Interv *2;267-276, 2009. Reprinted with permission from Elsevier.)*

11. Once the decision is made to treat the PVS, an exchange length Amplatz extra stiff 0.035-inch wire is advanced into the PV distal to the stenosis via the multipurpose catheter.

12. The multipurpose catheter is removed, an appropriately sized peripheral balloon is chosen (usually an 8- to 10-mm balloon is used), and balloon dilation is performed. Using a balloon larger than 12 mm significantly increases the risk of PV perforation or rupture, which may be catastrophic **(Figure 19–8, A).**

13. The balloon is removed, and a repeat selective angiography and reassessment of translesional gradient is performed with the multipurpose catheter. The decision to stent the residual PVS is made if there is still significant translesional gradient or if the residual stenosis is greater than 30%.

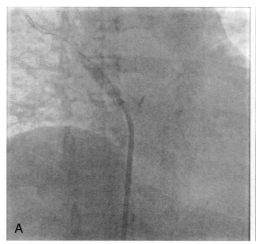 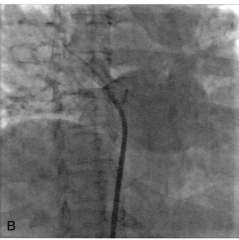

Figure 19–8 **A,** Ballooning of the right superior pulmonary vein. **B,** Final results post–stent placement.

14. If placement of a stent is deemed necessary, this is accomplished with the stiff Amplatz wire in the PV. Usually a 10-mm balloon expanded over the wire stents is used for PV that is 8 mm or larger in diameter; 10 × 18-mm or 10 × 29-mm Genesis stents (Cordis, Miami Lakes, Fla.) are routinely used. Smaller diameter PVs are usually left with a balloon-dilation result; occasionally drug-eluting stents are used to stent these smaller veins **(Figure 19–8, B).**

15. After stent deployment, a final translesional gradient is measured between the PV and the LA, and a final selective or subselective pulmonary venography is performed.

16. If there are other PVs in need of intervention, the procedure is repeated. Otherwise the procedure is completed, and all of the equipment is withdrawn from the LA into the right atrium (RA) and removed.

17. The sheaths are removed manually, and hemostasis is secured with manual pressure once the ACT is less than 180 seconds. **Videos 19–1 to 19–4** show the procedure involved and the result of stent placement for treatment of left superior PVS.

TIPS AND TRICKS FOR OPTIMAL PULMONARY VEIN DILATION AND STENT PLACEMENT

- A subselective pulmonary arteriogram with delayed filming is useful and may allow visualization of the venoatrial junction in cases where the PV orifice cannot be identified or accessed.
- Intracardiac ultrasound may also be used to guide engagement and access to the PV orifice.
- Pulmonary venography must be performed using at least two orthogonal views and is crucial in identifying the presence and extent of collateralization and involvement of significant side branches.
- Image set-up for treatment should allow visualization of the peripheral lung fields and adequate visualization of the plane of the ostium.

- Avoiding the use of hydrophilic wires when probing for the PV orifice reduces PV perforation that may lead to difficulty controlling hemorrhage. Soft-tip wires (e.g., the Storq wire) should be used.
- Occasionally the multipurpose catheter may be found to be quite stiff and inadequate for accessing the PV orifice. A soft catheter like the Glide catheter is usually helpful in this situation.
- The PV diameter should be measured using quantitative coronary angiography and confirmed with intracardiac ultrasound measurement before balloon dilation to determine the appropriate balloon size.
- The largest diameter of the dilation balloon should not exceed the largest pulmonary vein diameter by more than a 1.1:1 ratio.
- Intracardiac ultrasound is useful to achieve optimal stent positioning. It provides adequate visualization of the ostium, thus preventing too proximal a placement of the stent, which leads to the stent protruding into the LA.
- Occasionally bifurcation stenting techniques are necessary, especially in cases of common ostia/antrum seen with the left PVs. If a two-stent technique is required, this is achieved either with a second transseptal puncture and catheter set-up or with dilation performed through the side of one stent **(Figure 19–9).**
- Balloon diameters greater than 12 mm are usually too big and should be avoided during PV dilation.
- PVs less than 7 mm in diameter are usually left with a dilation result; occasionally drug-eluting stents are implanted, but their long-term outcomes have not been analyzed.
- After PV intervention, the stiff guide wire should always be withdrawn using fluoroscopy because the stiff wire can dislodge the freshly placed stent.

SPECIAL CIRCUMSTANCES

In cases where the preprocedural CT documents 100% occlusion of the PV, this occlusion is typically ostial. Left atrial angiography in the region of the ostium may reveal a dimple that can be probed with a stiffer

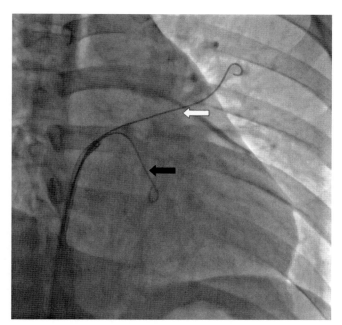

Figure 19–9 There is a common antrum between the left superior pulmonary vein (LSPV) and left inferior pulmonary vein (LIPV) with a tight stenosis. Two Amplatz Extra Stiff wires have been placed in the LSPV *(white arrow)* and LIPV *(black arrow)* preintervention.

or hydrophilic wire to see if patency can be restored. Alternatively, subselective pulmonary artery angiography can be performed with delayed imaging to evaluate left atrial filling. If the vein is completely occluded and the occlusion is probed successfully, maintenance of long-term patency is low.

Sometimes the PVs are small and fibrotic as assessed by CT or ultrasound imaging. In this instance, balloon dilation is usually performed using 4- to 5-mm coronary balloon catheters. There is anecdotal information on the efficacy of cutting balloons in this situation.

Occasionally the stenosed PVs have active thrombi seen as filling defects on CT imaging. To avoid embolization during the procedure, anticoagulation is optimized with warfarin, aspirin, and clopidogrel, and the interventional procedure is postponed until there is no evidence of residual thrombus on repeat imaging.

Progression of severe PVS can be quite rapid, and once a severe lesion is detected, it should be treated promptly. Given the potential for rapid progression, the follow-up schedule should be adjusted. A 50% to 70% stenosis on initial postablation CT should be reevaluated in 3 to 6 months. If the stenosis is greater than 75%, repeat CT in 3 months is warranted unless symptoms develop sooner. If a stenosis is found to be approximately 90%, urgent treatment is indicated because the lesion can progress to occlusion in 3 to 6 weeks.

ADJUNCTIVE THERAPY

Before the procedure, patients are given 325 mg of aspirin; unfractionated heparin is administered after a successful transseptal puncture with the ACT maintained between 250 to 300 seconds. Newer anticoagulants like enoxaparin or bivalirudin are not used at the Mayo Clinic because they are not reversible. After the procedure, patients continue with warfarin to maintain an INR of 2 to 3 and prevent PV thrombosis, which has been known to occur. The optimal duration of warfarin therapy is unknown, but from a clinical standpoint it is usually continued indefinitely. Occasionally aspirin and clopidogrel are added empirically, especially in cases where a stent has been placed.

19.7 Complications

ACCESS SITE

Meticulous technique must be used when obtaining access for the procedure. Complications that could occur from the access site include significant hematoma and/or bleeding because these patients receive anticoagulation therapy after the procedure. There could be development of arteriovenous fistula, pseudoaneurysm formation, or leg ischemia. Occasionally there is some scarring in the groin site, particularly at the venous entry site, because these patients have undergone multiple AF ablation procedures. Sometimes the veins are thrombosed and may be difficult to access.

TRANSSEPTAL PUNCTURE

There is a steep learning curve associated with transseptal puncture. Ability to master the technique of transseptal catheterization will prevent many of the known complications associated with the procedure. Common complications include perforation of the LA or RA with formation of a pericardial effusion, entry into the aortic wall, air embolism, or clot formation in the LA. Commonly, entry into the surrounding structures around the LA with the 18-gauge Brockenbrough needle does not lead to significant problems, but if the dilator is inadvertently advanced into the atrial wall, aortic wall, or pericardial space, significant complications may ensue. The availability of intracardiac imaging with visualization of the atrial septum has led to significant decrease in complications and has made this a much safer procedure. Nevertheless, meticulous attention to detail and optimal techniques are necessary when performing this procedure.

AIR EMBOLISM AND CLOT FORMATION

Once entry into the LA is achieved and confirmed, there are two critical things that must be performed to avoid major complications. First, the sheath/catheter system must be deaired and purged thoroughly of air or debris to avoid air emboli into the LA and subsequently to the brain or coronary arteries. Subsequent manipulations of catheters into the LA should be done under a continuous flush. Second, once access to the LA is achieved, adequate amounts of unfractionated heparin must be administered to achieve an ACT of 250 to

300 seconds and avoid formation of clots in the LA. Pre-procedural imaging with CT/TEE and intraprocedural imaging with ICE are also useful in excluding preexisting thrombus within the left atrial appendage, PVs, or LA. If thrombus is discovered in the PV during the procedure, the procedure should be stopped and the patient should undergo anticoagulation therapy with warfarin for 4 to 6 weeks (until there is documentation of resolution of thrombus) before being brought back for the procedure. In case of air/clot embolism, the procedure should be stopped, and all efforts should be made to optimize the outcome.

PULMONARY VEIN DISSECTION/PERFORATION

This is rarely seen, but when it occurs it can be fatal. Hydrophilic wires are typically avoided during the intervention because these are likely to track distally and can lead to perforation of the PV. Similarly, during balloon dilation and stent placement, careful sizing of the balloon and stent is crucial to avoid overdilation of the PV, which may lead to dissection and/or perforation. Undersized balloons and stents are generally used. In cases of significant perforation when the bleeding is difficult to stop percutaneously, balloon tamponade and reversal of anticoagulation is usually the first step; if this does not work, surgical control is warranted. Alternatively, appropriately sized covered stents can be deployed to seal the perforation. The authors have used this technique on one occasion, and the stent was deployed under direct visualization in the operating room.

DISLODGED STENT

This is a rare complication that may occur after stent placement and usually during manipulation of equipment in and out of the stented PV. It can be prevented by careful manipulation of equipment near the freshly placed stent. Once the stent has been dislodged, it floats in the LA and can embolize into the left ventricle and out into the aorta. Embolization is prevented by maintaining a wire through the embolized stent, keeping it within the LA. Retrieval of the stent can be complicated. If the stent is maintained on a wire within the LA, a gooseneck snare can be advanced over the wire and around the stent, and the stent is crushed with the snare loop, reducing the stent diameter. Once adequately crushed, the stent can be retracted into the RA and removed via the femoral vein. In cases where the stent has embolized into the aorta, it usually embolizes to the distal abdominal aorta. A second arterial access site is obtained with a 10F sheath; the stent is crossed with a stiff 0.035-inch wire, and a slightly larger balloon is advanced into the stent. If the stent is in the abdominal aorta, the balloon is advanced through the stent where it is inflated, and the stent is gently retracted into the corresponding iliac artery with the inflated balloon. Once in the iliac artery, the balloon is deflated and carefully retracted and positioned within the stent. The stent is subsequently

deployed in the iliac artery with minimal sequelae. Occasionally the stent is unable to be deployed in the iliac artery; it may have to be crushed with a gooseneck snare as described and withdrawn into the 10F sheath with subsequent removal. **Videos 19–5 to 19–9** show a dislodged LIPV stent.

19.8 Outcomes

Outcomes of PV dilation and/or stenting are variable depending upon the therapeutic strategy—dilation alone or dilation and stenting—and the size of the PV. The long-term efficacy of PV dilation compared with stenting was evaluated by Prieto et al in their study.[11] Thirty-four patients with 55 stenotic veins were treated with either balloon dilation or stenting and studied over the course of 25 months. Restenosis rates were 72% for balloon dilation, compared with 33% for stent placement (p < 0.001), with a longer time free from restenosis in patients who were treated with stent placement as opposed to those with balloon dilation. They also noted that patients treated with larger stents (>9 mm) had significantly improved outcomes compared with those treated with smaller stents (<9 mm). Data from the Mayo Clinic institution,[13] in which 23 patients with PVS were treated and studied over time, showed that all patients had significant reduction of symptoms immediately postprocedure. However, 57% (14 patients) developed recurrent symptoms at a mean time of 3.2 ± 2.8 months after the procedure, with 13 patients requiring repeat intervention. Overall, after a follow-up period of 18 ± 12 months, 15 of 23 patients were asymptomatic, 4 patients had mild symptoms, and 3 patients had moderate symptoms.

The rates of restenosis vary substantially depending on the follow-up protocol used and definition of restenosis; in one study[13] there was a 50% restenosis rate in patients treated with PV stents.

19.9 Follow-Up Protocols

Follow-up protocols vary depending on the institution. The authors typically perform CT imaging of the PVs the day after the procedure to document initial baseline improvement **(Figure 19–10)**. Afterwards follow-up care includes careful monitoring for recurrent symptoms with prompt evaluation if symptoms recur. Follow-up CT may also be performed, even though the patient is asymptomatic.

19.10 Summary

PVS after ablation for AF remains a significant but rare complication of AF ablation with incidence of 1% to 3% in experienced centers. The combination of clinical vigilance and use of multimodality diagnostic imaging has led to earlier diagnosis and treatment of these patients. The clinical presentation of these patients is quite variable, and treatment of PVS involves both anatomic and

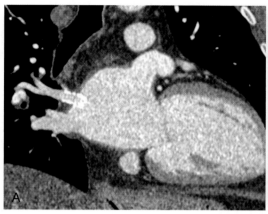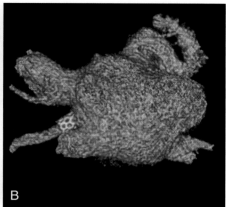

Figure 19–10 Follow-up computed tomography scan after stent placement in the right middle pulmonary vein (PV). The stent is patent and is well placed, covering the ostium of the right middle PV. **A** is 2D image, and **B** is a 3D reconstruction.

clinical consideration. Treatment includes PV dilation with or without stent placement or observation and close follow-up study in asymptomatic patients. Interventional cardiologists who wish to undertake intervention of PVs must be comfortable working in the LA, have a good understanding of left atrial anatomy, and have experience with various techniques to ensure procedural success and also manage potential complications that may arise.

REFERENCES

1. Lloyd-Jones D, Adams R, Carnethon M, et al: Heart disease and stroke statistics—2009 update: a report from the American Heart Association Statistics Committee and Stroke Statistics Subcommittee, *Circulation* 119:480–486, 2009.
2. Haissaguerre M, Jais P, Shah DC, et al: Electrophysiological endpoint for catheter ablation of atrial fibrillation initiated from multiple pulmonary venous foci, *Circulation* 101:1409–1417, 2000.
3. Calkins H, Brugada J, Packer DL, et al: HRS/EHRA/ECAS expert consensus statement on catheter and surgical ablation of atrial fibrillation: recommendations for personnel, policy, procedures and follow-up. A report of the Heart Rhythm Society (HRS) Task Force on Catheter and Surgical Ablation of Atrial Fibrillation developed in partnership with the European Heart Rhythm Association (EHRA) and the European Cardiac Arrhythmia Society (ECAS); in collaboration with the American College of Cardiology (ACC), American Heart Association (AHA), and the Society of Thoracic Surgeons (STS). Endorsed and approved by the governing bodies of the American College of Cardiology, the American Heart Association, the European Cardiac Arrhythmia Society, the European Heart Rhythm Association, the Society of Thoracic Surgeons, and the Heart Rhythm Society, *Europace* 9:335–379, 2007.
4. Thomas SP, Lim TW, McCall R, et al: Electrical isolation of the posterior left atrial wall and pulmonary veins for atrial fibrillation: feasibility of and rationale for a single-ring approach, *Heart Rhythm* 4:722–730, 2007.
5. Oral H, Knight BP, Tada H, et al: Pulmonary vein isolation for paroxysmal and persistent atrial fibrillation, *Circulation* 105:1077–1081, 2002.
6. Chen SA, Hsieh MH, Tai CT, et al: Initiation of atrial fibrillation by ectopic beats originating from the pulmonary veins: electrophysiological characteristics, pharmacological responses, and effects of radiofrequency ablation, *Circulation* 100:1879–1886, 1999.
7. Cappato R, Calkins H, Chen SA, et al: Worldwide survey on the methods, efficacy, and safety of catheter ablation for human atrial fibrillation, *Circulation* 111:1100–1105, 2005.
8. Kato R, Lickfett L, Meininger G, et al: Pulmonary vein anatomy in patients undergoing catheter ablation of atrial fibrillation: lessons learned by use of magnetic resonance imaging, *Circulation* 107:2004–2010, 2003.
9. Marom EM, Herndon JE, Kim YH, et al: Variations in pulmonary venous drainage to the left atrium: implications for radiofrequency ablation, *Radiology* 230:824–829, 2004.
10. Saad EB, Marrouche NF, Saad CP, et al: Pulmonary vein stenosis after catheter ablation of atrial fibrillation: emergence of a new clinical syndrome, *Ann Intern Med* 138:634–638, 2003.
11. Prieto LR, Schoenhagen P, Arruda MJ, et al: Comparison of stent versus balloon angioplasty for pulmonary vein stenosis complicating pulmonary vein isolation, *J Cardiovasc Electrophysiol* 19:673–678, 2008.
12. Qureshi AM, Prieto LR, Latson LA, et al: Transcatheter angioplasty for acquired pulmonary vein stenosis after radiofrequency ablation, *Circulation* 108:1336–1342, 2003.
13. Packer DL, Keelan P, Munger TM, et al: Clinical presentation, investigation, and management of pulmonary vein stenosis complicating ablation for atrial fibrillation, *Circulation* 111:546–554, 2005.
14. Yamaji H, Hina K, Kawamura H, et al: Prone position is essential for detection of pulmonary vein pseudostenosis by enhanced multidetector computed tomography in patients who undergo pulmonary vein isolation, *Circ J* 72:1460–1464, 2008.
15. Lickfett L, Dickfeld T, Kato R, et al: Changes of pulmonary vein orifice size and location throughout the cardiac cycle: dynamic analysis using magnetic resonance cine imaging, *J Cardiovasc Electrophysiol* 16:582–588, 2005.
16. Kluge A, Dill T, Ekinci O, et al: Decreased pulmonary perfusion in pulmonary vein stenosis after radiofrequency ablation: assessment with dynamic magnetic resonance perfusion imaging, *Chest* 126:428–437, 2004.
17. Berkowitsch A, Neumann T, Ekinci O, et al: A decrease in pulmonary vein diameter after radiofrequency ablation predicts the development of severe stenosis, *Pacing Clin Electrophysiol* 28(Suppl. 1):S83–S85, 2005.
18. Jander N, Minners J, Arentz T, et al: Transesophageal echocardiography in comparison with magnetic resonance imaging in the diagnosis of pulmonary vein stenosis after radiofrequency ablation therapy, *J Am Soc Echocardiogr* 18:654–659, 2005.
19. Nanthakumar K, Mountz JM, Plumb VJ, et al: Functional assessment of pulmonary vein stenosis using radionuclide ventilation/perfusion imaging, *Chest* 126:645–651, 2004.
20. Neumann T, Sperzel J, Dill T, et al: Percutaneous pulmonary vein stenting for the treatment of severe stenosis after pulmonary vein isolation, *J Cardiovasc Electrophysiol* 16:1180–1188, 2005.
21. Bedogni F, Brambilla N, Laudisa ML, et al: Acquired pulmonary vein stenosis after radiofrequency ablation treated by angioplasty and stent implantation, *J Cardiovasc Med (Hagerstown)* 8:618–624, 2007.
22. Di Biase L, Fahmy TS, Wazni OM, et al: Pulmonary vein total occlusion following catheter ablation for atrial fibrillation: clinical implications after long-term follow-up, *J Am Coll Cardiol* 48:2493–2499, 2006.

Chapter 20

Patent Foramen Ovale

JOHN M. LASALA • SHABANA SHAHANAVAZ

20.1 Embryology and Anatomy

The foramen ovale is pivotal during intrauterine life and facilitates the passage of oxygenated blood from the placenta to the fetal circulatory system. The blood flow from the umbilical veins enters the right atrium through the inferior vena cava (IVC) and bypasses the nonfunctional lungs across the foramen to enter the systemic circulation. Most blood flow from the superior vena cava (SVC) is routed through the tricuspid valve and enters the right ventricle. At birth, right heart pressure and pulmonary vascular resistance (PVR) drop, and there is increased pulmonary blood flow. Left atrial pressure may also rise as pulmonary venous return increases and there is a decrease in left ventricular compliance. Either or both of these mechanisms may result in functional closure of the foramen ovale by apposition of the septum primum against the septum secundum **(Figure 20–1).** In most people, the caudal portion of the septum primum on the left side and the cranial portion of the septum secundum on the right side fuse permanently in the ensuing months.[1] In 25% of the population, both parts of the interatrial septum remain separable.[2] The patent foramen ovale (PFO) is positioned caudally in the septum secundum and cranially in the septum primum, forming a slit valve, and the channel may open either when the right atrial pressure overrides the left atrial pressure (e.g., during a Valsalva maneuver), or merely from the inferior venacaval blood stream directed towards the fossa ovalis. This could provide an opportunity for small, otherwise undetectable clots to cross into the arterial system, bypassing the filter of the pulmonary vasculature and leading to a paradoxical embolism.

20.2 Incidence

The incidence of a PFO decreases with age, whereas the average diameter slightly increases. This could be because there may be closure of small PFOs later in life. The prevalence of PFO declines from 34% during the first three decades, to 25% during the fourth to eighth decade, and to 20% in the ninth decade and beyond.[2] Selective mortality

or spontaneous closure even late in life may be reasons for the decrease. An autosomal dominant inheritance has been demonstrated. There is no gender preference.[3]

20.3 Associations of Patent Foramen Ovale

ATRIAL SEPTAL ANEURYSM

Atrial septal aneurysm (ASA) is a congenital abnormality of the interatrial septum characterized by a redundant, amuscular membrane in the region of the fossa ovalis that corresponds to a sector of the central part of the septum primum **(Figure 20–2).**[4,5] The prevalence of ASA in the general population was about 1% in autopsy series and 2.2% in a population-based transesophageal echocardiography (TEE) study.[6,7] ASA is associated with a PFO in 50% to 85% of cases. ASA is generally diagnosed if the diameter of the base of the flimsy portion of the interatrial septum exceeds 15 mm and if the excursion of the aneurysmal membrane exceeds 10 mm in either the left or right atrium, or if the sum of the total excursion is greater than 10 mm.[8] ASA has been hypothesized to act as facilitator for paradoxical embolism via the following mechanisms: (1) by increasing the PFO diameter because of the highly mobile atrial septal tissue, leading to a more frequent and wider opening of an otherwise small channel[9]; (2) promoting right-to-left shunting by redirecting flow from the IVC toward the PFO[10]; and (3) acting as a nidus for local thrombus formation with subsequent embolization.[11]

CHIARI NETWORK

A Chiari network is an embryologic remnant of the right venous sinus valve **(Figure 20–3).**[12,13] In a study of 1436 consecutive adult patients, there was a Chiari network prevalence of 2% with a common association between Chiari networks and PFO in 83% of patients. Large right-to-left shunting was found significantly more often in patients with Chiari networks than in patients who were part of a control group (55% vs. 12%, p = 0.001). This

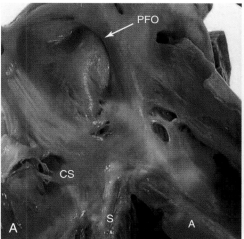
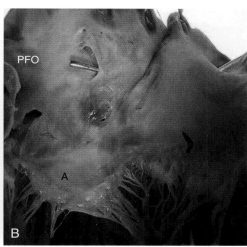

Figure 20–1 Patent forman ovale (PFO). A, Right atrial view of the atrial septum showing the PFO. *CS,* Coronary sinus; *S,* septal leaflet of the tricuspid valve; *A,* anterior leaflet of the tricuspid valve. **B,** Left atrial view of the atrial septum showing the probe patent PFO. *A,* Anterior mitral leaflet.

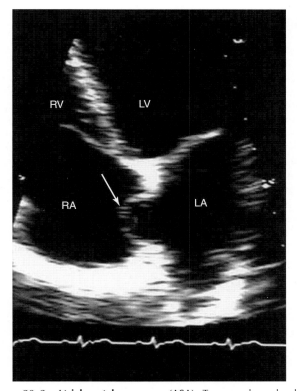

Figure 20–2 Atrial septal aneurysm (ASA). Transesophageal echocardiography showing an ASA bulging into the right atrium.

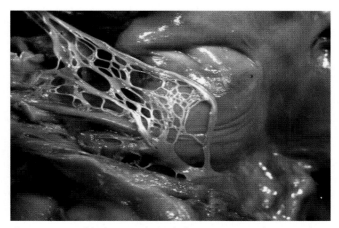

Figure 20–3 Chiari network. Pathology specimen showing Chiari network in the right atrium.

study also found Chiari networks associated with ASA in 24% of patients. The Chiari network is more common in cryptogenic stroke patients than in patients evaluated for other indications (4.6% vs. 0.5%), and it may also facilitate paradoxical embolism.[14]

20.4 Diagnosis of Patent Foramen Ovale

A number of ultrasound-guided options are available to diagnose a PFO. Imaging modalities such as contrast-enhanced transmitral Doppler, transthoracic echocardiography (TTE), TEE, and transcranial Doppler are established methods to detect a PFO with an active right-to-left shunt.[15] TTE and TEE are also able to detect potential cardiac sources of embolism other than PFO, including benign cardiac tumors (myxoma, papillary fibroelastoma), valvular strands (Lambl excrescences), mitral valve prolapse, left atrial spontaneous echo contrast or left atrial appendage thrombus, vegetations, and aortic arch and thoracic aortic atheroma.

Imaging should be repeated until the operator is confident that the existence of a PFO has been ruled out. Given the importance of coordinating these factors for diagnosing a PFO, bubble contrast studies, in which no sedation is necessary, are initially performed during TTE. Bubble contrast echocardiography requires an experienced operator who is aware of the potential pitfalls of misdiagnosis, which include the difficulty in distinguishing a pulmonary-level shunt from a cardiac-level shunt. Contrast from a cardiac shunt usually appears within three cardiac cycles. Various classification schemes have been proposed to standardize the grading of the size of the shunt according to the number of bubbles shunting, although none are, as yet, predominant. If analysis with

TTE bubble contrast shows a right-to-left shunt, TEE is necessary to confirm the presence and define the anatomy of the PFO, as well as to exclude the presence of other potential shunts.[16]

During the diagnostic work-up in patients with cryptogenic stroke and presumed paradoxical embolism, the diagnosis of PFO is or has usually been made with contrast TEE echocardiography. The sensitivity of TTE for detection of a PFO is lower. Therefore the assessment of the number of high-intensity transient signals by means of transcranial Doppler recordings is highly sensitive for right-to-left shunting but is not as specific as transesophageal contrast echocardiography.[17-19] Contrast transcranial Doppler ultrasonography is a highly sensitive and noninvasive method to screen for right-to-left shunting and shows close agreement with contrast echocardiography in shunt detection. This technique uses ultrasound to quantify the number of bubbles that reach the cerebral circulation. Patients with microemboli detected with contrast transcranial Doppler ultrasonography are more likely to have a history of cerebral ischemia. However, transcranial Doppler ultrasonography does not provide the anatomic information that can be derived from echocardiography and therefore cannot be used in isolation.[20] Alternative methods for the detection of PFO include computed tomography (CT) and magnetic resonance imaging (MRI). These techniques are likely to be as specific as TEE but far more expensive and not as readily available.[21,22]

20.5 Clinical Problems Associated with Patent Foramen Ovale

PATENT FORAMEN OVALE AND STROKE

Several observations have confirmed the concept of a thrombus trapped in the PFO tunnel and its ability to embolize to the brain, as in the first report by Cohnheim in 1877.[23] Zahn first used the term *paradoxical embolus* in 1881 to describe a branched thrombus from a uterine vein caught in a PFO on a postmortem examination.[24] Paradoxical embolism is proposed as a mechanism for cryptogenic stroke and occurs when a thrombus from the systemic venous circulation passes to the systemic arterial circulation via a right-to-left shunt, usually a PFO. A stroke is considered "cryptogenic" when no source of embolism is detectable.[25] This may be the case in up to 40% of strokes in young adults. In adults with cryptogenic strokes who are younger than 55 years of age, a PFO is found with a higher prevalence than in patients age 55 years and older. Retrospective analysis suggested an association between PFO, cryptogenic stroke, and young age. Some questions are unresolved: cryptogenic stroke is a complex diagnosis, not just related to PFO. A high percentage of the young and healthy population has a PFO without stroke. The association of both pathologies, PFO and cryptogenic stroke, may be incidental and is no proof that PFO is the cause of stroke.[26-28] In a meta-analysis of case-control studies, the association between ischemic stroke and PFO was confirmed. In the same overview, the role of an ASA was assessed. An ASA is 10 times less common than a PFO. Initially, an ASA was considered a risk factor for left-sided embolic events.[29] Recently, however, the Stroke Prevention Assessment of Risk in a Community study and the data of the Patent Foramen Ovale and Atrial Septal Aneurysm Study Group proved that an ASA enhances the risk of recurrent cerebrovascular events in the presence of a PFO but does not represent an independent source of embolism.[30] The latter study also challenged the role of a PFO as a mediator of paradoxical emboli in general. Coagulation disorders, such as prothrombotic genetic polymorphisms (factor V Leiden mutation, protein C or S deficiencies, anticardiolipin antibodies, and prothrombin G20210A mutation) or thrombocytosis may also play a role in the pathogenesis of paradoxical embolism.

THE PLATYPNEA–ORTHODEOXIA SYNDROME

The platypnea–orthodeoxia syndrome (POS) comprises both dyspnea (platypnea) and arterial desaturation (orthodeoxia) in the upright position with improvement in the supine position. It is uncommon, but several dozen cases are reported. Two components must coexist to create this syndrome. One is an anatomic defect, and the other is functional. The anatomic component must consist of an interatrial shunt, such as an atrial septal defect (ASD), PFO, fenestrated ASA, or intrapulmonary shunting. A functional component induces the deformity at the atrial level and may occur while the patient is rising to an upright from a recumbent position. Cardiac causes also exist, including pericardial effusion, constrictive pericarditis, and toxicity from drugs such as amiodarone. In this syndrome there is elevation of right atrial pressure, causing right-to-left shunt. Interestingly, blood may flow from right to left at the atrial level even when right heart pressure is normal, as typically occurs with persistent eustachian valves. Diagnosis of PFO with POS should be by tilt test, measuring arterial saturation in different positions, and contrast echocardiography, which should show intracardiac shunting. Note that the majority of right-to-left shunts in POS may be derived from IVC blood flow, and injection from an antecubital vein with return via the SVC may show less prominent shunting. The definitive treatment for POS is closure of the atrial shunt.[31,32]

EMBOLISM FROM DECOMPRESSION SICKNESS

Arterial gas embolism through an ASD was reported first in a scuba diver in 1986. Type 1 decompression sickness (DCS) is composed of localized joint pain, musculoskeletal pain, and skin rash, and type 2 DCS consists of neurologic symptoms (limb tingling, paresthesias, severe headache with mental confusion, paraplegia, loss of consciousness, audiovestibular symptoms, and dyspnea with chest pain). The PFO at rest is significantly associated with type 2 DCS. A recent study found a strong relationship between PFO size and DCS in a study of 230 divers. Another study demonstrated the functional and anatomic characteristics of PFO with and without DCS. This study suggested that DCS was associated with right-to-left shunting at rest. Atrial septal mobility and PFO diameter are also associated with the risk of developing DCS.[33-35] There are no society guidelines governing the role of PFO closure in divers, and the decision to proceed should be based on best clinical judgment.

MIGRAINE AND VASCULAR HEADACHE

Migraine and vascular headache may be related to PFO, according to an interesting series of studies. Migraines affect approximately 13% of the population aged 20 to 64 years, with 36% of migraines preceded by aura. Migraine with aura is associated with PFO and other causes of right-to-left shunting. It is hypothesized that a bloodborne substance that would ordinarily be filtered out by the lungs is delivered to the cerebral circulation via the shunt. However, the mechanisms that trigger migraines are unknown, and this theory remains unproven. Patients undergoing PFO closure for nonmigraine indications (e.g., paradoxical emboli) have reported an improvement in their migraine symptoms.[36] Migraine is a risk factor for cryptogenic stroke, especially in young patients without atherosclerotic risk factors.[36-38]

20.6 Indications for Patent Foramen Ovale Closure

The main indication for PFO closure is the prevention of recurrent paradoxical embolic cryptogenic stroke in younger patients (<55 years). This is done after an extensive work-up, including a complete neurologic examination and screening blood tests for thrombophilia. The American Academy of Neurology considers that evidence is insufficient for them to take a position on the efficacy of percutaneous or surgical closure, and American Heart Association (AHA)/American Stroke Association guidelines consider data insufficient to recommend PFO closure in patients with a first episode but recommend considering closure in patients who, although receiving medical treatment, experience a second episode (class IIb, evidence C).[39,40] In the absence of abnormal results of several tests, including cerebral MRI (except for ischemic lesions), angio-MRI of the circle of Willis, echo Doppler of extracranial cervical arteries, 12-lead electrocardiograph, 24-hour Holter monitoring, and echocardiography, controversial data are available in the literature about PFO closure for cryptogenic stroke prevention.[41] However, patient selection criteria, duration of follow-up study, definition of cryptogenic stroke, residual shunt after the procedure, different properties of the devices, and antithrombotic treatment remain unclear and make clinical trial design very complex. PFO closure was also proposed in the prevention of decompression illness in divers and to treat POS. Finally, prevention of migraine by PFO closure was investigated in

a randomized study without clinical evidence of benefit as compared with medical treatment.

The CLOSURE I trial enrolled 909 patients randomized equally to PFO closure using the STARFlex closure device (NMT Medical, Lowell, Mass.) with 24 months of aspirin and 6 months of clopidogrel or to best medical therapy—aspirin, warfarin, or a combination. There were no differences between the two groups with regard to their baseline features. At 2 years, there was no significant difference between the two treatment groups in the rate of recurrent stroke or TIA. Periprocedural major vascular complications occurred in 3.2% of patients in the closure group (13 of 402). Within 6 months, thrombus was found in the left atrium in 1.1% of patients in this group (4 of 366); 2 of the 4 patients with thrombus had a recurrent stroke.[42]

The RESPECT PFO clinical trial is another randomized control study to investigate whether percutaneous PFO closure using the Amplatzer PFO occluder is superior to current standard-of-care medical treatment in the prevention of recurrent paradoxical embolic stroke. Patient enrollment has been completed, but at the time of this writing, final results have not yet been published in a peer-reviewed journal.

20.7 Patent Foramen Ovale Devices

Bridges and Lock reported the use of the Clamshell septal umbrella (C.R. Bard Inc., Billerica, Mass.) for closure of PFO in 36 patients after a presumed paradoxical embolism during a multicenter clinical trial that was initiated in February 1989 and ended in June 1991.[43] Percutaneous PFO closure is now possible with different devices, depending upon availability.

AMPLATZER PATENT FORAMEN OVALE OCCLUDER AND SEPTAL OCCLUDER

The Amplatzer (St. Jude Medical, St. Paul, Minn.) family of devices includes the Amplatzer PFO occluder **(Figure 20–4)**, the multifenestrated (Cribriform) septal occluder **(Figure 20–5)**, and the Amplatzer atrial septal occluder **(Figure 20–6)**. All of these occluders are double-disc devices comprised of nitinol mesh and polyester fabric. Although the atrial septal occluder (ASO, or sometimes known as ASD *occluder*) was originally designed to close ASDs, it is occasionally implanted in large PFOs. The ASD and PFO occluders are very similar, but there are two important differences between them. The first is that whereas on the ASO the left atrial disc is larger, on the PFO occluder the right atrial disc is larger (except for the 18-mm PFO device, on which both discs are the same size). The other difference is in the diameter of the waist connecting the two discs. In the ASO, the broad connecting waist varies in diameter by device size (up to 40 mm). By contrast, the PFO occluder has a 3-mm connecting waist in each of its three currently available sizes: 18, 25, and 35 mm. The Cribriform device, like the PFO occluder, has a narrow waist, and like the PFO occluder, is available between 18 and 35 mm and is specifically designed

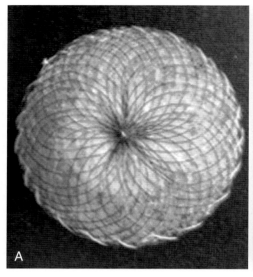
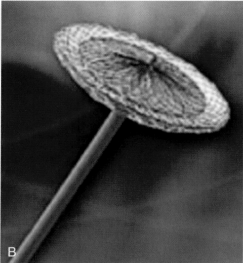

Figure 20–4 Amplatzer patent foramen ovale (PFO) occluder device. The Amplatzer PFO occluder is a double-disc device comprised of nitinol mesh and polyester fabric with a larger right atrial disc. *(Image courtesy St. Jude Medical, St. Paul, Minn.)*

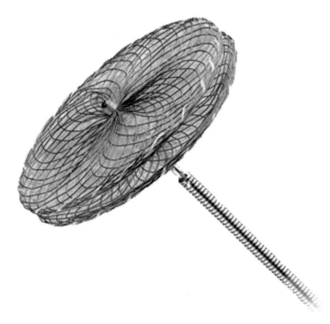

Figure 20–5 Amplatzer Cribriform device. The Amplatzer Cribriform device is a double-disc device comprised of nitinol mesh and polyester fabric. *(Image courtesy St. Jude Medical, St. Paul, Minn.)*

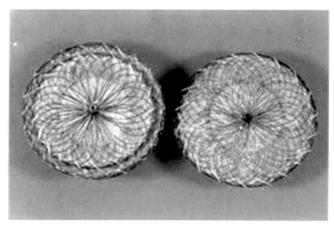

Figure 20–6 Amplatzer atrial septal occluder (ASO). The Amplatzer ASO is a double-disc device comprised of nitinol mesh and polyester fabric with a smaller right atrial disc. *(Image courtesy St. Jude Medical, St. Paul, Minn.)*

to meet multiple needs when occluding multifenestrated ASDs. All the devices can be expanded and collapsed throughout the entire procedure, thereby allowing for complete retrieval up to the point of final detachment from the delivery cable. The PFO occluder is not currently available in the United States.[44,45]

Fischer et al reported on 114 patients with PFO (60 men; age: 47 ± 13 years) and at least one thromboembolic event whose PFO closures were done with the Amplatzer PFO occluder.[46] Other causes for embolism were excluded. PFO closure was successful in all patients. After a mean of 10 months, no patient had either a significant residual shunt or a suspected thrombus formation on the occluder. During follow-up study five patients suffered from neurologic events (one stroke, two TIAs, and two epileptic seizures), although complete closure of the PFO was documented by TEE. One patient suffered from bleeding complications (upper gastrointestinal bleeding).[46]

CARDIOSEAL/STARFLEX

The CardioSEAL septal occluder (NMT Medical, Boston, Mass.) is no longer produced and was a modified version of the initial clamshell device **(Figure 20–7)**. It consisted of two square Dacron patches, mounted between four spring arms composed of a cobalt-based alloy that bent independently, and were therefore designed to enhance adherence to the interatrial septum. The device was available in diameter sizes from 17 to 40 mm. The STARFlex septal occluder represented a further revision of the CardioSEAL in that it had small microsprings attached at the end of each opposing arm **(Figure 20–8)**. These arms were designed to further enhance positioning in

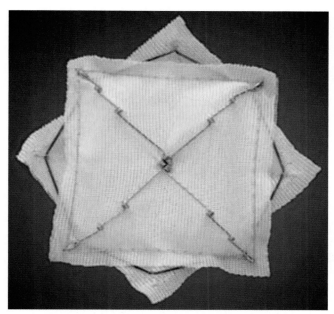

Figure 20–7 CardioSEAL septal occluder. The CardioSEAL septal occluder consists of two square Dacron patches mounted between four spring arms. *(Image courtesy Nitinol Medical Technologies, Boston, Mass.)*

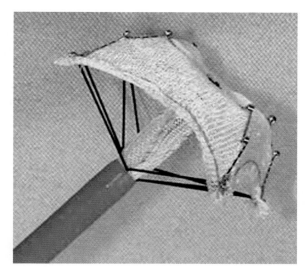

Figure 20–8 STARFlex device. The third-generation STARFlex device has major enhancements with a self-centering mechanism, improved pin-to-pin delivery, and a smaller delivery profile. *(Image courtesy Nitinol Medical Technologies, Boston, Mass.)*

the center of an ASD or PFO. They also provided a closer fit to the septum, thereby decreasing the device profile. To accommodate large-diameter PFOs and ASDs, the STARFlex was also available in a version with six, as opposed to four, arms (device diameter 38 mm), and the system was implanted through a 10F to 12F transseptal sheath. These devices have been discontinued. The prospective FORECAST registry involved 272 patients with presumed paradoxical embolism and PFO who underwent closure with the CardioSEAL and STARFlex devices. The devices were successfully implanted in 99.3% of the patients, with a procedural complication rate of 6.6%. Importantly, stroke or TIA occurred in 1.8% of the patients and device embolization occurred in 0.7%.[47]

NMT Medical further refined these devices and introduced the BioSTAR septal occluder. This innovative device utilizes the STARFlex scaffolding, but the polyester patches have been replaced with a heparin-coated, acellular, porcine-derived intestinal collagen matrix (Organogenesis, Canton, Mass.). This matrix allows absorption and replacement of the membranes with native human tissue up to 95%, leaving almost only the metal spring arms behind, which are also eventually endothelialized.

The theoretical advantages of this matrix are particularly relevant with reference to late complications seen with the earlier devices, such as inflammation and thrombus formation.[48-50] The BioSTAR device was investigated in the multicenter, prospective, randomized BEST trial evaluating safety and efficacy. The newest development, the BioTREK device, is based on the CardioSEAL BioSTAR technique but is completely resorbable. BioTREK uses a novel bioabsorbable, biosynthetic polymer known

as TephaFLEX (Tepha, Lexington, Mass.), a poly-4-hydroxybutyrate (P4HB) that is manufactured by a proprietary biotechnology process utilizing recombinant deoxyribonucleic acid technology. P4HB degrades via a combination of surface erosion and bulk hydrolysis to a natural metabolite (4HB) that is well tolerated and has a short half-life (35 minutes). It is ultimately broken down into carbon dioxide and water via the Krebs cycle, similar to other commonly used bioabsorbable polymers. Similar to BioSTAR, the BioTREK is a platform technology for delivering biological response modifiers. Over time, the patches and the connecting hub disappear, leaving the fibrous septum.[51,52]

GORE HELEX SEPTAL OCCLUDER

The HELEX septal occluder (WL Gore and Associates, Flagstaff, Ariz.) is a single, super-elastic, spiral-shaped, nitinol wire covered with a biocompatible membrane that is composed of expanded polytetrafluoroethylene (PTFE) **(Figure 20–9).** After deployment, the nitinol wire forms two flexible, round, equal-sized discs that are fixed by an integral locking system passing through the center of the device from left to right. The wire frame has three eyelets that act as markers and provide good visibility and positioning under fluoroscopic guidance. A locking mechanism connects the right-to-left atrial discs at their respective centers and stabilizes the position of the occluder within the atrial septum. The diameter of the discs ranges from 15 to 35 mm.

The HELEX device is implanted through a 9F delivery catheter. This feature spares the use of a long transseptal sheath and likely decreases the risk of air embolism. Advantages of this device are the ease of deployment and the ability to retrieve it throughout the entire procedure and even after release from the delivery catheter via a retrieval cord. In addition, if device embolization occurs after release, retrieval with a snare is easier than with other devices. The new version of this device includes a monorail delivery system and an improved locking mechanism. These two improvements further facilitate delivery and minimize device embolization.[53]

Ponnuthurai et al reported a study in which 75 adult patients (44.0 ± 11.7 years; 45.3% male) were referred for PFO closure. PFO was found in 69 patients, of whom 68/69 (98.6%) underwent closure with the GORE HELEX device (no PFO was found in five patients, and one patient had an atrial secundum defect closed with the Amplatzer septal occluder). Six of 69 cases required device retrieval, and five of six had successful replacement with a second GORE HELEX device. One of the six had a large PFO associated with atrial septal aneurysm, which was closed with the Amplatzer septal occluder. There were no major complications. At 3-month follow-up, 65/68 (95.6%) had no residual shunt on TTE, and three patients had small residual shunts believed to be related to incomplete endothelialization at 3 months.[54]

PREMERE PATENT FORAMEN OVALE CLOSURE SYSTEM

The Premere PFO occluder (St. Jude Medical, St. Paul, Minn.) is specifically designed for PFO closure. The device is composed of two cross-shaped nitinol anchors connected over a flexible polyester braided tether **(Figure 20–10)**. Important features of this device include a variable tether length that can be adjusted according to the thickness of the interatrial septum and tunnel length. Additionally, in an effort to limit foreign material and decrease the device profile, the left atrial side is uncovered, and only the right atrial anchor of the device is covered with a knitted polyester membrane. It is available in diameters

of 20 and 25 mm. A 30-mm device is under evaluation. This device is not available in the United States. Rigatelli et al[55] reported on 70 patients (48 females and 22 males, mean age 38 ± 6.7 years) with previous stroke who were referred for transcatheter closure of PFO with the Premere occlusion system on the basis of absence of moderate or severe ASA. Forty-six 20-mm and 24 25-mm Premere devices were implanted. Rates of procedural success, predischarge occlusion, and complication were 100%, 95.7%, and 0%, respectively. On mean follow-up time of 40 ± 10.9 months (range 6 to 54), the follow-up occlusion rate was 98.5%. During follow-up study, no cases of permanent atrial fibrillation, aortic/atrial erosion, device thrombosis, or atrioventricular (AV) valve inferences were noted.[55]

THE COHEREX FLATSTENT

The first use of the Coherex FlatStent PFO occluder (Coherex Medical, Inc., Salt Lake City, Utah) in a human was performed in October 2007 **(Figure 20–11)**. Whereas all other available occluders extend into both atria, this novel device leaves only a minimal amount of surface area exposed in the left atrium. The occluder consists of a super-elastic nitinol lattice with integrated polyurethane foam in the intratunnel cells of the device. This foam is intended to stimulate tissue growth inside the tunnel. The delivery catheter has a monorail design for rapid exchange functionality and is designed to be used by a single operator. The tip of the

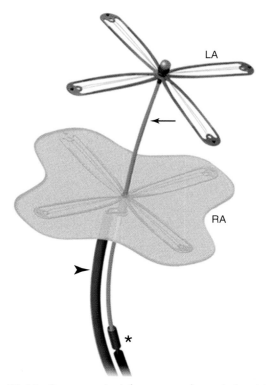

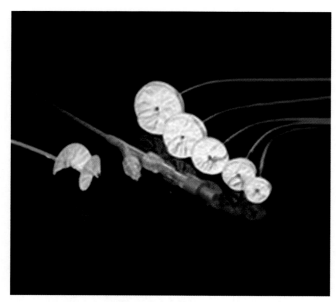

Figure 20–9 GORE HELEX septal occluder. The occluder is comprised of a nitinol wire frame covered with expanded polytetrafluoroethylene. *(Image courtesy WL Gore and Associates, Flagstaff, Ariz.)*

Figure 20–10 Premere patent foramen ovale occluder. *LA,* Left atrial disc; *RA,* right atrial disc; *horizontal arrow,* central flexible tether; *solid arrowhead,* advancing tool; *,* locking mechanism. *(Image courtesy St. Jude Medical, St. Paul, Minn.)*

catheter is shaped to simplify crossing of the PFO. The body of the device expands within the tunnel, drawing the septum primum and the septum secundum into contact without a significant change of the structure of the septum primum. Proximal anchors open into the right atrium, and strategically placed microtines are designed to ensure that the device cannot migrate or

embolize. The device can be resheathed and repositioned as necessary until it is detached.

The device is designed to ensure long-term closure and to have a reduced risk of thrombus formation. There is one size of the FlatStent available for stretched diameters from 4 to 10 mm with a tunnel length of 4 mm or larger. A second device in larger sizes is in development.[56]

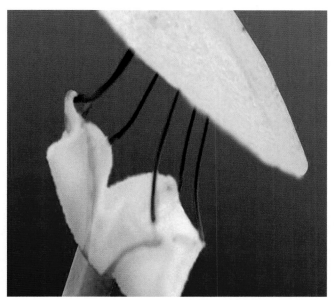

Figure 20–11   Coherex FlatStent patent foramen ovale occluder. The occluder consists of a super-elastic nitinol lattice with integrated polyurethane foam in the intratunnel cells of the device. *(Image courtesy Coherex Medical, Inc., Salt Lake City, Utah.)*

CARDIA ULTRASEPT PATENT FORAMEN OVALE OCCLUDER

The Cardia family of PFO occluders (Cardia, Burnsville, Minn.) consists of four generations of devices comprised of two Ivalon discs mounted and expanded by nitinol arms **(Figure 20–12).** The first two generations consist of square discs on four arms, and the second two incorporate hexagonal discs on six nitinol arms. Unique to the current iteration, the Intrasept has a dual articulating sail at the center of the device, which allows for a very low profile against the interatrial septum. The device is available in 5-mm increments from 20 to 35 mm, is delivered through a 9F to 11F transseptal sheath, and is fully retrievable throughout the procedure.[57] This device is currently not available in the United States.

SOLYSAFE SEPTAL OCCLUDER

The Solysafe septal occluder (Swiss Implant, Solothurn, Switzerland) is a self-centering ASD closure device consisting of two synthetic patches that are attached to wires made of a cobalt-based alloy called *Phynox* (a material similar to nitinol by virtues of elasticity and memory retention) **(Figure 20–13).** The wires are maintained in place by two wire holders on each side of the atrial septum. A major advantage of this new system is that it is delivered over a guidewire as opposed to a long transseptal sheath. This innovative technique involves the utilization of two control catheters that enable positioning of this device across the PFO and anchoring it against the interatrial septum. Even after complete deployment, the device is fully retrievable up to the point that the guidewire is removed.[58] Marketing and distribution of this product ceased on August 2010, in part because of a high rate of wire fracture.

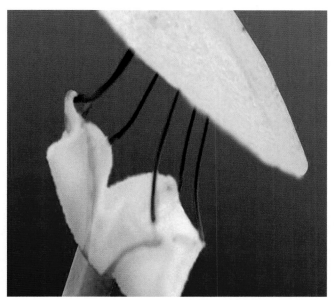

Figure 20–12   Cardia Ultrasept patent foramen ovale occluder. The first two generations consist of square discs on four arms, and the second two incorporate hexagonal discs on six nitinol arms. *(Image courtesy Cardia, Burnsville, Minn.)*

Figure 20–13 Solysafe Septal occluder. The device consists of two synthetic patches that are attached to wires made of a cobalt-based alloy called *Phynox. (Image courtesy Swiss Implant, Solothurn, Switzerland.)*

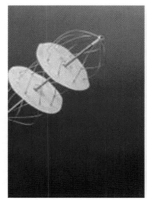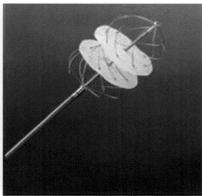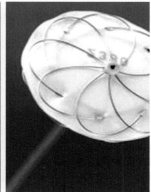

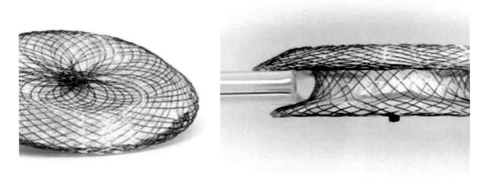

Figure 20–14 **OccluTech.** This is a double-disc device made of a self-expanding nitinol wire mesh. *(Image courtesy OccluTech, Jena, Germany.)*

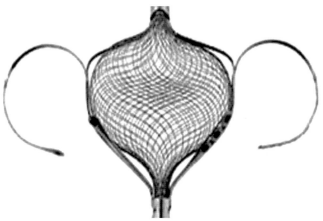

Figure 20–15 **SeptRx occluder.** The SeptRx device is a unique device in that it targets only the patent foramen ovale tunnel as opposed to the right and left atrial borders. *(Image courtesy Secant Medical, Perkasie, Penn.)*

OCCLUTECH

The OccluTech device (OccluTech, Jena, Germany) is technically similar to the Amplatzer devices; it is a double-disc device made of a self-expanding nitinol wire mesh **(Figure 20–14).** Distinguishing it from the Amplatzer devices, there is no hub on the left atrial side. In addition, the Dacron patch on the left side is on the outer surface covering the wire mesh and not inside of the wire mesh.[59]

SEPTRX OCCLUDER

The SeptRx (Secant Medical, Perkasie, Penn.) device is a unique device in that it targets only the PFO tunnel as opposed to the right and left atrial borders **(Figure 20–15).** It is implanted into the flap of the PFO and stretches the defect in an anterior–posterior direction, causing an approximation of septum primum and secundum. Potential advantages of this approach relate to the fact that it does not significantly change the configuration of septum primum and that it minimizes foreign material in the left atrium. This last feature may possibly decrease the risk of thrombus formation.[60]

HEARTSTITCH

HeartStitch (Sutura, Inc., Fountain Valley, Calif.) is a transcatheter polypropylene suture system to close PFOs that is based on the SuperStitch technology (used as a closure technique for femoral vessels) **(Figure 20–16).** The device consists of individually deployable needles, and its sutures pose no risk of erosion or embolization. The procedure is relatively simple: the HeartStitch system is introduced and deployed into the left atrium. Sequentially, the septum primum and secundum are then sutured and the HeartStitch system is withdrawn. Early investigation is under way.[61]

PFx

The PFx closure system (Cierra Inc., Redwood City, Calif.) **(Figure 20–17)** is another unique concept in that it is the only non–device-based approach for percutaneous PFO closure. The system is delivered into the overlapping part of septum primum and secundum via the right side of the atrial septum. A vacuum pump functions to hold both septa in place while radiofrequency is applied over an electrode, effectively "welding" the membranes together. The device is then withdrawn from the right atrium, and no foreign material is left behind.[62,63]

20.8 Implantation Technique

Techniques may vary among different hospitals and individual operators. Echocardiographic guidance (intracardiac echocardiography [ICE], TEE, or in some cases TTE) is helpful in most patients. Balloon sizing of the PFO is not required in the vast majority of cases.

The steps of the procedure are the same for most devices that are currently used (e.g., Amplatzer, CardiaStar, GORE HELEX) but not for older devices that were used earlier in this series (e.g., Das Angel Wings [Microvena Corporation, White Bear Lake, Minn.], atrial septal defect occluder system [ASDOS], Sideris buttoned device).

PROCEDURE

Initial procedure for PFO closure is similar to ASD closure. The timing of the heparin bolus may be delayed if

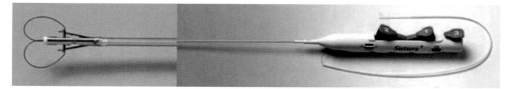

Figure 20–16   HeartStitch. The device consists of individually deployable needles, and its sutures pose no risk of erosion or embolization. *(Image courtesy Sutura, Fountain Valley, Calif.)*

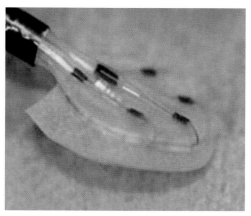

Figure 20–17   PFx. This is a non–device-based approach for percutaneous patent foramen ovale closure. A vacuum pump functions to hold both septa in place while radiofrequency is applied over an electrode, effectively "welding" the membranes together.

a transseptal needle puncture is needed to gain entry into the left atrium when the PFO is associated with a slitlike tunnel.

A baseline right-heart catheterization with measurement of pressure to exclude unexpected pulmonary hypertension is a reasonable diagnostic study to perform before all PFO closures. Oximetry measurement to quantify left-to-right or right-to-left shunts is recommended along with measuring right- and left-sided filling pressure. The measurement of pulmonary venous saturation is necessary to evaluate patients who are referred for PFO closure to rule out other sources of right-to-left shunting like pulmonary arteriovenous malformations (AVMs). Measurement of pulmonary capillary wedge pressure or direct left-atrial pressure measurement to determine the patient's volume status may be helpful. The routine performance of preclosure injection of agitated saline/blood/contrast for detection of right-to-left shunting through the PFO can be performed to confirm a right-to-left shunt but might not be necessary if a shunt was previously documented. In addition, agitated saline injection can be performed easily into the pulmonary artery to assess for a shunt through a pulmonary AVM. Angiography may provide additional information on anatomy of the septum primum and the septum secundum, as well as the length and the orientation of the PFO channel. A power injection can be performed in the right atrium, especially if there is a right-to-left shunt. Some operators routinely perform angiograms in the tunnel of the PFO for anatomic delineation. A power injection in the main pulmonary artery (MPA) during the levo phase

can delineate the left atrial side of the septum. This is best outlined by left anterior oblique (LAO)–cranial angulation, approximately LAO 30 and cranial 30. The ultrasound visualization of the interatrial septum with a TEE probe or an ICE catheter completes the diagnostic phase of the procedure. Imaging should verify the location and the nature of the PFO, determine the presence or absence of an ASA, and exclude the coexistence of an ASD. The ICE catheter tip is placed in the lateral aspect of the right atrium, manipulated to provide an optimal image of the PFO, and positioned and then placed in locked position to guide the subsequent steps during device placement.

A multipurpose catheter can be used to cross the septum and is then positioned in the left upper pulmonary vein with fluoroscopic guidance. A small subset of PFOs may be more challenging to cross because of an abnormal plane of the interatrial septum with the presence of an ASA or a complex tunnel PFO. A Judkins right coronary catheter tip shape may be useful in some of these patients. A hydrophilic guidewire also may allow easier crossing of these anatomic variants of PFO position and type. TEE or ICE imaging provides useful visual guidance in crossing some PFOs. Making a transseptal needle puncture is an option for PFO closure in some complex PFOs; with presence of a tunnel, the transeptal approach can be performed under ICE guidance with subsequent placement of the PFO closure device.

SIZING OF PATENT FORAMEN OVALE AND SELECTION OF DEVICE SIZE

The use of a sizing balloon during the PFO closure procedure is common, although it is of uncertain value in the opinion of some experts. Balloon sizing is performed by slowly and gently inflating a manufacturer's sizing balloon in the PFO using a stiff guidewire across the PFO with its distal end in a left pulmonary vein. The waist that appears with balloon inflation can be measured by ultrasound or digital fluoroscopic images with appropriate calibration. The device size is chosen, using the manufacturer's recommendations, based on the measured diameter of the opened PFO. Finally, the waist may be discrete, which indicates a simple PFO, or more lengthy, which suggests a tunnel-like PFO. The finding of a tunnel PFO leads some operators to perform a transseptal needle puncture to place a more centrally located perpendicular device that overlaps the PFO, rather than using the PFO itself for the location of the center connection of the device, which may be tilted by the tunnel. Other measurements of the patient's atrial anatomy can be made to estimate where the edge of the device will reach. The additional presence of an ASA often prompts the selection of a larger closure device.

Correct position is verified if tissue is seen between the left atrial and right atrial umbrella/discs on all sides of the PFO. Some operators use angiography along with ultrasound for confirmation of position. Agitated saline and color-flow Doppler interrogation of PFO closure can be performed at this time; however, the device is attached to the delivery cable and this often distorts the interatrial septal anatomy to preclude an assessment of final device effectiveness in PFO closure. A gentle push-and-pull test of the device provides further assurance of a proper and stable device position.

The device is released per the manufacturer's instructions. Traction or excessive push on the whole assembly during the release of the device should be avoided. By either ultrasound or fluoroscopy, the release of the device is accompanied immediately by a reorientation of the device after the tethering effect of the attachment is no longer present. Angiography, agitated saline with ultrasound, and color-flow Doppler interrogation of PFO closure can be performed at this point. The immediate effectiveness of the device in PFO closure can be assessed best with the ultrasound bubble test using an agitated mixture of saline and a small amount of blood. This is injected directly into the delivery catheter with its tip at the IVC–right atrial junction. Persistent right-to-left shunting may be seen in approximately one third of patients; in most patients this usually disappears in the subsequent months, presumably as a result of device endothelialization. Final measurements are made if indicated and venous access is then exited. Hemostasis can be achieved via manual compression or other mechanisms ("Z" stitch).

Final TEE and ICE images are acquired, and the respective devices are removed. Cinefluoroscopy of the device also can be performed to document the device placement. The best projection is a cranial LAO.

POSTINTERVENTIONAL TREATMENT AND FOLLOW-UP STUDY

Usually, patients can be discharged from the hospital the next day. The position of the device is confirmed by chest X-ray and TTE. For the prophylaxis of thromboembolic events after device implantation, patients are treated with 75 mg/day of clopidogrel for 4 weeks to 3 months and with 81 mg/day aspirin for 6 months. If the indication for device closure was paradoxical embolism, aspirin may be continued indefinitely. Standard bacterial endocarditis prophylaxis is recommended for 6 to 12 months. After 6 months, contrast echocardiography should be performed for detection of residual shunting.

PATENT FORAMEN OVALE WITH LONG TUNNEL

Long tunnels represent a particular problem for devices with a fixed distance between the right and left atrial components because there is the potential for both discs to be partially deployed within the tunnel. This can

result in a poorly conformed device. Techniques advocated to facilitate successful closure include balloon pull-through, transseptal puncture through the foraminal flap, and delivery of the device though the transseptal puncture site rather than via the tunnel. However, this has the additional risk associated with transseptal puncture, and its success is dependent on precise puncture through the foraminal flap, which can be challenging. It also has a higher residual shunt rate. Another technique that has been described is the balloon pull-through to render the septum primum incompetent and improve the final device position. The balloon pull-through has the disadvantage of being traumatic, and balloon pull-back cannot be fully controlled. Spence et al reported balloon detunnelization, in which a compliant balloon was used to dilate the PFO in a stepwise fashion until the PFO entrance and exit constraint sites approximated and merged on the fluoroscopic image.[64] Another method is to use a device such as the Premere occluder for long-tunnel PFOs with an adjustable distance between the left and right atrial discs or a distensible neck, on the basis of its strength and distensible neck rendering it resistant to trapping in long tunnels. Reports on the interventional closure of PFO in combination with ASA showed an increased risk for thrombus formation as well as for incomplete closure. Some operators recommend using a larger device to prevent malposition.

Lipomatous hypertrophy of the interatrial septum has a prevalence of 2% and is typically composed of both white and brown fat. The pathognomonic "dumb-bell" shape is caused by hypertrophy of the septum primum and secundum with sparing of the fossa ovalis. A septum secundum more than 15 mm thick has been the predominant defining criterion. Transcatheter closure of a PFO in the setting of lipomatous hypertrophy can be difficult because of the requirement of a device with a long transverse axis. Devices with short waists can result in either inability to capture the septum secundum, leading to incomplete apposition of the device and allowing continued shunt or device embolization. In one case series by Rigatelli et al, eight patients underwent closure via a Premere device and two via the Amplatzer Cribriform device.[65] Both patients who underwent closure with the Amplatzer devices continued to have residual shunt resulting from inadequate transverse waist length and malapposition.[65] For septa more than 20 mm thick, the Amplatzer muscular ventricular septal defect closure device (AGA Medical, Plymouth, Minn.) has been used to achieve successful closure.[66]

20.9 Atrial Septal Defect

ASD is a common congenital heart disease (CHD) that accounts for 8% to 10% of all CHDs and is considered to be the most common type of CHD in adults.[67,68] There are four types of ASDs with different anatomic and clinical features, and subsequently there are unique therapeutic approaches: ostium secundum, ostium primum, coronary sinus defects, and sinus venosus ASDs. The ostium secundum defect is the most common and is a generally suitable for device closure. In the ostium secundum ASD, there is a pathologic deficiency of septal tissue in the region of the fossa ovalis. These defects can be thought of as a continuum from a small intermittent shunt through a PFO with right-to-left shunting that is only demonstrable on echocardiographic contrast studies with the Valsalva maneuver, to ASA with associated PFO, to large and stretched PFOs with resting interatrial shunting, and finally to large or multiple secundum ASDs with hemodynamically significant left-to-right shunting.[69,70] As a result, the indications for closure are diverse and may include paradoxical embolism, POS, decompression illness, migraine headache, or significant shunts with or without pulmonary hypertension.[71,72] The magnitude of the shunt and direction of flow through any ASD depend on the size of the defect and the relative diastolic filling properties of the left and right ventricles. Under normal physiologic conditions, there is net left-to-right shunting across an ASD because the left ventricle is far less compliant than the right ventricle. This shunt of fully oxygenated blood back to the right atrium results in a volume load to the right-sided heart chambers and to the pulmonary vasculature; if left untreated, large-volume left-to-right shunting can result in atrial arrhythmias, right ventricular diastolic and systolic failure, worsened functional class, decreased exercise capacity, left ventricular diastolic failure, and, uncommonly, development of pulmonary arterial hypertension (PAH).[71,72]

Many patients with ASDs are free of overt symptoms, although most become symptomatic at some point in their lives. The age at which symptoms appear is highly variable and is not exclusively related to the size of the shunt. Exercise intolerance in the form of exertional dyspnea or fatigue is the most common initial presenting symptom. Atrial fibrillation or flutter is an age-related reflection of atrial dilation and stretch that seldom occurs in patients younger than 40 years of age; its arrival usually causes substantial symptoms because of both the tachycardia and the underlying hemodynamics governed by impaired left ventricular filling and reduced systemic cardiac output. Less commonly, decompensated right heart failure may occur, almost always in the older patient. This is often in the presence of substantial tricuspid regurgitation secondary to severe right heart and tricuspid annular dilation with coexistent PAH of variable severity (developing slowly in response to excessive pulmonary blood flow over a long period of time). Occasionally, a paradoxical embolus or TIA may be the first clue to the presence of an ASD.[73-79]

TTE may rarely in a thin adult document the type(s) and size of the ASD(s), the direction(s) of the shunt, and, in experienced hands, the presence of anomalous pulmonary venous return. TTE in adults usually detects an enlarged right side, which prompts further workup such as TEE. The functional importance of the defect can be estimated by the size of the right atrium and ventricle, the presence/absence of paradoxical septal motion (right ventricular volume overload), ventricular septal orientation in diastole (volume overload) and systole (pressure overload), and an estimation of the shunt ratio (based on pulmonary and aortic flows). Pulmonary artery systolic pressures may be estimated from the Doppler velocity of tricuspid regurgitation.[80,81]

TEE may be useful to confirm the type of ASD and to delineate the pulmonary venous return. If a patient presents with poor acoustic windows, the cause of right atrial and right ventricular enlargement may not be readily apparent using TTE. In such situations, TEE may help to define better the presence of one or more defects, as well as to accurately size the defect before repair. ASD shape and size can vary significantly, and may be elliptical, complex (irregularly shaped), or circular. Thus imaging the septum from several planes is crucial. Nonetheless, two-dimensional (2D) TEE can underestimate the area of complex shaped ASDs. Therefore real-time three-dimensional (3D) echocardiography can be used to delineate the size, shape, and number of defects better and is particularly relevant for irregular and complex shaped ASDs. It is also commonly used in support of device closure of ASDs.[82-86]

Cardiac MRI may be useful and may give the same type of information that echocardiography can provide, although the anatomy of the ASD might not be well defined in smaller defects. It is seen as providing the gold standard for the assessment of right ventricular size and function, and it may help define whether the right heart chambers are in fact enlarged. MRI is also excellent at assessing pulmonary venous return. Small ASDs might not be well seen.[87,88] In patients who cannot have an MRI, CT scanning and angiography can offer similar information.[89]

PROPER PATIENT SELECTION AND INDICATIONS FOR THE PROCEDURE

The indication to treat an ASD is typically related to its hemodynamic significance and its effects on the right ventricle. The beneficial effects of ASD closure include positive right and left heart remodeling,[90-97] improvement in symptoms, increase in exercise capacity,[98,99] reduction in tendency to develop atrial arrhythmias,[100-102] and decrease in pulmonary arterial pressures.[103,104] Furthermore, when comparing a catheter-based approach with ASD closure with a surgical approach, transcatheter closure may offer more rapid improvement in right ventricular remodeling and differences in periprocedural morbidity.[101,105-107] King and Mills in 1974 were the first to develop transcatheter closure of ASD. Because of the large-profile delivery system required, technical difficulties, and a high rate of residual shunting, their device was not accepted for general clinical use.[108] In recent decades, many devices have been developed for percutaneous closure of ASD; most of these have high success rates.

Patients with a stretched secundum ASD larger than 36 mm, those with inadequate atrial septal rims to permit stable device deployment, or those with proximity of the defect to the AV valves, the coronary sinus, or the vena cavae are usually referred for surgical repair. Presence of other associated defects like partial anomalous pulmonary veins or concurrent ASDs in the nonsecundum location are also usually surgical referrals. Absolute contraindications include sinus venosus, coronary sinus defects or primum ASD, intracardiac thrombi, sepsis, or associated cardiac lesions that require surgical repair.

Device closure is a safe and effective procedure in experienced hands, with major complications such as cardiac perforation or device embolization occurring in less than 1% of patients. The presence of an ASD also does not always necessitate closure, and there are specific clinical scenarios in which ASD repair or closure should be considered as either not indicated or contraindicated. In some cases, the defect may be too small to be considered hemodynamically significant, and patients should be monitored both clinically and via imaging modalities to watch for progressive right heart dilation, remodeling, and/or dysfunction. Exercise testing might also provide insight regarding functional ability of the patient in the presence of vague symptoms. In patients with either advanced pulmonary hypertension or severe left ventricular dysfunction, the ASD may be physiologically required to act as a "pop-off valve" for either the right or left ventricle, respectively, and defect repair is relatively contraindicated in such patients if they are nonreactive to pulmonary vasodilators or afterload reduction.

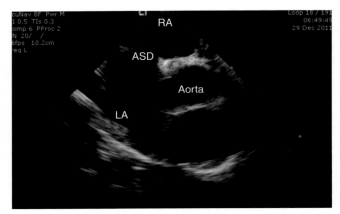

Figure 20–18 Intracardiac echocardiography image of an atrial septal defect (ASD). Two-dimensional evaluation shows an ASD with some deficiency of the aortic rim.

20.10 Implantation Procedure

The procedure is performed under fluoroscopic and echocardiographic guidance in a still patient. TEE might require general anesthesia, whereas ICE guidance allows a more simple procedure under sedation. The advantages of ICE are multiple. The quality of the images may be superior to TEE because the transducer is within the cardiac chambers, enabling high resolution and close-up visualization of structures; accurate assessment of the interatrial septum, position and size of the defects, adequacy of the rims, and drainage of the pulmonary veins is then possible. ICE also retains an advantage over TEE in imaging the posteroinferior portion of the interatrial septum **(Figures 20–18 and 20–19, Videos 20–1 and 20–2).** Disadvantages of ICE include the need for insertion of a second venous sheath, the requirement for supplemental training, the expense of ultrasound catheters that can be used only twice with need for resterilization after the initial use, and potential provocation of transient atrial arrhythmias. In addition, ICE has a more limited field of view than TEE and thus is less suited for the evaluation of far-field device complications.[109,110]

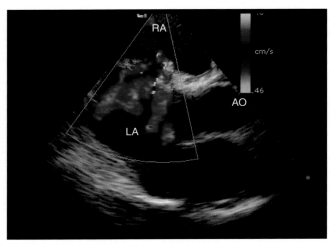

Figure 20–19 Color Doppler evaluation of an atrial septal defect (ASD) on intracardiac echocardiography imaging showing left-to-right flow across the ASD.

PREMEDICATION

Aspirin therapy should be started at least 3 days before implantation. Patients taking warfarin (Coumadin) may be transitioned to enoxaparin (Lovenox) or intravenous heparin for the procedure.

PROCEDURE

Many centers using TEE for implantation perform the procedure with the patient under general anesthesia. If ICE is used, the procedure is performed with moderate conscious sedation and local anesthesia with lidocaine infiltration of the groin region. One or two sheaths are inserted in the femoral vein after gaining access. An 8.5F or 10F short sheath is used for the ICE catheter, and a 7F or 8F sheath is used for the initial right heart catheterization. Both sheaths can be placed in the same femoral vein or bilateral veins per operator preference. After sheath placement into the femoral vein, unfractionated heparin is administered at 75 to 100 units per kg body weight. Anticoagulation during the ASD closure procedure is important. The goal is an activated clotting time (ACT) of approximately 250 seconds, although no studies have been done to determine the optimal level of anticoagulation. The chief concerns are thrombus formation on intracardiac guidewires, catheters, and devices during the implantation. One dose of an intravenous antibiotic like cephalosporin (or clindamycin if the patient is allergic to cephalosporins) is administered during device implantation in many institutions. This may be followed by a second dose in 6 to 8 hours, but protocols differ among institutions. Continuous monitoring of electrocardiographic leads, noninvasive systemic arterial pressure monitoring, noninvasive oxygen saturation monitoring, and neurologic mental status observation should be performed in all cases.

Initial hemodynamic evaluation is performed with an end-hole catheter. Oxygen saturation in the SVC and the pulmonary artery is obtained, allowing the interventionist to calculate a Qp:Qs ratio if there is a net left-to-right shunt. In the presence of systemic desaturation, oxygen saturations in the pulmonary veins should be obtained to differentiate between right-to-left shunting at the atrial level versus pulmonary venous desaturation caused by lung disease. Evaluation of a right-to-left shunt at the atrial level is especially important in the presence of pulmonary hypertension because it can dictate closure. Right heart pressures are documented, after which the defect is crossed and left atrial and ventricular pressures are recorded. PVR is calculated. In patients with left ventricular dysfunction where the ASD might function as a pop off, documentation of left-sided filling pressures is assessed both at baseline and with balloon occlusion.

It is recommended to perform an angiogram in the MPA with an angiographic catheter to exclude partial anomalous pulmonary venous return to the right heart on levophase **(Video 20–3).** Complete echocardiographic evaluation of the septum, AV valves, and pulmonary veins is recommended before crossing the defect so as to not create artifact with the catheter or wire during evaluation of the septum. The septum is evaluated for presence of additional defects, adequacy of rims, and proximity to AV valves or coronary sinus. Documentation of normal pulmonary venous return should be done as well.

A multipurpose catheter is then advanced across the defect and positioned in the left upper pulmonary vein on fluoroscopy. Entry into the left atrial appendage typically is recognized by either tactile resistance to further advancement or the tip of the catheter never advancing beyond the fluoroscopic border of the heart and the production of premature atrial contractions with catheter advancement. The catheter is torqued clockwise to direct it superiorly and away from the left atrial appendage. Advancement of the tip of the guidewire or any catheter excessively deep into the pulmonary venous system with accompanying resistance should be avoided. Deep penetration of a pulmonary vein may provoke coughing, which can cause the generation of negative intrathoracic pressures with the accompanying risk of air entry into a catheter or delivery sheath. In addition, perforation of a pulmonary vein is a potential complication. A stiff guidewire is then parked in the pulmonary vein. A sizing balloon is advanced over the stiff exchange wire. Sizing of the defect can be performed by dynamic or static balloon occlusion with echocardiography and/or fluoroscopic imaging. The safest approach is probably to use both and to measure the waist on the balloon to select the appropriate size of the device. For dynamic balloon sizing, the Meditech balloon (Boston Scientific, Watertown, Mass.), sized 20, 27, 33, or 40 mm depending on the estimated ASD size, is passed into the left atrium over the guidewire and inflated to a diameter of approximately 5 mm greater than the estimated ASD diameter using dilute contrast (30%). Under TEE

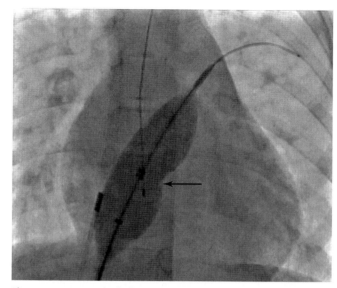

Figure 20–20 **Static balloon sizing of the atrial septal defect.** A stiff wire has been positioned in the left upper pulmonary vein with a NuMED sizing balloon (NuMED Canada, Inc., Cornwall, Ontario, Canada) across the defect. There is an intracardiac echocardiography probe positioned in the right atrium to evaluate for stop flow.

guidance, the balloon is then gently pulled onto the atrial septum, at which stage color flow on the TEE should be completely eliminated. While maintaining firm but not undue pressure on the septum and under continuous TEE guidance, the balloon is slowly deflated until it pops through the defect into the right atrium. The diameter at which this occurs is the stretched balloon diameter of the ASD, which in essence is the diameter of the firm margins of the ASD. The balloon is deflated, withdrawn from the body, and reinflated using the prerecorded volume and measured against a sizing plate.

For static balloon sizing, either the Amplatzer sizing balloon or NuMED sizing balloon (NuMED Canada, Inc., Cornwall, Ontario, Canada), both of which are highly compliant balloons, can be used **(Figure 20–20).** The Amplatzer sizing balloon is available in three diameters—18, 24, and 34 mm with a shaft size of 6F to 8F—and can be used to measure maximum defect sizes of 20, 27, and 40 mm respectively. The NuMED sizing balloon ranges from 20 to 40 mm and has a shaft size of 8F to 9F. Two methods can be used to size ASDs using a compliant balloon. Some operators inflate the balloon until a waist is visible, and others inflate it only until no shunting is demonstrable by echocardiogram.[111-113] Echocardiography has the advantage of providing the "stop flow" diameter, using color Doppler to evaluate the size of the waist when the shunt disappears. The sizing balloon is inflated until a waist is seen and echocardiographic evaluation by color is performed to look for residual shunt **(Video 20–4).** If no residual shunt is seen, then the balloon is deflated slightly until the first sign of a shunt is seen. This technique decreases the risk of oversizing as compared with the stretched diameter. A thorough echocardiographic evaluation of the septum should be repeated with balloon inflation to exclude additional defects. The gantry can then be angulated to right anterior oblique and LAO projections with cranial angulation on both the PA and lateral intensifiers respectively. In a single-plane lab, LAO with cranial projection outlines the balloon without significant foreshortening. The balloon stop flow diameter should be measured with both imaging modalities. It is sometimes difficult on echocardiography to visualize the balloon waist in relation to the septum.

Device selection depends on the sizing and the characteristics of the septum. For ASD closure, a device size that is 2 mm greater than the stop flow diameter is usual for Amplatz septal occluders. For the GORE HELEX devices, the device size used is twice the stop flow diameter. The GORE HELEX septal occluder is not recommended for defects larger than 18 mm and for patients with a septal thickness of greater than 8 mm in the area of the occluder placement.

For the Amplatzer device delivery, the delivery sheath is advanced over the stiff exchange wire into the left atrium. The insertion of the delivery catheter or sheath is a critical step and is guided by fluoroscopy. Typically, the tip of the guidewire is placed in a left upper pulmonary vein for stability. The catheter is rotated gently during advancement into the right atrium to allow it to assume the typical appearance aimed at the septum. Once the dilator of the delivery sheath is advanced into the left atrium, the sheath is advanced into the pulmonary vein holding the dilator steady. The dilator and wire are then removed carefully so as not to cause vacuum and introduce air into the sheath. This can be done during simultaneous flushing of the sheath. The sheath is aspirated carefully, retracting slowly until there is no air in the sheath. The sheath is then flushed slowly with a good volume of saline and preferably under fluoroscopy to look for any air being advanced into the left atrium. Alternatively many operators intentionally remove the dilator when the tip of the catheter is in the upper IVC. This is done to flush the catheter and to minimize the chance of air entry. The delivery cable and device are connected, the device is retracted into a loading tube with vigorous flushing to remove all air, and the device is loaded into the delivery catheter. The keys to optimal device preparation and loading include inspection to detect any abnormalities, verification that the attachment between the device and delivery cable is secure and capable of being unlocked, and confirmation that all air has been removed. When introduced into the sheath, the device along with cable should be accompanied by continuous flushing. Device delivery generally is straightforward for most ASDs. For ICE guidance, the catheter tip is deflected to the lateral wall of the right atrium and adjusted such that the entire device deployment can be observed from this parked position. The next key step is the advancement of the device to the end of the delivery catheter that is now usually pulled back into the midleft atrium. The next step is the deployment of the left atrial disc that is achieved by pulling back on the delivery catheter and exposing the device so that it expands. If the delivery catheter is too deep in the left atrium, the left atrial portion of the device will not deploy fully until the whole assembly is retracted further. Using TEE or ICE, the left atrial disc is pulled against the septum using gentle traction. There is slight resistance as the left atrial disc touches the left side on the atrial septum. In the presence of a large ASD, the device may prolapse to the right side during this and different maneuvers to be discussed subsequently. With fluoroscopic, echocardiographic, and tactile confirmation of the correct position of the left atrial umbrella/disc, the deployment of the right atrial side of the device immediately follows by once again pulling back the delivery catheter while keeping the device–cable system fixed in space. The deployment of the right atrial portion follows, and the delivery catheter is pulled back further, to allow the closure device to rest in place, but is still attached to the delivery cable. Final inspection of the location of the device by fluoroscopy and TEE or ICE is key. Before release of the device, it can be pushed and pulled gently to verify the correct position and stability. The device position is also assessed on fluoroscopy (on a left oblique cranial projection); the discs should be parallel to each other and separated from each other by the atrial septum. Echo should also be used to evaluate the relationship of the device to the right upper pulmonary vein, AV valves, coronary sinus, and aortic root; to verify the absence of pericardial effusion; and to exclude a significant residual shunt using color Doppler. "Minnesota wiggle" and "push-and-pull" techniques are routinely performed by some operators to check for device stability before release of the device. After device release, the position of the device is again checked using fluoroscopy and echocardiography. The device position can change with release of tension from the delivery cable, and therefore it is critical for detailed echocardiographic evaluation before leaving the catheterization lab.

20.11 Atrial Septal Devices

AMPLATZER SEPTAL OCCLUDER

The Amplatzer septal occluder is a double-disc device formed of a 0.005-inch nitinol mesh and was first described in 1997.[109] It consists of two discs that are linked to each other through a central connecting waist. Dacron fabric is incorporated into each disc and the connecting waist to enhance thrombosis. The device size is defined by the diameter of the connecting waist and is available from 4 to 38 mm. A 40-mm device is available outside the United States and has completed tests under an investigational device exemption. It is currently awaiting U.S. Food and Drug Administration (FDA) approval. The connecting waist has a length between 3 and 4 mm, with the diameter of the left atrial disc exceeding the connecting waist by 12 to 16 mm and the diameter of the right atrial disc exceeding the connecting waist by 8 to 10 mm.

The device has a low risk of procedure- or device-related complications. Closure rates at 12 months postprocedure are 98% to 100%, and device embolization is rare (<1%), usually only occurring during the procedure itself. Electrophysiologic abnormalities are often seen in the first 24 hours after device implantation but usually do not require any treatment. These abnormalities usually resolve quickly; rhythm or conduction abnormalities 1 year after device occlusion are extremely rare. A release of nickel from the device with a peak at 1 month post-implantation has been described. However, its clinical significance is questionable, and reports of clinically significant allergic reactions to nickel after device implantation are rare. A rare but serious complication is the erosion of the device through the anterior atrial wall and into the aortic root. Its incidence is estimated at approximately 0.1%, and most of the described cases have occurred in older, female patients. Even though oversizing of the device has been implicated as a potential causal factor, it could not be documented in all affected patients and therefore the exact etiology and disposition of this serious complication remain unclear.[114-117]

CARDIOSEAL AND STARFLEX SEPTAL OCCLUSION SYSTEM

The CardioSEAL and STARFlex septal occlusion devices represent second- and third-generation modifications of the original Clamshell device that was withdrawn due to the occurrence of stress fractures in some of the device's arms. Both devices were classical double-umbrella devices, with the umbrella frame being composed of four arms made of 0.009-inch MP35n, a cobalt-based alloy that is more flexible and less corrosive than stainless steel. Each arm contained two hinges, with the umbrella material itself being woven Dacron fabric. The two umbrellas were attached to each other at the center, and the devices are available in sizes of 17, 23, 28, and 33 mm; these sizes represent the maximum diagonal diameter of the expanded umbrellas. The STARFlex device, introduced in 1999, differed from the CardioSEAL device in that it had four central nitinol springs that facilitated a "self-centering" mechanism of the device. The main disadvantage of this group of devices was related to the implantation process, which did not allow repositioning of the device. Device retrieval was cumbersome and often impossible.[118-120] The devices have been discontinued.

In 2000, Carminati and colleagues reported on the European multicenter experience of using the Cardio-SEAL and STARFlex double-umbrella devices to close intraatrial communications in 334 patients with a mean age of 12 years. Implantation was achieved in 97% of patients, with early device embolization being seen in 4% of procedures, most of which subsequently underwent surgical ASD closure and removal of the device. Residual shunting was observed more often when compared with the Amplatzer septal occluder. Immediately after the procedure, 41% of patients had a detectable residual shunt that decreased gradually to 21% at a 12-month follow-up study. However, when excluding trivial leaks, the rate of complete closure was as high as 93% at a 1-year follow-up examination. Two patients required late explantation of the device: one because of malposition and one because of late embolization. Fractures of the device arms were observed in 6% of patients, none of which were associated with a clinically significant adverse event. Device erosions into adjacent structures

were not observed, and no patient died as a result of the device implantation.[121,122]

The buttoned device developed by Sideris consisted of a square-shaped rectangular left atrial umbrella and a right atrial counteroccluder. A new version of this occluder is the ButtonSeal Centering on Demand device, and occlusion rates up to 95% have been reported. The ASDOS, consisting of two self-opening umbrellas made of a nitinol wire skeleton, has also been used in some centers. The Das-AngelWings atrial septal occlusion device was the first self-centering device but has been withdrawn from the market. A new version, the Guardian Angel ASO is being already been tested in experimental animals, and clinical trials are planned.[123-127]

GORE HELEX SEPTAL OCCLUDER

The HELEX septal occluder was first described by Zahn and colleagues in 2001.[53] Its frame is made of a long nitinol wire, with a strip of PTFE fabric attached alongside. Three "eyelets" are embedded along the device to facilitate accurate positioning—one at each end and one in a central position between both discs. In its deployed status, the device forms two circular discs that are composed by the spiraling nitinol wire with its attached PTFE membrane. The device is available in sizes from 15 to 35 mm (diameter of discs) in 5-mm increments; a device-to-unstretched defect ratio of 1.7:2.1 is recommended. This device is not recommended for defects larger than 18 mm or with a septal thickness of greater than 8 mm in the area of the occluder placement. When compared with the ASO, the device has a lower profile and a more atraumatic contour. It is delivered through a 9F catheter system that is advanced via a 10F short sheath (internal diameter [ID] ≥ 0.131 inch or 3.33 mm) without a wire. It can also be as a monorail over a wire via a 13F sheath (ID ≥ 0.171 inch or 4.33 mm), rather than relying on a long sheath. This creates less distortion of the atrial septum before its release. The HELEX delivery sheath can be advanced across the septum in the absence of a wire by direct manipulation using echo and fluoroscopic guidance or by using a 0.035-inch wire as a monorail. The device is positioned as per company specifications, and cine is performed to document the locking loop across all the islets before its release **(Videos 20–5 and 20–6).**

Jones et al reported on the results of 143 patients in whom delivery of the HELEX septal occluder was attempted in 135 (94.4%) of the enrolled patients.[128] The eight patients with no delivery attempt were found during catheterization to have a balloon-occlusion defect size greater than 22 mm. Successful device delivery was achieved in 88.1%. Device delivery was not successful because of anatomical considerations in 10 of the 16 patients in whom the attempt failed; in the six remaining patients, the investigator was unable to achieve satisfactory device placement. Major adverse events were reported in 5.9% of patients. In the device arm, removal of the device was required in five of those seven patients. Minor adverse events were reported in 27.7% of patients, with the most common events being arrhythmias (5.0%) and headaches (4.2%). Fractures in the wire frame of the device were reported in six patients through the 12-month series of visits. None of these patients required intervention, and the Data Safety Monitoring Board adjudicated these as minor adverse events. At 12 months postprocedure, 98.1% of patients were determined to have had successful defect closure.[128] Serious complications, such as erosions into the aortic root that have been described with the Amplatzer devices, have not been observed with the HELEX septal occluder thus far.[129]

20.12 Closure of Large Defects

A large defect (>30 mm), especially associated with deficient rims (a distance of less than 5 mm from the defect to the wall of atrium), is still challenging. In such circumstances, there is often prolapse of the device into the right atrium, typically because of the failure of the left atrial disc to align in the plane of the atrial septum. There are several techniques that can be used to overcome such difficulties in aligning the left atrial disc parallel to the atrial septum and will result in a successful procedure. These techniques are discussed in the following sections.

HAUSDORF SHEATH/MODIFIED SHEATH

The Hausdorf sheath (Cook, Bloomington, Ind.) is a specially designed long sheath that has two posterior curves at the tip of the sheath that help align the left atrial disc parallel to the septum **(Figure 20–21)**. This sheath is available in sizes from 10F to 12F. In some cases, counterclockwise rotation of the sheath will orient the tip posterior and allow deployment of the left disc parallel to the septum to prevent prolapsing into the right atrium. If the Hausdorf sheath is not available, the same result can be achieved by cutting the distal tip of a Mullins sheath at a bevel to improve device orientation.[130,131]

RIGHT UPPER PULMONARY VEIN TECHNIQUE

The right upper pulmonary vein approach may allow better alignment of the left atrial disc along the plane of the atrial septum at the time of the device deployment **(Figure 20–22)**. The delivery sheath is carefully positioned in the right upper pulmonary vein, and then the device is advanced to the tip of the sheath. The left atrial disc is partially deployed in the right upper pulmonary vein. The sheath is then quickly retracted to deploy the remainder of the left disc; this will result in the disc jumping from that location to be parallel to the atrial septum. Quick and successive deployment of the connecting waist and the right disc is carried out before the sheath has the opportunity to change its position or before the left disc prolapses through the defect to the right atrium.[130-132]

LEFT UPPER PULMONARY VEIN TECHNIQUE

The delivery sheath is carefully positioned in the left upper pulmonary vein, and the device is then advanced to the tip of the sheath before starting to deploy the left disc inside the vein. Deployment of the waist and right disc

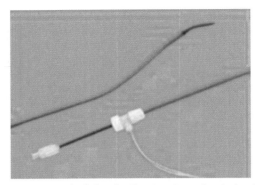

Figure 20–21 Hausdorf sheath. This is a long sheath that has two posterior curves at the tip of the sheath that help align the left atrial disc parallel to the septum.

is continued, which essentially appears as a lengthened device. As the sheath reaches the right atrium, the left disc disengages from the pulmonary vein and reforms its inherent shape to be parallel to the atrial septum. Continuous retraction of the sheath over the cable by pulling the entire assembly towards the right atrium will result in parallel alignment of the left disc to the septum[130-133] **(Video 20–7).**

DILATOR-ASSISTED TECHNIQUE (WAHAB TECHNIQUE)

After deployment of the left atrial disc, a long dilator (usually the length of the delivery sheath being used) is advanced into the left atrium by an assistant to hold the superior anterior part of the left atrial disc and prevent it from prolapsing into the right atrium, while the operator continues to deploy the waist and right atrial disc in their respective locations. Once the right disc is deployed in the right atrium, the assistant withdraws the dilator back to the right atrium.[134]

BALLOON-ASSISTED TECHNIQUE

Dalvi et al reported a new balloon-assisted technique to facilitate device closure of large ASDs and to prevent prolapsing of the left disc into the right atrium **(Figure 20–23)**.[135] In essence, it is similar in concept to the dilator technique. In this technique a second wire is placed in the left upper pulmonary vein, and a Meditech balloon (Boston Scientific, Natick, Mass.) or Equalizer balloon (Boston Scientific) is positioned in the right atrial side of the atrial septum. During device deployment, the balloon catheter is used to support the left atrial disc of the ASO, preventing its prolapse into the right atrium. The right atrial disc is then deployed, and the balloon is deflated and retracted along with the second wire. All 14 patients in this report with the median ASD stretched size of 32 mm (range 26 to 40 mm) had successful deployment of the device using this technique.[135]

ATRIAL SEPTAL DEFECT AND PULMONARY HYPERTENSION

Evaluation of PVR is an important step before ASD closure. PVR is calculated using the ratio of the transpulmonary

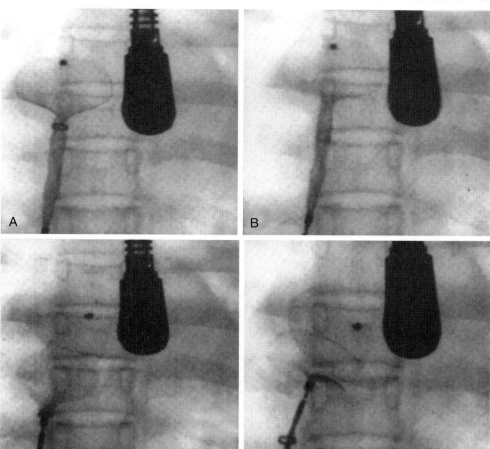

Figure 20–22 Right upper pulmonary vein technique. Deployment of the atrial septal defect device is initiated in the right upper pulmonary vein to obtain better alignment with the atrial septum.

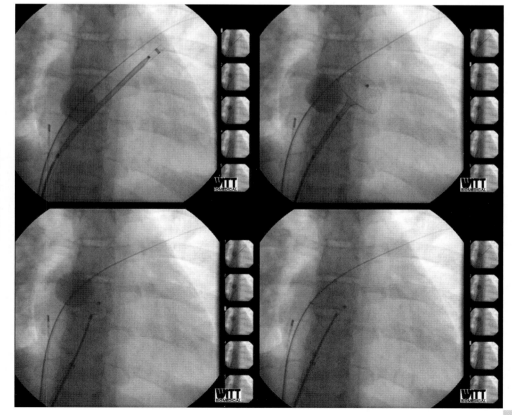

Figure 20–23 Balloon-assisted technique. Sequential deployment of the atrial septal defect device with the use of an Equalizer balloon. The balloon is positioned in the atrial septum over a second wire. Once the device is deployed and before release, the balloon and wire are retracted across the atrial septum and position is confirmed.

gradient to the indexed pulmonary blood flow and is depicted in Woods Units/m^2

$$\frac{\text{Mean pulmonary artery pressure (mmHg)} - \text{Mean pulmonary capillary wedge pressure (mmHg)}}{\text{Indexed Qp L/m}^2}$$

ASD closure is indicated for all symptomatic patients with net left-to-right shunt and resting O_2 saturations greater than 92%. If there is a bidirectional shunt, then pulmonary vasodilator testing should be performed. If there is a net left-to-right shunt on vasodilation or test occlusion of ASD shows a favorable response with a fall in mean PA pressures with no decrease in cardiac output and no increase in right atrial pressures, then the ASD should be closed. In the absence of a favorable response, the patient can be given pulmonary vasodilators and reassessed in the cardiac catheterization lab after 6 months. Borderline cases may benefit from fenestrated ASD device closure, although there are no studies to document improved survival with this approach. The fenestration can be achieved by perforating the polyester fabric of the Amplatzer ASO device before implantation. A 4F-5F dilator can be used to achieve an adequate fenestration. Another technique that has been used is to perforate the Amplatzer ASO device with a stiff wire and run a coronary wire through the perforation before loading. The device is then loaded with the wire in place and deployed in the ASD. Then a coronary stent is advanced over the wire and deployed within the device to create a fenestration **(Figure 20–24)**.

Balint et al reported a study in 2008 in which 54 patients with moderate (50 to 59 mmHg) (n = 34) or severe PAH (60 mmHg) (n = 20) underwent successful device implantation between 1999 and 2004.[136] At the early follow-up examination (mean 2.3 months) all patients were alive, and the baseline right ventricular systolic pressure (RVSP) decreased from 57 mmHg to 51 mmHg (p = 0.003). At the late follow-up examination (n = 39, mean [SD] duration 31 [15] months), two patients had died, and the baseline RVSP decreased from 58 mmHg to 44 mmHg (p = 0.004). Although the overall mean RVSP decreased at a later follow-up examination, only 43.6% (17/39) of patients had normalization (<40 mmHg) of the RVSP and 15.4% (6/39) had persistent severe PAH.[117,137]

MULTIPLE ATRIAL SEPTAL DEFECTS AND MULTIFENESTRATED DEFECTS

It is common to encounter either multiple small ASDs or a multifenestrated defect. The technique of closure varies slightly for these defects. In the presence of multiple ASDs it is necessary to evaluate the distance between the defects in multiple planes by echocardiography. This helps in assessing their spatial relationship to attempt closure with a single device versus multiple devices. Most defects within 7 mm of each other can be closed by a single device. Balloon sizing of individual defects can be performed to help with closure **(Figure 20–25)**. In the presence of a floppy septum between two defects, balloon stretching/device placement in a defect might cause the septum to shift and effectively close the other defect. If the two defects are in remote locations, more than one device can be used **(Figures 20–26 and 20–27, Video 20–8)**. These defects can be closed in succession or assessed with simultaneous balloon sizing and closure of the defect. It is advisable to first close the smaller defect but not release the device, and then close the larger defect with the aim of overlapping the smaller device with the larger device. It is also recommended that wire access be maintained through both defects during the

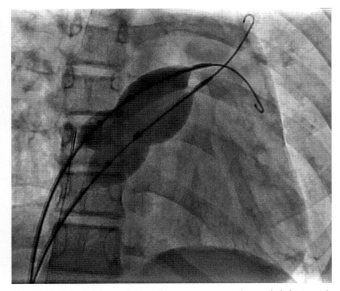

Figure 20–24 Fenestrated atrial septal defect creation with premounting a coronary stent within an Amplatzer device. Color Doppler shows flow through the stent.

Figure 20–25 Balloon sizing of two remote atrial septal defects with two separate balloons.

procedure because closure of one defect may make reaccessing the second defect difficult. The smaller device is released before the larger device. Multiple fenestrations are commonly encountered along the posteroinferior portion of the atrial septum. If the fossa ovalis itself has multiple fenestrations, then use of a non–self-centering device such as the HELEX device or the Amplatz Cribriform device is appropriate. In some ASDs, part of the margin can be thin and flimsy and contain perforations or even small ASDs. Provided there is sufficient firm septal tissue to anchor an ASO, this is of little consequence because the thin septal tissue is pushed aside and contained between the two atrial discs, thus occluding any small adjacent ASDs.

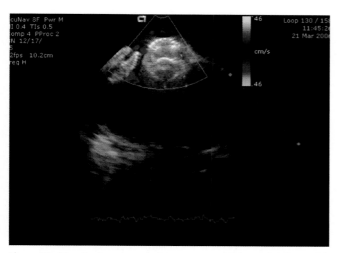

Figure 20–26 Device closure of two remote atrial septal defects with two separate Amplatzer atrial septal occluder devices. Color Doppler evaluation shows no residual shunt.

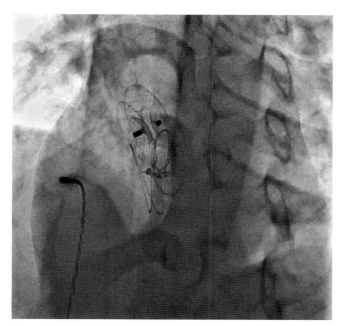

Figure 20–27 Fluoroscopy image in left anterior oblique cranial projection shows an Amplatzer atrial septal occluder device and a HELEX device used to close two separate atrial septal defects.

20.13 Deployment Problems with the Atrial Septal Occluder Device

There can be herniation of a Chiari network into the left atrium during advancement of the delivery sheath across the ASD. If unrecognized, this complication can result in difficulties in deploying the device. If this complication is suspected, the guidewire and sheath should be pulled back into the right atrium with subsequent recrossing of the ASD. Another potential problem is entrapment of a redundant eustachian valve by the occluder device. A redundant eustachian valve may extend between the IVC and the ASD and interfere with deployment of the device. McMahon et al[138] reported four cases where this problem was overcome by placing a steerable radiofrequency ablation catheter into the right atrium from the femoral vein. Under TEE guidance, the tip of the steerable catheter was deflected anteriorly and laterally to displace the eustachian valve against the lateral right atrial wall, thereby allowing free passage of the septal occluder.

TWISTING OF DEVICE: COBRA HEAD MALFORMATION

During deployment of the ASO, the left atrial disc rotates as it exits the delivery sheath and returns to its inherent shape. Likewise, the central waist and right atrial disc rotate as they exit the catheter. If these rotatory movements are impeded in any way, such as by opening the left atrial disc in the left atrial appendage or in the orifice of a pulmonary vein, the device may twist and assume a "cobra head" appearance as the delivery sheath is withdrawn. This is recognized by a distortion of the left atrial pin away from the axis of the left atrial disc and by failure of the left atrial arm to flatten as it is pulled into the septum; the device should be withdrawn back into the delivery sheath, and redeployment should be attempted. This can happen with the right atrial disc as well, in which case the relaxation technique of releasing tension might help reform the device. There might be failure of the device to collapse into the delivery sheath. This might warrant changing to a large bailout sheath over the delivery cable to enable recapture. The Amplatzer exchange system is intended for removal of an Amplatzer delivery sheath and subsequent exchange of an Amplatzer delivery sheath of equal or larger diameter. This bail-out mechanism is a delivery system especially adapted for use in conjunction with the Amplatzer family of occlusion devices. The system components are identical to the Amplatzer delivery system, with the exception of the dilator, which incorporates an enlarged inner lumen for passage over an Amplatzer delivery cable. The bail-out system consists of a delivery sheath, a dilator, and a delivery cable. The cable consists of a thread-on capsule located on the proximal end of the cable and permits connection of two delivery cables, thus lengthening the system for exchange of the existing delivery sheath with the bail-out sheath. The bail-out sheath can then be used for device recapture and delivery.

20.4 Complications

AIR EMBOLISM

Several important complications that may be seen with ASD/PFO are air embolism during the procedure, device positioning problems, device embolization, postprocedure device thrombosis, and atrial arrhythmias. Air embolism can be rare but is potentially lethal. The use of large-bore catheters placed in the pulmonary vein or left atrium have the potential to introduce air. This is especially true in a sedated adult with obstructive sleep disease causing high negative inspiratory pressure in the atrium. These patients might need continuous positive airway pressure or bilevel positive airway pressure during the procedure to avoid this complication. Embolization of air occurs immediately with clinical manifestations that most commonly are coronary but also can involve the central nervous system circulation. Air embolism is more likely to the right coronary artery because of the anterior and superior nature in a supine patient. The most common manifestation of air embolism is ST elevation on monitored electrocardiographic leads. Other manifestations of ischemia may follow immediately, including chest pain (unless the patient is under general anesthesia), sinus bradycardia, heart block, and other arrhythmias. Confusion or focal neurologic deficits may indicate air embolism to the brain. Although permanent sequelae are rare, the rapid transition from a coherent, calm, and comfortable patient to one who has severe pain and life-threatening arrhythmia is dramatic. The duration of the ischemia is brief; improvement is apparent within a few minutes, and complete resolution occurs in 5 to 10 minutes. Supplemental oxygen, analgesia, and volume expansion are general measures that may be beneficial. In the case of air embolism to the right coronary artery, some operators recommend transitioning the patient to prone position. In the presence of significant air embolism, there is role for air embolectomy using an end-hole catheter. Treatment of arrhythmias should follow standard practices. Atropine for severe sinus bradycardia or heart block is the main medication that should be readied after the initial ST elevation is recognized. Prompt defibrillation should be available. Some additional technical tips can minimize air embolism during the insertion of the delivery catheter or sheath. The first is preprocedure hydration for the patient who is fasting. The second tip is to keep the proximal end of the delivery catheter/sheath below the level of the left atrium if possible. This adds hydrostatic pressure to the column of fluid and blood in the catheter and prevents air entry. Flushing of the side port of a delivery sheath during withdrawal of the dilator is used by some cardiologists to reduce the chance of air entry during the negative pressure in the catheter that can be created by the removal of the dilator. Fluoroscopy can be performed briefly to see if an air bubble is being pushed during flushing of the sheath or during advancement of the device in the delivery catheter.

POSITIONING PROBLEMS AND EMBOLIZATION

Device positioning problems during deployment include prolapse of a portion of the device to the incorrect side of the interatrial septum, incomplete expansion of the device, poor coaptation of the device to the interatrial septum, and tunnel-related incomplete expansion of both sides of the device during closure of PFO. These problems can be recognized with a combination of fluoroscopic and echocardiographic images during deployment. Removal of the device may be necessary.

Device embolization is rare with PFO closure; it has been reported most commonly in the setting of large ASDs, with undersized ASD devices, and in malfunction of the device-delivery cable attachment. Device embolization is more commonly into right-sided chambers, given the interatrial pressure gradient. All operators who use the ASO should be prepared to perform percutaneous device retrieval in the event of a device embolization. After device embolization, the first objective is simply to get the device into a position in which it will not cause harm. The device may be stabilized and moved with a snare or a bioptome. Most commonly, the device is malpositioned in the atrial septum or in one of the atria. For select cases of devices embolized to the left atrium or malpositioned in the atrial septum, it may be possible to reposition the device into proper position by pulling the right atrial disc into the right atrium with a snare. In general, devices that embolize to the atria should be stabilized to prevent migration to the ventricles either using a wire or bioptome. The next objective is to snare the microscrew on the ASO right atrial disc. Retrieval is not possible via snaring the knob on the left atrial disc. The device must be oriented such that the right atrial disc is accessible, and a gooseneck snare should be secured around the base of the screw mechanism. A bioptome cannot pull the right atrial disc screw with enough force to pull a device into a sheath but may aid retrieval if used to place tension from above (via a right internal jugular sheath) on the left atrial disc. A 15- or 20-mm snare (Amplatz Gooseneck Snare Kit, ev3, Plymouth, Minn.) may be advanced through the long sheath alongside the bioptome, or an additional venous sheath may be placed. Once the microscrew is snared, the bioptome may be removed, and the device can be pulled into the sheath. Some operators recommend pulling the device from the right atrium into the IVC below the kidneys to elongate the device and limit the migration. Once in the low IVC, a stiff wire can be placed via the implant sheath through the device, and its tip can be carefully advanced into the SVC to further stabilize it and limit the device's ability to migrate. The retrieval sheath chosen should be at least 2 F sizes larger than the implant sheath. One can also use a sheath 1 F size larger and then modify the tip by cutting a bevel at the tip of the sheath to increase its circumference. Once engaging the snared device, care should be taken to rotate the sheath so it will engage the screw better, or use a bioptome from the internal jugular vein to better orient, elongate, and place tension on the device. If a device migrates across the tricuspid valve or mitral valve, it is not recommended to pull the device retrograde across an AV valve. In order to avoid entangling the device in the valve apparatus, it may be removed through a long sheath within the ventricle, or it may be moved antegrade across the semilunar valve and retrieved through a long sheath in the pulmonary artery or through a sheath in the systemic artery using the technique described previously. Orientation of the microscrew may be improved by snaring it with two loop snares through the long sheath, allowing easier retraction into the sheath. Furthermore, although bare venous retrieval of a device has been successfully performed, it is not recommended because of the risks involved to the iliac and femoral veins as well as the risk of retroperitoneal hemorrhage. Amplatzer devices may be reused after retrieval and inspection.

The first step in the retrieval strategy for CardioSEAL and STARFlex devices is similar to that previously described for the various Amplatzer devices. The embolized device should be stabilized with the use of a wire, snare, or bioptome to prevent passage through the AV valves. A 90% retrieval rate, either through a sheath or via cut-down, has been reported. The HELEX device has a white retrieval cord that allows for easy retrieval of a device that does not lock appropriately. A device that is not locked can also be easily retrieved with a snare and the HELEX delivery sheath. Devices that are locked are much more difficult to retrieve. Snaring of the left atrial eyelet, which is attached to the locking loop, is necessary for successful retrieval. The locking loop that holds the device together originates from the left atrial side; thus pulling the device from this side unlocks the lock mechanism and permits the device to unravel. When this strategy is used for device retrieval, the right atrial eyelet is the last part of the device to be pulled into the rescue sheath. The right atrial eyelet wire loop, per benchtop reports, can get caught on the end of the sheath in many of the retrieval attempts.

POSTPROCEDURE ARRHYTHMIAS

Postprocedure atrial arrhythmias occur in 3% to 4% of patients. Routine monitoring probably would detect more. Most patients who have this complication detected have symptoms that require medical attention. Palpitations and an irregular pulse are the most common symptoms. Some reports suggest that this complication occurs most commonly 4 to 6 weeks postoperatively. Other patients may have immediate postprocedure premature atrial contractions that often are asymptomatic and resolve spontaneously. The atrial arrhythmias that occur later often are symptomatic, include atrial fibrillation, and may not resolve spontaneously. Management is routine and may include β-blockers, cardioversion, or other medications to manage ventricular response and to maintain normal sinus rhythm. Cardioversion before endothelialization of the device has the potential risk of device embolization.

DEVICE THROMBOSIS

Device thrombosis is a major complication that can lead to catastrophic events such as embolization of

thrombus, the need for open heart surgery for device removal, and prolonged hospitalization for thrombolysis. It remains a rare and poorly understood complication. The unresolved issues include the frequency of this complication, whether underlying hypercoagulable states increase its frequency, whether the different devices have a different thrombogenicity, and whether more aggressive postimplantation anticoagulation regimens should be used routinely. Thrombi on right and left atrial sides of the device have been reported. A large and loose-appearing left-sided thrombus may prompt a surgical removal approach, whereas a right-sided thrombus may lead to a pharmacologic route of treatment. The management of device thrombosis is similar to that of prosthetic valve thrombosis. Only isolated case studies have been reported; therefore management remains highly individualized. In the presence of prothrombotic conditions special attention should be paid to anticoagulation with use of dual agents: warfarin and an antiplatelet drug.

DEVICE EROSION

A total of 28 cases (14 in the United States) of adverse events were reported to AGA Medical. All erosions occurred at the dome of the atria near the aortic root. Deficient aortic rim (<5 mm) was seen in 89%, and the defect was described as high ASD, suggesting deficient superior rim. The device-to-unstretched ASD ratio was significantly larger (148% larger) in the adverse event group when compared with the FDA trial group (138% larger).[117,139] The incidence of device erosion in the United States was 0.1%. The risk of device erosion with the ASO is low, and complications can be decreased by identifying high-risk patients and monitoring their conditions closely. This review suggested that the anterosuperior atrial walls and/or adjacent aorta are uniquely vulnerable; the side of the larger ASO disc does not predict site of cardiac perforation; and trauma over multiple cardiac cycles can damage even the thicker, more resilient aortic wall. Patients with deficient aortic rim and/or superior rim may be at higher risk for device erosion. An oversized ASO may increase the risk of erosion. The defect should not be overstretched during balloon sizing. Patients with small pericardial effusion at 24 hours should have closer follow-up examination. The rounded design and flexibility of the ASO are speculated to minimize risk of cardiac perforation, even when oversized. An occlusion device within confines of the anteroposterior septal length is subjected to deformation forces.

FATIGUE FRACTURES

Fatigue fractures are not reported with the ASO, and the discs retain their preformed shape; Fagan et al reported a study examining the factors associated with, and clinical effects of, wire frame fractures (WFFs) of the GORE HELEX septal occluder.[140] Of the 298 HELEX implants, 90% of subjects were studied for more than 12 months, 19/298 (6.4%) patients with the HELEX device implanted were found to have WFF. Univariate predictors of WFF were large device size ($p = .0003$) and balloon defect size ($p = .001$); however, large device size ($p = .0003$) was the only significant predictor of WFF by multivariate analysis. WFFs of the 30-mm and 35-mm HELEX accounted for 84% (16/19) of all WFFs. Review of HELEX images with WFFs revealed all WFFs except one (straight portion of locking loop) occurred along the circumferential wire. There were no clinical sequelae resulting from WFF; however, secondary to right atrial disc mobility, the HELEX with locking loop WFF was percutaneously removed 6 weeks after implantation.[140]

20.5 Summary

Transcatheter closure of most ASDs and PFOs in adults has been demonstrated to be a feasible and safe alternative to surgical closure. Although transcatheter closure should be considered the treatment of choice in most cases of intracardiac defect repair in adults, there are special circumstances in which either surgical repair or deferral of any repair should be strongly considered. Furthermore, thorough preprocedural planning and defect evaluation with both 2D and 3D imaging techniques, advances in device and delivery system design, increased operator experience through both simulation training and live cases, and utilization of novel technologies such as rapid prototyping will hopefully continue to advance the field and ultimately allow transcatheter closure of most intracardiac defects in adults to become a mainstay of interventional laboratories.

REFERENCES

1. Hara H, Virmani R, Ladich E, et al: Patent foramen ovale: current pathology, pathophysiology, and clinical status, J Am Coll Cardiol 46(9):1768–1776, 2005 Nov 1.
2. Hagen PT, Scholz DG, Edwards WD: Incidence and size of patent foramen ovale during the first 10 decades of life: an autopsy study of 965 normal hearts, Mayo Clin Proc 59:17–20, 1984.
3. Wilmshurst PT, Pearson MJ, Nightingale S, et al: Inheritance of persistent foramen ovale and atrial septal defects and the relation to familial migraine with aura, Heart 90(11):1315–1320, 2004 Nov.
4. Kerut EK, Norfleet WT, Plotnick GD, et al: Patent foramen ovale: a review of associated conditions and the impact of physiological size, J Am Coll Cardiol 38:613–623, 2001.
5. Ho SY, McCarthy KP, Rigby ML: Morphological features pertinent to interventional closure of patent oval foramen, J Interv Cardiol 16:33–38, 2003.
6. Olivares-Reyes A, Chan S, Lazar EJ, et al: Atrial septal aneurysm: a new classification in two hundred five adults, J Am Soc Echocardiogr 10:644–656, 1997.
7. Marazanof M, Roudaut R, Cohen A, et al: Atrial septal aneurysm: morphological characteristics in a large population—pathological associations. A French multicenter study on 259 patients investigated by transoesophageal echocardiography, Int J Cardiol 52:59–65, 1995.
8. Homma S, Di Tullio MR, Sacco RL, et al: Characteristics of patent foramen ovale associated with cryptogenic stroke: a biplane transesophageal echocardiographic study, Stroke 25:582–586, 1994.
9. Schuchlenz HW, Weihs W, Horner S, et al: The association between the diameter of a patent foramen ovale and the risk of embolic cerebrovascular events, Am J Med 109:456–462, 2000.
10. De Castro S, Cartoni D, Fiorelli M, et al: Morphological and functional characteristics of patent foramen ovale and their embolic implications, Stroke 31:2407–2413, 2000.
11. Silver MD, Dorsey JS: Aneurysms of the septum primum in adults, Arch Pathol Lab Med 102:62–65, 1978.
12. Werner JA, Cheitlin MD, Gross BW, et al: Echocardiographic appearance of the Chiari network: differentiation from right-heart pathology, Circulation 63:1104–1109, 1981.
13. Chiari H: About network development in the right side of the heart, Beitr Pathol Anat 22:1–10, 1897.
14. Schneider B, Hofmann T, Justen MH, et al: Chiari's network: normal anatomic variant or risk factor for arterial embolic events? J Am Coll Cardiol 26:203–210, 1995.
15. Pinto FJ: When and how to diagnose patent foramen ovale, Heart 91:438–440, 2005.
16. Pearson AC, Labovitz AJ, Tatineni S, et al: Superiority of transesophageal echocardiography in detecting cardiac source of embolism in patients with cerebral ischemia of uncertain etiology, J Am Coll Cardiol 17:66–72, 1991.
17. Teague SM, Sharma MK: Detection of paradoxical cerebral echo contrast embolization by transcranial Doppler ultrasound, Stroke 22:740–745, 1991.
18. Sloan MA, Alexandrov AV, Tegeler CH, et al: Assessment: transcranial Doppler ultrasonography: report of the Therapeutics and Technology Assessment Subcommittee of the American Academy of Neurology, Neurology 62:1468–1481, 2004.
19. Blersch WK, Draganski BM, Holmer SR, et al: Transcranial duplex sonography in the detection of patent foramen ovale, Radiology 225:693–699, 2002.
20. Kerr AJ, Buck T, Chia K, et al: Transmitral Doppler: a new transthoracic contrast method for patent foramen ovale detection and quantification, J Am Coll Cardiol 36:1959–1966, 2000.
21. Di Tullio M, Sacco RL, Venketasubramanian N, et al: Comparison of diagnostic techniques for the detection of a patent foramen ovale in stroke patients, Stroke 24:1020–1024, 1993.
22. Lynch JJ, Schuchard GH, Gross CM, Wann LS: Prevalence of right-to-left atrial shunting in a healthy population: detection by Valsalva maneuver contrast echocardiography, Am J Cardiol 53:1478–1480, 1984.
23. Cohnheim J: A general pathologic lecture. Thrombosis and Embolism, Berlin, 1877, Marzhouzer, pp 134–137.
24. Zahn FW: Thrombose de plusieurs branches de la veine cave inférieure avec embolies consécutives dans les artéres pulmonaire, splénique, rénale et iliaque droite [French], Rev Med Suisse Romande 1:227–237, 1881.
25. Lechat P, Mas JL, Lascault G, et al: Prevalence of patent foramen ovale in patients with stroke, N Engl J Med 318:1148–1152, 1988.
26. Lamy C, Giannesini C, Zuber M, et al: Clinical and imaging findings in cryptogenic stroke patients with and without patent foramen ovale: the PFO-ASA Study; atrial septal aneurysm, Stroke 33:706–711, 2002.
27. Cramer SC, Rordorf G, Maki JH, et al: Increased pelvic vein thrombi in cryptogenic stroke: results of the Paradoxical Emboli from Large Veins in Ischemic Stroke (PELVIS) study, Stroke 35:46–50, 2004.
28. Mas JL, Arquizan C, Lamy C, et al: Recurrent cerebrovascular events associated with patent foramen ovale, atrial septal aneurysm, or both, N Engl J Med 345:1740–1746, 2001.
29. Overell JR, Bone I, Lees KR: Interatrial septal abnormalities and stroke: a meta-analysis of case-control studies, Neurology 55:1172–1179, 2000.
30. Meissner I, Whisnant JP, Khandheria BK, et al: Prevalence of potential risk factors for stroke assessed by transesophageal echocardiography and carotid ultrasonography: the SPARC study, Mayo Clin Proc 74:862–869, 1999.
31. Medina A, de Lezo JS, Caballero E, et al: Platypneaorthodeoxia due to aortic elongation, Circulation 104:741, 2001.
32. Cheng TO: Mechanisms of platypneaorthodeoxia: what causes water to flow uphill? Circulation 105:e47, 2002.
33. Wilmshurst PT, Ellis BG, Jenkins BS: Paradoxical gas embolism in a scuba diver with an atrial septal defect, Br Med J (Clin Res Ed) 293:1277, 1986.
34. Torti SR, Billinger M, Schwerzmann M, et al: Risk of decompression illness among 230 divers in relation to the presence and size of patent foramen ovale, Eur Heart J 25:1014–1020, 2004.
35. Cartoni D, De Castro S, Valente G, et al: Identification of professional scuba divers with patent foramen ovale at risk for decompression illness, Am J Cardiol 94:270–273, 2004.
36. Wahl A, Praz F, Tai T, et al: Improvement of migraine headaches after percutaneous closure of patent foramen ovale for secondary prevention of paradoxical embolism, Heart 96(12):967–973, 2010 Jun.
37. Anzola GP, Magoni M, Guindani M, et al: Potential source of cerebral embolism in migraine with aura: a transcranial Doppler study, Neurology 52:1622–1625, 1999.
38. Morandi E, Anzola GP, Angeli S, et al: Transcatheter closure of patent foramen ovale: a new migraine treatment? J Interv Cardiol 16:39–42, 2003.
39. Reisman M, Christofferson RD, Jesurum J, et al: Migraine headache relief after transcatheter closure of patent foramen ovale, J Am Coll Cardiol 45:493–495, 2005.
40. Goldstein LB, Adams R, Alberts MJ, et al. Primary prevention of ischemic stroke: a guideline from the American Heart Association/American Stroke Association Stroke Council: cosponsored by the Atherosclerotic Peripheral Vascular Disease Interdisciplinary Working Group; Cardiovascular Nursing Council; Clinical Cardiology Council; Nutrition, Physical Activity, and Metabolism Council; and the Quality of Care and Outcomes Research Interdisciplinary Working Group [published correction appears in Circulation]. 114:e617, 2006.
41. Sacco RL, Adams R, Albers G, et al: Guidelines for prevention of stroke in patients with ischemic stroke or transient ischemic attack: a statement for healthcare professionals from the American Heart Association/American Stroke Association Council on Stroke: co-sponsored by the Council on Cardiovascular Radiology and Intervention, Circulation 113: 2006, e409–ee49.

42. Furlan AJ, Reisman M, Massaro J, et al: Closure or medical therapy for cryptogenic stroke with patent foramen ovale for the CLOSURE I investigators, N Engl J Med 366:991–999, 2012.
43. Bridges ND, Hellenbrand W, Latson L, et al: Transcatheter closure of patent foramen ovale after presumed paradoxical embolism, Circulation 86:1902–1908, 1992.
44. Maisel WH, Laskey WK: Patent foramen ovale closure devices: moving beyond equipoise, JAMA 294:366–369, 2005.
45. Hong TE, Thaler D, Brorson J, et al: Transcatheterclosure of patent foramen ovale associated with paradoxical embolism using the Amplatzer PFO occluder: initial and intermediate-term results of the U.S. multicenter clinical trial, Catheter Cardiovasc Interv 60:524–528, 2003.
46. Fischer D, Haentjes J, Klein G, et al: Transcatheter closure of patent foramen ovale (PFO) in patients with paradoxical embolism: procedural and follow-up results after implantation of the Amplatzer occluder device, J Interv Cardiol 24:85–91, 2011.
47. Alameddine F, Block PC: Transcatheter patent foramen ovale closure for secondary prevention of paradoxical embolic events: acute results from the FORECAST registry, Catheter Cardiovasc Interv 62(4):512–516, 2004 Aug.
48. Sigler M, Jux C: Biocompatibility of septal defect closure devices, Heart 93(4):444–449, 2007.
49. Sherman JM, Hagler DJ, Cetta F: Thrombosis after septal closure device placement: a review of the current literature, Catheter Cardiovasc Interv 63(4):486–489, 2004.
50. Krumsdorf U, Ostermayer S, Billinger K, et al: Incidence and clinical course of thrombus formation on atrial septal defect and patient foramen ovale closure devices in 1,000 consecutive patients, J Am Coll Cardiol 43(2):302–309, 2004.
51. Jux C, Bertram H, Wohlsein P, et al: Interventional atrial septal defect closure using a totally bioresorbable occluder matrix: development and preclinical evaluation of the BioSTAR device, J Am Coll Cardiol 48(1):161–169, 2006.
52. Jux C, Wohlsein P, Bruegmann M, et al: A new biological matrix for septal occlusion, J Interv Cardiol 16(2):149–152, 2003.
53. Zahn EM, Wilson N, Cutright W, et al: Development and testing of the Helex septal occluder: a new expanded polytetrafluoroethylene atrial septal defect occlusion system, Circulation 104(6):711–716, 2001 Aug 7.
54. Ponnuthurai FA, van Gaal WJ, Burchell A, et al: Single centre experience with GORE-HELEX septal occluder for closure of PFO, Heart Lung Circ 18:140–142, 2009.
55. Rigatelli G, Cardaioli P, Dell'avvocata F, et al: Premere occlusion system for transcatheter patent foramen ovale closure: midterm results of a single-center registry, Catheter Cardiovasc Interv 77(4):564–569, 2011 Mar 1.
56. Reiffenstein I, Majunke N, Wunderlich N, et al: Percutaneous closure of patent foramen ovale with a novel FlatStent, Expert Rev Med Devices 5(4):419–425, 2008 Jul.
57. Spies C, Strasheim R, Timmermanns I, et al: Patent foramen ovale closure in patients with cryptogenic thromboembolic events using the Cardia PFO occluder, Eur Heart J 27(3):365–371, 2006.
58. Kretschmar O, Sglimbea A, Daehnert I, et al: Interventional closure of atrial septal defects with the Solysafe Septal Occluder: preliminary results in children, Int J Cardiol 143(3):373–377, 2010 Sep 3.
59. Krizanic F, Sievert H, Pfeiffer D, et al: The Occlutech Figulla PFO and ASD occluder: a new nitinol wire mesh device for closure of atrial septal defects, J Invasive Cardiol 22(4):182–187, 2010 Apr.
60. Zimmermann WJ, Heinisch C, Majunke N, et al: Patent foramen ovale closure with the SeptRx device initial experience with the first "In-Tunnel" device, JACC Cardiovasc Interv 3(9):963–967, 2010 Sep.
61. Ruiz CE, Kipshidze N, Chiam PT, et al: Feasibility of patent foramen ovale closure with no device left behind: first-in-man percutaneous suture closure, Catheter Cardiovasc Interv 71:921–926, 2008.
62. Majunke N, Sievert H: ASD/PFO devices: what is in the pipeline? J Interv Cardiol 20:517–523, 2007.
63. Sievert H, Ruygrok P, Salkeld M, et al: Transcatheter closure of patent foramen ovale with radiofrequency: acute and intermediate term results in 144 patients, Catheter Cardiovasc Interv 73:368–373, 2008.
64. Spence MS, Khan AA, Mullen MJ: Balloon assessment of patent foramen ovale morphology and the modification of tunnels using a balloon detunnelisation technique, Catheter Cardiovasc Interv 71:222–228, 2008.
65. Rigatelli G, Dell'Avvocata F, Giordan M, et al: Transcatheter patent foramen ovale closure in spite of interatrial septum hypertrophy or lipomatosis: a case series, J Cardiovasc Med (Hagerstown) 11:91–95, 2010.
66. Lin CH, Balzer DT, Lasala JM: Defect closure in the lipomatous hypertrophied atrial septum with the Amplatzer muscular ventricular septal defect closure device: a case series, Catheter Cardiovasc Interv 78(1):102–107, 2011 Jul 1.
67. Hoffman JL: Incidence of congenital heart disease. I. Postnatal incidence, Pediatr Cardiol 16:103–113, 1995.
68. Hoffman JI, Kaplan S, Liberthson RR: Prevalence of congenital heartdisease, Am Heart J 147:425–439, 2004.
69. English RF, Anderson RH, Ettedgui JA: Interatrial communications. In Anderson RH, Baker EJ, Redington A, et al, editors: Paediatric Cardiology, ed 3, London: Churchill Livingstone, 2010, pp 523–546.
70. Ferreira MJ, Anderson RH: The anatomy of interatrial communications: what does the interventionist need to know? Cardiol Young 10:464–473, 2000.
71. Rigatelli G, Rigatelli G: Congenital heart diseases in aged patients: clinical features, diagnosis, and therapeutic indications based on the analysis of a twenty five-year Medline search, Cardiol Rev 13:293–296, 2005.
72. Warnes CA, Williams RG, Bashore TM, et al: Writing Committee to Develop Guidelines on the Management of Adults With Congenital Heart Disease. Atrial septal defect. In ACC/AHA 2008 guidelines for the management of adults with congenital heart disease: report of the American College of Cardiology/American Heart Association Task Force on Practice Guidelines, Circulation 118:e714–e833, 2008.
73. Webb G, Gatzoulis MA: Atrial septal defects in the adult: recent progress and overview, Circulation 114:1645–1653, 2006.
74. Sommer RJ, Hijazi ZM, Rhodes JF Jr: Pathophysiology of congenital heart disease in the adult. I. Shunt lesions, Circulation 117:1090–1099, 2008.
75. Gatzoulis MA, Redington AN, Somerville J, et al: Should atrial septal defects in adults be closed? Ann Thorac Surg 61(2):657–659, 1996 Feb.
76. Berdjis F, Brandl D, Uhlemann F, et al: [Adults with congenital heart defects: clinical spectrum and surgical management], Herz 21(5):330–336, 1996 Oct.
77. Craig RJ, Selzer A: Natural history and prognosis of atrial septal defect, Circulation 37:805–815, 1968.
78. Booth DC, Wisenbaugh T, Smith M, et al: Left ventricular distensibility and passive elastic stiffness in atrial septal defect, J Am Coll Cardiol 12:1231–1236, 1988.
79. Benefit of atrial septal defect closure in adults: impact of age, Eur Heart J 32:553–560, 2011.
80. Delgado V, van der Kley F, Schalij MJ, et al: Optimal imaging for planning and guiding interventions in structural heart disease: a multimodality imaging approach, Eur Heart J Suppl 12(suppl E):E10–E23, 2010.
81. Mehta RH, Helmcke F, Nanda NC, et al: Uses and limitations of transthoracic echocardiography in the assessment of atrial septal defect in the adult, Am J Cardiol 67(4):288–294, 1991 Feb 1.
82. Hausmann D, Daniel WG, Mügge A, et al: Value of transesophageal color Doppler echocardiography for detection of different types of atrial septal defect in adults, J Am Soc Echocardiogr 5(5):481–488, 1992 Sep-Oct.
83. Masani ND: Transoesophageal echocardiography in adult congenital heart disease, Heart 86(Suppl 2):II30–II40, 2001.
84. Chen FL, Hsiung MC, Hsieh KS, et al: Real time three-dimensional transthoracic echocardiography for guiding Amplatzer septal occluder device deployment in patients with atrial septal defect, Echocardiography 23(9):763–770, 2006 Oct.
85. Johri AM, Passeri JJ, Picard MH: Three dimensional echocardiography: approaches and clinical utility, Heart 96:390–397, 2010.
86. Johri AM, Witzke C, Solis J, et al: Real-time three-dimensional transesophageal echocardiography in patients with secundum atrial septal defects: outcomes following transcatheter closure, J Am Soc Echocardiogr 24:431–437, 2011.
87. Holmvang G, Palacios IF, Vlahakes GJ, et al: Imaging and sizing of atrial septal defects by magnetic resonance, Circulation 92:3473–3480, 1995.
88. Kilner PJ, Geva T, Kaemmerer H, et al: Recommendations for cardiovascular magnetic resonance in adults with congenital heart disease from the respective working groups of the European Society of Cardiology, Eur Heart J 31(7):794–805, 2010 Apr. Epub 2010 Jan 11.
89. Johri AM, Rojas CA, El-Sherief A, et al: Imaging of atrial septal defects: echocardiography and CT correlation, Heart 97(17):1441–1453, 2011 Sep.
90. Kort HW, Balzer DT, Johnson MC: Resolution of right heart enlargement after closure of secundum atrial septal defect with transcatheter technique, J Am Coll Cardiol 38:1528–1532, 2001.
91. Schussler JM, Anwar A, Phillips SD, et al: Effect on right ventricular volume of percutaneous Amplatzer closure of atrial septal defect in adults, Am J Cardiol 95:993–995, 2005.
92. Teo KS, Dundon BK, Molaee P, et al: Percutaneous closure of atrial septal defects leads to normalisation of atrial and ventricular volumes, J Cardiovasc Magn Reson 10:55, 2008.
93. Sun P, Wang ZB, Xu CJ, et al: Echocardiographic and morphological evaluation of the right heart after closure of atrial septal defects, Cardiol Young 18:593–598, 2008.
94. Salehian O, Horlick E, Schwerzmann M, et al: Improvements in cardiac form and function after transcatheter closure of secundum atrial septal defects, J Am Coll Cardiol 45:499–504, 2005.
95. Patel A, Lopez K, Banerjee A, et al: Transcatheter closure of atrial septal defects in adults ≥ 40 years of age: immediate and follow-up results, J Interv Cardiol 20:82–88, 2007.
96. Schoen SP, Kittner T, Bohl S, et al: Transcatheter closure of atrial septal defects improves right ventricular volume, mass, function, pulmonary pressure, and functional class: a magnetic resonance imaging study, Heart 92:821–826, 2006.
97. Wu ET, Akagi T, Taniguchi M, et al: Differences in right and left ventricular remodeling after transcatheter closure of atrial septal defect among adults, Catheter Cardiovasc Interv 69:866–887, 2007.
98. Brochu MC, Baril JF, Dore A, et al: Improvement in exercise capacity in asymptomatic and mildly symptomatic adults after atrial septal defect percutaneous closure, Circulation 106:1821–1826, 2002.
99. Giardini A, Donti A, Specchia S, et al: Recovery kinetics of oxygen uptake is prolonged in adults with an atrial septal defect and improves after transcatheter closure, Am Heart J 147:910–914, 2004.

100. Silversides CK, Siu SC, McLaughlin PR, et al: Symptomatic atrial arrhyth- mias and transcatheter closure of atrial septal defects in adult patients, Heart 90:1194–1198, 2004.
101. Murphy JG, Gersh BJ, McGoon MD, et al: Long-term outcome after surgical repair of isolated atrial septal defect: follow-up at 27-32 years, N Engl J Med 323:1645–1650, 1990.
102. Gatzoulis MA, Freeman MA, Siu SC, et al: Atrial arrhythmia after surgical closure of atrial septal defects in adults, N Engl J Med 340:839–846, 1999.
103. Steele PM, Fuster V, Cohen M, et al: Isolated atrial septal defect with pul- monary vascular obstructive disease: long-term follow-up and prediction of outcome after surgical correction, Circulation 76:1037–1042, 1987.
104. Frost AE, Quinones MA, Zoghbi WA, et al: Reversal of pulmonary hyperten- sion and subsequent repair of atrial septal defect after treatment with con- tinuous intravenous epoprostenol, J Heart Lung Transplant 24:501–503, 2005.
105. Suchon E, Pieculewicz M, Tracz W, et al: Transcatheter closure as an alterna- tive and equivalent method to the surgical treatment of atrial septal defect in adults: comparison of early and late results, Med Sci Monit 15(12):CR612– CR617, 2009 Dec.
106. Du ZD, Hijazi ZM, Kleinman CS, et al: Comparison between transcatheter and surgical closure of secundum atrial septal defect in children and adults: results of a multicenter nonrandomized trial, J Am Coll Cardiol 39(11):1836– 1844, 2002 Jun 5.
107. Rosas M, Zabal C, Garcia-Montes J, Buendia A, et al: Transcatheter versus surgical closure of secundum atrial septal defect in adults: impact of age at intervention—a concurrent matched comparative study, Congenit Heart Dis 2(3):148–155, 2007 May-Jun.
108. King TD, Thompson SL, Steiner C, et al: Secundum atrial septal defect: non- operative closure during cardiac catheterization, JAMA 235:2506–2509, 1976.
109. Koenig P, Cao QL: Echocardiographic guidance of transcatheter closure of atrial septal defects: is intracardiac echocardiography better than trans- esophageal echocardiography? Pediatr Cardiol 26(2):135–139, 2005 Mar-Apr.
110. Boccalandro F, Baptista E, Muench A, et al: Comparison of intracardiac echocardiography versus transesophageal echocardiography guidance for percutaneous transcatheter closure of atrial septal defect, Am J Cardiol 93(4):437–440, 2004 Feb 15.
111. Helgason H, Johansson M, Söderberg B, et al: Sizing of atrial septal defects in adults, Cardiology 104(1):1–5, 2005. Epub 2005 May 24.
112. Carlson KM, Justino H, O'Brien RE, et al: Transcatheter atrial septal defect closure: modified balloon sizing technique to avoid overstretching the de- fect and oversizing the Amplatzer septal occluder, Cathet Cardiovasc Intervent 66:390–396, 2005.
113. Krishnamoorthy KM, Tharakan JA, Ajithkumar AK, et al: Balloon sizing of atrial septal defects, Tex Heart Inst J 29(1):73–74, 2002.
114. Masura J, Gavora P, Formanek A, et al: Transcatheter closure of secundum atrial septal defects using the new self-centering Amplatzer septal occluder: initial human experience, Cathet Cardiovasc Diagn 42:388–390, 1997.
115. Everett AD, Jennings J, Sibinga E, et al: Community use of the amplatzer atrial septal defect occluder: results of the multicenter MAGIC atrial septal defect study, Pediatr Cardiol 30(3):240–247, 2009 Apr.
116. Divekar A, Gaamangwe T, Shaikh N, et al: Cardiac perforation after device closure of atrial septal defects with the Amplatzer septal occluder, J Am Coll Cardiol 45:1213–1218, 2005.
117. Amin Z, Hijazi ZM, Bass JL, et al: Erosion of Amplatzer septal occluder de- vice after closure of secundum atrial septal defects: review of registry of complications and recommendations to minimize future risk, Catheter Car- diovasc Interv 63:496–502, 2004.
118. Rome JJ, Keane JF, Perry SB, et al: Double-umbrella closure of atrial defects: initial clinical applications, Circulation 82:751–758, 1990.
119. Latson LA: The CardioSEAL device: history, techniques, results, J Interv Car- diol 11:501–505, 1998.
120. Rao PS, Berger F, Rey C, et al: Results of transventral defects with the fourth generation buttoned device: comparison with first, second and third gen- eration devices. International Buttoned Device Trial Group, J Am Coll Cardiol 36(2):583–592, 2000.
121. Carminati M, Chessa M, Butera G, et al: Transcatheter closure of atrial septal defects with the STARFlex device: early results and follow-up, J Interv Cardiol 14(3):319–324, 2001 Jun.
122. Carminati M, Giusti S, Hausdorf G, et al: A European multicentric experience using the CardioSeal and Starflex double umbrella devices to close interatri- al communications holes within the oval fossa, Cardiol Young 10(5):519–526, 2000 Sep.
123. Rickers C, Hamm C, Stern H, et al: Percutaneous closure of secundum atrial septal defect with a new self centering device ("angel wings"), Heart 80:517– 521, 1998.
124. Sideris EB, Kaneva A, Haddad J, et al: The centering on demand device: early results in atrial septal defect occlusion, Cardiol Young 9(Suppl):91, 1999.
125. Sideris EB, Sideris SE, Fowlkes JP, et al: Transvenous septal defect occlusion in piglets with a "buttoned" double-disc device, Circulation 81:312–318, 1990.
126. O'Laughlin MP: Microvena atrial septal defect occlusion device: update 2000, J Interv Cardiol 14(1):77–80, 2001.
127. Hausdorf G, Schneider M, Franzbach B, et al: Transcatheter closure of se- cundum atrial septal defects with the atrial septal defect occlusion system (ASDOS): initial experience in children, Heart 75(1):83–88, 1996.
128. Jones TK, Latson LA, Zahn E, et al: Multicenter pivotal study of the HELEX Septal occluder investigators: results of the U.S. multicenter pivotal study of the HELEX septal occluder for percutaneous closure of secundum atrial septal defects, J Am Coll Cardiol 49:2215–2221, 2007.
129. Vincent RN, Raviele AA, Diehl HJ: Single-center experience with the HELEX septal occluder for closure of atrial septal defects in children, J Interv Cardiol 16(1):79–82, 2003 Feb.
130. Hamden MA, Cao QL, Hijazi ZM: Amplatzer septal occluder. In Rao PS, Kern MJ, editors: Catheter-based devices for the treatment of noncoronary cardiovascular disease in adults and children: for the treatment of noncoronary cardiovascular disease in adults and children, Philadelphia, 2003, Lippincott, Williams and Wilkins, pp 51–60.
131. Kannan BRJ, Francis E, Sivakumar K, et al: Transcatheter closure of very large (≥25 mm) atrial septal defects using the Amplatzer septal occluder, Cathet Cardiovasc Interv 59:522–527, 2003.
132. Berger F, Ewert P, Abdul-Khaliq H, et al: Percutaneous closure of large atrial septal defects with the Amplatzer septal occluder: technical overkill or rec- ommendable alternative treatment? J Interv Cardiol 14:63–67, 2001.
133. Varma C, Benson LN, Silversides C, et al: Outcomes and alternative tech- niques for device closure of the large secundum atrial septal defect, Catheter Cardiovasc Interv 61:131–139, 2004.
134. Wahab HA, Bairam AR, Cao QL, et al: Novel technique to prevent prolapse of the Amplatzer septal occluder through large atrial septal defect, Catheter Cardiovasc Interv 60:543–545, 2003.
135. Dalvi BV, Pinto RJ, Gupta A: New technique for device closure of large atrial septal defects, Catheter Cardiovasc Interv 64:102–107, 2005.
136. Balint OH, Samman A, Haberer K, et al: Outcomes in patients with pul- monary hypertension undergoing percutaneous atrial septal defect closure, Heart 94(9):1189–1193, 2008 Sep.
137. Yong G, Khairy P, De Guise P, et al: Pulmonary arterial hypertension in pa- tients with transcatheter closure of secundum atrial septal defects: a longi- tudinal study, Circ Cardiovasc Interv 2(5):455–462, 2009 Oct. Epub 2009 Sep 22.
138. McMahon CJ, Pignatelli RH, Rutledge JM, et al: Steerable control of the eu- stachian valve during transcatheter closure of secundum atrial septal de- fects, Catheter Cardiovasc Interv 51:455–459, 2000.
139. Zahid Amin MD, Ziyad M, Hijazi MD, John L, Bass MD, John P, Cheatham MD, William Hellenbrand MD, Charles S, Kleinman MD: PFO closure com- plications from the AGA registry, Catheter Cardiovasc Interv 72:74–79, 2008.
140. Fagan T, Dreher D, Cutright W, et al: Fracture of the GORE HELEX septal occluder: associated factors and clinical outcomes, Catheter Cardiovasc Interv 73:941–948, 2009.

Chapter 21

Atrial Septal Defect Creation

JEFFERY MEADOWS • PHILLIP MOORE

Pulmonary hypertension (HTN) with end-stage pulmonary vascular disease results in right heart failure, low output, and death, with few therapeutic options other than lung transplantation. Opening of the atrial septum (most common), ventricular septum, or ductus arteriosus allows for right-to-left shunt decompression of the right heart volume and pressure at the expense of systemic desaturation. Opening of the atrial septum is the preferred approach in most patients because of the relative ease and safety. Despite the decrease in systemic saturation with opening of the atrial septum, left heart loading is augmented, enhancing cardiac output and improving peripheral O_2 delivery.[1-4] An optimal balance must be struck, because too much right-to-left shunting (too large a defect) results in profound desaturation with a marked decrease in tissue O_2 delivery and exacerbates symptoms severely, to the point of death. After creation of a right-to-left shunt resulting in this physiologic trade-off, clinical evidence has shown an improvement in symptoms,[1,3,5] exercise tolerance,[6-7] right ventricular function,[5] and possibly improved survival.[7-8] Clinical improvement can be sustained for many years.[5] Interventional techniques now allow for an easy, safe nonsurgical option for this palliative therapy in patients.

Nonsurgical opening of the atrial septum was first described in 1966 by Rashkind and Miller[9] for palliative treatment of neonates with transposition of the great arteries, creating a left-to-right shunt at the atrial level to improve systemic saturations. This treatment remains in use for stabilization of neonates in anticipation of corrective surgical repair. The technique was expanded to treat older patients with transposition by the development of a "blade" catheter by Park et al in 1975.[10] These techniques rapidly expanded to treat a variety of infants and children who had congenital defects with atrial septal restriction, such as mitral atresia and anomalous pulmonary venous return.[11,12] In 1983, Rich and Lam[13] applied the Park blade followed by a Rashkind atrial septostomy to a 28-year-old patient with end-stage pulmonary HTN for symptomatic palliation. Since then, newer techniques, including oversized static balloon dilation,[14] cutting balloon dilation,[15] stent implantation,[16-18]

and fenestrated device implantation[19,20] have been used. This chapter details preferred techniques for atrial septal defect (ASD) creation, including cutting balloon dilation with large static balloon postdilation, stent implantation, and fenestrated device implantation.

21.1 Patient Selection/Indications

Patients receiving medical therapy for symptomatic end-stage pulmonary HTN who are awaiting transplant remain the primary group who benefits from opening of the atrial septum **(Table 21–1)**. Syncope in the setting of severe pulmonary HTN carries a significant mortality risk. Wait times for lung transplantation remain long with limited survival to transplant. Patients who have pulmonary HTN but are not transplant candidates yet are symptomatic while receiving maximal medical therapy may also benefit from atrial septal opening with improvement in symptoms.

A second group of patients, much less common, are those who develop severe pulmonary HTN in the setting of a large secundum ASD. Most of these patients should have their ASD closed completely, but there are a select few whose limited response to maximal medical therapy and test balloon occlusion suggest a small residual defect may be beneficial. Definitive indications for this subset of patients remains in evolution, but ASD closure with creation of a residual fenestration may be considered in those with a minimal pulmonary vascular resistance (PVR) of more than 4 Wood units and an ASD larger than 10 to 15 mm in diameter.

Creation of a right-to-left shunt at the atrial level is also used in congenital cardiac patients with failing single ventricle physiology. These patients are typically surgically corrected with a total cavopulmonary connection, commonly referred to as a *Fontan repair*. In this setting the inferior vena cava (IVC) and superior vena cava (SVC) are directly connected to the pulmonary arteries for passive flow through the lungs. Cardiac or pulmonary failure results in IVC pressure elevation, causing a condition

TABLE 21–1

Indications for Atrial Septal Defect Creation

Group	Shunt	Indications	Goal
Symptomatic Pulmonary HTN	R to L	PVR > 4 on 3 agents, syncope	Sat 80-85
Pulmonary HTN + ASD	R to L	Minimum PVR > 4, ASD > 15 mm	Sat 90-95
Failing Fontan	R to L	PLE on maximum medical therapy	Sat 80-85
LVAD support	L to R	LAp > 20, LA distension on echo	LAp < RAp + 5

ASD, Atrial septal defect; *HTN,* hypertension; *L,* left; *LA,* left atrial; *LAp,* left atrial pressure; *LVAD,* left ventricular assist device; *PLE,* protein losing enteropathy; *PVR,* pulmonary vascular resistance; *R,* right; *RAp,* right atrial pressure; *Sat,* saturation.

known as *protein-losing enteropathy.* When medical management fails, cardiac transplant is the only option. The creation of a communication between the Fontan circuit (physiologically the right atrium) and the left atrium with the development of a right-to-left shunt is an effective palliative treatment in some patients to improve protein-losing enteropathy. Clinical indications in this group of patients include the diagnosis of protein-losing enteropathy (low serum albumin and elevated stool α-1-antitrypsin) despite maximal medical therapy (e.g., diuretics, afterload reduction, pulmonary vasodilators) in patients whose saturations are greater than 90%.

Lastly, patients with severe left ventricular (LV) dysfunction on ventricular assist device with left atrial (LA) HTN will benefit substantially from the creation of an atrial communication.[21] In this setting, unlike others, the intent is for an adequate but transient atrial communication to allow a left-to-right shunt for LA decompression. The goal of defect patency is short, only a few weeks at most, while the ventricular-assist support is needed. To that end the favored technique for defect creation in this subgroup of patients would be cutting balloon with static balloon dilation to allow adequate immediate shunting, with a greater chance of spontaneous closure once the ASD is no longer needed.

21.2 Technique

Interventional techniques have evolved and are still evolving with regard to ASD creation. The goal in the majority of patients is a small, controlled, permanent defect between the left and right atrium that allows a modest consistent right-to-left shunt. Too large a defect results in too much desaturation (<80%), and too small a defect gives no benefit. Because many of these patients have no alternative therapies or must wait months for transplant, the defect must remain patent with minimal change in diameter for months to years. The most commonly used techniques currently include (1) cutting balloon atrial septostomy followed by post–high-pressure balloon dilation, (2) atrial septal stent implantation, and (3) fenestrated device implantation.

CUTTING BALLOON/HIGH-PRESSURE BALLOON DILATION

This technique has evolved as a result of the disappointingly high incidence of spontaneous closure of

atrial septal communication with static balloon dilation alone.[5,7,22] The technique is simple but requires an intact septum that is crossed solely with a transseptal needle or radiofrequency (RF) perforation wire, so the initial cutting balloon dilation will result in true scoring of the septum before large static balloon dilation (because of current limitation in maximum cutting balloon sizes at 8 mm diameter). The procedure is performed with the patient under moderate sedation with intracardiac echocardiography (ICE) guidance or if preferred, anesthesia with transesophageal echocardiography. Although echo guidance is not required, it does allow for more exact positioning of the defect creation and can be very useful in the setting of an existing patent foramen ovale (PFO) to assure the septum is crossed away from the PFO and not through it. Preferably the septum should be crossed inferior and posterior in the region of the fossa. Cutting balloon with large static balloon dilation through a PFO is ineffective at producing a persistent opening because of the distensibility of the PFO limiting the size of the tear in the septal tissue. This results in the creation of a small defect at most that has a high rate of spontaneous closure.

A 7F or 8F transseptal sheath is placed in a femoral vein, preferably the right. The left vein can be used but may then necessitate adjusting the shape of the transseptal needle by adding a proximal bend of 30 to 45 degrees 10 to 15 cm along the needle from the hub **(Figure 21–1).** Monitoring of arterial pressure and saturations is needed to assess adequacy of the ASD size, so an arterial cannula is placed. For more accurate assessment, a 5F to 6F sheath is placed so direct LV pressure can be monitored. Complete right heart hemodynamics are obtained with a wedge or thermodilution catheter. Mixed venous saturations, both SVC and branch pulmonary artery (PA) samples, as well as arterial saturation (PaO$_2$ as well if the patient is breathing supplemental O$_2$) should be obtained at baseline and after ASD creation to determine shunting and guide defect size. Left heart pressure measurements with monitoring of left ventricle end-diastolic (LVED) pressure during ASD creation can also be helpful to assess adequacy of defect size. The hemodynamic changes shown in **Table 21–2** with the creation of a 7-mm ASD (6-mm cutting balloon followed by a 7-mm diameter stent) in this 4-year-old child with severe pulmonary HTN but preserved LV function are typical. The acute creation of a significant right-to-left shunt increasing cardiac output results in a large decrease in aortic saturation with only a modest increase in LV filling

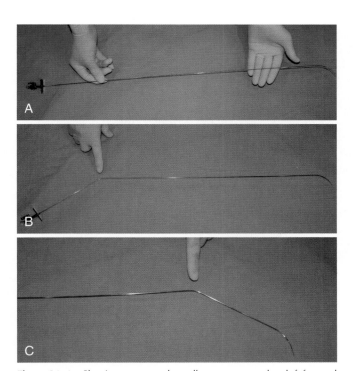

Figure 21–1 Shaping transseptal needle to accommodate left femoral vein access. **A,** Normal needle, **B,** Needle shaped for LFV approach, and **C,** Additional bend if the right atrium is dilated.

TABLE 21–2

Hemodynamic Changes with ASD Creation in a Patient with Pulmonary Hypertension

	Before	After
Pressures		
RA	24	22
LVED	10	12
Ao	92/52	91/51
Saturations		
PA	74	69
Ao	92	81
Cardiac Outputs		
Qs	2.8	4.9
Qp	2.8	2.7
Qp:Qs	1.0	0.6

Ao, Aorta; *LVED,* left ventricle end-diastolic; *PA,* pulmonary artery; *Qp,* pulmonary flow in liters/min/meters squared; *Qs,* systemic flow in liters/min/meters squared; *RA,* right atrial.

pressure. This may not be the case in a diseased non-compliant left ventricle where creation of the same-sized ASD may result in a larger increase in LV filling pressure.

After initial hemodynamic assessment, transseptal puncture is performed centrally in the septum, preferably through the area of the fossa ovalis, if intact **(Figure 21–2).** If there is a PFO, the transseptal puncture should be performed slightly posterior and inferior, taking care not to slip thru the foramen but instead puncturing the septum primum. Once through the septum the dilator and sheath are advanced across the puncture into the

left atrium, and pressure and saturation obtained. A shaped directional catheter such as a 5F JR4, multipurpose, or JB1 is used to position a stiff 0.014-inch wire or a stiff 0.018-inch wire in a left pulmonary vein, preferably the upper vein. An 8 mm × 2 cm cutting balloon is then advanced over the wire to the tip of the sheath in the left atrium. The sheath is pulled back to the right atrium and then advanced back to the septum, and a hand injection angiogram through the side-arm of the sheath is performed **(Figure 21–3).** This, together with ICE imaging, confirms septal location for exact balloon positioning. The balloon should be centered on the septum and fully inflated to a maximum of 8 atm using an insufflator to minimize risk of balloon rupture. Removal of a ruptured cutting balloon poses challenges with risks of vascular injury and blade embolization. As the balloon expands, a mild waist is often, but not always, seen **(Figure 21–4 and Video 21–1).** Repeat dilation should be performed with adjustment of balloon position if there is any concern that the balloon was not centered on the atrial septum based on angiographic and ICE landmarks.

The balloon is removed, and the directional catheter is advanced over the small wire into the left atrium with a Y-adapter to allow for pressure monitoring. Simultaneous LA and right atrial (RA) pressures, systemic saturation measurement, and ICE imaging should be performed to assess the newly created defect. As noted, the goal is for a reduction in systemic saturations by at least 5% but no lower than the mid to low 80s, and an increase in LA or LVED pressures by 2 to 10 mmHg. It may be prudent to target a maximum LVED pressure of 16 or less to avoid the risk of subsequent pulmonary edema. This latter change depends on the compliance of the left ventricle, so even with a significant right-to-left shunt, the LVED may increase only slightly if the left ventricle is healthy. Most often, 8-mm (max size) cutting balloon dilation alone gives an inadequately sized atrial communication, so postdilation with a larger static balloon is required. High-pressure balloons that have low profiles and long shoulders allow use of the already positioned 7F or 8F sheath and ease of positioning for dilation. The 0.018-inch wire in the left pulmonary vein is exchanged through the directional catheter for a stiff 0.035-inch soft-tipped wire (Bard Atlas PTA dilation catheter; Bard Peripheral Vascular, Inc., Tempe, Ariz.). A 12-mm to 20-mm balloon is advanced over the wire across the septum and inflated fully to resolution of the waist **(Figure 21–5 and Video 21–2).** The size of the balloon is chosen based on post–cutting balloon measurements and ultimate defect size goal. In adult patients starting with a 14-mm balloon, reassessing hemodynamics and saturations and serially enlarging is a prudent strategy. Acute creation of too large a defect results in severe desaturation and can rapidly progress to hemodynamic instability and death, so stepwise defect enlargement and reassessment is strongly recommended. Final complete hemodynamic assessment is performed after final dilation and includes ICE imaging and angiography (optional) before sheath removal **(Figure 21–6).**

Careful postprocedural observation is required, including continuous cardiac and saturation monitoring.

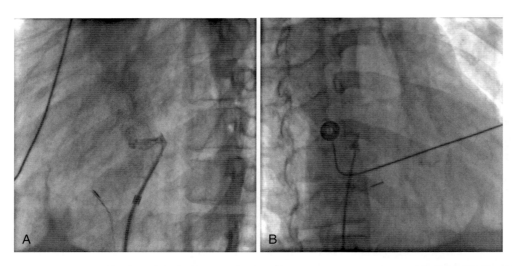

Figure 21–2 Anteroposterior (**A**) and lateral (**B**) angiographic views of the intact fossa ovalis as seen by contrast injection through transseptal sheath in the right atrium.

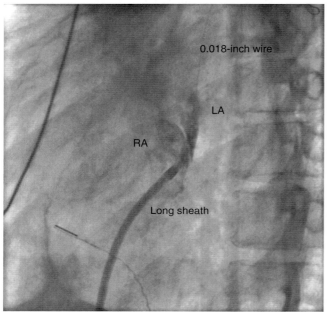

Figure 21–3 Angiogram through side-arm of sheath, defining RA septal location before insertion of the cutting balloon. *LA,* Left atrium; *RA,* right atrium.

If systemic saturations have decreased significantly (<80%) despite supplemental oxygen with creation of the septal defect, measurement of hemoglobin (Hgb) with transfusion recommended if the level is less than 10 g/dL. Optimal Hgb level postprocedure is 12 g/dL or more. Once groin sites are stable, the patient should resume preprocedure anticoagulation therapy or antiplatelet strategy. If the patient was not taking any anticoagulation or antiplatelet medications preprocedure, the patient should start taking at least 81 mg acetylsalicylic acid (ASA) daily for a minimum of 6 months.

ATRIAL SEPTAL STENT IMPLANTATION:

Septal stent placement has the advantage of optimizing long-term patency of the hole and is the authors' preferred approach if long-term decompression is needed,

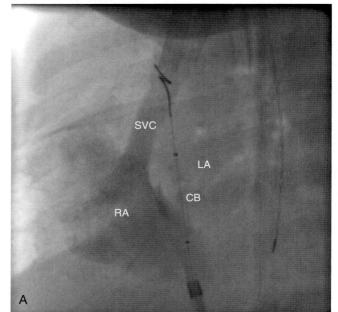

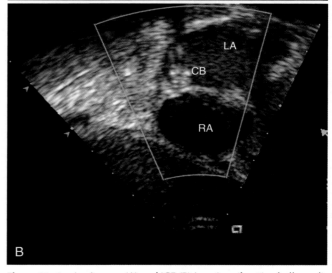

Figure 21–4 Angiogram (**A**) and ICE (**B**) imaging of cutting balloon dilation of the atrial septum. *CB,* Cutting balloon; *ICE,* intracardiac echocardiography; *LA,* left atrium; *RA,* right atrium; *SVC,* superior vena cava.

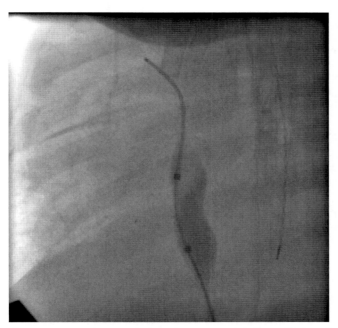

Figure 21–5 Angiogram of a large (18-mm) static balloon dilation of the atrial septum after cutting with an 8-mm cutting balloon.

such as with palliation for patients with severe pulmonary HTN. In addition to the benefit of longer defect patency, stent implantation allows very controlled and precise defect size creation. The risk, of course, is that size adjustment is possible only in one direction: gradual enlargement by serially larger balloon dilations. Too large a stented defect does not decrease spontaneously in size over time and is challenging to make significantly smaller, so it would need to be completely closed and the process repeated with a smaller stent.

As with cutting balloon dilation, it is critical to cross through septal tissue and not a PFO. There are reports, both published and personal communication, of stent embolization when placement was attempted in a patent foraminal tunnel at target diameters of 6 to 12 mm. Although larger stent diameters might stay in a foraminal tunnel, the size of the defect would be too large in most applications to make the approach useful. Crossing of the septum for stent placement is best done superior and posterior to a PFO, through thicker septum secundum tissue to allow for easier more stable placement.

This procedure is identical to that described for the preliminary hemodynamic assessment and atrial septal crossing. If transseptal puncture is not possible because there is a thick fibrotic resistant septum, a radiofrequency transseptal needle can be useful (NRG RF transseptal needle; Baylis Medical, Montreal, Quebec, Canada). The transseptal technique is similar to that already described with ICE guidance; however, the preferred location is either the fossa ovalis or slightly superior and posterior through the thicker septum secundum.

Once the transeptal needle has passed to the left atrium, the sheath is advanced and LA saturation and pressure measurements are obtained. Using a directional catheter an 0.018-inch stiff wire is positioned in the left

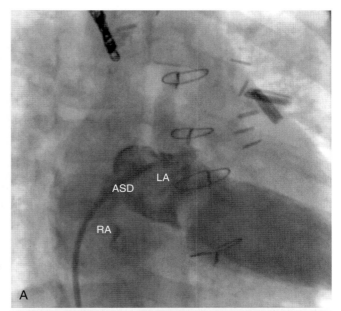

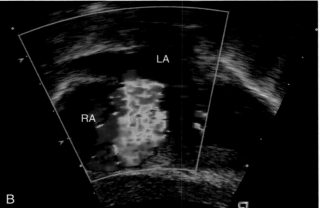

Figure 21–6 Final ASD postcutting with static dilation. **A,** Angiogram, and **B,** ICE imaging. *ASD,* Atrial septal defect; *ICE,* intracardiac echocardiography; *LA,* left atrium; *RA,* right atrium.

upper pulmonary vein. The authors prefer using a premounted peripheral vascular balloon expandable stent with diameters of 5 to 7 mm and a length of either 18 or 24 mm (such as the Cordis Palmaz Blue, Bridgewater, N.J.). A longer stent should be used if the stent will be through a thick portion of the septum, and a shorter stent if it will go through a thin portion. The maximal achievable diameter of these peripheral stents is 12 mm. Shortening of stent length will begin when dilated above a diameter of 10 mm, with an approximate 20% foreshortening at 12 mm. These stents are delivered through a 6F multipurpose guide advanced into the left atrium through the transseptal sheath. Place a Y adapter on the back of the guide so angiography can be performed through the guide to assist with stent positioning during delivery. Remember that the initial implant diameter choice should err on the small side. Serial dilations to achieve the final desired size is quite straightforward, whereas initial oversizing is much more problematic. The delivery technique is to advance 40% of the stent out the end of the guide catheter in the left atrium. While maintaining stent position across the septum, withdraw the guide back until the guide just crosses the septum, reaching the right atrium. Perform a hand angiogram through the guide in this position to confirm that the stent is centered on the septum **(Figure 21–7, A).** The position should be confirmed with ICE **(see Figure 21–7, B).** While keeping the guide covering the proximal portion of the stent in the right atrium, fully inflate the balloon to expand the distal half of the stent in the left atrium. Keep slight withdrawal tension on the delivery balloon–stent system while inflating the LA portion of the stent; then withdraw the guide off the proximal balloon stent, allowing for expansion of the proximal RA portion of the stent. Inflate the balloon fully to maximal

recommended atmospheres. Use an insufflator with a gauge to prevent overdilation and balloon rupture that can increase the risk of embolization. Deflate the balloon completely and advance the guide to the proximal RA edge of the stent for support as the balloon is withdrawn, leaving the wire in position in the left upper pulmonary vein. Reassess hemodynamics and arterial saturations. If there is not an adequate decrease in arterial saturations and increase in LVED pressure, then post–implant dilation should be performed. Do not postdilate with a balloon more than 2 mm larger than the implant balloon to avoid oversizing the defect. (The authors prefer to postdilate serially with balloons that are progressively 1 mm larger and reassess hemodynamics until the desired result is achieved.)

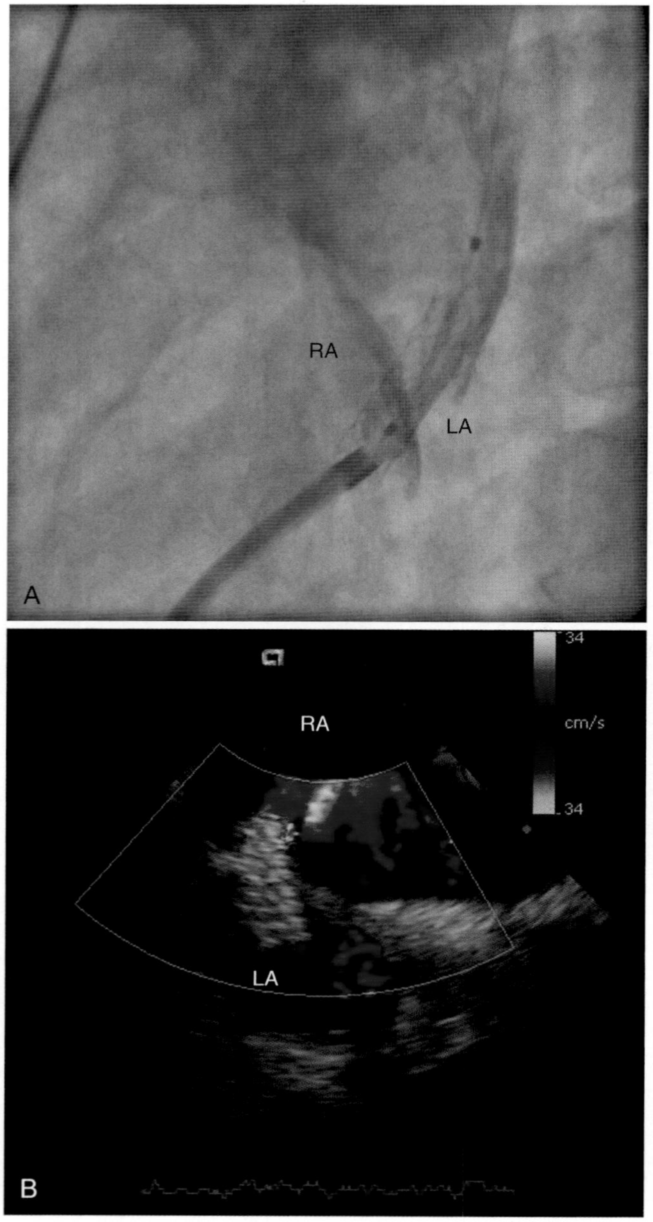

Some authors have advocated a "butterfly" shape to atrial septal stents to fix the central portion at a desired diameter with the ends flared to appose the septal walls[23,24] **(Figure 21–8).** Although aesthetically pleasing, this more complicated technique is not necessary (there are neither reports of thrombus formation on atrial septal stents nor late embolization) as long as one delivers the stent through a transseptal puncture and not into an existing ASD or PFO and the appropriate length of stent produces very little protrusion into either the right or left atrium. In addition, the "butterfly" stent technique

Figure 21–7 Septal stent implantation delivery. **A,** RA angiogram through sheath to confirm placement. **B,** ICE imaging of septal stent positioning. *ICE,* Intracardiac echocardiography; *LA,* left atrium; *RA,* right atrium.

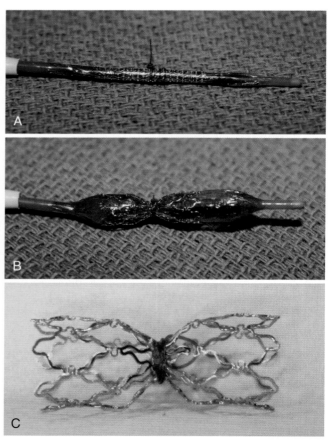

Figure 21–8 Butterfly stent in the atrial septum created by placing a Gore-Tex suture in the center of the stent **(A),** limiting expansion to targeted diameter **(B),** and mounting/delivering on a larger balloon to flare ends **(C).**

requires fixing the central stent diameter with a suture to achieve the desired shape. Although it is initially perhaps more attractive, this limits the ability to easily serially dilate to the desired diameter. Serial dilations can be easily performed by repeat catheterization 4 months after initial implant once the stent is fixed in the septum by endocardial ingrowth. The existing stent is crossed with a floppy 0.014-inch wire using a 5F JR4 catheter through a long (63 or 75 cm) 7F Mullins sheath. The wire should be positioned in the left upper pulmonary vein. An appropriately sized balloon (6 to 9 mm diameter × 2 cm) is advanced across the stent, inflated to complete dilation, and deflated with the long sheath advanced to the RA edge of the stent to support during balloon removal. This can be repeated if need be. It is preferable to err on the side of small increases in balloon diameter to minimize the risk of too large a right-to-left shunt.

As with the cutting balloon technique, careful postprocedural observation is required, including continuous cardiac and saturation monitoring. If systemic saturations have decreased significantly (<80%), Hgb should be checked, and if it is more than 10 g/dL, a packed red blood cell transfusion is recommended. The optimal postprocedure Hgb is 12 g/dL or greater. Once groin sites are stable, the patient should resume preprocedure anticoagulation therapy with warfarin (Coumadin) or begin dual antiplatelet therapy with 81 mg of ASA with 75 mg (clopidogrel) Plavix po daily for a minimum of 6 months.

FENESTRATED DEVICE PLACEMENT:

Although uncommon, there are patients with significant pulmonary HTN associated with a large ASD who will benefit from ASD closure (because of a predominant left-to-right shunt) but still may require a small residual defect (minimal PVR remains high despite maximal vasodilators). Several techniques have been described, ranging from cutting holes in the fabric of ASD devices before implantation to placing bare metal stents through devices after complete healing.[5,19,25,26] Devices have been developed with residual holes, but none are currently available in the United States.[19,20] The authors prefer stent placement through the ASD device at the time of implant, allowing for controlled sizing of the residual defect from the onset to minimize risk. The procedure includes standard baseline right and left heart hemodynamic assessment pre–ASD closure, in addition to pulmonary vasodilator testing (hemodynamic assessment after 5 minutes of 100% O_2 with 40 ppm NO inhalation). Balloon test occlusion of the ASD is performed with ICE guidance to assure that the device will be stable. It is important to remember that large ASD devices such as the Amplatzer atrial septal occluder (ASO) device have an LA disc that is larger (4 to 6 mm) than the RA disc. In the setting of significant pulmonary HTN, the RA pressures may transiently rise above LA pressures, exerting a right-to-left force on the device once it has been implanted, so device size should be chosen accordingly to assure stable position and minimize the risk of embolization.

Once the device is chosen, a 12F dilator is used to puncture through the RA and LA discs next to the central

pin (Figure 21–9, A). A delivery sheath one size larger than that recommended for the device size is positioned across the ASD into the left atrium. Using a directional catheter through the delivery sheath, a stiff exchange-length 0.014-inch wire is positioned across the ASD into the left upper pulmonary vein. The Amplatzer ASD device is screwed onto the delivery cable, and the proximal end of the 0.014-inch wire is slipped through the defect created in the ASO device (Figure 21–9, B). The device is then collapsed into the loader with the 0.014-inch wire through it and advanced through the delivery sheath, the compressed device sliding over the 0.014-inch wire. Using both fluoroscopic and ICE guidance, the device is positioned across the ASD in the usual manner. Once in position with the 0.014-inch wire through it, a push-pull test is performed to confirm stable position. While still connected to the delivery cable, a premounted peripheral or coronary balloon expandable stent (5 to 6 mm in diameter, 15 to 18 mm long) is advanced over the 0.014-inch wire and centered through the ASD device (Figure 21–9, C and Video 21–3, A). Inflation is with an insufflator to assure complete expansion but minimize risk of balloon rupture (Figure 21–9, D and Video 21–3, B). Once stent position is confirmed, the ASD device cable is unscrewed, and the system is permanently implanted (Figure 21–9, E and Video 21–3, C). Repeat right and left heart hemodynamic assessment is performed, including SVC and PA saturation measurements to calculate the residual degree of atrial shunting.

If on follow-up examination with ongoing aggressive pulmonary HTN management there is improvement in the patient's PVR and the residual shunting through the fenestration is all left to right, interventional closure is straightforward. A small ASO device or vascular plug II is easily placed in the stent fenestration for closure (Figure 21–10 and Video 21–4).

21.3 Postprocedure Management/ Complications

Care must be taken when creating an ASD in a patient with severe pulmonary HTN not to overachieve. Too large of a defect will result in profound right-to-left shunt, marked desaturation, and can lead to progressive decreasing O_2 delivery and death.[2,13,27] Procedural mortality has decreased because of increasing knowledge and experience, as well as improved techniques. Blade septostomy and balloon septostomy alone historically reported procedural mortality of 7% to 18%.[4,7,8,22,28] Recent reports of atrial stent implantation and fenestrated device placement have not described procedural deaths. If O_2 saturations decrease to less than 80%, transcatheter reduction in defect size or complete closure is indicated urgently. This is done through ASD device closure technique if a cutting balloon with static dilation approach was used to create the defect. A fenestrated device can be placed (as described) to create a smaller defect.[29] If an atrial septal stent was placed, defect size reduction can be achieved by implanting a covered stent (iCast covered stent; Atrium Medical, Hudson, N.H.) that is limited in

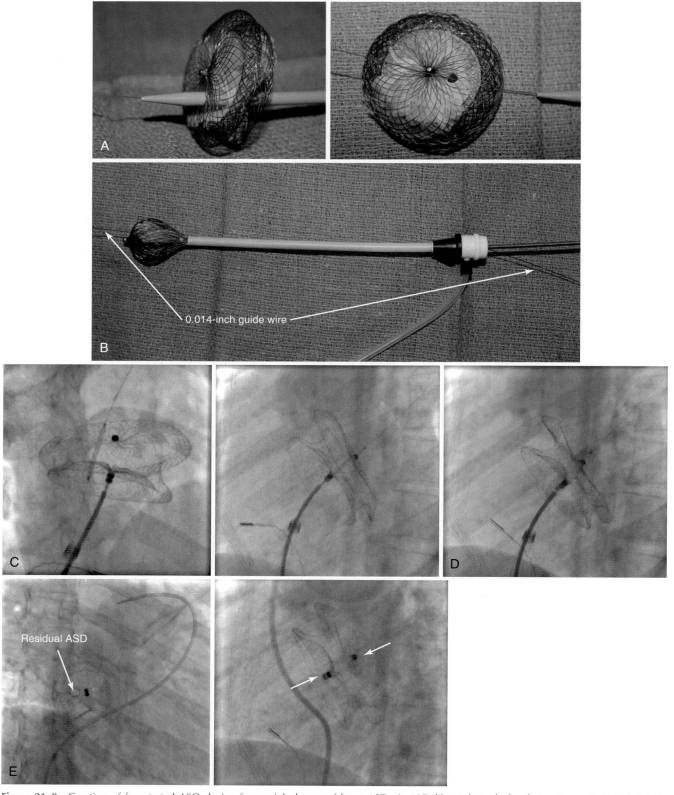

Figure 21–9 Creation of fenestrated ASO device for partial closure of large ASD. **A,** 12F dilator through the device to create initial defect. **B,** Threaded 0.014-inch wire through the device before loading. **C,** Stent positioning through the device. **D,** Stent delivery. **E,** After implantation, residual ASD is shown by arrows. *ASD,* Atrial septal defect; *ASO,* atrial septal occluder.

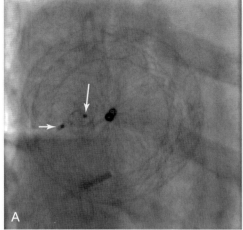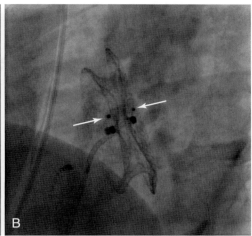

Figure 21–10 Vascular plug II closure of fenestrated atrial septal defect device after improvement of pulmonary hypertension. A, Right anterior oblique and caudal projection. **B,** Left anterior oblique and cranial projection.

central expansion by a suture. The covered stent is balloon-expanded to the desired diameter on the table and a Gore-Tex suture is sewn around the center of the stent by weaving it through the covering and tying it to a strut. The stent is compressed on a delivery balloon the size of the existing defect and inserted centered on the existing stent. This produces a butterfly shape to the system, reducing the cross-sectional area of the communication to the predetermined sutured diameter. This suture can be broken at a later time with a very high-pressure balloon (20 to 25 atm; e.g., Cordis Powerflex Extreme, Bridgewater, N.J.; Bard Peripheral Vascular, ConQuest, Tempe, Ariz.), and the communication can be enlarged if needed.

Postprocedure management should focus on close cardiac and systemic saturation monitoring. Pulmonary hypertensive crisis postcatheterization is possible, so intensive care unit support, mechanical ventilation, and inhalable nitric oxide should be available if needed. Liberal use of supplemental O_2 and intravenous fluids postcatheterization is needed to minimize PVR and support preload to maintain output with optimal O_2 delivery. An adequate Hgb after the procedure is critical, so a postprocedure complete blood count should be obtained. Echocardiogram before discharge is recommended to document patency and size of shunt for comparison on follow-up evaluations.

Late complications include infection of the implant, thrombus, and spontaneous closure of the defect. In this population, this procedure by design creates a right-to-left shunt, resulting in the potential for paradoxical embolic event. Therefore, aggressive postprocedure and long-term thrombosis prevention with medical prophylaxis is required. There are not comparative data to determine the best approach in this setting, but the authors prefer long-term anticoagulation therapy with warfarin (Coumadin) and an International Normalized Ratio (INR) target of 2.0 to 2.5.

21.4 Summary

Procedural success is high, with early reports suggesting a 5% to 10% failure rate resulting either from procedural

death or inability to cross the septum.[2,4,7,8] Recent reports and experience would suggest that with current techniques, including ICE guidance and RF perforation if needed, procedural success should be close to 100%. If an appropriate degree of right-to-left shunting is created (generally a systemic saturation decrease to 84% to 89% with a defect size of 5 to 8 mm), then significant improvement in cardiac index (15% to 20%) and O_2 delivery (5% to 15%) will result.[1-3] Improvement in functional class by 1 grade[1,3] and increase in 6-minute walk test distance by greater than 20% are reported.[6,7] No comparative data are available to evaluate potential benefit for survival, and all series reported are quite small, making the use of historical controls problematic. The larger series conclude a survival advantage over historical controls,[7,8] but more study is indicated.

REFERENCES

1. Kurzyna M, Dabrowski M, Bielecki D, et al: Atrial septostomy in treatment of end-stage right heart failure in patients with pulmonary hypertension, *Chest* 131(4):977–983, 2007.
2. Reichenberger F, Pepke-Zaba J, McNeil K, et al: Atrial septostomy in the treatment of severe pulmonary arterial hypertension, *Thorax* 58(9):797–800, 2003.
3. Rothman A, Sklansky MS, Lucas VW, et al: Atrial septostomy as a bridge to lung transplantation in patients with severe pulmonary hypertension, *Am J Cardiol* 84(6):682–686, 1999.
4. Rich S, Dodin E, McLaughlin VV: Usefulness of atrial septostomy as a treatment for primary pulmonary hypertension and guidelines for its application, *Am J Cardiol* 80(3):369–371, 1997.
5. Micheletti A, Hislop AA, Lammers A, et al: Role of atrial septostomy in the treatment of children with pulmonary arterial hypertension, *Heart* 92(7):969–972, 2006.
6. Troost E, Delcroix M, Gewillig M, et al: A modified technique of stent fenestration of the interatrial septum improves patients with pulmonary hypertension, *Catheter Cardiovasc Interv* 73(2):173–179, 2009.
7. Sandoval J, Gaspar J, Pulido T, et al: Graded balloon dilation atrial septostomy in severe primary pulmonary hypertension: a therapeutic alternative for patients nonresponsive to vasodilator treatment, *J Am Coll Cardiol* 32(2):297–304, 1998.
8. Kothari SS, Yusuf A, Juneja R, et al: Graded balloon atrial septostomy in severe pulmonary hypertension, *Indian Heart J* 54(2):164–169, 2002.
9. Rashkind WJ, Miller WW: Creation of an atrial septal defect without thoracotomy: a palliative approach to complete transposition of the great arteries, *JAMA* 196(11):991–992, 1966.

10. Park SC, Zuberbuhler JR, Neches WH, et al: A new atrial septostomy technique, *Cathet Cardiovasc Diagn* 1(2):195–201, 1975.
11. Park SC, Neches WH, Zuberbuhler JR, et al: Clinical use of blade atrial septostomy, *Circulation* 58(4):600–606, 1978.
12. Perry SB, Lang P, Keane JF, et al: Creation and maintenance of an adequate interatrial communication in left atrioventricular valve atresia or stenosis, *Am J Cardiol* 58:622–626, 1986.
13. Rich S, Lam W: Atrial septostomy as palliative therapy for refractory primary pulmonary hypertension, *Am J Cardiol* 51:1560–1561, 1983.
14. Ballerini L, di Carlo DC, Cifarelli A, et al: Oversize balloon atrial septal dilatation: early experience, *Am Heart J* 125(6):1760–1763, 1993.
15. Coe JY, Chen RP, Timinisky J, et al: A novel method to create atrial septal defect using a cutting balloon in piglets, *Am J Cardiol* 78(11):1323–1326, 1996.
16. O'Laughlin MP: Stent fenestration of hemi-Fontan baffles: an intriguing addition to the armamentarium, *Cathet Cardiovasc Diagn* 43:433, 1998.
17. Miga DE, Clark JM, Cowart KS, et al: Transcatheter fenestration of hemi-Fontan baffles after completion of Fontan physiology using balloon dilatation and stent placement, *Cathet Cardiovasc Diagn* 43:429–432, 1998.
18. Pedra CA, Pihkala J, Benson LN, et al: Stent implantation to create interatrial communications in patients with complex congenital heart disease, *Cathet Cardiovasc Interv* 47:310–313, 1999.
19. Fraisse A, Chetaille P, Amin Z, et al: Use of Amplatzer fenestrated atrial septal defect device in a child with familial pulmonary hypertension, *Pediatr Cardiol* 27(6):759–762, 2006.
20. O'Loughlin AJ, Keogh A, Muller DW: Insertion of a fenestrated Amplatzer atrial septostomy device for severe pulmonary hypertension, *Heart Lung Circ* 15(4):275–277, 2006.
21. Seib PM, Faulkner SC, Erickson CC, et al: Blade and balloon atrial septostomy for left heart decompression in patients with severe ventricular dysfunction on extracorporeal membrane oxygenation, *Catheter Cardiovasc Interv* 46(2):179–186, 1999.
22. Kerstein D, Levy PS, Hsu DT, et al: Blade balloon atrial septostomy in patients with severe primary pulmonary hypertension, *Circulation* 91(7):2028–2035, 1995.
23. Stumper O, Gewillig M, Vettukattil J, et al: Modified technique of stent fenestration of the atrial septum, *Heart* 89(10):1227–1230, 2003.
24. Prieto LR, Latson LA, Jennings C: Atrial septostomy using a butterfly stent in a patient with severe pulmonary arterial hypertension, *Catheter Cardiovasc Interv* 68(4):642–647, 2006.
25. Schneider HE, Jux C, Kriebel T, et al: Fate of a modified fenestration of atrial septal occluder device after transcatheter closure of atrial septal defects in elderly patients, *J Interv Cardiol* 24(5):485–490, 2011.
26. Kretschmar O, Sglimbea A, Corti R, et al: Shunt reduction with a fenestrated Amplatzer device, *Catheter Cardiovasc Interv* 76(4):564–571, 2010.
27. Kurzyna M, Dabrowski M, Torbicki A, et al: Atrial septostomy for severe primary pulmonary hypertension: report on two cases, *Kardiol Pol* 58(1):27–33, 2003.
28. Moscucci M, Dairywala IT, Chetcuti S, et al: Balloon atrial septostomy in end-stage pulmonary hypertension guided by a novel intracardiac echocardiographic transducer, *Catheter Cardiovasc Interv* 52(4):530–534, 2001.
29. Baglini R, Scardulla C: Reduction of a previous atrial septostomy in a patient with end-stage pulmonary hypertension by a manually fenestrated device, *Cardiovasc Revasc Med* 11(4):264, 2010. e9–e11.

Chapter 22

Unwanted Vascular Communications: Patent Ductus Arteriosus, Coronary Fistulas, Pulmonary Arteriovenous Malformations, and Aortopulmonary Collaterals

C. HUIE LIN • NICOLAS T. RAMZI • JOSHUA MURPHY • DAVID T. BALZER

Patent ductus arteriosus (PDA), coronary fistulas, pulmonary arteriovenous malformations (PAVMs), and aortopulmonary collaterals (APCs) represent unwanted vascular communications that can potentially cause severe clinical sequelae such as heart failure, myocardial infarction, or even endarteritis. Although surgical ligation or expectant management have previously been the only available options, transcatheter techniques have evolved to become a powerful and minimally invasive method for managing these vessels. This chapter will present the clinical background, indications, and basic techniques for the transcatheter closure of these vessels, as well as potential pitfalls of these procedures.

22.1 Patent Ductus Arteriosus

BACKGROUND

The ductus arteriosus is derived from the left sixth embryologic arch and connects the origin of the left main pulmonary artery (MPA) to the aorta, just below the left subclavian artery.

During fetal life, the ductus carries the majority of the outflow of the right ventricle (RV) to the descending aorta. Spontaneous functional closure of the ductus arteriosus usually occurs after delivery by approximately 15 hours of age,[1] with permanent closure occurring within several weeks. Persistent PDA is estimated to occur in approximately 0.8/1000 live births,[2] exclusive of silent PDA. The prevalence of PDAs decreases with age, but the true prevalence in the adult population is unknown because many cases of hemodynamically insignificant PDA have no signs or symptoms and patients remain undiagnosed. Silent PDAs (those in whom no pathologic murmur is audible) are estimated to occur in up to 0.5% of patients referred for echocardiographic evaluation of an innocent murmur[3]; however, the clinical significance of these is controversial.

The clinical manifestations of a PDA are dependent upon the direction and degree of shunting across the PDA. Factors that control the direction and magnitude of the shunt across the PDA include the diameter and length of the ductus arteriosus, the pressure difference between the aorta and pulmonary artery (PA), and the systemic and pulmonary vascular resistances.[4]

The physiologic effects of the PDA are related to the left-to-right shunt. Normally if the pulmonary vascular resistance is low, oxygenated blood from the aorta crosses the PDA into the PA. This lowers the systemic diastolic pressure and widens the pulse pressure. There is increased pulmonary blood flow with resulting increased pulmonary venous return. The left atrium (LA) may become dilated from the volume load, as may the left ventricle (LV). Dilation of the LV may result in increased ventricular end-diastolic pressure and subsequently secondary elevation in the left atrial and pulmonary venous pressures. With large left-to-right shunts, this may result in left heart failure with pulmonary edema. If untreated, a subgroup of patients may develop progressive elevation in pulmonary vascular resistance and ultimately develop irreversible pulmonary vascular disease and Eisenmenger physiology with a right-to-left shunt at the PDA.

DIAGNOSIS AND CLINICAL PRESENTATION

If the shunt across the PDA is small, no signs or symptoms may be present, or a murmur heard during physical examination might be the only abnormality. Patients are typically asymptomatic. The murmur may be a soft systolic murmur best heard at the left upper sternal border or a continuous murmur. The murmur is often harsh and may have a "machinery" quality. The presence of the murmur does not necessarily imply that the PDA is hemodynamically significant, because the murmur most likely results from the jet from the PDA striking the anterior aspect of the PA.[5] Likewise the absence of a murmur does not imply that the PDA is hemodynamically insignificant, because left heart dilation has been found even in the absence of a murmur.[6] Chest x-ray findings may be normal with a small PDA, as may the electrocardiograph (ECG). Echocardiography in a parasternal short-axis view is diagnostic with color Doppler demonstrating the left-to-right shunt **(Video 22–1).** Echocardiography is also used to assess the hemodynamic significance of the PDA by measuring the size of the LA and LV and to assess for signs of pulmonary hypertension. Other testing such as a computed tomography (CT) scan or magnetic resonance imaging (MRI) are usually not necessary to diagnose a PDA[7] (although they may be helpful in situations in which the echocardiographic assessment is suboptimal) and often leads to overestimation of the size of the PDA.

Patients with moderately sized PDAs may complain of dyspnea on exertion and easy fatigability. Moderately sized PDAs result in widened pulse pressure and the continuous murmur, as described. The chest x-ray may be normal or demonstrate mild cardiomegaly. The ECG may demonstrate left ventricular hypertrophy (LVH). The echocardiogram demonstrates the PDA, as well as left atrial and ventricular dilation.

Patients with large PDAs also complain of dyspnea on exertion and fatigability and may have overt signs of left heart failure. Large PDAs result in a wide pulse pressure with a continuous murmur. A thrill from the PDA may be palpable, and the second heart sound may be accentuated. The chest x-ray demonstrates cardiomegaly and increased pulmonary vascularity. The ECG demonstrates LVH. The echocardiogram demonstrates the PDA with a dilated LA and LV. There is a low velocity diastolic flow jet in the PA, and there may be diastolic flow reversal in the descending aorta.

Large PDAs associated with the development of pulmonary vascular disease lead to a decrease in left-to-right shunt across the PDA and eventually a right-to-left shunt. This is manifest by a soft systolic or no murmur and a loud P2. The chest x-ray demonstrates findings of pulmonary vascular disease with a normal heart size and prominent central pulmonary arteries. The ECG shows right ventricular hypertrophy. There may be clubbing and cyanosis of the lower extremities because the desaturated blood from the PA is directed across the PDA into the descending aorta. Echocardiography may demonstrate a right-to-left shunt across the PDA with evidence of pulmonary hypertension. The right-to-left shunt may be difficult to appreciate on transthoracic echocardiography, and a cardiac catheterization may be indicated.

MANAGEMENT

The only potential indication to close a small hemodynamically insignificant PDA is prevention of endarteritis. This is a controversial topic. A recent review on this subject by Fortescue et al[8] estimated that the risk of endarteritis associated with this type of a PDA is between 0.01% and 0.001% per year. These authors also reviewed 10 published papers on transcatheter PDA closure as well as their own institutional experience. They reported a major overall adverse event rate of 1.5%, with a minor adverse event rate of 8%. Their conclusion was that "there is no evidence to support a superior risk/benefit balance for routine closure of the very small hemodynamically insignificant PDA, and accordingly, it is difficult to justify closure of such defects simply to reduce the risk of infective endocarditis and its complications."

According to 2008 guidelines from the American College of Cardiology/American Heart Association (ACC/AHA),[9] routine follow-up examination every 3 to 5 years is recommended for patients with a small PDA and no evidence of left heart enlargement (Class I recommendation; **Box 22–1).**

PROCEDURAL TECHNIQUE

PDAs of 2 mm or smaller at the narrowest portion are suitable for coil embolization. Coils are available in a variety of shapes and sizes **(Figure 22–1).** PDAs larger than 2 mm in diameter may be closed with coils, but the embolization risk is higher, and multiple coils and specialized techniques may be required. Therefore for larger PDAs, device closure using the Amplatzer ductal occluder (ADO; St. Jude Medical, St. Paul, Minn.) is preferred. Ductal morphology is important, in addition to size of the ductus. The Krichenko classification is generally used for PDA morphology **(Figure 22–2).**[10]

Coil Occlusion

Multiple techniques for transcatheter coil occlusion of PDAs have been described. This chapter covers the basic technique and briefly mentions some of the modifications that have been used.

1. Establish femoral venous and arterial access. Perform a right and left heart catheterization to assess the degree of shunt and pulmonary pressures and resistance.
2. Perform an aortogram. The straight lateral projection usually profiles the PDA quite well. Steep right anterior oblique ($\approx$45 degrees) can also be used to elongate the ductus. The catheter should be positioned in the descending aorta near the left subclavian artery.
3. Assess the morphology of the PDA from the angiogram **(see Figure 22–2).** Measure the narrowest portion of the PDA. If the PDA is 2 mm or smaller in diameter, coil embolization may be performed. If the diameter is larger than 2 mm, device deployment is easiest.
4. Using an angled catheter such as a Judkins right coronary catheter, a soft-tipped 0.018-inch or 0.035-inch floppy wire is advanced retrograde across the ductus from the aorta. The catheter is then advanced over the wire and into the MPA, and the wire is subsequently removed.
5. A coil that has a diameter of at least twice the narrowest diameter of the ductus is chosen. The length of the coil should be such that approximately 4 loops of coil will form. This allows one loop to be placed in the MPA side and the remaining loops within the aortic ampulla. A quick way

to determine this is to divide the length of the coil in millimeters (mm) by (π ($\approx$3) × the coil diameter loop in mm). For example, if a 0.035-5-5 coil is chosen, the length is 5 cm (50 mm). 50 is divided by 15 (3 × 5), which yields approximately 3.3 loops of coil. Thicker gauge coils such as 0.035-inch, 0.038-inch, or even 0.052-inch are generally preferred. The thicker coils have more radial strength and are less likely to embolize.

6. The coil is loaded into the delivery catheter and advanced by using the soft end of a straight wire. For example, if a 4F delivery catheter is chosen with an internal dimension of 0.038-inch, and a 0.038-inch coil is used, a 0.035-inch or 0.038-inch wire may be used to advance the coil.
7. One half to one loop of coil is extruded into the MPA, and the catheter and coil are pulled back as a unit toward the aorta until the coil loop is positioned at the MPA end of the ductus. This is best appreciated on the straight lateral projection. For most PDAs this is at the anterior aspect of the tracheal air column.
8. Once the coil is positioned at the MPA end of the PDA, the delivery catheter is pulled into the aorta. The push wire can be used to advance coil loops into the aortic ampulla as the catheter is pulled back. The goal is to deliver one half to one loop on the PA end of the PDA and 3 to 4 loops in the aortic ampulla **(Figure 22–3).**

This method of coil deployment does not allow proximal or distal control of the coil loop; therefore coil maldeployment or embolization are risks of the procedure. In order to have more controlled delivery of the coil, multiple techniques have been developed, including snaring the coil in the MPA,[11] the bioptome-assisted technique,[12] the balloon-occlusion technique,[13] and a combination of the snare and bioptome-assisted techniques.[14] For a full description of these techniques, please consult the referenced articles. In addition to these methods, controlled release or detachable coils such as the Flipper coil (**see Figure 22–1, B;** Cook Medical, Bloomington, Ind.) are available.[15,16] These coils are quite useful because they allow repositioning and decrease the risk of embolization.

Device Occlusion

The ADO **(Figure 22–4)** is the most commonly used device to close moderate to large PDAs since approval by the U.S. Food and Drug Administration in 2003. The ADO has an aortic retention disk with an attached slightly conical-shaped body. The body tapers in diameter away from the aortic retention disk. The device is intended for implantation from a transvenous approach and is deployed through a 5F to 7F long sheath.

1. Similar to coil delivery, an aortic angiogram is performed **(Figure 22–5).** The device is chosen so that the smaller end of the device is 2 mm larger than the narrowest diameter of the PDA. If the PDA is

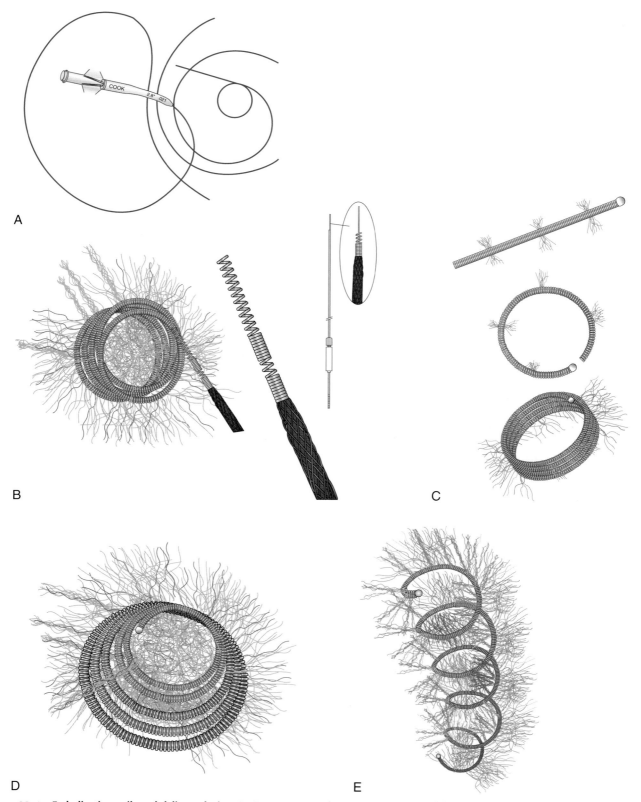

Figure 22–1 Embolization coils and delivery device. A, Cantata microcatheter (2.5F or 2.8F available). **B,** Flipper MREye 0.035 detachable coil and delivery system. **C,** Hilal 0.018-inch higher radial force microcoil. **D,** Tornado 0.018-inch and 0.035-inch soft coil. **E,** MREye Inconel 0.035-inch higher radial force coil. *(Permission for use granted by Cook Medical Incorporated, Bloomington, Ind.)*

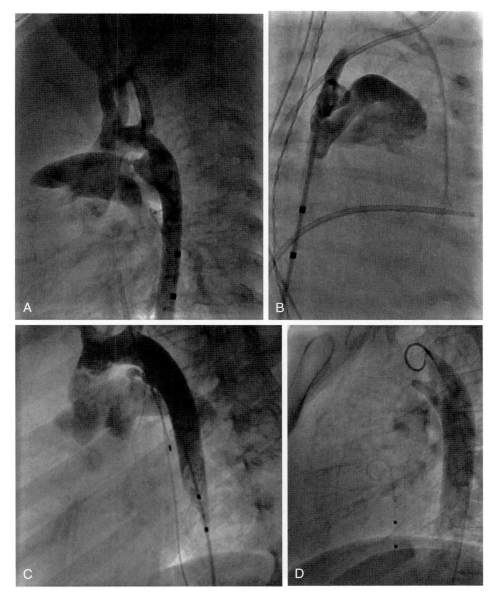

Figure 22–2 **Krichenko classification. A,** Type A ductus with narrowest insertion near the main pulmonary artery and short, conical-shaped ductus with well-developed aortic ampulla. A type B ductus is not shown; this patent ductus arteriosus (PDA) is short with the narrowest site at the aortic end. **B,** Right anterior oblique view of type C ductus, which is tubular and has no constriction. **C,** Type D PDA with multiple constrictions. **D,** Type E PDA is an elongated conical ductus with the narrowest insertion anterior to the anterior border of the airway on a lateral projection.

tubular in shape (Krichenko type C, **Figure 22–6, A**), an Amplatzer vascular plug II can be used, and also should be sized 2 mm bigger than the PDA diameter **(Figure 22–6, B)**.

2. After a device is chosen, the PDA is crossed from the PA end and an appropriately sized TorqVue delivery sheath (St. Jude Medical, Plymouth, Minn.) is placed over a wire across the PDA. In many adults it is very difficult or impossible to cross the PDA antegrade from the MPA because the ductus tends to be inserted in the roof of the PA. In this situation, the ductus is crossed retrograde from the aorta with a wire, and a snare is placed transvenously into the MPA. The wire is snared in the MPA, and then the wire is pulled into the descending aorta as the snare and catheter are advanced into the descending aorta. The snare is released and removed from the body, leaving the snare catheter in the descending aorta. A 0.035-inch exchange wire is advanced through the snare catheter into the aorta, and the snare catheter is then removed. The TorqVue sheath is advanced over the wire and into the descending aorta, the wire and dilator are removed, and the sheath is flushed with saline.

3. The ADO is threaded onto the delivery cable, loaded into the delivery system, and advanced through the long sheath. The aortic retention disk is delivered into the aorta. Attention should be made not to perforate the descending aorta while

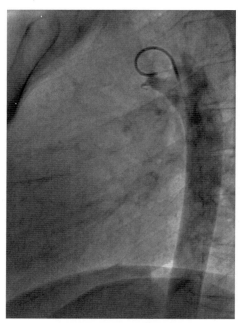

Figure 22–3   Lateral angiogram demonstrating proper positioning of a deployed coil. One half to one loop of coil should be deployed in the pulmonary artery with the remaining loops of coil in the aortic ampulla.

doing so. The sheath tip should not be against the back wall of the aorta during advancement of the device.

4. Once the retention disk is delivered, the whole delivery system is pulled back until the disk is well seated in the aortic ampulla, and then the remainder of the device is deployed. The airway often serves as a useful landmark for the PDA on the lateral view and positioning of the device.

5. An aortic angiogram is performed before releasing the device. This will confirm device position and assess for residual shunts. Once the device is in satisfactory position, it can be released from the delivery system **(Figure 22–7)**.

A dose of antibiotics is given 30 minutes before coil or device placement and then every 8 hours for two more doses. Prophylaxis for subacute bacterial endocarditis (SBE) is indicated for 6 months after successful transcatheter PDA closure. If a residual shunt is still present, life-long SBE prophylaxis is needed.

OUTCOME AND COMPLICATIONS

A recent review of transcatheter PDA closure was reported from Boston Children's Hospital.[8] The authors included their own institutional experience for a total of 1808 patients. Complete closure was reported in 94% of patients with follow-up periods ranging from 1 day to 1 year (86% to 100%). There were a total of 18 major adverse events (1.5%) and 169 minor adverse events (8%). Major adverse events occurred in 10 patients in whom the device/coil embolized and was

not retrieved and in six patients in whom an additional catheter or surgery was required for repair. In addition there was one patient death that was not related to the procedure and one case of endocarditis. Minor adverse events included 70 patients in whom a device embolized and was retrieved at the same procedure. For the overall series, device embolization occurred in 1.4% to 11.6% of patients. Other minor adverse events included mild aortic or left pulmonary artery (LPA) narrowing, arrhythmias, hemolysis, pulse loss, and the need for a blood transfusion.

SUMMARY

Persistent patency of the ductus arteriosus is a common congenital heart defect. In the current era, closure of the hemodynamically insignificant ductus is not indicated. For hemodynamically significant PDAs, transcatheter closure using either coils or devices is now the procedure of choice. Procedural outcomes are excellent, with complete closure rates of 94% and major adverse event rates of 1.5%.

22.2   Coronary Artery Fistulas

BACKGROUND

Coronary artery fistulas (CAFs) are a rare congenital or acquired abnormality in which a coronary artery branch terminates in a low-pressure vessel or chamber **(Figure 22–8 and Video 22–2)**. Although CAFs most commonly (up to 90%) terminate in right-sided chambers or vessels (including the right atrium [RA], RV, PA, coronary sinus, superior vena cava), termination in left-sided chambers has also been reported (LA and LV).[17] Coronary fistulas have been referred to as *coronary–cameral fistulas*; however, this phrase more appropriately describes the subset of fistulas that terminate in a cardiac chamber.[18] Coronary fistulas may arise from the right coronary, left coronary, or even both vessels in the same individual.[19]

CAFs were first described by Wilhelm Krause in 1865 in an otherwise healthy 53-year-old man who was ultimately found to have a large ramus intermedius-to-pulmonary artery fistula,[20] and successful surgical closure was first described by Biorck and Crafoord in 1947.[21] Interestingly, the first transcatheter closure was performed in 1981 by Reidy and colleagues[22] after successful angioplasty of a severe left anterior descending artery (LAD) lesion. The operators then directed a detachable balloon to the distal circumflex to occlude the fistula to the bronchial artery. Follow-up angiography approximately 7 months later demonstrated persistent occlusion of the CAF as well as patency of the circumflex and LAD.[22]

Since those historic milestones, the incidence of congenital CAFs in the general population has been estimated at 0.002%.[23] A systematic review of approximately 125,000 angiograms performed at the Cleveland Clinic during the years of 1960 to 1988 revealed an incidence of 0.12% "small coronary fistulas" and 0.05% "multiple

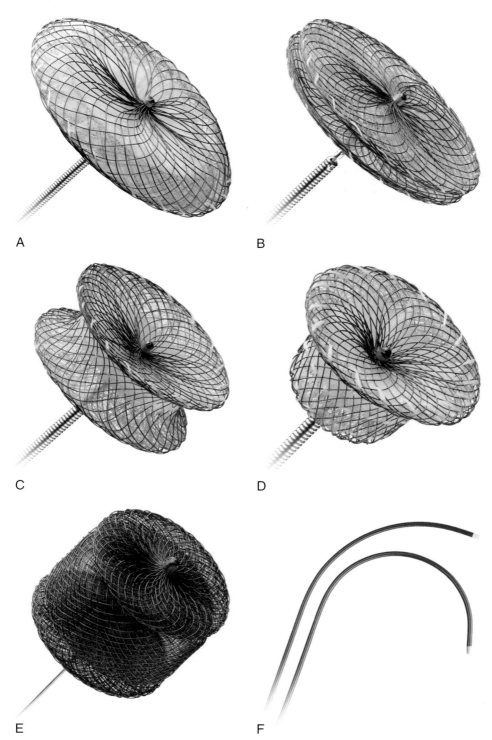

Figure 22–4 **Amplatzer occlusion devices. A,** Amplatzer septal occluder. **B,** Amplatzer multifenestrated septal occluder (Cribriform Amplatzer duct occluder). **C,** Amplatzer muscular ventral septal defect occluder. **D,** Amplatzer duct occluder. **E,** Amplatzer Vascular Plug II. **F,** Amplatzer TorqVue 45-degree and 180-degree delivery systems. *(Reprinted with permission of St. Jude Medical, St. Paul, Minn., 2012. All rights reserved.)*

or large-sized coronary fistulas"; however, patients with congenital heart disease or other coronary anomalies were excluded from analysis.[24] In contrast, acquired coronary fistulas are even rarer and can occur as a result of complications of cardiac surgery,[25] endomyocardial biopsy,[26,27] or coronary angioplasty.[28] Traumatic CAFs result most commonly from penetrating chest trauma involving the coronary artery and have a more acute natural history than coronary fistulas resulting from other etiologies.[29,30]

Coronary fistulas can also be associated with complex congenital heart disease, specifically single ventricle abnormalities such as pulmonary atresia with intact ventricular septum[31] or hypoplastic left heart syndrome.[32-34] These diffuse fistulas, often referred to as *sinusoids*, are associated with poor outcome caused by inadequate myocardial perfusion and additional

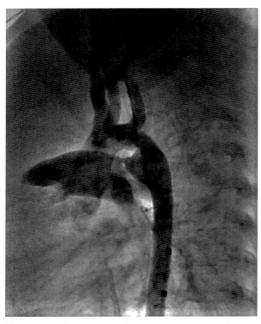

Figure 22–5 Lateral angiogram demonstrating type A ductus suitable for closure using the Amplatzer duct occluder.

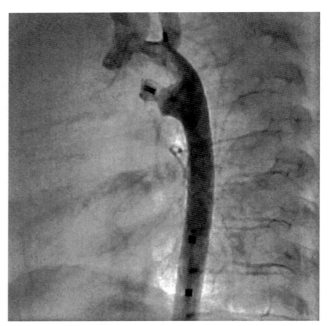

Figure 22–7 Angiogram demonstrating an appropriately placed Amplatzer duct occluder with no residual shunt.

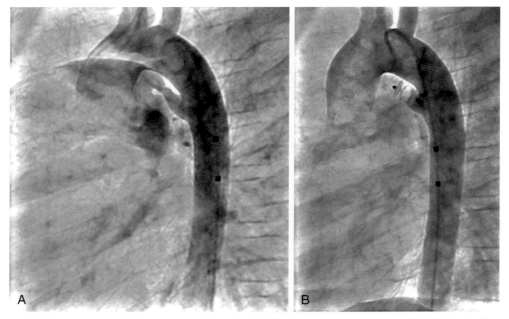

Figure 22–6 **A,** Krichenko type C ductus (tubular). This type of ductus is difficult to occlude with coils or the duct occluder and is most suitable for the Amplatzer vascular plug II. **B,** Lateral angiogram after closure of the tubular ductus demonstrating appropriate positioning and complete ductal closure.

volume load. The diffuse nature of these fistulas are also generally less amenable to closure or ligation **(Figure 22–9 and Video 22–3).**

DIAGNOSIS AND CLINICAL PRESENTATION

The pathophysiology and clinical presentation of a CAF results from the absence of an intervening capillary bed. Symptoms are largely dependent on the size of the vessel and the chamber with which it communicates. For example, large coronary fistulas that drain into right-sided chambers and systemic veins can cause a left-to-right shunt and volume overload with heart failure symptoms **(Table 22–1).** Alternatively, the high-flow run-off can produce steal from the myocardial capillary bed, producing myocardial ischemia with anginal symptoms such as chest pain or dyspnea on exertion. Myocardial infarction can result because the large caliber fistula can serve as a nidus for thrombus formation (especially

in aneurysmal vessels), which can either propagate retrograde into a branch coronary artery or embolize distally. Cerebral infarction has been reported as a result of thrombus embolization from a coronary fistula to the RA across a patent foramen ovale.[35]

Smaller fistulas are often asymptomatic and may be monitored; a 10-year follow-up study in one series demonstrated that these patients are unlikely to develop symptoms or enlargement of fistulas.[36] Finally, endocarditis may occur in up to 3% of medium and large coronary fistulas.[37]

Whereas small coronary fistulas are silent on physical examination, large coronary fistulas may result in both continuous systolic and diastolic murmurs and can often been identified on transthoracic echocardiography **(see Figure 22–8, *B* and *C*, and Video 22–2 *B* and *C*).** In contrast, small coronary fistulas may only be seen as an incidental finding on coronary angiography. Cardiac CT or MRI are generally not required for diagnosis, but they may be helpful for preprocedural planning. Nuclear

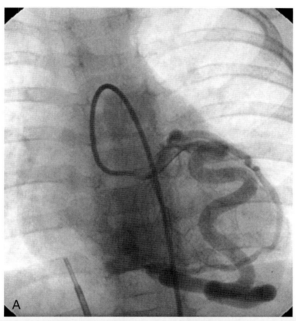

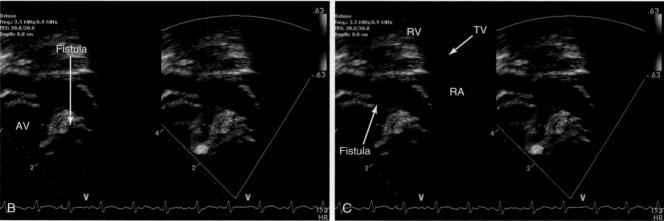

Figure 22–8 A, Angiogram of a large left coronary fistula to the right ventricle (RV) in an infant. **B,** Echocardiogram with color Doppler in modified apical five-chamber view. **C,** RV inflow view demonstrating the fistula opening under the tricuspid valve (TV).

myocardial perfusion may be helpful for evaluating for ischemia in the territory of the fistula resulting from coronary steal,[38] especially in patients with a history of atherosclerotic coronary disease. Cardiac catheterization and angiography is the gold standard for identification of the coronary fistula **(see Figure 22–8, A, and Video 22–4).** Most adult patients do not have a quantifiable left-to-right shunt by catheterization, whereas rarely, infants with an especially large coronary fistula may have a Qp:Qs greater than 1.

Aneurysm formation of the coronary fistula up to 4 or 5 cm in diameter has been reported,[19,39] with a rate of up to 26% in one series.[40] Aneurysm formation in coronary fistulas may be related to an underlying inflammatory

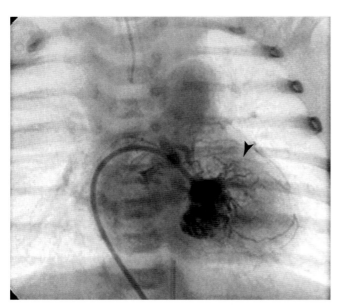

Figure 22–9 Left ventriculogram in hypoplastic left heart syndrome with diffuse coronary fistulas. Diffuse sinusoids can be seen from left ventricular injection with flow to coronary arteries (*arrowhead*).

process.[35] Increased shear stress caused by increased flow as well as turbulence may predispose the vessel to mural thinning as well as thrombus formation. Coronary fistula aneurysm rupture can occur, resulting in tearing chest pain (with or without radiation to the back), syncope, and, ultimately, tamponade.[41,42]

Rarely, mitral regurgitation can be seen as a result of a left circumflex to coronary sinus fistula.[43]

PATIENT SELECTION

Guidelines for the treatment of coronary fistulas were published by the ACC and the AHA in 2008[9] **(see Table 22–1).** Although this chapter focuses on transcatheter closure, surgical treatment of coronary fistulas continues to play an important role, especially in patients with other cardiovascular issues requiring surgical intervention. Surgical closure of large coronary fistulas has been safe and feasible. Approximately half of surgical procedures published were performed off cardiopulmonary bypass when taking an extracardiac approach, whereas intracardiac repair required cardiopulmonary bypass, but the rate of residual shunt has been reported to be lower. Regardless of approach, overall mortality has been about 1%.[18,44] Older adults were more likely to have complications such as arrhythmia (2% to 10%), myocardial ischemia (14%), infarction (2%), or postpericardiotomy syndrome (10%).[45,46] In addition, follow-up angiography in one series demonstrated that 19% of the parent coronary arteries had either thrombosed or become threadlike, and 19% had residual fistulous flow.[46] Two cases have resulted in aneurysmal dilation of the LAD with thrombus formation, myocardial infarction, or left ventricular aneurysm formation, and one patient has gone on to develop mitral regurgitation.[47] Finally, very late (up to 10 years) thrombus formation with myocardial infarction can occur after surgical closure.[48,49] Taken together, as with all cardiac surgery, patient-specific risks as well as procedural risks must be balanced against the risks of the coronary fistula.

TABLE 22–1 ∎

Definition of Size of Coronary Artery Fistulas, Pathophysiology, and ACC/AHA Guidelines for Management[9]

	Size	2008 ACC/AHA Guidelines
Small	<2 × reference vessel diameter	Class I: A small to moderate CAVF in the presence of documented myocardial ischemia, arrhythmia, otherwise unexplained ventricular systolic or diastolic dysfunction or enlargement, or endarteritis should be closed via either a transcatheter or surgical approach after delineation of its course and its potential to fully obliterate the fistula. (Level of Evidence: C)
		Class IIa: Clinical follow-up with echocardiography every 3 to 5 years can be useful for patients with small, asymptomatic CAVF to exclude development of symptoms or arrhythmias or progression of size or chamber enlargement that might alter management. (Level of Evidence: C)
		Class III: Patients with small, asymptomatic CAVF should not undergo closure of CAVF. (Level of Evidence: C)
Moderate	2-3 × reference vessel diameter	See above.
Large	>3 × reference vessel diameter	Class I: A large CAVF, regardless of symptomatology, should be closed via either a transcatheter or surgical route after delineation of its course and its potential to fully obliterate the fistula. (Level of Evidence: C)

ACC, American College of Cardiology; *AHA*, American Heart Association; *CAVF*, coronary arteriovenous fistula.

As such, the transcatheter approach to closure of coronary fistulas has become an appealing alternative. Although data are limited regarding outcomes related to patient factors in transcatheter closure,[50] factors that play a role in coronary interventional outcomes may be extrapolated and include renal insufficiency, congestive heart failure, diabetes mellitus, and peripheral arterial disease (especially involving the aortoiliofemoral system). Certainly, atherosclerotic coronary artery disease may interfere with or complicate transcatheter closure of the coronary fistula.

Lesion Characteristics

A number of specific features of the coronary fistula may present challenges for transcatheter closure: (1) If the coronary artery branch is near the occlusion site, placement of the occlusion device adjacent to the ostium of a branch coronary artery may lead to obstruction of the branch or propagation of thrombus into the branch; (2) although advances in coronary wire technology have made negotiation of extreme tortuosity feasible, advancing a sheath and device to the site can be severely challenging. In addition, the tortuosity may add length to the vessel, requiring longer delivery sheaths and catheters than available; (3) multiple drainage sites have previously been thought to be a contraindication to transcatheter closure because of difficulty in occluding all sites; however, with advances in delivery systems and closure devices, upstream fistula closure is now feasible.

TECHNIQUE

The approach to closure of a coronary fistula is dependent on the origin and termination of the fistula **(Figure 22–10).**[51] In the distal type of coronary fistula, the fistula is located at the distal end of the coronary artery, inducing dilation of the entire coronary vessel. Intuitively, closure should be directed toward the distal fistulous segment. In contrast, the proximal type of coronary fistula branches early from the main coronary artery, creating a large conduit vessel that terminates in the low-pressure chamber or vessel. Latson and coworkers have recommended closing this type of fistula at both the distal termination site as well as the near the proximal take-off of the fistula in order to prevent the formation of a large blind pouch and attendant nidus for thrombus with possible embolic complications from both the coronary end and the cardiac-chamber end.[17]

The shape and size of the fistula and its termination site also influence the choice of device. A long, narrow terminus may be treated with a Gianturco or detachable coils **(see Figure 22–1B;** Cook Medical, Bloomington, Ind).[52] A larger fistula or larger terminus may require larger devices such as the ADO, Amplatzer vascular plug, or the Grifka-Gianturco vascular occlusion device.[50,53] Massive fistulas without ideal distal closure sites may require larger devices such as the Amplatzer muscular ventricular septal defect occluder or the Amplatzer atrial septal occluder[54] **(see Figure 22–4).** Finally, covered stents have also been used to stent across the fistula, especially in the setting of atherosclerotic stenotic disease.[55]

In addition, direction of approach to the fistula can vary depending on the specific anatomy of the fistula. For example, closure of the fistula can be undertaken from the antegrade approach (from the aortic root and coronary ostium to the distal fistula) via arterial access only. In contrast, the terminal end of the fistula can be directly cannulated, and closure can be performed from venous access only. Thirdly, an arteriovenous loop can be created by advancing a guidewire through the coronary

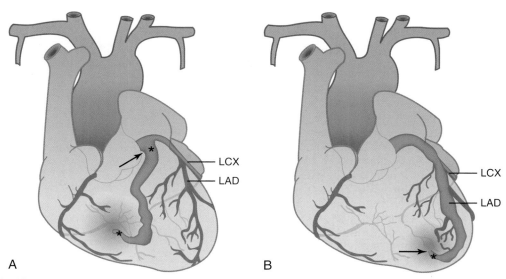

Figure 22–10 **Classification of coronary fistulas. A,** Proximal type coronary fistula. A vessel branches off the main coronary artery and terminates in the low-pressure chamber or vessel, becoming dilated while leaving the remainder of the main vessel normal caliber. **B,** Distal type coronary fistula. The distal end of the native coronary artery terminates in a low-pressure chamber or vessel, causing the entire main coronary artery to dilate. *LCX,* Left circumflex coronary artery; *LAD,* left anterior descending artery. *(Modified from Gowda ST, Latson LA, Kutty S, et al: Intermediate to long-term outcome following congenital coronary artery fistulae closure with focus on thrombus formation, The Am J Cardiol 2011;107:302-308.)*

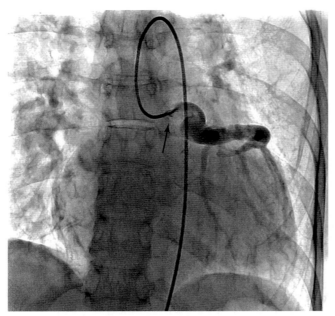

Figure 22–11 Guide catheter cannulation. A 6F VL-4 Wiseguide (Boston Scientific, Boston, Mass.; *arrow*) has been used to cannulate the left coronary fistula, giving excellent support and opacification of the vessel.

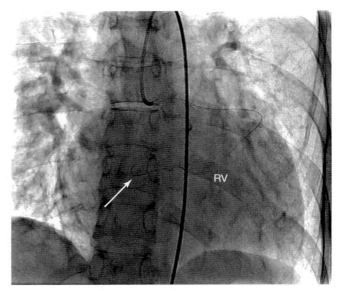

Figure 22–12 Guidewire advancement. A soft, hydrophilic 0.014-inch Intuition guidewire (Medtronic, Minneapolis, Minn.) has been advanced through the length of the fistula, right ventricle *(RV)*, and into the right atrium.

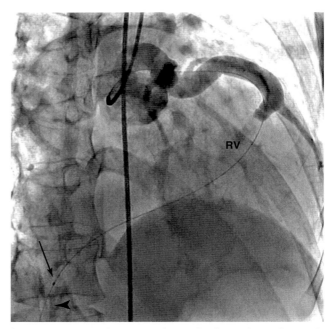

Figure 22–13 Arteriovenous wire and microcatheter loop. The 0.014-inch wire *(arrowhead)* has been advanced along with a microcatheter *(radiopaque mark, arrow)* through the length of the fistula through the right ventricle *(RV)*, snared and externalized through the venous access sheath. (Note: The snare has already been externalized and is not seen in this figure.) The microcatheter covers the length of the wire through the length of the fistula, protecting the vessel and adjacent structures from injury by excessive tension on the wire loop.

fistula and exteriorizing the wire to generate ultimate support for device delivery.[56]

The following list is a general outline of one approach to transcatheter closure of coronary fistulas.

1. Guide cannulation: Cannulation of the coronary ostium may be more straightforward, given the vast number of commercially available coronary guide catheters, than an attempt to cannulate the terminus of the fistula. In addition, once stable guide position has been established, antegrade coronary angiography can be performed by hand injection from the guide to visualize the vessel at any time during the procedure **(Figure 22–11 and Video 22–4).**

2. Guidewire placement: As with wiring any coronary lesion, care must be taken not to perturb the intima or produce possible mural thrombus. A large gentle curve on the tip of the wire will facilitate negotiating large tortuous fistulas, especially if using a soft, hydrophilic polymer-jacketed wire. A 300-cm wire should be used if an arteriovenous loop is planned, and the wire should be advanced out the fistula terminus to the chamber **(Figure 22–12).**

3. Snare and arteriovenous loop creation (coronary fistulas to left-sided structures may require a slightly different strategy): The creation of an arteriovenous loop is a powerful method to increase support for delivery of the occlusion device. Once the guidewire has been advanced through the fistula and out into the chamber or vessel, an appropriately sized snare and catheter is used to capture the guidewire and externalize it from the venous sheath **(Figure 22–13 and Video 22–5).** The MPA, superior vena cava, and inferior vena cava serve as ideal chambers to snare the guidewire because of the straight shape of the chambers.

4. Microcatheter/catheter protection: Once the arteriovenous wire loop has been created, care must

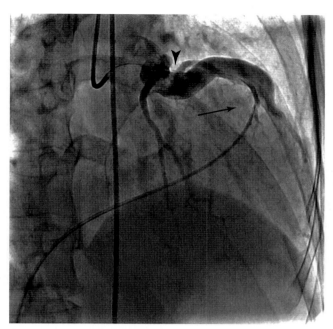

Figure 22–14   Test Occlusion. A 7F balloon-tipped end-hole catheter has been advanced over the arteriovenous loop *(arrowhead)* to the coronary fistula and inflated *(arrow)* to test-occlude the vessel given the proximity of the nearby coronary artery branch.

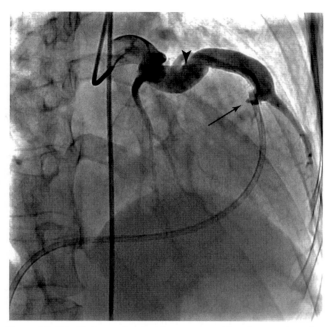

Figure 22–15   Delivery sheath advancement. After the creation of an arteriovenous wire loop, the device delivery sheath *(arrow)* has been advanced over the wire *(arrowhead)* from the venous access site to the coronary fistula.

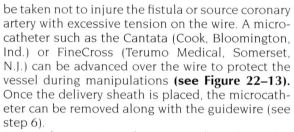

be taken not to injure the fistula or source coronary artery with excessive tension on the wire. A microcatheter such as the Cantata (Cook, Bloomington, Ind.) or FineCross (Terumo Medical, Somerset, N.J.) can be advanced over the wire to protect the vessel during manipulations **(see Figure 22–13).** Once the delivery sheath is placed, the microcatheter can be removed along with the guidewire (see step 6).

5. Test occlusion: Once the site to place the occlusion device has been identified, a balloon-tipped catheter such as a wedge catheter (Arrow, Garrycastle, Ireland) or angioplasty catheter is advanced to the site and inflated for approximately 15 minutes **(Figure 22–14 and Video 22–6).** The ECG is monitored for any evidence of ischemic changes, and additional angiography is performed to evaluate patency of nearby coronary artery branches. If no ischemic or hemodynamic compromise is evident, the procedure can proceed safely with device closure.

6. Delivery sheath advancement: The delivery sheath or guiding catheter for device deployment is then advanced over the arteriovenous wire loop, either antegrade or retrograde, depending on specific anatomic constraints **(Figure 22–15).** For example, to place an ADO with the retention disk on the fistula side, the delivery sheath is advanced retrograde into the fistula to deploy the device in the correct orientation. Some operators have suggested the use of a balloon-tipped catheter inside the delivery sheath rather than the stiff dilator given the fragile and thin-walled nature of the coronary fistula.[57]

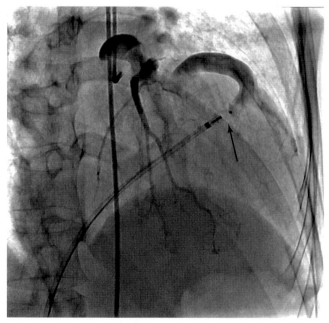

Figure 22–16   Device deployment. An Amplatzer ductal occluder has been deployed at the proximal take-off of the coronary fistula *(arrow)*. The nearest coronary artery branch can be seen proximal to, but distant from, the deployment position of the device.

7. Device deployment: After deployment of the device, the ECG, hemodynamics, and coronary artery flow should be monitored before device release. On occasion, coronary artery spasm can be seen and can be easily treated by intracoronary injection of up to 200 mcg of nitroglycerin or other vasodilator **(Figure 22–16 and Video 22–7).** If no ischemia

BOX 22–2
Coronary Artery Fistulas: Tips and Tricks

Guide selection: A medium support guide is likely adequate if arteriovenous loop is planned.
Arteriovenous loop: Maximizes support for device delivery. Use a microcatheter to protect fistula from wire trauma.
Antegrade and retrograde approach: Use an antegrade approach to wire lesion and perform angiography retrograde to efficiently deliver the device.
Guidewire selection: An atraumatic, polymer-jacketed hydrophilic wire is recommended for tortuous fistulas.
Coronary spasm: Coronary spasm can occur as a result of manipulation, and intracoronary nitroglycerin and other vasodilators should be available and used if the patency of a nearby coronary branch is in question **(Figure 22–17 and Video 22–8).**

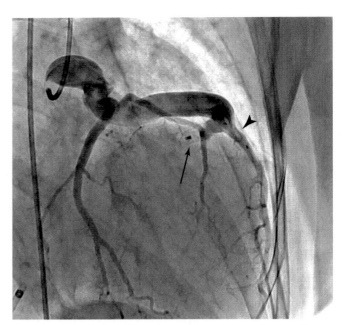

Figure 22–17 Spasm of the coronary branch immediately adjacent to the occlusion point of the fistula has been treated by advancing a coronary angioplasty balloon catheter *(arrowhead)* over a 0.014-inch coronary wire to the distal segment of the vessel. Nitroglycerin was then given directly through the angioplasty catheter to successfully treat the spasm. Angiography demonstrates brisk, normal flow after direct administration of a vasodilator. The occlusion device can be seen stably positioned in the background, without evidence of compromising the ostium of the coronary branch *(arrow).*

or hemodynamic compromise is seen, the device is released, and final angiography is performed to confirm position.

8. Postprocedure: Anticoagulation is a necessity; however, the regimen and time frame remain highly controversial.[51,58] Whereas some operators recommend immediate anticoagulation with heparin and then warfarin for at least 1 year postprocedure, others recommend the use of aspirin and warfarin for at least 6 months. Although there remains minimal data to support a specific regimen, the patient, lesion, and procedural characteristics should play a role. For example, in a patient with an atherosclerotic disease, a complex fistula with a residual large blind pouch and sluggish flow in the fistula proximal to multiple coronary branches should receive more aggressive anticoagulation with warfarin (or some other antithrombotic) and at least one antiplatelet drug. Follow-up imaging also remains undefined, although regular noninvasive evaluation by CT or MR angiography, as well as functional evaluation by way of treadmill stress with echocardiography or nuclear perfusion, has been proposed. In patients who remain at higher risk, follow-up invasive angiography may also be considered[59] **(Box 22–2).**

COMPLICATIONS

Overall, transcatheter closure of coronary fistulas is safe and feasible, with an excellent rate of acute procedural success.[50-53,56,57] No mortalities have been reported, although some case series report a small number of serious complications. Coronary thrombosis and myocardial infarction occurred in 3% to 10% of cases, whereas residual shunt requiring subsequent reintervention was seen in 22% with follow-up angiography.[56,60] Device embolization occurred in 6% to 23% of cases, transient ischemic ECG changes in 10%, atrial arrhythmias in 15%, coronary spasm in one patient, and clinically silent dissection in two patients.

When considered with the surgical literature, Gowda and coworkers[51] have proposed three risk factors for thrombotic occlusion of the parent or branch coronary artery: (1) occlusion of the distal type coronary fistula **(see Figure 22–10);** (2) closure in an older patient; and (3) absence of anticoagulation after closure. In addition, placement of a closure device as close to the take-off of the branch-vessel type of coronary fistula may prevent formation of a blind pouch and resulting nidus of thrombus.[59]

Long-term complications, including coronary thrombosis and recurrent fistula, have been well-documented in the surgical literature; however, long-term complication remains incompletely studied in transcatheter closures. The Congenital Cardiovascular Interventional Study Consortium is developing an outcomes registry for transcatheter closure of coronary fistulas.[59] Additional work will be required to define optimal follow-up assessment, anticoagulation strategies, and long-term complication rates after transcatheter coronary fistula closure.

22.3 Pulmonary Arteriovenous Malformations

BACKGROUND

PAVMs are high-flow, low-pressure communications between pulmonary arteries and pulmonary veins, allowing deoxygenated blood to bypass the pulmonary capillary bed and return to the LA. PAVMs were first described at autopsy in 1897 by Churton.[61] PAVMs are not only a cause of cyanosis and exercise intolerance but also a source for thromboemboli resulting in cerebrovascular accident or brain abscess. The size and number of these PAVMs determine the degree of cyanosis and the risk for embolic events. PAVMs can be either congenital or acquired, with the majority of congenital PAVMs found in individuals with hereditary hemorrhagic telangiectasia (HHT).[62]

HHT is a genetic disorder caused by gene mutations in the transforming growth factor-beta pathway. Three genes' mutations have been identified that account for 85% to 90% of individuals that have a clinical diagnosis of HHT. HHT-1 is caused by a mutation in ENG, the gene encoding the endothelial cell surface-binding protein Endoglin. The Endoglin gene mutation has been mapped to chromosome 9q3. HHT-2 is caused by a mutation in the gene for activin receptor-like kinase 1 (ACVRL1 or ALK1), also an endothelial cell-binding protein, which has been mapped to chromosome 12q. SMAD4, a gene encoding an intracellular signaling protein, has been identified as an additional mutation in some patients with HHT.[62]

PAVMs may also be found in a variety of acquired conditions. Right-to-left shunting as a result of communications between pulmonary arteries and pulmonary veins has been reported in hepatic cirrhosis[63] and rarely in schistosomiasis.[64] Mitral stenosis, trauma, actinomycosis,[65] and Fanconi syndrome[66] have also been implicated in intrapulmonary shunting. Cardiologists specializing in congenital heart disease encounter PAVMs that are more commonly associated with single ventricle physiology such as following the Glenn shunt, a superior cavopulmonary anastamosis,[67] or following the Fontan, a total cavopulmonary connection.[68]

The distribution of pulmonary blood flow has been shown to affect the angiogenesis and vascular remodeling of the pulmonary vasculature.[69-71] As with hepatopulmonary syndrome, PAVMs can develop if the pulmonary arterial bed has received deficient hepatic venous blood flow. The direct mechanism by which these PAVMs develop is unclear. The generally accepted theory is that there is a "hepatic factor" in the hepatic venous return that is involved in vascular apoptosis or pulmonary vasoconstriction. If the hepatic venous-to-pulmonary artery connection is diverted, 25% to 30% of individuals develop PAVMs within 3 to 5 years. These PAVMs may involute over time once adequate hepatic venous flow is reestablished to the pulmonary vascular bed, as in a Fontan completion after a classic Glenn shunt.[72-74]

CLINICAL PRESENTATION AND DIAGNOSIS

PAVMs are a rare but treatable cause of cryptogenic stroke. A contrast echocardiogram or echo bubble study is a sensitive test for diagnosing PAVMs. Injecting agitated saline via a peripheral vein while simultaneously imaging the right and left atria by ultrasound is a quick and sensitive test to diagnose intracardiac or intrapulmonary shunting.[75,76] In the case of intracardiac shunting such as from a patent foramen ovale or atrial septal defect, the LA and RA almost simultaneously fill with contrast bubbles, whereas in the case of PAVMs there is a delay of three to five cardiac cycles before contrast bubbles are seen in the LA **(Video 22–9)**. Near-simultaneous right atrial and left atrial filling may represent a proximal PAVM and not an intracardiac shunt. Shunt quantification and PAVM localization based on bubble studies and other contrast media is somewhat limited and much less sensitive compared to pulmonary angiography.[75]

PAVMs are of significant clinical concern because of their relative high-flow nature. If left untreated, 25% to 35% of individuals with PAVMs will have a stroke or brain abscess.[77-79] Evaluation of this data by Rosenblatt and White and the HHT Center at Yale found that individuals who had a neurologic event had a PAVM with a feeding artery of 3 mm or greater in diameter.[80] This single observational abstract was the basis for the guidelines that all PAVMs should be embolized if the feeding artery is 3 mm or greater. Despite this data, however, smaller feeding arteries are not free from risk for an embolic event,[81,82] and as such many centers are now taking the approach of embolizing all PAVMs that can be accessed without regard to feeding-artery size.[83]

EMBOLIZATION THERAPY

Embolization therapy has become the standard approach for treating PAVMs. The first case of embolization therapy of PAVM was reported by Porstman in 1977 using handmade steel coils in Germany.[84] Since then embolization with coils, detachable balloons, or devices has been well documented and has become the standard of care for treatment of PAVMs. It is thought that the arterial occlusion of a simple PAVM is technically easier and less time-consuming than that of complex PAVM, but that it involves a greater risk for paradoxical embolization.[85] The technique of coil embolotherapy involves localization of the PAVM by angiography followed by selective catheterization of the feeding artery. The catheter tip is advanced past the point of any proximal vessels that supply normal lung parenchyma and positioned as close to the neck of the PAVM as possible. The camera angles need to be set such that the feeding artery and aneurysmal sac are seen as they come together. Improper, overlapping images could lead to improper coil position and potential coil embolization. Often, several angiographic images need to be taken in subsegmental branches in order to obtain optimal angles for proper coil or device positioning. A coil is advanced through the catheter and released at this point, angiography is repeated, and additional coils are positioned if needed until blood flow to the PAVM has ceased. Gaining stable guide-catheter position can be one of the more challenging aspects of this procedure, given the multiple angulations involved traversing the RA, RV, PA, and multiple segmental PAs. Often, a "nested" catheter technique with two or more guides and catheters may be required, especially for lower-lobe PAVMs. With smaller, distal PAVMs

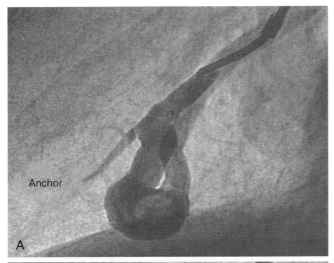

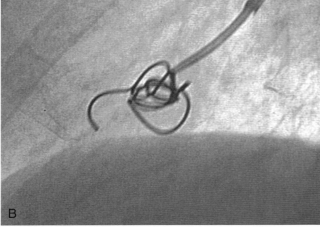

Figure 22–18 The Anchor technique described by White et al,[85] in which a small segment of the distal coil is placed in a small side branch and the remaining coil is deployed in the main, feeding artery of the pulmonary arteriovenous malformation.

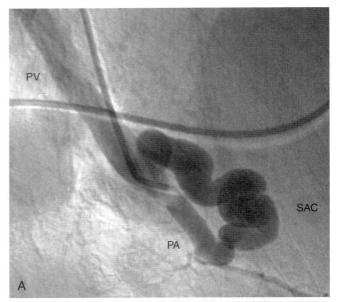

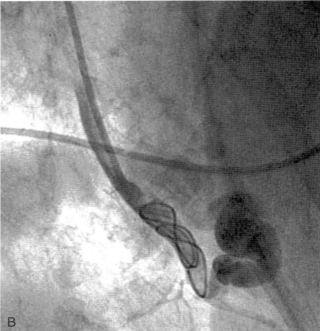

Figures 22–19 The scaffold technique described by White et al,[85] in which a larger, oversized coil is placed in the feeding artery of the pulmonary arteriovenous malformation as a base structure to hold the softer and more flexible coils. **A,** An Amplatzer vascular plug has been deployed proximal to a large AVM. **B,** Coils have been deployed proximal to a deployed Amplatzer vascular plug to completely occlude the AVM. *PA,* Pulmonary artery; *PV,* pulmonary vein.

stability can be achieved by advancing a microcatheter through a 4F multipurpose or Judkins right catheter that is advanced together through a guide catheter or long sheath. Positioning the guide catheter or long sheath in the mid right or LPA will remove some of the movement caused by cardiac motion and allow for a more stable microcatheter.

White and colleagues[85] have developed two techniques for coil delivery to avoid coil embolization into the aneurysmal sac or to the pulmonary veins. The first technique, the "anchor" method, involves using a small proximal arterial branch to deliver a small segment of coil and then releasing the remaining coil in a slow stacking or weaving manner in the feeding artery **(Figure 22–18).**

The second method is the scaffold technique. This technique uses a larger diameter coil with a higher radial strength as a base for additional softer coils **(Figures 22–19).**

Another embolotherapy technique makes use of Amplatzer vascular plugs. After localization of the PAVM by angiography, a catheter is exchanged over a guidewire and positioned at the neck of the PAVM. The

vascular plug is delivered into the neck of the feeding artery, and angiography is repeated to ensure vessel occlusion. The advantage of the vascular plugs is that they can be recaptured and repositioned if they are not properly seated. For PAVM with feeding vessels greater than 7 to 10 mm in diameter, a combination of plugs and coils is commonly used to achieve total cross-sectional occlusion[86] **(Figure 22–20).** The disadvantage of vascular plugs is that they are more expensive than coils, large, and may be difficult to place in a

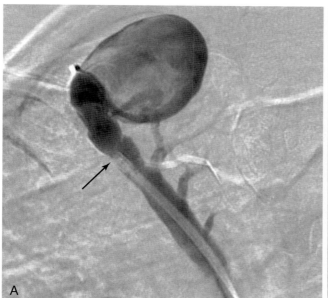 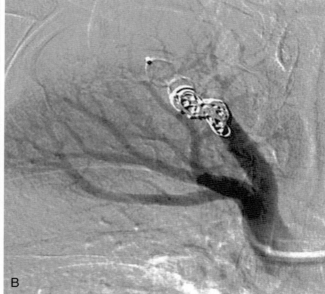

Figure 22–20 Amplatzer vascular plugs in addition to coils are needed to ensure complete cross-sectional occlusion of the pulmonary arteriovenous malformations.

distal feeding artery without compromising surrounding parenchymal tissue.

Embolization Risks and Pitfalls

The most common complication of embolization of a PAVM is coil embolization into the systemic circulation. Typically, the PAVM sacs are relatively wide, open vessels that empty freely into the pulmonary veins. A malpositioned coil can easily embolize to the systemic circulation. Additionally, care must be taken to avoid proximal PA embolization because viable lung tissue may be sacrificed and bronchial artery dilation may occur. Systemic collateralization via bronchial arteries increases the risk of pulmonary hemorrhage.

PAVMs with short feeding arteries may be embolized by placement of large coils in the venous sac; however, this technique damages viable lung tissue. Follow-up studies have shown that once a PAVM has been embolized, the aneurysmal sac involutes and normal lung tissue fills in.[87] As such, large embolization coils or occluding devices within the PAVM aneurysmal sacs are not only unnecessary, but may be harmful.

White and coworkers have reviewed the technical details of coil and embolotherapy extensively.[80,87] The general results of embolotherapy are excellent, with a technical success rate of over 95%.[87] Unfortunately, many individuals with macroscopic PAVMs with feeding arteries greater than 3 mm also have smaller microscopic or diffuse PAVMs. Embolization therapy does not remove all PAVMs and does not completely remove the risk of an embolic event. No mortality has been reported to date with embolization of PAVM, and complications have in general been rare and self-limited. Pleuritic chest pain is a relatively common finding and is seen in the first 24 to 48 hours after embolization.[80,88] Pulmonary infarction

may occur secondary to occlusion of normal pulmonary arterial branches. Procedural risks and complications include air embolism or thromboembolism, transient symptoms of angina, bradycardia, perioral paresthesias, aphasia, stroke, and seizures. Deep venous thrombosis of the lower extremity used for catheterization was reported in 1.6% of patients. Device migration has been reported in fewer than 2% of cases overall; however, this complication may be more common in larger PAVMs, because it was reported in 4% of those patients.[80,89]

FOLLOW-UP CARE AND LONG-TERM MONITORING

An echo bubble study is too sensitive for monitoring the response to embolotherapy because intrapulmonary shunting persists through microscopic PAVMs despite successful occlusion of all angiographically visible vessels. These microscopic PAVMs may be difficult to identify on CT scan or angiography. Patients with persistent markedly positive bubble studies after embolotherapy may have a previously unrecognized PAVM.[76,85] Follow-up monitoring is critical for patients with PAVMs and should be done with high resolution chest CT scans every 3 to 5 years, as should functional pulse oxygen testing such as an exercise stress test or the 6-minute walk test.[90]

Long-term follow-up study of patients treated with embolotherapy has been variable. Potentially serious complications have been seen in up to 5% of patients, including brain abscesses and strokes.[77,78,80] These were presumably caused by paradoxical embolization either from a treated PAVM or the development of a new PAVM.

In summary, treatment of PAVM with embolization therapy is very successful and is associated with minimal morbidity and mortality. Therefore it is recommended that all symptomatic individuals with PAVM be treated by embolization therapy to minimize the risk for thromboembolic events. All identified PAVMs should be approached with caution and care to protect viable lung tissue and avoid coil or device embolization. Any identified PAVM should be embolized regardless of the size of the feeding artery because recent data demonstrate several cases of serious neurologic sequelae that have occurred in individuals with small or asymptomatic PAVM.[77-79,91] Caution must be taken to avoid proximal PA embolization to avoid the risk of systemic collateralization and possible pulmonary hemorrhage. Additionally, the anchoring and scaffolding techniques described are two methods to help avoid coil embolization in small distal vessels.

22.4 Aortopulmonary Collaterals

BACKGROUND

 APCs **(Figure 22–21 and Video 22–10),** also known as systemic-to-pulmonary collaterals, are most commonly found in congenital heart diseases in which there is obstructed pulmonary blood flow, such as tetralogy of Fallot or single ventricle lesions, or less commonly they are the result of acquired etiologies such as chronic alveolar hypoxia, very low–birth-weight infants,[92] trauma (e.g., from an anteriorly directed chest tube[93] or resulting from coronary artery bypass grafting after use of an in situ left internal mammary artery graft), infection such as tuberculosis,[94] or tumor (Hodgkin disease[95]). Typically, a major arterial branch from the subclavian artery or descending aorta forms microvascular communications with pulmonary arterioles (potentially related to elevated angiogenic factors such as vascular endothelial

growth factor [VEGF][96]), resulting in a left-to-right shunt. Although they are a potential source of significant morbidity in children with congenital heart disease, APCs may be asymptomatic in adult patients. The indications for catheterization of APCs are limited[9] **(Table 22–2),** and transcatheter closure should be reserved primarily for collaterals of clinical significance.

The most common indications for closure of APCs are in the setting of single-ventricle physiology of congenital heart disease. In single-ventricle physiology, APCs may add an additional volume load to the single ventricle because of the left-to-right shunt, resulting in futile blood flow of oxygenated blood recirculating to the lungs. This additional volume load is thought to increase filling pressures and contribute to diastolic dysfunction, adverse ventricular remodeling, systemic ventricular dilation, and ultimately ventricular failure. In addition, APCs may contribute to increased pulmonary arterial pressure, contributing to pulmonary flow energy loss equivalent to the square of the difference of the venous and systemic arterial flow velocities.[97] In the single ventricle palliation strategies involving passive pulmonary blood flow such as the Glenn (superior cavopulmonary connection) or Fontan procedures, this loss of flow energy can impede effective pulmonary blood flow (flow of deoxygenated blood to the lungs) and increasing pulmonary pressures. Taken together, APCs are thought by many operators to be a source of significant pathology in single ventricle physiology.

The deleterious effects of APCs are most evident in the postoperative period after a Glenn or Fontan procedure,

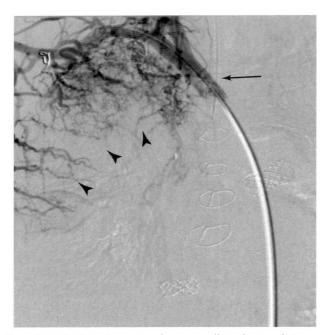

Figure 22–21 Extensive aortopulmonary collateral network *(arrowhead)* in a patient after Fontan palliation for a single ventricle coming off the right innominate and subclavian artery *(arrow).*

TABLE 22–2

Indications for Closure of Aortopulmonary Collaterals from ACC/AHA Guidelines for Care of the Adult with Congenital Heart Disease[9]

	2008 ACC/AHA Guidelines[9]
Before Fontan procedure	Class I: Evaluation of hemodynamics to assess the potential for definitive palliation of unoperated or shunt palliated adults with univentricular hearts; catheterization is indicated to assess and eliminate systemic-to-pulmonary artery connections (especially in evaluation of patients with protein-losing enteropathy). (Level of Evidence: C)
Tetralogy of Fallot, after repair	Class IIb: Catheterization may be considered to better define potentially treatable causes of otherwise unexplained LV or RV dysfunction, fluid retention, chest pain, or cyanosis. In these circumstances, transcatheter interventions may include elimination of residual shunts or APC vessels. (Level of Evidence: C)

ACC, American College of Cardiology; *AHA,* American Heart Association; *APC,* aortopulmonary collateral; *LV,* left ventricle; *RV,* right ventricle.

potentially related to increased angiogenic factors such as the VEGF after surgery.[96] The incidence and duration of pleural effusions after the Fontan procedure are related to increased grade of APCs.[98] In addition, the presence of APCs are associated with increased duration of inotropic support, postoperative ventilation, intensive care unit stay, and postoperative hospitalization after Fontan palliation.[99] Management of APCs, however, remains controversial,[100] and there is wide variation in management strategies of APCs in the single ventricle.[101]

Irrespective of these controversies, it should be noted that in the adult with normal two ventricle physiology, APCs may cause little or no hemodynamic impact, and there are a few indications for closure that will be discussed in the next section. Coronary-to-pulmonary arterial fistulas are described in a different section of this chapter.

DIAGNOSIS AND CLINICAL PRESENTATION

Although symptomatic APCs are rare in the adult with two-ventricle physiology, patients can have with hemoptysis,[102,103] congestive heart failure, endarteritis, vessel degeneration, or even rupture,[104] although these episodes are rare and nearly nonexistent in contemporary literature. In contrast, many patients seek care for nonrelated complaints and the APC is identified as an incidental finding.

In contrast, APCs are common in patients with single-ventricle physiology after Glenn or Fontan palliation—up to 36% in one series.[105] However, transcatheter closure in a large, multicenter study with more than 500 patients demonstrated no significant difference in hospital length of stay in patients who underwent APC closure before Fontan surgery,[101] resulting in significant controversy regarding management of these vessels.

Putting aside the controversies of pre-Fontan treatment of APCs, the physiology of these vessels is thought to result in left-to-right shunt at the level of the pulmonary arteries. As a result, if large in size and/or number, the left-to-right shunt can induce left-sided ventricular volume overload and contribute to the development of a number of poor outcomes such as elevated pulmonary or Fontan pressures, postoperative pleural effusions, protein-losing enteropathy, low cardiac output syndrome, congestive heart failure, and systemic ventricular failure. As such, many operators continue to advocate a high index of suspicion to identify and low threshold for intervening on APCs.[106]

APCs may be identified on physical examination and can be mistaken for PDAs given the physiology and similar machinelike murmur. The vast majority, however, require cardiac catheterization, which also allows transcatheter closure during the same session. Nonselective ascending aortography, however, may be limited in sensitivity (only 9% in one series), requiring selective angiography of head and neck vessels for definitive identification.[105] An important limitation of invasive angiography is the inability to quantitate the extent of APC flow, which intuitively should relate to the clinical significance of these lesions. Indeed, differences in total contribution

to ineffective pulmonary blood flow may account for the variation in results of the previously described studies.

Definitive quantitation during cardiopulmonary bypass by measurement of pulmonary venous blood flow during aortic cross-clamp has been described[100,107] and has provided prognostic guidance; however, the invasive nature of this technique renders it impractical for transcatheter procedural planning. Inuzuka and coworkers have described a combination of invasive hemodynamic measurement and lung scintigraphy to accurately quantitate extent of aortopulmonary flow.[108] Finally, phase contrast MRI has allowed fully noninvasive quantitation of APC flow by pulmonary venous minus pulmonary arterial flow[109] or aorta minus systemic venous flow,[110] leading some investigators to suggest that pre-Glenn cardiac catheterization may be unnecessary.[111] Irrespective of management strategy, quantitative imaging may aid in risk stratification and precardiac catheterization procedural planning.

PATIENT SELECTION

Patients referred for cardiac catheterization for evaluation of APCs should be considered only if symptoms are a result of volume overload, elevated pulmonary pressures, or other more unusual symptoms such as hemoptysis. In addition, in the adult with single-ventricle palliation, femoral arterial access cannot be taken for granted because during the rocky course of management of the single ventricle from birth to adulthood, the femoral arteries may have become occluded. The operator must be prepared for this and consider alternative access sites (e.g., radial or brachial).

TECHNIQUE

Each transcatheter closure should be preceded by hemodynamic evaluation to rule out additional etiologies of pathophysiology such as pulmonary vascular disease, primary pulmonary hypertension, venovenous collaterals and pulmonary venous desaturation, or PAVMs. Once accomplished, the following list is a rough outline that must be tailored to the individual anatomy of the patient.

1. Visualization: Ascending aortography is initially performed by power injection to give a general sense of the burden and extent of APCs. From there, a Judkins right catheter is used to access the right subclavian artery, which is subsequently exchanged for a cut pigtail catheter over a 0.018-inch wire to perform semiselective angiography of the vessels off the right subclavian artery, preferably with digital subtraction **(see Figure 22–21 and Video 22–10).** The left subclavian system can be similarly visualized. In one report, 34% of APCs arose from the internal mammary, 22% from the thyrocervical trunk, and 8% from lateral thoracic and thoracodorsal arteries[105] **(Figure 22–22).** Angiography should confirm that the segment of lung has dual supply and that intervention will not cause pulmonary infarct. Although rare, some collaterals do

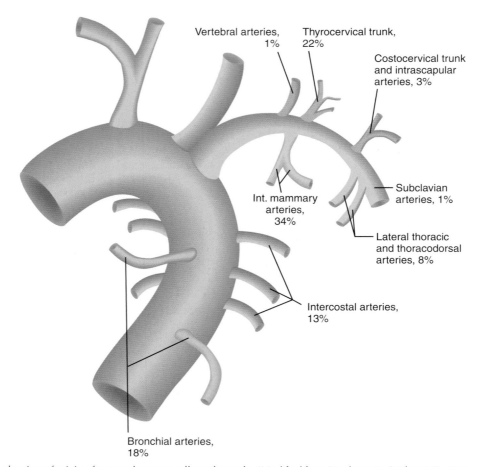

Figure 22–22 Vascular sites of origin of aortopulmonary collateral vessels. *(Modified from Triedman JK, Bridges ND, Mayer Jr JE, et al: Prevalence and risk factors for APC vessels after Fontan and bidirectional Glenn procedures,* J Am Coll Cardiol *1993;22:207-215.)*

arise from the descending aorta, and if suspicion is high, an addition digital subtraction angiogram can be performed to identify any of these vessels.

2. Coaxial system: Once a roadmap has been created by angiography, a coaxial system is used to cannulate and deliver the embolic device. Typically the same 4F Judkins right catheter, loaded with a microcatheter (**see Figure 22–1, A;** Cantata 2.5 or 2.8F) that has been loaded with a steerable 0.014-inch or 0.018-inch guidewire is brought to the target vessel.

3. Cannulate collateral: Using the coaxial system, the target vessel is cannulated, and the wire and microcatheter are advanced as deeply as possible into the vessel. At this time, additional angiography is performed to confirm the position of the microcatheter.

4. Particle versus coil embolization: Depending on the anatomy of the APC, microparticles can be injected via the microcatheter to occlude the microvasculature, giving a more durable result **(Figures 22–23 and 22–24, and Video 22–11).** It is imperative that a complete understanding of the collateral size and anatomy is obtained before using particle embolization to exclude any large communications that

would allow embolization of the particles into the pulmonary vascular bed or into the systemic circulation. EmboGold (Merit Medical, South Jordan, Utah) particles are available in a variety of sizes, and care must be taken when choosing a size to be certain that the chosen size will lodge in the distal portion of the target vessel. It is recommended that operators not familiar with the use of particulate embolization utilize an interventional radiologist or pediatric interventional cardiologist for assistance during the procedure.

5. Alternatively, 0.018-inch coils can be delivered via the microcatheter **(Figure 22–25 and Video 22–12);** however, care should be taken to pack the coil mass tightly to achieve complete occlusion. Otherwise the collateral may recanalize late after occlusion. It is recommended that a coil that has a diameter 20% to 30% larger than the target vessel be chosen for delivery. If the coaxial system is not used, the guide catheter itself can be used to deliver the coils if the target vessel can be intubated distally enough to allow distal placement of the coil. Use of the guide catheter as a delivery catheter allows large coils such as 0.035-inch or 0.038-inch sizes, depending on the type of guide used.

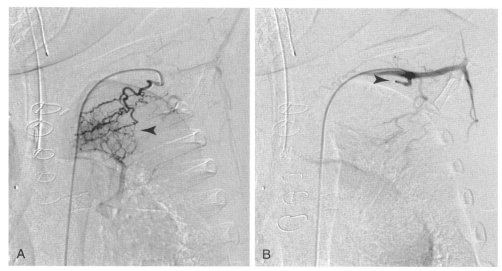

Figure 22–23   Particle embolization of superior thoracic artery to pulmonary collaterals. A, Digital subtraction angiography via Judkins right catheter injection of the superior thoracic artery demonstrating extensive pulmonary collaterals *(arrowhead)* before particle embolization. **B,** Angiography after particle embolization demonstrating no run-off from superior thoracic artery *(arrowhead).*

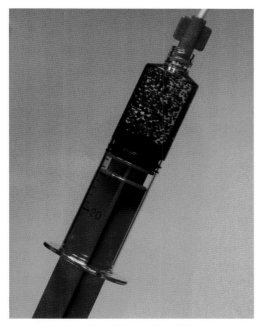

Figure 22–24   EmboGold particle embolization system.

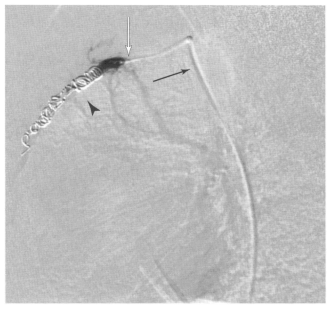

Figure 22–25   Digital subtraction angiography demonstrating coil occlusion *(arrowhead)* of an internal mammary artery delivered through a microcatheter *(white arrow)* and Judkins right catheter *(black arrow).*

6. Postprocedural care: Pre- and postprocedural antibiotics may be considered. In addition, position of any deployed coils or other devices should be confirmed by chest x-ray on the day after the procedure.

A wide range of devices and coils have been described in the closure of APCs. The selection of these should be based on the anatomy of the collateral and its parent vessel. For example, Goldstein and coworkers have reported successful use of the AZUR Hydrogel expandable coil system (Terumo Medical, Somerset, N.J.) for closure of APCs.[112] Hijazi and coworkers have described use of the

Amplatzer vascular plug.[113] Additional devices and techniques are certainly feasible; however, further discussion is beyond the scope of this chapter **(Box 22–3).**

COMPLICATIONS

Although reported complications of APC closure are rarely described in the literature, anecdotal reports have described device/coil embolization (with infarction of the downstream tissue), particle embolization complicated by cerebrovascular infarct, late recanalization of collateral, and rarely, endarteritis and hemolysis

BOX 22–3 ■■■■■■■■■■■■■■■■■■■■■■■■■■■
Tips and Tricks

- Selective angiography of the vessel is often needed to identify a collateral.
- Before closure, confirm dual supply to the segment of lung.
- Optimize secure deployment by using a detachable coil if position appears potentially unstable with potential to embolize device.
- There is a preference for particle embolization because of recanalization of collateral after coil embolization.
- The inner diameter of the lumen of the delivery catheter should be slightly larger than the coil caliber to prevent the device from coiling inside the delivery catheter.
- With large vessels, consider scaffolding using a higher tensile-strength coil and then packing within using a soft coil.
- Administer antibiotics after the procedure.

resulting from incomplete closure. The ratio of risks and benefits of APC closure may be improved in the future as noninvasive quantitation of APC flow gains acceptance and becomes a routine part of preprocedural planning and risk stratification.

REFERENCES

1. Moss AJ, Emmanouilides G, Duffie ER: Closure of the ductus arteriosus in the newborn infant, Pediatrics 32:25–30, 1963.
2. Hoffman JIE, Kaplan S: The incidence of congenital heart disease, J Am Coll Cardiol 39:1890–1900, 2002.
3. Houston AB GJ, Lim MK, Doig WB, et al: Doppler ultrasound and the silent ductus arteriosus, Br Heart J 65:97–99, 1991.
4. Heymann MA: Heart disease in infants, children, and adolescents. In Adams FH EG, Riemenschneider TA, editors: Heart disease in infants, children and adolescents, 4th ed, Baltimore, 1989, Williams & Wilkins, p 210.
5. Bennhagen RG, Benson LN: Silent and audible persistent ductus arteriosus: an angiographic study, Pediatr Cardiol 24:27–30, 2003.
6. Thilen U, Åstrom-Olsson K: Does the risk of infective endarteritis justify routine patent ductus arteriosus closure? Eur Heart J 18:503–506, 1997.
7. Schneider DJ, Moore JW: Patent ductus arteriosus, Circulation 114:1873–1882, 2006.
8. Fortescue EB, Lock JE, Galvin T, et al. To close or not to close: the very small patent ductus arteriosus. Congenit Heart Dis 5:354–365.
9. Warnes CA, Williams RG, Bashore TM, et al: ACC/AHA 2008 Guidelines for the management of adults with congenital heart disease, Circulation 118:e714–e833, 2008.
10. Krichenko A, Benson LN, Burrows P, et al: Angiographic classification of the isolated, persistently patent ductus arteriosus and implications for percutaneous catheter occlusion, The Am J Cardiol 63:877–880, 1989.
11. Sommer RJ, Gutierrez A, Lai WW, et al: Use of preformed nitinol snare to improve transcatheter coil delivery in occlusion of patent ductus arteriosus, Am J Cardiol 74:836–839, 1994.
12. Hays MD, Hoyer MH, Glasow PF: New forceps delivery technique for coil occlusion of patent ductus arteriosus, Am J Cardiol 77:209–211, 1996.
13. Berdjis F, Moore JW: Balloon occlusion delivery technique for closure of patent ductus arteriosus, Am Heart J 133:601–604, 1997.
14. Ing MDFF, Recto MDMR, Saidi MDA, et al: A method providing bidirectional control of coil delivery in occlusions of patent ductus arteriosus with shallow ampulla and Pott's shunts, Am J Cardiol 79:1561–1563, 1997.
15. Akagi T, Hashino K, Sugimura T, et al: Coil occlusion of patent ductus arteriosus with detachable coils, Am Heart J 134:538–543, 1997.
16. Podnar T, Masura J: Percutaneous closure of patent ductus arteriosus using special screwing detachable coils, Catheter Cardiovasc Diagn 41:386–391, 1997.
17. Latson LA: Coronary artery fistulas: how to manage them, Catheter Cardiovasc Interv 70:110–116, 2007.
18. Mavroudis C, Backer CL, Rocchini AP, et al: Coronary artery fistulas in infants and children: A surgical review and discussion of coil embolization, Ann Thorac Surg 63:1235–1242, 1997.
19. Renard C, Chivot C, Jarry G, et al: Communicating bilateral coronary artery to pulmonary artery fistula with aneurysm in asymptomatic patient: successful conservative management with selective coil embolization of the aneurysm, Int J Cardiol 150:e107–e109, 2011.
20. Krause W: Ueber den Ursprung einer accessorischen A. Coronaria Cordis aus der A, Pulmonalis. Zeitschrift fuer Rationelle Medizin 24:225–227, 1865.
21. Biorck G, Crafoord C: Arteriovenous aneurysm on the pulmonary artery simulating patent ductus arteriosus botalli, Thorax 2:65–74, 1947.
22. Reidy JF, Sowton E, Ross DN: Transcatheter occlusion of coronary to bronchial anastomosis by detachable balloon combined with coronary angioplasty at same procedure, Br Heart J 49:284–287, 1983.
23. Luo L, Kebede S, Wu S, et al: Coronary artery fistulae, Am J Med Sci 332:79–84, 2006.
24. Yamanaka O, Hobbs RE: Coronary artery anomalies in 126,595 patients undergoing coronary arteriography, Cathet Cardiovasc Diagn 21:28–40, 1990.
25. Mavroudis C, Backer CL, Muster AJ, et al: Expanding indications for pediatric coronary artery bypass, J Thorac Cardiovasc Surg 111:181–189, 1996.
26. Sandhu JS, Uretsky BF, Zerbe TR, et al: Coronary artery fistula in the heart transplant patient: a potential complication of endomyocardial biopsy, Circulation 79:350–356, 1989.
27. Pophal SG, Sigfusson G, Booth KL, et al: Complications of endomyocardial biopsy in children, J Am Coll Cardiol 34:2105–2110, 1999.
28. Saad RM, Jain A: Coronary artery fistula related to dilatation of totally occluded vessel, Clin Cardiol 16:835–836, 1993.
29. Lowe JE, Adams DH, Cummings RG, et al: The natural history and recommended management of patients with traumatic coronary artery fistulas, Ann Thorac Surg 36:295–305, 1983.
30. Hancock Friesen C, Howlett JG, Ross DB: Traumatic coronary artery fistula management, Ann Thorac Surg 69:1973–1982, 2000.
31. Calder AL, Co EE, Sage MD: Coronary arterial abnormalities in pulmonary atresia with intact ventricular septum, Am J Cardiol 59:436–442, 1987.
32. O'Connor WN, Cash JB, Cottrill CM, et al: Ventriculocoronary connections in hypoplastic left hearts: an autopsy microscopic study, Circulation 66:1078–1086, 1982.
33. Sauer U, Gittenberger-de Groot AC, Geishauser M, et al: Coronary arteries in the hypoplastic left heart syndrome: histopathologic and histometrical studies and implications for surgery, Circulation 80:1168–1176, 1989.
34. Baffa JM, Chen SL, Guttenberg ME, et al: Coronary artery abnormalities and right ventricular histology in hypoplastic left heart syndrome, J Am Coll Cardiol 20:350–358, 1992.
35. Preiss M, Habicht J, Bongartz G, et al: Aneurysmal and partially thrombosed orifice of a coronary artery fistula into the right atrium combined with patent foramen ovale, Thorac Cardiovasc Surg 49:120–121, 2001.
36. Hobbs RE, Millit HD, Raghavan PV, et al: Coronary artery fistulae: a 10-year review, Cleve Clin Q 49:191–197, 1982.
37. Liberthson RR, Sagar K, Berkoben JP, et al: Congenital coronary arteriovenous fistula: report of 13 patients, review of the literature and delineation of management, Circulation 59:849–854, 1979.
38. Hiraishi S, Misawa H, Horiguchi Y, et al: Effect of suture closure of coronary artery fistula on aneurysmal coronary artery and myocardial ischemia, Am J Cardiol 81:1263–1267, 1998.
39. Krishnamoorthy KM, Rao S: Saccular aneurysm of congenital coronary arteriovenous fistula, Interact Cardiovasc Thorac Surg 2:295–297, 2003.
40. Said SA, el Gamal MI: Coronary angiographic morphology of congenital coronary arteriovenous fistulas in adults: report of four new cases and review of angiograms of fifteen reported cases, Cathet Cardiovasc Diagn 35:29–35, 1995.
41. Misumi T, Nishikawa K, Yasudo M, et al: Rupture of an aneurysm of a coronary arteriovenous fistula, Ann Thorac Surg 71:2026–2027, 2001.
42. Bauer HH, Allmendinger PD, Flaherty J, et al: Congenital coronary arteriovenous fistula: spontaneous rupture and cardiac tamponade, Ann Thorac Surg 62:1521–1523, 1996.
43. Said SA, Austermann-Kaper T, Bucx JJ: Congenital coronary arteriovenous fistula associated with atrioventricular valvular regurgitation in an octogenarian, Int J Cardiol 38:96–97, 1993.
44. Lowe JE, Oldham HNJ, Sabiston DCJ: Surgical management of congenital coronary artery fistulas, Ann Surg 194:373–380, 1981.
45. Urrutia SC, Falaschi G, Ott DA, et al: Surgical management of 56 patients with congenital coronary artery fistulas, Ann Thorac Surg 35:300–307, 1983.
46. Cheung DLC, Au W-K, Cheung HHC, et al: Coronary artery fistulas: long-term results of surgical correction, Ann Thorac Surg 71:190–195, 2001.
47. Wang NK, Hsieh LY, Shen CT, et al: Coronary arteriovenous fistula in pediatric patients: a 17-year institutional experience, Taiwan Yi Xue Hui Za Zhi 101:177–182, 2002.
48. Mesko ZG, Damus PS: Myocardial infarction in a 14-year-old girl, ten years after surgical correction of congenital coronary artery fistula, Pediatr Cardiol 19:366–368, 1998.
49. Hamada M, Kubo H, Matsuoka H, et al: Myocardial infarction complicating surgical repair of left coronary-right ventricular fistula in an adult, Am J Cardiol 57:372–374, 1986.
50. Armsby LR, Keane JF, Sherwood MC, et al: Management of coronary artery fistulae: patient selection and results of transcatheter closure, J Am Coll Cardiol 39:1026–1032, 2002.
51. Gowda ST, Latson LA, Kutty S, et al: Intermediate to long-term outcome following congenital coronary artery fistulae closure with focus on thrombus formation, Am J Cardiol 107:302–308, 2011.
52. Qureshi SA, Reidy JF, Alwi MB, et al: Use of interlocking detachable coils in embolization of coronary arteriovenous fistulas, Am J Cardiol 78:110–113, 1996.

53. Behera SK, Danon S, Levi DS, et al: Transcatheter closure of coronary artery fistulae using the Amplatzer duct occluder, *Catheter Cardiovasc Interv* 68:242–248, 2006.

54. Ascoop AK, Budts W: Percutaneous closure of a congenital coronary artery fistula complicated by an acute myocardial infarction, *Acta Cardiol* 59:67–69, 2004.

55. Balanescu S, Sangiorgi G, Medda M, et al: Successful concomitant treatment of a coronary-to-pulmonary artery fistula and a left anterior descending artery stenosis using a single covered stent graft: a case report and literature review, *J Interv Cardiol* 15:209–214, 2002.

56. Jama A, Barsoum M, Bjarnason H, et al: Percutaneous closure of congenital coronary artery fistulae: results and angiographic follow-up, *JACC* 4:814–821, 2011.

57. Bruckheimer E, Harris M, Kornowski R, et al: Transcatheter closure of large congenital coronary-cameral fistulae with Amplatzer devices, *Catheter Cardiovasc Interv* 75:850–854, 2010.

58. Kharouf R, Cao QL, Hijazi ZM: Transcatheter closure of coronary artery fistula complicated by myocardial infarction, *J Invasive Cardiol* 19:E146–E149, 2007.

59. Latson L: Coronary fistulae: proficient plugging proliferates, but don't forget the follow-up, *Catheter Cardiovasc Interv* 75:855–856, 2010.

60. Valente AM, Lock JE, Gauvreau K, et al: Predictors of long-term adverse outcomes in patients with congenital coronary artery fistulae, *Circ Cardiovasc Interv* 3:134–139, 2010.

61. Churton T: Multiple aneurysms of the pulmonary artery, *Br Med J* 1:1223–1225, 1897.

62. Faughnan ME, Palda VA, Garcia-Tsao G, et al: International guidelines for the diagnosis and management of hereditary haemorrhagic telangiectasia, *J Med Genet* 48:73–87, 2011.

63. Hoffbauer FW, Rydell R: Multiple pulmonary arteriovenous fistulas in juvenile cirrhosis, *Am J Med* 21:450–460, 1956.

64. De Faria JL, Czapski J, Leite MO, et al: Cyanosis in Manson's schistosomiasis: role of pulmonary schistosomatic arteriovenous fistulas, *Am Heart J* 54:196–204, 1957.

65. Prager RL, Laws KH, Bender HW Jr: Arteriovenous fistula of the lung, *Ann Thorac Surg* 36:231–239, 1983.

66. Taxman RM, Halloran MJ, Parker BM: Multiple pulmonary arteriovenous malformations in association with Fanconi's syndrome, *Chest* 64:118–120, 1973.

67. Glenn WW: Circulatory bypass of the right side of the heart. IV. Shunt between superior vena cava and distal right pulmonary artery: report of clinical application, *N Engl J Med* 259:117–120, 1958.

68. Fontan F, Baudet E: Surgical repair of tricuspid atresia, *Thorax* 26:240–248, 1971.

69. Samanek M, Oppelt A, Kasalicky J, et al: Distribution of pulmonary blood flow after cavopulmonary anastomosis (Glenn operation), *Br Heart J* 31:511–516, 1969.

70. McFaul RC, Tajik AJ, Mair DD, et al: Development of pulmonary arteriovenous shunt after superior vena cava-right pulmonary artery (Glenn) anastomosis: report of four cases, *Circulation* 55:212–216, 1977.

71. Glenn WW: Superior vena cava–pulmonary artery anastomosis, *Ann Thorac Surg* 37:9–11, 1984.

72. Cloutier A, Ash JM, Smallhorn JF, et al: Abnormal distribution of pulmonary blood flow after the Glenn shunt or Fontan procedure: risk of development of arteriovenous fistulae, *Circulation* 72:471–479, 1985.

73. Srivastava D, Preminger T, Lock JE, et al: Hepatic venous blood and the development of pulmonary arteriovenous malformations in congenital heart disease, *Circulation* 92:1217–1222, 1995.

74. Gomes AS, Benson L, George B, et al: Management of pulmonary arteriovenous fistulas after superior vena cava-right pulmonary artery (Glenn) anastomosis, *J Thorac Cardiovasc Surg* 87:636–639, 1984.

75. Seward JB, Tajik AJ, Spangler JG, et al: Echocardiographic contrast studies: initial experience, *Mayo Clin Proc* 50:163–192, 1975.

76. Barzilai B, Waggoner AD, Spessert C, et al: Two-dimensional contrast echocardiography in the detection and follow-up of congenital pulmonary arteriovenous malformations, *Am J Cardiol* 68:1507–1510, 1991.

77. Thompson RL, Cattaneo SM, Barnes J: Recurrent brain abscess: manifestation of pulmonary arteriovenous fistula and hereditary hemorrhagic telangiectasia, *Chest* 72:654–655, 1977.

78. Roman G, Fisher M, Perl DP, et al: Neurological manifestations of hereditary hemorrhagic telangiectasia (Rendu-Osler-Weber disease): report of 2 cases and review of the literature, *Ann Neurol* 4:130–144, 1978.

79. Suresh CG, Coupe MO, Jegarajah S: Recurrent cerebral abscesses 20 years before recognition of multiple pulmonary arteriovenous malformations, *Br J Clin Pract* 49:105–106, 1995.

80. White RI Jr, Lynch-Nyhan A, Terry P, et al: Pulmonary arteriovenous malformations: techniques and long-term outcome of embolotherapy, *Radiology* 169:663–669, 1988.

81. Todo K, Moriwaki H, Higashi M, et al: A small pulmonary arteriovenous malformation as a cause of recurrent brain embolism, *AJNR Am J Neuroradiol* 25:428–430, 2004.

82. Shovlin CL, Jackson JE, Bamford KB, et al: Primary determinants of ischaemic stroke/brain abscess risks are independent of severity of pulmonary arteriovenous malformations in hereditary haemorrhagic telangiectasia, *Thorax* 63:259–266, 2008.

83. Trerotola SO, Pyeritz RE, Bernhardt BA: Outpatient single-session pulmonary arteriovenous malformation embolization, *J Vasc Interv Radiol* 20:1287–1291, 2009.

84. Portsmann W: Therapeutic embolization of arteriovenous pulmonary fistula by catheter technique, *Curr Concepts Pediatr Radiol* 23–31, 1977.

85. White RI Jr: Pulmonary arteriovenous malformations and hereditary hemorrhagic telangiectasia: embolotherapy using balloons and coils, *Arch Intern Med* 156:2627–2628, 1996.

86. Trerotola SO, Pyeritz RE: Does use of coils in addition to Amplatzer vascular plugs prevent recanalization? *AJR Am J Roentgenol* 195:766–771, 2010.

87. White RI Jr, Pollak JS, Wirth JA: Pulmonary arteriovenous malformations: diagnosis and transcatheter embolotherapy, *J Vasc Interv Radiol* 7:787–804, 1996.

88. Lee DW, White RI Jr, Egglin TK, et al: Embolotherapy of large pulmonary arteriovenous malformations: long-term results, *Ann Thorac Surg* 64:930–939, 1997. discussion 9–40.

89. White RI Jr, Mitchell SE, Barth KH, et al: Angioarchitecture of pulmonary arteriovenous malformations: an important consideration before embolotherapy, *AJR Am J Roentgenol* 140:681–686, 1983.

90. Murphy J, Pierucci P, Chyun D, et al: Results of exercise stress testing in patients with diffuse pulmonary arteriovenous malformations, *Pediatr Cardiol* 30:978–984, 2009.

91. Dines DE, Arms RA, Bernatz PE, et al: Pulmonary arteriovenous fistulas, *Mayo Clin Proc* 49:460–465, 1974.

92. Acherman RJ, Siassi B, Pratti-Madrid G, et al: Systemic-to-pulmonary collaterals in very low birth weight infants: color Doppler detection of systemic to pulmonary connections during neonatal and early infancy period, *Pediatrics* 105:528–532, 2000.

93. Edmiston WA, Walters JR, Finck EJ, et al: Angiographic demonstration of an acquired internal mammary-to-pulmonary artery fistula, *Angiology* 28:712–719, 1977.

94. Denlinger CE, Egan TM, Jones DR: Acquired systemic-to-pulmonary arteriovenous malformation secondary to mycobacterium tuberculosis empyema, *AnnThorac Surg* 74:1229–1231, 2002.

95. Dunn RP, Wexler L: Systemic-to-pulmonary fistula in intrapulmonary Hodgkin's disease, *Chest* 66:590–594, 1974.

96. Mori Y, Shoji M, Nakanishi T, et al: Elevated vascular endothelial growth factor levels are associated with aortopulmonary collateral vessels in patients before and after the Fontan procedure, *Am Heart J* 153:987–994, 2007.

97. Ascuitto RJ, Ross-Ascuitto NT: Systematic-to-pulmonary collaterals: a source of flow energy loss in Fontan physiology, *Pediatr Cardiol* 25:472–481, 2004.

98. Spicer RL, Uzark KC, Moore JW, et al: Aortopulmonary collateral vessels and prolonged pleural effusions after modified Fontan procedures, *Am Heart J* 131:1164–1168, 1996.

99. Kanter KR, Vincent RN, Raviele AA: Importance of acquired systemic-to-pulmonary collaterals in the Fontan operation, *Ann Thorac Surg* 68:969–974, 1999.

100. Bradley SM, McCall MM, Sistino JJ, et al: Aortopulmonary collateral flow in the Fontan patient: does it matter? *Ann Thorac Surg* 72:408–415, 2001.

101. Banka P, Sleeper LA, Atz AM, et al: Practice variability and outcomes of coil embolization of aortopulmonary collaterals before Fontan completion: a report from the Pediatric Heart Network Fontan Cross-Sectional Study, *Am Heart J* 162:125–130, 2011.

102. Suda K, Matsumura M, Sano A, et al: Hemoptysis From collateral arteries 12 years after a Fontan-type operation, *Ann Thorac Surg* 79:e7–e8, 2005.

103. Pate GE, Carere RG: Percutaneous occlusion of a pulmonary aneurysm causing hemoptysis in a patient with pulmonary atresia and aortopulmonary collaterals, *Catheter Cardiovasc Interv* 65:310–312, 2005.

104. Shumacker HB Jr: Aneurysm development and degenerative changes in dilated artery proximal to arteriovenous fistula, *Surg Gynecol Obstet* 130:636–640, 1970.

105. Triedman JK, Bridges ND, Mayer JE Jr, et al: Prevalence and risk factors for aortopulmonary collateral vessels after Fontan and bidirectional Glenn procedures, *J Am Coll Cardiol* 22:207–215, 1993.

106. Stern HJ: The argument for aggressive coiling of aortopulmonary collaterals in single ventricle patients, *Catheter Cardiovasc Interv* 74:897–900, 2009.

107. Ichikawa H, Yagihara T, Kishimoto H, et al: Extent of aortopulmonary collateral blood flow as a risk factor for Fontan operations, *Ann Thorac Surg* 59:433–437, 1995.

108. Inuzuka R, Aotsuka H, Nakajima H, et al: Quantification of collateral aortopulmonary flow in patients subsequent to construction of bidirectional cavopulmonary shunts, *Cardiol Young* 18:485–493, 2008.

109. Grosse-Wortmann L, Al-Otay A, Yoo S-J: Aortopulmonary collaterals after bidirectional cavopulmonary connection or Fontan completion: clinical perspective, *Circ Cardiovasc Imaging* 2:219–225, 2009.

110. Whitehead KK, Gillespie MJ, Harris MA, et al: Noninvasive quantification of systemic-to-pulmonary collateral flow: clinical perspective, *Circ Cardiovasc Imaging* 2:405–411, 2009.

111. Brown DW, Gauvreau K, Powell AJ, et al: Cardiac magnetic resonance versus routine cardiac catheterization before bidirectional Glenn anastomosis in infants with functional single ventricle, *Circulation* 116:2718–2725, 2007.

112. Goldstein BH, Aiyagari R, Bocks ML, et al: Hydrogel expandable coils for vascular occlusion in congenital cardiovascular disease: a single center experience, *Congenit Heart Dis*, 7:212–218, 2011.

113. Hijazi ZM: New device for percutaneous closure of aortopulmonary collaterals, *Catheter Cardiovasc Interv* 63:482–485, 2004.

Chapter 23

Percutaneous Relief of Vascular Obstruction: Potpourri

DHAVAL PAREKH • FRANK ING

23.1 Key Points

1. Cardiovascular obstructions in adult congenital heart disease (CHD) often involve branch pulmonary artery stenosis and postsurgical baffles, homografts, and conduits.
2. Stenting various cardiovascular obstructions in adult CHD requires a good understanding of available stents and balloons of all sizes and all of their unique characteristics.
3. Intravascular stenting should accommodate for adult growth potential of the patient.
4. Accurate measurements and basic techniques of angioplasty and stenting of large pulmonary and systemic vessels are essential in the management of adult CHD.

Relief of vascular obstruction initially described by Dotter and Judkins[1] for peripheral atherosclerotic disease is now routinely applied to a variety of cardiovascular obstructions found in congenital and postsurgical heart disease. Advances in catheters, wires, stents, and therapeutic techniques allow for advanced interventions to relieve these obstructions from the newborn infant to the elderly adult. Although pediatric interventionists manage the majority of these lesions, as CHD patients survive to adulthood and enter into the adult clinics and hospitals, adult interventional cardiologists should become familiar with the diagnosis and management of these lesions as well.

This chapter discusses the diagnosis and interventional management of some commonly encountered cardiovascular obstructions seen in CHD that present in both the pediatric and adult patient. In particular, available balloons and stents as well as techniques and potential complications are reviewed.

Main interventional options for treating CHD obstructions include balloon dilation using standard-pressure balloons, cutting balloons or high-pressure balloons. When angioplasty fails and when the anatomy permits, stent implantation is another option.

23.2 Basic Concepts

BALLOON ANGIOPLASTY

Much procedural knowledge, technique development, and refinement in the use of static balloon angioplasty can be traced to the results of the Valvuloplasty and Angioplasty of Congenital Heart Disease Registry (VACA).[2] Although there are many manufacturers of balloons who use different materials, sizes, and lengths, all balloons impart a certain advantage or disadvantage for specific lesions. It is imperative for an active catheterization lab to carry and become familiar with a wide array of inventoried balloons. An ideal balloon has a low profile and folds tightly over a catheter shaft with short shoulders.[3] It should dilate to a predetermined diameter at maximal pressure without overexpanding and then deflate rapidly so as to assume its original native configuration for retrieval. The effectiveness of angioplasty is caused by appropriately tearing tunica intima and distention of the medial vascular layer,[4] which at times requires high-pressure balloons usually made of thicker material and having larger profiles.

The suspect vessel is visualized on angiogram using contrast injection with biplane imaging profiling the lesion to allow for accurate calibrated measurements of length and diameter, as well as any important side branches. Occasionally, multiple angles are needed to best profile a vascular stenosis, especially if it is located adjacent to a superimposed larger structure (**Figure 23–1).** The standard practice of using the French size of a catheter as a measurement reference should be avoided. Whereas this technique is acceptable for comparable

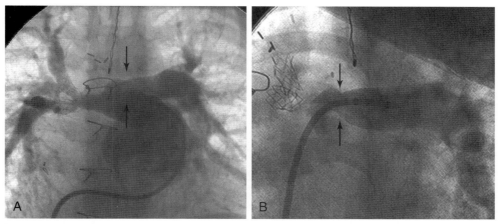

Figure 23–1 **A,** Bilateral pulmonary artery stenosis in anteroposterior projection; left pulmonary artery (LPA) stenosis (arrows) is not well seen because of superimposition of the dilated main pulmonary artery. **B,** At 30 degrees left anterior oblique/30 degrees cranial angulation, the LPA orifice stenosis is profiled.

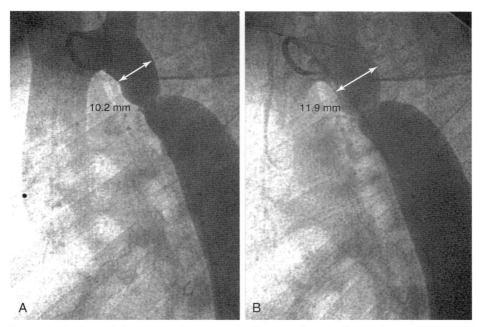

Figure 23–2 **Proper frame selection is needed to accurately measure the diameter of a pulsatile vessel. A,** Coarctation of the aorta: it is tempting to select the frame with the most contrast. The diameter of this frame measures 10.2 mm (double-headed arrow). **B,** In the same angiogram, this frame shows less contrast, but the diameter measures 11.9 mm, a 20% increase.

coronary diameters, the larger sizes of major vessels involved in CHD render this technique too inaccurate. A 10% error in the reference measure could result in a miscalculation of several millimeters. Choosing the proper frame for measurement is also important. Although it is natural to select the frame with the best contrast outlining the target vessel, it is actually more important to select the frame with the largest diameter. Because of the pulsatility of some vessels, there may be a significant difference between the largest and smallest diameters during systole and diastole of a cardiac cycle **(Figure 23–2).** This is especially true for systemic arteries such as the aorta. Introduction of dynamic angiography and three-dimensional (3D) rendering adds another important modality for better understanding the anatomy before an intervention.

Once measurements are made, the lesion is crossed with an end-hole catheter and placed as far distal as possible. In adults with branch pulmonary artery stenosis and a dilated right atrium and ventricle, passage of any catheter across the right heart may be challenging and require all kinds of techniques to avoid catheter and wire buckling within the atrium or ventricle. A very useful technique is to shape a "left pulmonary artery (LPA)" or "right pulmonary artery (RPA)" curve with the stiff end of a guidewire to help guide the catheter into position. Once this is achieved, a stiff wire is introduced in a manner maximally accommodated by the lumen of the balloon catheter so as to allow for appropriate support and maintain balloon position for dilation. A commonly used wire is an Amplatz Super Stiff "short tip" (Boston Scientific, Natick, Mass.). These have only a 2-cm floppy tip at the end to maximize the length of stiff wire crossing the right ventricular outflow tract. The chosen length and diameter of a balloon that will not impinge on smaller caliber vessels undergoes a "negative prep" to remove all air while not altering the tight factory folding with a large syringe of 1:3 to 1:5 dilute contrast/saline, a three way stopcock, and a pressure monitor inflation device. The larger the balloon, the less concentration of contrast to saline is needed to visualize the inflation, and the quicker the inflation and deflation.

Once the balloon is prepared, it is advanced over the stiff wire to the target lesion. A second sheath on the contralateral femoral vein is often placed to advance a catheter to the site of interest for angiography to determine exact positioning. Keep in mind that it is not uncommon for the native geometry to be altered by the combination of a balloon catheter and stiff wire. Whereas incorrect positioning from altered geometry only results in a repeat dilation, an incorrectly positioned stent after implantation can lead to disastrous results. When the desired position is achieved, an inflation device with a pressure gauge is used until the waist is relieved or maximal inflation pressure is achieved. Depending on the vessel, cardiac output may be completely obscured, and inflation and deflation should be carried out quickly. In the presence of calcium, care should be taken to avoid vessel dissection. In general, the target diameter should be the diameter of the normal adjacent vessel, or no more than 3 to 4 times the minimal diameter, whichever is less.

STENTING

Clinical use of intravascular stents has grown since its early use in peripheral and branch pulmonary arteries in humans.[5,6] Stents are indicated when vascular elastic recoil or external compression results in restenosis in spite of adequate angioplasty. Since the early days of stenting using the Palmaz stents (Johnson and Johnson, Bridgewater, N.J.), stents are now available in a wide variety of materials, tensile strength, or cell design; self-expanding or balloon-expandable; and in various diameters and lengths. Unlike coronary artery disease, in which most vessels are similar in size, vascular obstructions in CHD can vary widely in location and size and present in all ages from infancy to adulthood. Hence it is prudent to use a stent that can be serially dilated to the normal adult size of the vessel in which it is implanted.

Even in adult patients, it may be necessary to stage a serial dilation in severely stenotic vessels, especially those that are calcified and in the systemic circulation.

As with balloons, a functional catheterization lab should stock a full assortment of stent types for specific lesions. In general, stents used for CHD are broken into four broad categories based on maximal diameters. "Small" stents are coronary stents that can be dilated to 4 or 5 mm and used to maintain shunt or ductal patency in lesions with ductal dependency for systemic or pulmonary flow. "Medium" stents can be expanded to 12 mm and should be used in small lobar and segmental pulmonary arteries or to maintain Fontan fenestration

patency. "Large" stents can be expanded to a diameter of 18 mm and should be used in proximal branch and large lobar pulmonary arteries. "Extra-large" stents are expandable to 24 mm and should be used in coarctation of the aorta and right ventricular outflow tract conduits. Although most small and medium sized stents are available premounted, most large and extra-large stents are hand-mounted and balloon-expanded. Specific features of various commercially available stents are beyond the scope of this chapter.

General Techniques for Stent Implantation

After accurate measurements are made of the lesion to be stented, an end hole is introduced past the area of narrowing and placed far distally. The 0.035-inch Amplatz Super Stiff "short-tip" exchange guidewire is most commonly used because it has only a 2-cm floppy tip that allows for more stiff wire to traverse the stenotic area, which improves the trackability for the stiff long sheath and subsequent stent/balloon catheter combination, especially across dilated chambers in pulmonary artery stenting. Careful attention is paid to the wire tip in the distal small branches to avoid perforation. A balloon with short shoulders is preferred to avoid pinhole perforation by the stent edge, but newer stents with rounded edges have reduced this complication. Predilation before stenting has advantages of allowing the vessel compliance to be tested and making sure the balloon does not slip during expansion, but testing may also reduce the radial force to hold a stent and is an added step that is not necessary for all cases. The chosen sheath should have a French size large enough to accommodate delivery of the balloon and stent (usually 1F to 2F larger than needed for the balloon alone) and long enough to traverse the lesion. Although some have advocated delivery of a premounted stent without long sheaths, this technique carries risks, because there is no sheath to prevent the stent from slipping backwards when the balloon is withdrawn from the stent. The exact stent and balloon size are chosen to allow for relief of the present obstruction but so as to not limit future expansion to appropriate adult vessel caliber. The stent is hand crimped on the balloon using umbilical tape to facilitate even circumferential compression **(Figure 23–3)**. Some interventionists add a small amount of contrast on the stent/balloon unit to enhance "stickiness" and try to minimize any stent shifts while it is advanced through the long sheath. The balloon and stent system are then advanced through the long sheath and positioned over the stiff wire using a roadmap from prior angiograms.

Once the balloon and stent are centered on the lesion with the sheath tip just distal to the lesion, the sheath is withdrawn slowly over the balloon/stent. Exact positioning is ensured by an angiogram from a second catheter, and adjustments are made for appropriate centering of the stent. For initial deployment greater than 15 mm in diameter, the BIB balloon (NuMED, Hopkinton, N.Y.) is ideal. This balloon has an inner and outer balloon for expansion. The inner balloon has a diameter one half the size of the outer balloon and is several millimeters

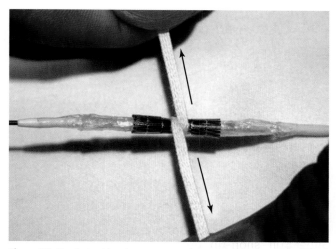

Figure 23–3 A stent has been mounted onto a balloon, and umbilical tape is wrapped around the stent once and pulled in opposite directions *(arrows)*. This technique provides even circumferential pressure to crimp the stent and minimize the profile of the stent/balloon unit for delivery.

shorter in length. The inner balloon is inflated first, and then the outer balloon is inflated. The design of this balloon allows for a more even stent expansion and minimizes foreshortening in larger diameters. Another advantage of this balloon is that small stent adjustments can be made for optimal positioning even after inner balloon expansion but before outer balloon expansion.

23.3 Angioplasty and Stenting of Pulmonary Artery Branch Stenosis

Branch pulmonary artery stenoses are now routinely addressed in the catheterization lab. They occur in multiple settings, including discreet or long-segment stenosis in sites of old shunt insertions (Blalock-Taussig, Waterston and Potts), pulmonary artery bands, conduits, or postsurgical repairs. They can occur with geometric aberrations such as folds, kinks, or twists or as a result of external compression by adjacent structures. They can be congenital with multiple stenoses and diffuse hypoplasia (i.e., Williams or Alagille syndrome). In general, indications for relief of obstruction include greater than one half to two thirds systemic right ventricular pressure, hypertension in unaffected portions of the vascular bed, or marked decrease in flow to an affected portion or clinical symptoms.[7] More recent American Heart Association (AHA) guidelines[8] for angioplasty include:

Class I: 1. Pulmonary angioplasty is indicated for the treatment of significant peripheral branch pulmonary artery stenosis (see text for definition of "significant" stenosis) or for pulmonary artery stenosis in very small patients in whom primary stent implantation is not an option (Level of Evidence: B).

Class IIa: 1. Pulmonary angioplasty is reasonable to consider for treatment of significant distal arterial stenosis (as defined in the introduction to *Pulmonary Artery Angioplasty and Stent Placement*) or for stenosis in larger, more proximal branch pulmonary arteries that do not appear to be amenable to primary stent implantation (Level of Evidence: B).

Class IIb: 1. Pulmonary angioplasty may be considered for treatment of significant main pulmonary artery stenosis that results in an elevation of pressure to more than two thirds of systemic pressure in the proximal pulmonary artery segment or in the right ventricle (in the absence of pulmonary valve stenosis). This stenosis is usually a form of supravalvar pulmonic stenosis, which is not particularly responsive to balloon dilation alone (Level of Evidence: C).

For stent implantation, the AHA guidelines are:

Class I: 1. Primary intravascular stent implantation is indicated for the treatment of significant proximal or distal branch pulmonary artery stenosis when the vessel/patient is large enough to accommodate a stent that is capable of being dilated to the adult diameter of that vessel (Level of Evidence: B).

Class IIa: 1. It is reasonable to consider pulmonary artery stent implantation in critically ill postoperative cardiac patients when it has been determined that significant branch pulmonary artery stenosis is resulting in a definite hemodynamic compromise in a patient/vessel of any size, particularly if balloon dilation is unsuccessful (Level of Evidence: B). 2. Primary intravascular stent implantation is reasonable in the treatment of significant stenosis of the main pulmonary artery segment that results in elevation of the right ventricular pressure, provided that the stent definitely will not compromise a functioning pulmonary valve and will not impinge on the pulmonary artery bifurcation (Level of Evidence: B).

Class IIb: 1. It may be reasonable to implant small pulmonary artery stents that lack the potential to achieve adult size in small children as part of a cooperative surgical strategy to palliate severe branch pulmonary artery stenosis. These stents may need to be enlarged surgically or removed during a future planned operation (e.g., conduit replacement, Fontan completion) (Level of Evidence: C).

Balloon dilation remains the preferred treatment of choice in very small infants where a large enough stent to dilate to adult size may be technically difficult if not impossible, in patients with anticipated surgery, and in patients with highly resistant lesions that do not respond to even high-pressure balloons and require specialized cutting balloons. Most of the other lesions are amenable to stenting of the branch pulmonary arteries to allow complete relief of obstruction without eventual recoil **(Figure 23–4).** The technique for single-vessel stenting is described earlier under the section entitled "General Techniques for Stent Implantation."

Pulmonary artery dilation and stenting, given its circuitous route through the right ventricle, may be one of the most challenging interventional procedures. Because of its complexity and high-risk nature, it is preferred to do these procedures with patients under general anesthesia.

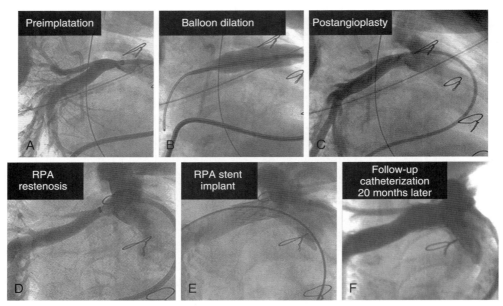

Figure 23–4 **A,** Severe proximal right pulmonary artery (RPA) stenosis. **B,** Angioplasty of RPA stenosis. **C,** Postangioplasty angiogram show improvement in stenosis. **D,** At 4-month follow-up catheterization, angiogram showing restenosis of RPA orifice. **E,** Angiogram after stenting of RPA. **F,** 20-month follow-up angiogram showing persistent in-stent patency.

Usually two venous sheaths are placed: one for balloon dilation or stent deployment, and another for angiography to assure positioning and as a central line for medications as needed. Once the lesion of interest is engaged by the angiographic catheter, selective biplane imaging is obtained in angulations that permit optimal profiling of the stenosis (i.e., right anterior oblique [RAO]/cranial [CR] for the RPA, left anterior oblique [LAO]/CR or caudal [CAU] for the LPA). For dilation only, the balloon size chosen is 3 to 4 times the narrowing or no more than 120% of the adjacent normal vessel. The dilation balloon is advanced and positioned across the stenosis using an angiographic roadmap. Precise manipulations can be accomplished by advancing the balloon over a fixed wire; advancing the wire slightly allows for the balloon to move back. The balloon is typically inflated to burst pressure or until the waist disappears. If hemodynamics are stable, the balloon is held up for 15 to 30 seconds. It is important to observe the deflation as well to evaluate recoil. The authors routinely save the fluoroscopy of the inflations for future review. A careful review of follow-up angiography is needed postdilation to look for signs of residual stenosis and more importantly, any aneurysms or tears.

Some very tight lesions may require special cutting balloons to adequately relieve the waist. Unfortunately, the maximal size of cutting balloons is limited to 8 mm in diameter and for balloon withdrawal to avoid separation of the blades from the balloon. Careful review of the angioplasty is required to measure the diameter of the residual waist. The cutting balloon selected should be no more than 1 to 2 mm larger than the residual waist. The purpose of the cutting balloon is to "score" the intima and media and allow for more effective dilation with larger regular balloons and/or additional stenting **(Figures 23–5 and 23–6).** Repeated angiography is crucial to evaluate for aneurysms and dissections.

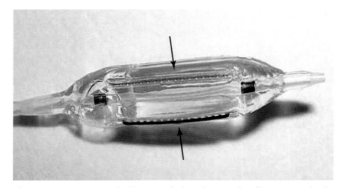

Figure 23–5 Cutting balloon with four longitudinally mounted atherotomes and a working height of 0.005 inch.

Because of the high incidence of recoil or restenosis, balloon dilation rarely results in long-term "normalization" of vessel size and often requires placement of a stent to provide structural support. The optimal stent should be able to be dilated to accommodate the size of the most normal adjacent adult-size vessel with a length that does not "jail" adjacent side branches. If jailing a side branch is unavoidable because of the stenosis spanning across the orifice of a side branch, using a stent with an "open-cell" design (i.e., IntraStent Max LD stent; eV3, Plymouth, Minn.) is preferred. This strategy can be used in both the pulmonary and systemic arterial systems **(Figures 23–7 through 23–9).** Such stents allow dilation of its side cells to accommodate up to a 12-mm diameter balloon.

In bilateral ostial stenoses that are closely related, stenting in one branch may jail the contralateral branch. This can also occur at the lobar level, usually in patients who underwent unifocalization of aortopulmonary collaterals. In this scenario, simultaneous bilateral stenting

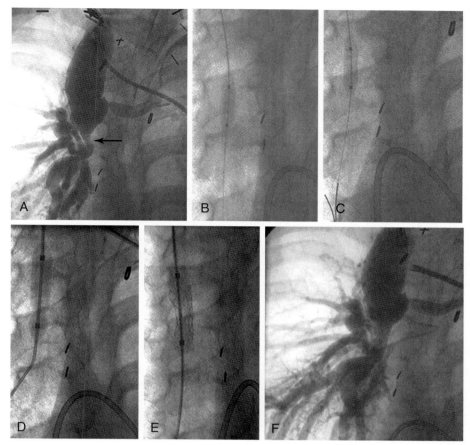

Figure 23–6 **A,** Severe hypoplastic segment of a right lower lobe (arrow) found years after unifocalization of aortopulmonary collaterals in a patient with pulmonary atresia/ventral septal defect. **B,** and **C,** Cutting balloon used to predilate this hypoplastic segment. **D,** Further dilation using a conventional balloon. **E,** Implantation of medium size stent. **F,** Poststent angiogram.

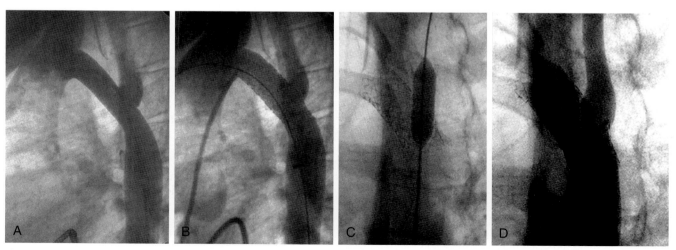

Figure 23–7 **A,** Coarctation of the aorta involving the distal arch spanning across the orifice of the left subclavian artery. **B,** After stent implantation, the left subclavian artery is jailed by the stent. **C,** Balloon dilation of side cell of stent. **D,** Postdilation angiogram.

offers another technique to eliminate the stenoses and maintain patency to both branches.⁹ In borderline cases, the adjacent contralateral branch should have a guidewire positioned during the stenting procedure just in case jailing occurs. If that happens, the guideline can be used to position a sheath, and a second stent can be implanted in the contralateral branch. In order to avoid pinhole rupture of the balloon by the contralateral stent, both stents are expanded simultaneously. It is also important to deflate the balloons simultaneously to avoid compression of the stent by late deflation of the contralateral balloon **(Figure 23–10).** Multiple operators and good communication are required for this technique.

A major complication specific to pulmonary manipulation is vessel tear or rupture. Most small tears are

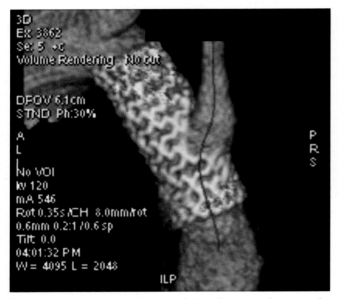

Figure 23–8 Three-dimensional rendering of computed tomography angiogram demonstrating good flow through side cell of the implanted stent into the left subclavian artery.

"confined" by the adjacent postsurgical scars and do not require further intervention. Small distal perforations can be managed with temporary occlusion of the affected branch with a balloon long enough for clot formation at the puncture site, but a large rupture may demonstrate hemoptysis, pleural effusion, and possibly hemodynamic compromise, thereby requiring surgical repair. Covered stents (Atrium iCAST stents; Hudson, N.H.) are self-expanding and limited in size but may be lifesaving in the case of distal perforations and dissections. Newer and larger sized covered stents (e.g., Numed CP stent, Hopkinton, N.Y.) are only available for compassionate use in trials. Stenting of the pulmonary arteries is associated with many potential pitfalls, resulting in various degrees of adverse events and complications including partial stent deployment, balloon rupture, and stent migration. In general, if a stent is not in a good position, the first option is to try to reposition it back into a good position. If that is not possible, the next option is to implant the stent in a safe position, doing neither harm nor good. This can be achieved by implanting the stent in an adjacent normal segment of the pulmonary artery without obstructing major side branches or withdrawing it into the inferior vena cava (IVC). Care must be taken, however, to not pull a partially deployed stent with flared sharp edges across the pulmonary and tricuspid valves, creating more harm. If implanting a stent in a safe position is not possible, surgical retrieval and repair is the final course. A full discussion of how to avoid and how to manage various complications during pulmonary artery stenting is available in the literature.¹⁰

Published reports of angioplasty for pulmonary artery stenosis indicate success rates of 50% to 60% with a recurrence rate of 15% and complication rate of 6% to 12%.⁷,¹¹,¹² On the contrary, published data on stent implantation for pulmonary artery stenosis indicate success rates as high as 90% with restenosis rates of 3.9%.¹³⁻¹⁸ In summary, it is generally accepted that pulmonary artery stenting provides better relief of stenosis in the

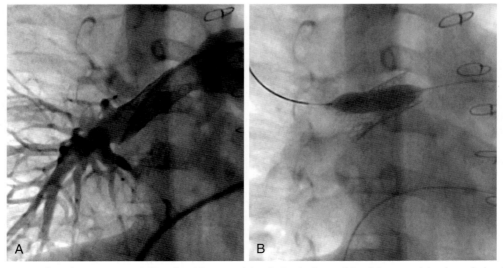

Figure 23–9 **A,** Stent in right pulmonary artery jailing the right upper lobe. **B,** Angioplasty of the right upper lobe through the side cell of a Mega LD stent.

short and long term, but in certain discrete lesions, angioplasty may provide equal relief. For small infants in whom transcatheter stenting may be technically difficult, angioplasty may provide temporary relief until there is adequate somatic growth to permit stenting, or the patient may undergo a hybrid stent procedure intraoperatively. For distal branches where stenting may not be possible, a combination of high-pressure and cutting balloons may provide adequate relief.[19]

23.4 Angioplasty and Stenting for Coarctation of the Aorta

Coarctation of the aorta occurs in approximately 7% of all CHD and 0.04% of live births and involves an anatomic narrowing of the aorta.[20] There are multiple types reported, but important to the technician are the type (discreet or tubular), location (juxtaductal, abdominal), and morphology of the lesion (arch hypoplasia). Additional considerations are the size of the patient, associated congenital anomalies or syndromes (e.g., bicuspid aortic valve, Shone syndrome, Turner syndrome), and a history of previous coarctation repair. Recent AHA guidelines for indications for angioplasty include:[8]

Class I: 1. Balloon angioplasty of recoarctation is indicated when associated with a transcatheter systolic coarctation gradient of greater than 20 mmHg and suitable anatomy, irrespective of patient age (Level of Evidence: C). 2. Balloon angioplasty of recoarctation is indicated when associated with a transcatheter systolic coarctation gradient of less than 20 mmHg and in the presence of significant collateral vessels and suitable angiographic anatomy, irrespective of patient age, as well as in patients with univentricular heart or with significant ventricular dysfunction (Level of Evidence: C).

Class IIa: 1. It is reasonable to consider balloon angioplasty of native coarctation as a palliative measure to stabilize a patient irrespective of age when extenuating circumstances are present such as severely depressed ventricular function, severe mitral regurgitation, low cardiac output, or systemic disease affected by the cardiac condition (Level of Evidence: C).

Class IIb: 1. Balloon angioplasty of native coarctation may be reasonable in patients beyond 4 to 6 months of age when associated with a transcatheter systolic coarctation gradient greater than 20 mmHg and suitable anatomy (Level of Evidence: C).

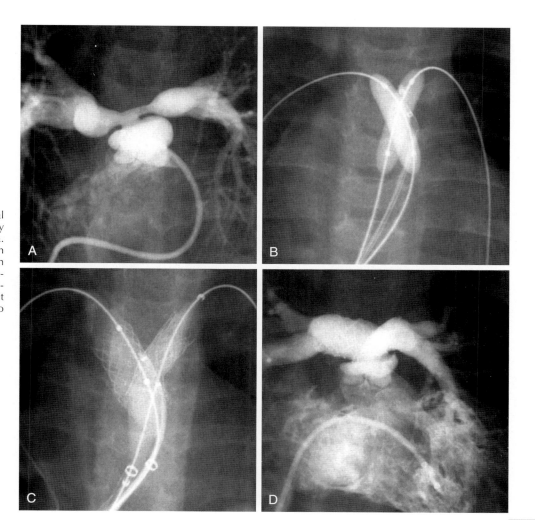

Figure 23–10 A, Severe bilateral proximal branch pulmonary artery stenosis with closely related ostia. **B,** Simultaneous double-balloon angioplasty of right and left branch pulmonary arteries. **C,** Simultaneous double stenting to avoid jailing of either branches. **D,** Poststent angiograms showing good flow to both branches.

2. Balloon angioplasty of native or recurrent coarctation of the aorta might be considered in patients with complex coarctation anatomy or systemic conditions such as connective tissue disease or Turner syndrome but should be scrutinized on a case-by-case basis (Level of Evidence: C).

For stenting, the indications are:

Class I: 1. Stent placement is indicated in patients with recurrent coarctation who are of sufficient size for safe stent placement, in whom the stent can be expanded to an adult size, and who have a transcatheter systolic coarctation gradient greater than 20 mmHg (Level of Evidence: B).

Class IIa: 1. It is reasonable to consider placement of a stent that can be expanded to an adult size for the initial treatment of native or recurrent coarctation of the aorta in patients with: a transcatheter systolic coarctation gradient of greater than 20 mmHg (Level of Evidence: B); a transcatheter systolic coarctation gradient of less than 20 mmHg but with systemic hypertension associated with an anatomic narrowing that explains the hypertension (Level of Evidence: C); a long-segment coarctation with a transcatheter systolic coarctation gradient greater than 20 mmHg (Level of Evidence: B). 2. Stent implantation for the treatment of coarctation (native or recurrent) is reasonable in patients in whom balloon angioplasty has failed, as long as a stent that can be expanded to an adult size can be implanted (Level of Evidence: B).

Class IIb: 1. It may be reasonable to consider stent implantation for the treatment of coarctation in infants and neonates when complex aortic arch obstruction exists despite surgical or catheter-mediated attempts to relieve this obstruction and when further surgery is regarded as high risk. Implantation of a stent with less than adult-sized potential implies a commitment on the part of the surgical team to remove or enlarge this stent at a later date when the final diameter of this device is no longer adequate to maintain unobstructed aortic flow (Level of Evidence: C). 2. It may be reasonable to consider placement of a stent that can be expanded to an adult size for the initial treatment of native or recurrent coarctation of the aorta in patients with: a transcoarctation gradient of less than 20 mmHg but with an elevated left ventricular end-diastolic pressure and an anatomic narrowing (Level of Evidence: C); a transcoarctation gradient of less than 20 mmHg but in whom significant aortic collaterals exist, which results in an underestimation of the coarctation (Level of Evidence: C).

Percutaneous balloon angioplasty of a coarctation was first described in 1982[21] and along with stenting has become the preferred treatment of choice in adults with primary coarctation of the aorta and in patients with surgical recoarctation. As with all balloon dilation techniques, tearing of intima and media dilation is required for relief of obstruction. In infants younger than 6 months, primary

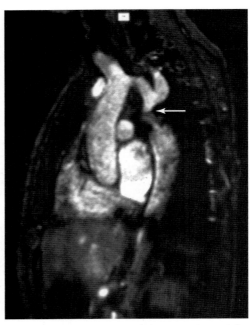

Figure 23–11 Severe coarctation of the aorta *(arrow)* found in a 25-year-old female during her second trimester of pregnancy.

surgical repair is still preferred, but with improvement in newer low profile balloons and stents as well as more experience, boundaries for primary coarctation stenting are being pushed to the lower age and weight groups.

Although patients with coarctation of the aorta may never reach normal diameters, the normal mean diameters of distal aortic arches in fully grown adults are 21.1 mm for women and 26.1 mm for men.[22] Hence "extra-large" stents should be used for coarctation of the aorta to allow for further dilation to adulthood **(Figures 23–11 and 23–12).**

After obtaining a detailed angiogram profiling the coarctation via a retrograde or a transseptal prograde approach, careful and calibrated measurements are made of the diameter and length of the coarctation, as well as diameters of the adjacent normal vessel and distance to the brachiocephalic branches. Selecting the proper frame for measurements is important, because arterial pulsatility can result in a 20% difference between the largest and smallest diameters measured. Usually the frame with the most contrast and hence the most clear luminal edge is not the one with the largest diameter, resulting in undersizing the balloon and stent and subsequent stent migration. The interventionist must be careful to select the frame with the largest possible aortic diameter as reference for balloon and stent selection. In general, the first option for discrete "membranous" coarctations should be angioplasty. If angioplasty is inadequate, then the interventionist should proceed to stenting. Some interventionists prefer to test vessel compliance and balloon stability with angioplasty before stenting, but this technique is not universal.

After careful evaluation of the aortic arch, an appropriately sized stent and balloon are chosen. An Amplatz Super Stiff "short-tip" wire is placed distally over a catheter, ideally deep in the right subclavian artery or down into

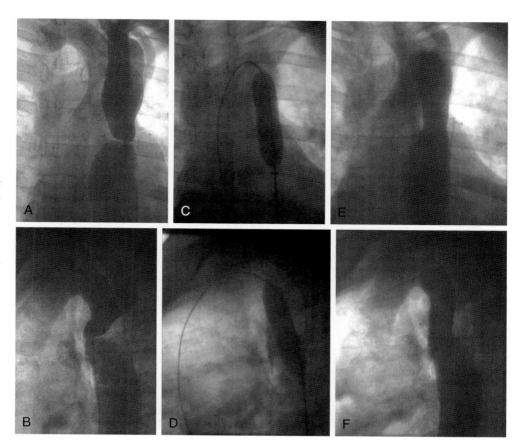

Figure 23–12 A, Anteroposterior and lateral **(B)** projection of severe discrete coarctation of the aorta at the isthmus. **C,** Stent implantation at the coarctation site in anteroposterior and lateral **(D)** projections. **E,** Poststent angiogram in anteroposterior and lateral **(F)** projections with elimination of coarctation.

the ascending aorta. In some lesions, it is reasonable to test vascular compliance with a soft balloon at low atmospheres (<4 atm) to determine the need for staged dilation and decrease the small risk for vascular complications.[23] Additionally, placement of a catheter in the aortic arch via a transseptal puncture from a second femoral venous access or radial approach to monitor proximal aortic pressures and for repeat angiograms is useful to avoid wire exchanges and to minimize further trauma to the recently dilated coarctation site. The ultimate final size of the balloon or stent varies with centers and experience, but typically the stent is expanded to match the normal adjacent vessel caliber or three to four times the narrowest area, whichever is less. In general, extra-large stents that can expand to 24 mm in diameter should be used. Occasionally, a large stent that expands to 18 mm can be selected for a small adult. As mentioned earlier, typically with large diameter balloons, a BIB balloon is chosen to expand the stent. The process of mounting the stent and delivering it to the target is similar to pulmonary artery stenting described previously under the section entitled "General Techniques for Stent Implantation." Because of the high pressure of the aortic flow that could theoretically cause the stent and balloon to shift distally during inflation, some have advocated the use of right ventricular pacing to decrease the stroke volume and systolic blood pressure in order to stabilize the stent during implantation.[24] The authors have not found this to be necessary during stent deployment for coarctation of the aorta. Because coarctation of the aorta can be located next to the left subclavian

artery orifice or even span across it, stenting may jail the orifice. If that is a risk, an open-cell stent such as the IntraStent Max LD stent should be used. Opening the side of the stent cell can be performed if flow to the left subclavian artery is compromised **(see Figure 23–8).**

Technically, stenting a coarctation of the aorta is simpler than pulmonary artery stenosis, because it is not necessary to traverse two chambers of the heart and two valves. However, the procedure is performed in the largest systemic artery under high pressures and any complication can be catastrophic, with significant morbidity and mortality when it occurs. Calcifications may be present in older adults, which increase the risk for dissections. Conservative gentle testing with low pressure dilations (<4 atm) is highly recommended. Some have advocated stent implantation with an initial conservative dilation, leaving a residual stent waist at the coarctation site. The patient is brought back to the catheterization lab in a few months, and the waist is serially dilated to the normal adult caliber. Theoretically this strategy allows for proper endothelialization and vessel growth to accommodate the increase in circumference at the coarctation site and to minimize risk of vascular tears.

It is important to carefully evaluate the stent after implantation to look for aortic dissection and aneurysm formation, which may be surgical emergencies. Angiograms in biplane and even multiple angulations should be used for this evaluation, with careful comparison to preintervention angiograms. Overnight observation with careful monitoring of any signs and symptoms of aortic

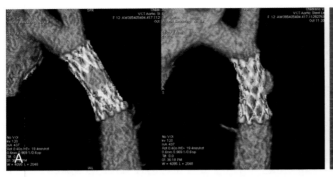
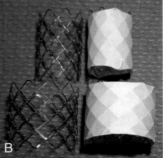

Figure 23–13 **A,** 5-year follow-up computed tomography angiograms showing a small aneurysm at the side of a stented coarctation site. **B,** Example of a NuMED covered stent that can be used to treat these aneurysms. At publication, this stent was in the trial phase.

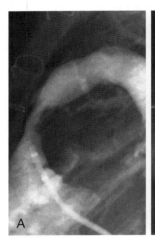
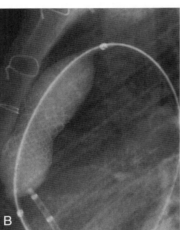
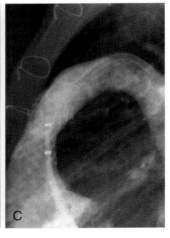

Figure 23–14 **A,** Lateral projection of severely stenotic right ventricle-to-pulmonary artery conduit. **B,** Stent implantation in conduit. **C,** Post-stent angiogram showing excellent relief of conduit stenosis.

dissection is mandatory. Although it would be ideal to have large-caliber covered stents available, they are only available in a clinical trial in selected large pediatric centers. Some have used implantable aortic grafts as an off-label bail-out device. Overall, stenting a coarctation of the aorta is very gratifying with a high technical success rate and a low rate of complications. A large multiinstitutional study showed stenting was superior to balloon angioplasty with gradients decreasing from 36.7 mmHg to 4.8 mmHg in the stent group, as compared to the angioplasty group, whose gradients decreased from 38.8 mmHg to 10.3 mmHg. Furthermore, the stent group had lower complication rates (2.3% vs. 9.8%).[25]

Many other publications have confirmed the safety and efficacy of stent treatment for coarctation of the aorta.[26,27] Multiinstitutional trials using a new platinum–iridium stent are underway, and preliminary results are promising.[28] Other advancements include use of a covered stent to avoid and treat aortic dissections and aneurysms[29-32] **(Figure 23–13).**

23.5 Angioplasty and Stenting of Surgical Conduits, Baffles, and Homograft

Conduits and baffles are routinely placed surgically to divert blood or to create new pathways. The materials used, either synthetic (e.g., Gore-Tex, Dacron) or homograft, usually become sclerosed or even calcified over time. However, many of these conduits and baffles can be dilated or even stented, although it is important to remember that circular synthetic conduits generally cannot be dilated past their native diameter **(Figure 23–14).** Stenoses found in right ventricle-to-pulmonary artery conduits (either valved or not) are routinely stented, but depending on adjacent contractile tissues and the retrosternal space, stents implanted in this area may be prone to fracture. Follow-up studies found stents placed in conduits in the right ventricle-to-pulmonary artery position to have a fracture rate of 25% to 43% out to 15-year follow-up. It was thought that repetitive stent compression in the retrosternal position was a major cause, but stent fracture, although it resulted in restenosis, did not cause acute hemodynamic consequences.[33,34] Fractured stent fragments may rarely embolize to the distal pulmonary arteries, but they do not result in obstruction to downstream flow.

Overall, stents in these conduits can extend the lifespan of the patient and help the patient avoid surgery by an average of 4 years. In growing children, palliative stenting in the conduit can delay surgery until the child grows further and thereby minimize the total number of conduit replacements over a lifetime. Implantation of multiple stents may add enough structural support to avoid stent fractures.[35]

Predilation is highly recommended not only to determine compliance of the stenotic conduit, but more

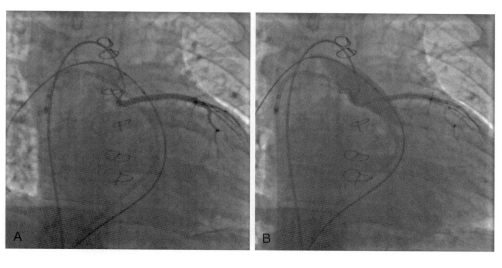

Figure 23–15 **A,** Initial left coronary artery injection showing normal flow. **B,** With test-balloon inflation within right ventricle-to-pulmonary artery conduit, repeat left coronary artery injection now demonstrates coronary artery compression. This is a contraindication for stent or Melody valve implantation.

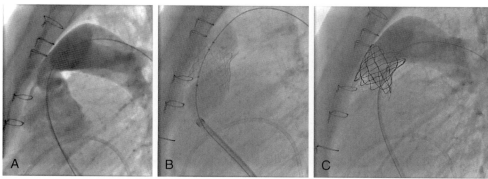

Figure 23–16 **A,** Right ventricle-to-pulmonary artery conduit stenosis just behind the sternum. **B,** Initial implantation of Palmaz XD stent for added structural support to prevent recoil and stent fracture. **C,** Final implantation of Melody valve.

importantly to assess for potential compression of an adjacent coronary artery if a stent is implanted **(Figure 23–15).** This is the most important complication to avoid. It is not uncommon for patients with CHD to also have abnormal coronary artery courses or to have prominent conal branches off the right coronary artery lying in the region of the right ventricular outflow tract.

It should be kept in mind that valved conduits that are stented may relieve the obstruction but result in pulmonary insufficiency if the stent straddles the conduit valve as in most cases. Fortunately, insufficiency can be tolerated more easily than stenosis. Currently available transcatheter valves (i.e., the Medtronic Melody valve; Minneapolis, Minn.) can be used to restore valve function and is discussed in Chapter 8. Many high-volume centers implanting the Melody valve are prestenting as a way of preventing stent fracture of the Melody valve, but data about longer term follow-up care using this strategy are not available at this time **(Figure 23–16).**

Systemic venous baffles (i.e., Mustard and Senning) placed in infancy, as in the case of d-transposition of the great arteries, after atrial switch can become obstructed over time **(Figure 23–17).** Both the superior limb and the inferior limb can become obstructed. Interestingly, many of these patients are relatively asymptomatic because of adequate collateral venous flow and azygous "pop off." However, these patients can experience varying degrees of superior vena cava and/or IVC syndrome. When an

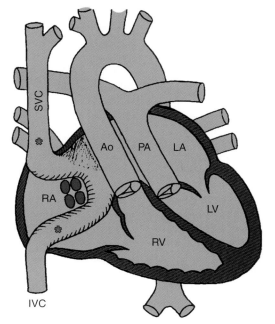

Figure 23–17 **Diagram of the Mustard operation (atrial switch) for d-transposition of the great arteries.** The superior vena cava *(SVC)* and inferior vena cava *(IVC)* are baffled into the left atrium *(LA).* Systemic venous blood is passed through the left ventricle *(LV)* and into the pulmonary arteries *(PA)* for oxygenation. The four pulmonary veins are directed into the right atrium *(RA)* to the right ventricle *(RV)* and out of the aorta *(Ao).* Common areas of obstruction are found in the SVC and IVC baffle *(red asterisks).*

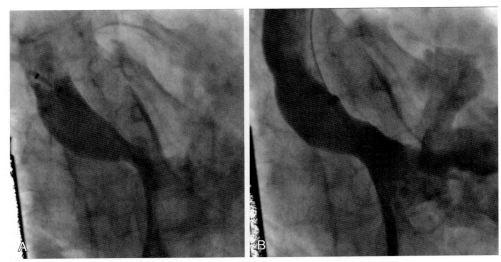

Figure 23–18 **A,** Stenosis of superior limb of Mustard baffle in a patient with d-transposition of the great arteries. **B,** Angiogram after stent implantation.

intervention is planned, stenting is almost always the primary option, because angioplasty is usually inadequate. Alternatively, these baffles can have residual leaks causing varying degrees of left-to-right shunting or even right-to-left shunting if there is combined baffle obstruction. Published reports using stents, covered stents, and occlusion devices indicated excellent results.[36-40]

Cardiac imaging with magnetic resonance imaging or computed tomography angiography may help to elucidate the adjacent anatomy to facilitate the interventional plan. Biplane angiography with accurate assessment of the anatomy is essential for successful stenting. Techniques are not dissimilar to stenting other large cardiovascular structures. A super-stiff wire provides the primary rail for the delivery system, stent, and balloon to be positioned across the stenosis. Because of the large dimensions of this area, large and extra-large stents are usually selected. The most important consideration in systemic venous baffle stenting is to avoid compression of the adjacent pulmonary venous baffle. This requires a second venous sheath and transbaffle access into the pulmonary venous confluence for angiography with temporary balloon dilation within the systemic venous baffle. Alternatively, a pulmonary artery angiogram can be performed to assess pulmonary venous return during the levophase. However, if there is pulmonary venous compression, additional stenting of the pulmonary venous baffle may be required. Rarely, both the systemic and pulmonary venous baffles are obstructed, requiring simultaneously stenting of both baffles. These interventions are quite complicated technically and should be reserved for the most experienced centers treating CHD. Some have advocated the hybrid approach to simplify the approach.[41]

One additional factor to consider is that older patients with this operation often have varying degrees of sick sinus syndrome and heart block, requiring pacemakers. If a transvenous pacing wire is inserted across a systemic venous baffle, a collaborative strategy with the electrophysiologist is required to treat the dysfunctional baffle and the arrhythmias. Scant reports of these collaborations have proven to be successful, although long-term data is unknown[42,43] **(Figures 23–18 and 23–19).**

Adults with single ventricle variants after palliation with a Glenn and Fontan baffle may develop stenosis that requires stenting. These patients can have protein-losing enteropathy (PLE) and pleural/pericardial effusions, requiring aggressive treatment. Interestingly, many of these stenoses are subtle with very low gradients. Stenting of these baffles requires large to extra-large stents, and implantation techniques are similar to those described previously in the section entitled "General Techniques for Stent Implantation." **(Figures 23–20 and 23–21).**

Occasionally, Fontan baffle leaks cause significant right-to-left shunting and require closure. New advances in covered stents may be an excellent way of eliminating these types of leaks.[44]

In summary, adults with CHD can had a variety of vascular stenoses that require angioplasty and/or stenting for adequate relief. Interventions to treat these stenoses require not only a good fund of knowledge of the congenital cardiac defect and surgical repairs, but also the techniques of how to perform angioplasty and stenting in medium and large sized vessels. The ideal setting for these procedures is one where there is close collaboration with pediatric interventional cardiologists.

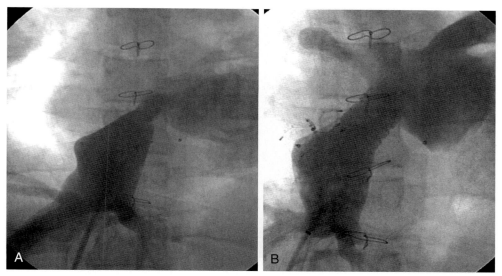

Figure 23–19 **A,** Stenosis of inferior limb of Mustard baffle in another patient with d-transposition of the great arteries. **B,** Angiogram after stent implantation.

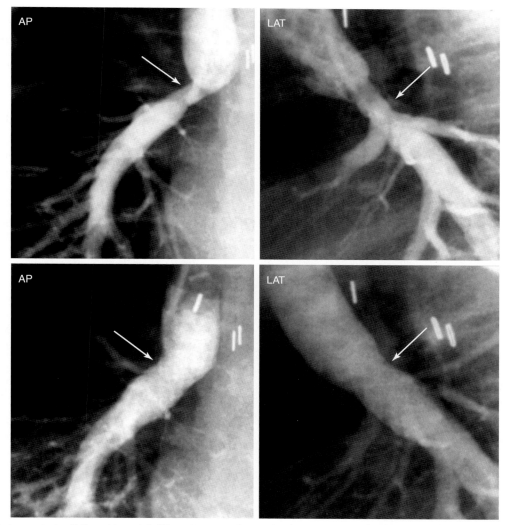

Figure 23–20 Anteroposterior (AP) and lateral (LAT) angiograms of stenosis of a superior caval-pulmonary (Glenn) shunt in a single ventricle (upper panels) patient with a Fontan physiology and same angiograms after stent implantation (lower panels).

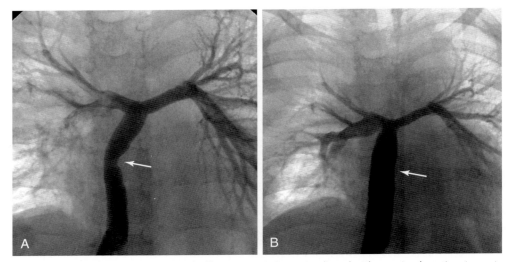

Figure 23–21 **A,** Stenosis in a Fontan baffle *(arrow).* **B,** Stenosis relieved with stent implantation *(arrow).*

REFERENCES

1. Dotter CT, Judkins MP: Transluminal treatment of arteriosclerotic obstruction: description of a new technic and a preliminary report of its application, *Circulation* 30:654–670, 1964.
2. Allen HD, Mullins CE: Results of the valvuloplasty and angioplasty of congenital anomalies registry, *Am J Cardiol* 65(11):772–774, 1990.
3. Mullins CE: *Cardiac catheterization in congenital heart disease: pediatric and adult.* Oxford: Blackwell, 2006.
4. Casteneda-Zuniga WR, Formanek A, Tadavarthy M, et al: The mechanism of balloon angioplasty, *Radiology* 135(3):565–571, 1980.
5. Sigwart U, Puel J, Mirkovitch V, et al: Intravascular stents to prevent occlusion and restenosis after transluminal angioplasty, *N Engl J Med* 316(12):701–706, 1987.
6. O'Laughlin MP, Perry SB, Lock JE, et al: Use of endovascular stents in congenital heart disease, *Circulation* 83(6):1923–1939, 1991.
7. Rothman A, Perry SB, Keane JF, et al: Early results and follow-up of balloon angioplasty for branch pulmonary artery stenoses, *J Am Coll Cardiol* 15(5):1109–1117, 1990.
8. Feltes TF, Bacha E, Beekman RH 3rd, et al: Indications for cardiac catheterization and intervention in pediatric cardiac disease: a scientific statement from the American Heart Association, *Circulation* 123(22):2607–2652, 2011.
9. Stapleton GE, Hamzeh R, Mullins CE, et al: Simultaneous stent implantation to treat bifurcation stenoses in the pulmonary arteries: initial results and long-term follow-up, *Catheter Cardiovasc Interv* 73(4):557–563, 2009.
10. Ing FF: Stenting branch pulmonary arteries. In Hijazi Z, Feldman T, Cheatham JP, editors: *Complications in percutaneous interventions for congenital and structural heart disease,* London: Informa Healthcare, 2009.
11. Trant CA Jr, O'Laughlin MP, Ungerleider RM, et al: Cost-effectiveness analysis of stents, balloon angioplasty, and surgery for the treatment of branch pulmonary artery stenosis, *Pediatr Cardiol* 18(5):339–344, 1997.
12. Kan JS, Marvin WJ Jr, Bass JL, et al: Balloon angioplasty-branch pulmonary artery stenosis: results from the valvuloplasty and angioplasty of congenital anomalies registry, *Am J Cardiol* 65(11):798–801, 1990.
13. Law MA, Shamszad P, Nugent AW, et al: Pulmonary artery stents: long-term follow-up, *Catheter Cardiovasc Interv* 75(5):757–764, 2010.
14. Spadoni I, Giusti S, Bertolaccini P, et al: Long-term follow-up of stents implanted to relieve peripheral pulmonary arterial stenosis: hemodynamic findings and results of lung perfusion scanning, *Cardiol Young* 9(6):585–591, 1999.
15. Kenny D, Amin Z, Slyder S, et al: Medium-term outcomes for peripheral pulmonary artery stenting in adults with congenital heart disease, *J Interv Cardiol* 24(4):373–377, 2011.
16. Ing FF, Grifka RG, Nihill MR, et al: Repeat dilation of intravascular stents in congenital heart defects, *Circulation* 92:893–897, 1995.
17. McMahon CJ, El-Said H, Grifka RG, et al: Redilation of endovascular stents in congenital heart disease: factors implicated in the development of restenosis and neointimal proliferation, *J Am Coll Cardiol* 38:521–526, 2001.
18. Shaffer KM, Mullins CE, Grifka RG, et al: Intravascular stents in congenital heart disease: short- and long-term results from a large single-center experience, *J Am Coll Cardiol* 31(3):661–667, 1998.
19. Bergersen L, Gauvreau K, Lock JE, et al: Recent results of pulmonary arterial angioplasty: the differences between proximal and distal lesions, *Cardiol Young* 15(6):597–604, 2005.
20. Fyler D: Report of the New England Regional Infant Cardiac Program, *Pediatrics* 65(2):375–461, 1980.
21. Singer MI, Rowen M, Dorsey TJ: Transluminal aortic balloon angioplasty for coarctation of the aorta in the newborn, *Am Heart J* 103(1):131–132, 1982.
22. Garcier JM, Petitcolin V, Filaire M, et al: Normal diameter of the thoracic aorta in adults: a magnetic resonance imaging study, *Surg Radiol Anat* 25(3.4):322–329, 2003.
23. Golden AB, Hellenbrand WE: Coarctation of aorta: stenting in children and adults, *Catheter Cardiovasc Interv* 69(2):289–299, 2007.
24. Daehnert I, Rotzsch C, Wiener M, et al: Rapid right ventricular pacing is an alternative to adenosine in catheter interventional procedures for congenital heart disease, *Heart* 90(9):1047–1050, 2004.
25. Forbes TJ, Kim DW, Du W, et al: Comparison of surgical, stent, and balloon angioplasty treatment of native coarctation of the aorta: an observational study by the CCISC (Congenital Cardiovascular Interventional Study Consortium), *J Am Coll Cardiol* 58(25):2664–2674, 2011.
26. Hamdan MA, Maheshwari S, Fahey JT, et al: Endovascular stents for coarctation of the aorta: initial results and intermediate-term follow-up, *J Am Coll Cardiol* 38:1518–1523, 2001.
27. Mahadevan VS, Vondermuhll IF, Mullen MJ: Endovascular aortic coarctation stenting in adolescents and adults: angiographic and hemodynamic outcomes, *Catheter Cardiovasc Interv* 67:268–275, 2006.
28. Ringel RE, Gauvreau K, Moses H, et al: Coarctation of the Aorta Stent Trial (COAST): study design and rationale, *Am Heart J* 164(1):7–13, 2012.
29. Goldstein BH, Hirsch R, Zussman ME, et al: Percutaneous balloon-expandable covered stent implantation for treatment of traumatic aortic injury in children and adolescents, *Am J Cardiol* 110(10): 1541–1545, 2012.
30. Martins JD, Cabanelas N, Pinto FF: Repair of near-atretic coarctation of the aorta in children with a new low-profile covered stent, *Congenit Heart Dis* 7(6):E89–E90, 2012.
31. Butera G, Piazza L, Chessa M, et al: Covered stents in patients with complex aortic coarctations, *Am Heart J* 154(4):795–800, 2007.
32. Butera G, Dua J, Chessa M, et al: Covered Cheatham-Platinum stents for serial dilatation of severe native aortic coarctation, *Catheter Cardiovasc Interv* 75(3):472, 2010.

33. Peng LF, McElhinney DB, Nugent AW, et al: Endovascular stenting of obstructed right ventricle-to-pulmonary artery conduits: a 15-year experience, *Circulation* 113(22):2598–2605, 2006.

34. Breinholt JP, Nugent AW, Law MA, et al: Stent fractures in congenital heart disease, *Catheter Cardiovasc Interv* 72(7):977–982, 2008.

35. Aggarwal S, Garekar S, Forbes TJ, et al: Is stent placement effective for palliation of right ventricle to pulmonary artery conduit stenosis? *J Am Coll Cardiol* 49(4):480–484, 2007.

36. Hill KD, Fleming G, Curt Fudge J, et al: Percutaneous interventions in high-risk patients following mustard repair of transposition of the great arteries, *Catheter Cardiovasc Interv* 80(6):905–914, 2012.

37. Daehnert I, Hennig B, Wiener M, et al: Interventions in leaks and obstructions of the interatrial baffle late after Mustard and Senning correction for transposition of the great arteries, *Catheter Cardiovasc Interv* 66(3):400–407, 2005.

38. Sharaf E, Waight DJ, Hijazi ZM: Simultaneous transcatheter occlusion of two atrial baffle leaks and stent implantation for SVC obstruction in a patient after Mustard repair, *Catheter Cardiovasc Interv* 54(1):72–76, 2001.

39. Schneider DJ, Moore JW: Transcatheter treatment of IVC channel obstruction and baffle leak after Mustard procedure for d-transposition of the great arteries using Amplatzer ASD device and multiple stents, *J Invasive Cardiol* 13(4):306–309, 2001.

40. Okubo M, Benson LN: Intravascular and intracardiac stents used in congenital heart disease, *Curr Opin Cardiol* 16(2):84–91, 2001.

41. Sareyyupoglu B, Burkhart HM, Hagler DJ, et al: Hybrid approach to repair of pulmonary venous baffle obstruction after atrial switch operation, *Ann Thorac Surg* 88(5):1710–1711, 2009.

42. Chintala K, Forbes TJ, Karpawich PP: Effectiveness of transvenous pacemaker leads placed through intravascular stents in patients with congenital heart disease, *Am J Cardiol* 95(3):424–427, 2005.

43. Ing FF, Mullins CE, Grifka RG, et al: Stent dilation of superior vena cava/innominate vein obstructions permits transvenous pacing lead implantation, *Pacing Clin Electrophysiol* 21:1517–1530, 1998.

44. Choi EY, Lee KS, Song JY: The use of a self-expandable stent with a self-expandable stent graft in a Fontan baffle, *Cardiol Young* 23:125–128, 2013.

Index

Page numbers followed by *f* indicate figures; *t*, tables; *b*, boxes.